Oral Histology and Oral Histopathology

S R Prabhu • Nagamani Narayana • Norman A Firth
David F Wilson
Editors

Oral Histology and Oral Histopathology

A Practical Guide for Dental Students and a Companion to Pathologists

Springer

Editors
S R Prabhu
School of Dentistry
The University of Queensland
Brisbane, QLD, Australia

Norman A Firth
Clinipath Pathology, Perth,
and Dental School
The University of Western Australia
Perth, Australia

Nagamani Narayana
College of Dentistry
University of Nebraska
Lincoln, NE, USA

David F Wilson
Charles Sturt University Centre for Rural
Health, Orange NSW and Dental School
University of Adelaide
Adelaide, SA, Australia

ISBN 978-3-031-77483-6 ISBN 978-3-031-77481-2 (eBook)
https://doi.org/10.1007/978-3-031-77481-2

This Springer imprint is published by the registered company Springer Nature Switzerland AG
The registered company address is: Gewerbestrasse 11, 6330 Cham, Switzerland

In memory of Newell Johnson, who has contributed enormously to the field of Oral and Maxillofacial Pathology

Foreword

I am delighted to write the foreword for *Oral Histology and Oral Histopathology*. There is a tendency to regularly pronounce the textbook dead and assume that web-based resources and even social media might replace it. This text proves otherwise; there is no substitute for a book of combined factual knowledge and interpretation. It is often the latter that students have most difficulty with, and it can be difficult to find sources that go beyond the facts to their application in the clinical world. The incorporation of normal histology, development and general pathological principles into the text will also find favour with students. Often, teaching of these topics is separated in the curriculum by one or more years and teachers of sciences in the early years are rarely involved in teaching of pathological topics. Bringing both together in one book is best practice and should be more widespread. I wish the authors and editors success with the project.

E. W. Odell
King's College London and Guy's Hospital
London, UK

Preface

In most parts of the world, oral histology is taught in the early years of the dental training programme, and the subject of oral pathology, including oral histopathology, is dealt with later when students enter clinics. The time gap between these two compartmentalised training programmes is several months to a year, during which students will likely have forgotten a considerable amount of knowledge of the histological features of oral structures. To align with the course structure and delivery, most available books separately deal with oral histology and oral histopathology. The editors identified the need for a comprehensive resource that covers these two essential aspects in one volume, providing a link between the two critical aspects of the learning process at the microscopic level and ensuring that students are well-informed about the histological and histopathological features of oral structures and diseases.

To fulfil this aim, the book *Oral Histology and Oral Histopathology—A Practical Guide for Dental Students and a Companion to Pathologists* is meticulously designed to meet the global curricular requirements of dental training programmes. It is structured into three parts, encompassing 36 chapters. Chapters in Part I delve into the histological features of the teeth, oral mucosa, jawbone, temporomandibular joint, and salivary glands. Part II provides a comprehensive overview of key clinical features of oral diseases, presenting their histopathological features in greater detail. Part III is dedicated to oral soft tissue biopsy techniques and laboratory diagnostic methods available in oral and maxillofacial pathology. The text is enriched with a wealth of photomicrographic images. To maintain its unique focus, clinical and radiographic images are intentionally omitted. Twenty-nine international experts have lent their expertise as chapter contributors to this book, which we believe is a testament to our commitment to delivering a resource that meets the highest academic standards. Dental students, pathologists, and clinicians are expected to find this book helpful in their diagnostic workup.

S R Prabhu
Brisbane, QLD, Australia

Nagamani Narayana
Lincoln, NE, USA

Norman A Firth
Perth, WA, Australia

David F Wilson
Adelaide, SA, Australia

Acknowledgements

Editors thank Professor Emeritus Edward Odell for his foreword, in which he emphasises the fact that there is no substitute for a book of combined factual knowledge and interpretation. Chapter contributors deserve our special appreciation, and thanks to them for making this a reality. We also thank those international colleagues who shared their photomicrographic material for this book. We have made every effort to acknowledge the copyrighted material for photomicrographs used. We thank the staff of Springer Nature, who offered editorial guidance while preparing the manuscripts and for producing excellent print and electronic versions of this book.—Editors.

Contents

Editors and Contributors

About the Editors

S R Prabhu is an Honorary Associate Professor at the School of Dentistry, Brisbane. His expertise is in Oral and Maxillofacial Pathology and Oral Medicine. Professor Prabhu formerly held academic positions in Oral Medicine and Oral Pathology at university dental schools in India, Kenya, Sudan, Australia, Trinidad and Tobago, Malaysia, Saudi Arabia, and UAE, and administrative positions as Director and Dean of Dental Schools in Trinidad and Tobago West Indies, and the UAE, respectively. Professor Prabhu is a Fellow of the dental faculties of all four Royal Colleges of Surgeons in the UK and Ireland and the International College of Dentists. He was an external examiner for the Royal College of Surgeons of Edinburgh, UK dental membership examinations. He received the Commonwealth Medical Scholarship awarded by the British Council and the Rotary Foundation award for teaching in developing countries. Professor Prabhu has conducted workshops on HIV/AIDS for oral healthcare professionals in several countries in the Asian and Caribbean regions. He has published numerous papers in refereed journals, edited/co-edited, and authored/co-authored several books. Some prominent book titles include *Oral Diseases in the Tropics* (Oxford University Press), *Textbook of Oral Medicine* (Oxford University Press), *Textbook of Oral Anatomy Histology and Embryology* (Oxford University Press), *Textbook of Oral Diagnosis* (Oxford University Press), *HIV/AIDS for Dental Practice* (Dental Council of India), *Handbook of Oral Pathology and Oral Medicine* (Wiley Blackwell), *Oral Diseases for Medical Practitioners* (Oxford University Press), *Clinical Diagnosis in Oral Medicine* (Jaypee Bros. Medical Publishers), and *Sexually Transmissible Oral Diseases* (Wiley Blackwell). Professor Prabhu is on the *International Dental Journal* (IDJ) editorial board, published by the FDI World Dental Federation, Geneva.

Nagamani Narayana is a Professor in Oral Pathology and Oral Medicine at UNMC, College of Dentistry. In addition to her training in India, Nagamani is dually trained in Oral Medicine and Oral and Maxillofacial Pathology from UMKC, School of Dentistry, Kansas City, and New York Hospital, Queens. She obtained her DMD from Temple University School of Dentistry. She is a diplomate of the American Academy of Oral Medicine and American Academy of Oral Pathology. Presently, Nagamani teaches Oral Pathology and Oral Medicine at the school; in addition she sees patients in the University Dental Associates and is the Director of the oral biopsy service of the UNMC College of Dentistry. She is a member of the American Academy of Oral and Maxillofacial Pathology, American Academy of Oral Medicine, American Board of Oral and Maxillofacial Pathology, NDA, and ADA. She is a past President of the American Board of Oral Medicine. She is active in providing continuing education programs locally, nationally, and internationally.

Norman A Firth is currently an Oral Medicine Specialist with the CCDHB in New Zealand and Consultant Histopathologist with Clinipath WA in Australia. He is also currently a Consultant Oral Pathologist with Sullivan Nicolaides Pathology (Qld) and Adjunct Associate Professor at University of Queensland (UQ) and University of Western Australia (UWA). Dr Firth is a registered specialist in Oral Medicine and Oral Pathology in both New Zealand and Australia and an experienced Forensic Odontologist. His undergraduate training was at the University of Adelaide and postgraduate training at University of Melbourne. Dr Firth currently serves on committees with both the Royal Australasian College of Dental Surgeons (RACDS) and Royal College of Pathologists of Australasia. He is an examiner for the RACDS Primary Examinations. In addition to UQ and UWA, he has been a full-time academic staff member at the University of Otago and University of Melbourne. His research interests include oral cancer and immune-mediated oral mucosal diseases.

David F Wilson was formerly a registered Specialist in Oral and Maxillofacial Pathology, Fellow of the Faculty of Oral and Maxillofacial Pathology, Royal College of Pathologists of Australasia, and Fellow of the Royal College of Physicians and Surgeons, Glasgow. His academic career spanned over 40 years with academic posts in Australia (University of Adelaide and Charles Sturt University), Canada, Saudi Arabia, United Arab Emirates, and Malaysia. He is a holder of a variety of senior academic and academic-administrative positions, including Head/Dean of School of Dentistry (United Arab Emirates and Australia). He is involved in the establishment of new dental schools in the United Arab Emirates, Malaysia, and Australia. His principal career activities centered on teaching, research, and oral and maxillofacial pathology practice. The latter included oral and maxillofacial pathology diagnostic histopathology, patient consultations, and forensic odontology. His research and scholarship includes circa 95 journal and book chapter publications and 121 conference and professional conference presentations. He is the co-editor and contributor to the textbook *Oral Diseases in the Tropics*, Oxford University Press (790pp) revised and reprinted in 2017 by Jaypee Brothers Medical Publishers, New Delhi.

Contributors

Sadeq Ali Al-Maweri Department of Preclinical oral Health Sciences, College of Dental Medicine, QU Health, Qatar University, Doha, Qatar

Radhika Manoj Bavle Krishnadevaraya College of Dental Sciences, Bengaluru, India

Ying Shi Chang Discipline of Oral Surgery, Medicine and Diagnostics, School of Dentistry, Faculty of Medicine and Health, The University of Sydney, Sydney, NSW, Australia

Nepean Centre for Oral Health, Nepean Blue Mountains Local Health District, NSW Health, Sydney, NSW, Australia

Hardeep Chehal Faculty of Dentistry, Creighton University, Omaha, NE, USA

Janina Christoforou University of Western Australia School of Dentistry, Perth, WA, Australia

G. S. Deepak Pateel Faculty of Dentistry, MAHSA University, Jenjarom, Selangor, Malaysia

Kshipra Deshpande Department of Oral Pathology, Dr. Hedgewar Dental College, Hingoli, Maharashtra, India

Norman A Firth Clinipath Pathology, Perth, and Dental School, The University of Western Australia, Perth, Australia

Nidhi Handoo University of Iowa School of Dentistry, Iowa City, IA, USA

Vinay K. Hazarey Oral and Maxillofacial Pathology, Datta Maghe Institute of Medical Sciences, Wardha, India

H. M. Hussaini Department of Diagnostic and Surgical Sciences, Faculty of Dentistry, University of Otago, Dunedin, New Zealand

Tabita Joy Department of Oral Pathology and Microbiology, Government Dental College and Hospital, Mumbai, India

Ooi Der Jiun Faculty of Dentistry, Department of Preclinical Sciences, MAHSA University, Jenjarom, Selangor, Malaysia

Juma Alkhabuli Faculty of Dentistry, University of Qatar, Doha, Qatar

Omar Kujan Oral Pathology Discipline, UWA Dental School, The University of Western Australia, Perth, WA, Australia

Emily Ming-Chieh Lu Periodontology Unit, Centre for Host-Microbiome Interactions, Faculty of Dentistry, Oral and Craniofacial Sciences, Kings College London, Guy's Hospital, London, UK

Nagamani Narayana College of Dentistry, University of Nebraska, Lincoln, NE, USA

Shankargouda Patil College of Dental Medicine, Roseman University of Health Sciences, South Jordan, UT, USA

Ajith Polonowita Department of Diagnostic Surgical Sciences, Head of Oral Medicine, University of Otago School of Dentistry, Dunedin, New Zealand

S R Prabhu School of Dentistry, The University of Queensland, Brisbane, QLD, Australia

Yeshwant Rawal Marquette University School of Dentistry, Milwaukee, WI, USA

Benedict Seo Faculty of Dentistry, Department of Oral Diagnostic and Surgical Sciences, University of Otago, Dunedin, New Zealand

Vidya Gurram Shankar Department of Public Health, Texila American University, Georgetown, Guyana

Monica Charlotte Solomon Manipal College of Dental Sciences, Manipal Academy of Higher Education, Manipal, India

Devaki Sundararajan Division of Oral and Maxillofacial Pathology, Boston University Henry M. Goldman School of Dental Medicine, Boston, MA, USA

Avinash Tamgadge D Y Patil University School of Dentistry, Navi Mumbai, India

Sandhya Tamgadge D Y Patil University School of Dentistry, Navi Mumbai, India

Hannah Walsh School of Dentistry, University of Sheffield, Sheffield, UK

David F Wilson Charles Sturt University Centre for Rural Health, Orange NSW and Dental School University of Adelaide, Adelaide, SA, Australia

Muhammed Yakin Adelaide Dental School, University of Adelaide, Adelaide, SA, Australia

Oral Histology

Contents

The Human Cell

S R Prabhu

Contents

S R Prabhu et al. (eds.), *Oral Histology and Oral Histopathology*, https://doi.org/10.1007/978-3-031-77481-2_1

1

1.1 Introduction

Cells are the basic building blocks of living tissues and organs. Cells belong to two groups: eukaryotes and prokaryotes. A eukaryote has a nucleus and membrane-bound organelles, while a prokaryote lacks these structures. This chapter deals with the basics of eukaryote cell structure and its functions.

1.2 Human Cell Structure and Functions

The human cell has a plasma membrane, cytoplasm, nucleus, ribosomes, and other membrane-bound organelles that allow for the compartmentalisation of functions (◘ Fig. 1.1, ◘ Table 1.1).

1.2.1 Plasma Membrane

The plasma membrane is a tri-laminar membrane made up predominantly of lipids. It also contains several proteins and carbohydrates (◘ Fig. 1.2). It separates the cell from the external environment and controls the passage of organic molecules, ions, water, oxygen, and wastes into and out of the cell. The membrane is highly permeable to oxygen and water but has limited permeability to sodium and potassium ions.

1.2.2 Cytoplasm

Cytoplasm provides structure to the cell. It is the site of many metabolic reactions and is a medium in which

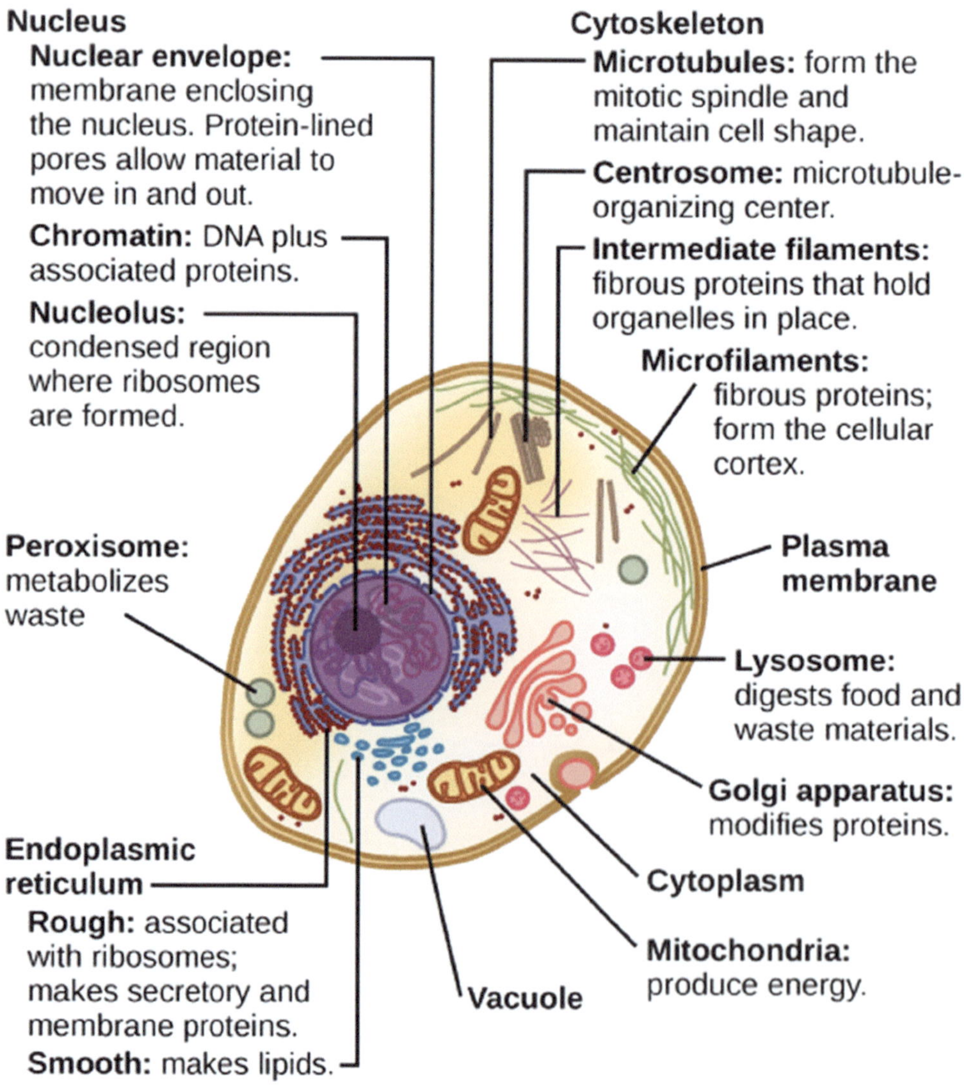

◘ **Fig. 1.1** The human cell. (*Source:* ► Concepts of Biology—1st Canadian Edition *by Charles Molnar and Jane Gair. Licensed under a* ► Creative Commons Attribution 4.0 International License*). Molnar, C., & Gair, J. (2015). Concepts of Biology—1st Canadian Edition. BCcampus. Retrieved from* ► https://opentextbc.ca/biology/ *Chapter 3.3. Eukaryotic cells. Pp 95-112. All images*)

Table 1.1 Summary of cell components and functions

Cell component	Functions
Cytoplasm	Provides structure to cell; site of many metabolic reactions; medium in which organelles are found
Nucleus	A cell organelle that houses DNA and directs the synthesis of ribosomes and proteins
Ribosomes	Protein synthesis
Mitochondria	ATP production/cellular respiration
Peroxisomes	Oxidises and breaks down fatty acids and amino acids and detoxifies poisons
Vesicles and vacuoles	Storage and transport; digestive function in plant cells
Centrosome	Unspecified role in cell division in animal cells; organising centre of microtubules in animal cells
Lysosomes	Digestion of macromolecules; recycling of worn-out organelles
Endoplasmic reticulum	Modifies proteins and synthesises lipids
Golgi apparatus	Modifies, sorts, tags, packages, and distributes lipids and proteins
Cytoskeleton	Maintains cell's shape, secures organelles in specific positions, allows cytoplasm and vesicles to move within the cell, and enables unicellular organisms to move independently

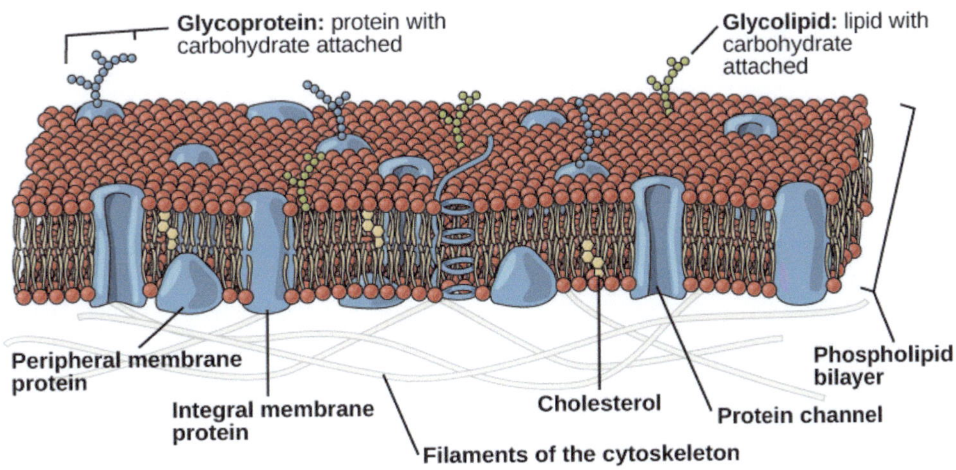

Fig. 1.2 Plasma membrane. (*Source:* ▶ Concepts of Biology—1st Canadian Edition *by Charles Molnar and Jane Gair. It is licensed under a* ▶ Creative Commons Attribution 4.0 International License*). Molnar, C., & Gair, J. (2015). Concepts of Biology—1st Canadian Edition. BCcampus. Retrieved from* ▶ https://opentextbc.ca/biology/ *Chapter 3.3. Eukaryotic cells. Pp 95-112. All images*)

organelles are found. The cytosol is the gel-like material of cytoplasm in which cell structures (organelles) are suspended.

1.2.3 Organelles

Organelles are cellular structures that perform specific functions within a cell (Fig. 1.3). Examples of organelles include the nucleus, nucleolus, ribosomes, endoplasmic reticulum, microtubules, mitochondria, lysosomes, Golgi body, centrioles, and cytoskeleton. The cytoskeleton is a network of fibres that help the cell maintain its shape and support organelles. All functions for cell expansion, growth, and replication are carried out in the cytoplasm of a cell.

1.2.3.1 Nucleus

All living human cells except red blood cells contain a nucleus. The nucleus has a double-layered membrane called a nuclear envelope (nuclear membrane) that shows perforations (Fig. 1.4). These pores are called nuclear pores, specialised to have selective permeability.

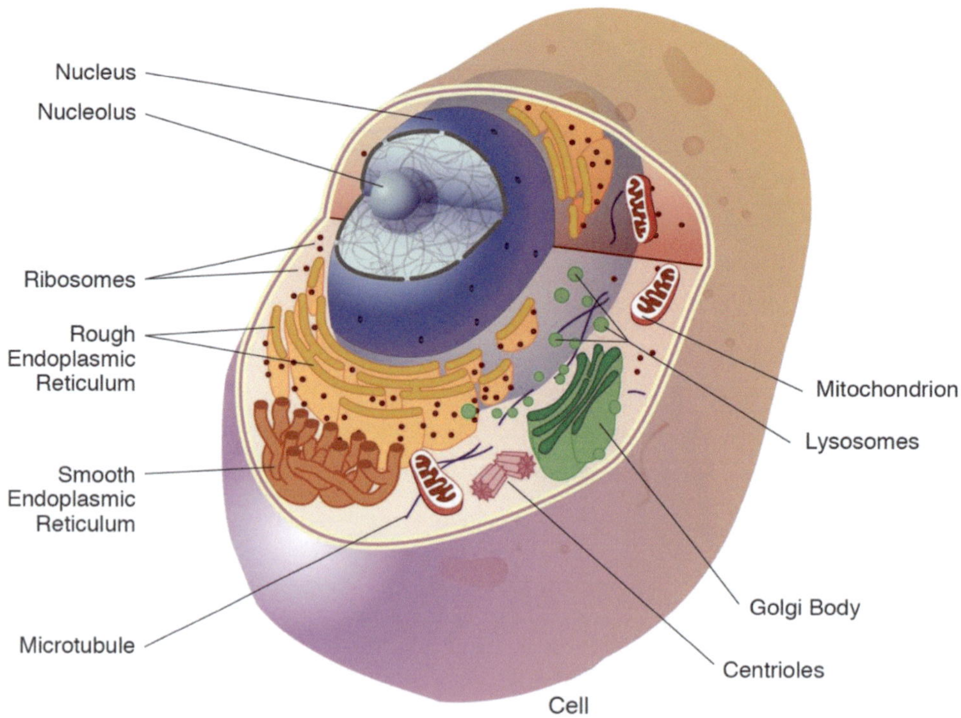

Fig. 1.3 Organelles showing nucleus, nucleolus, ribosomes, endoplasmic reticulum, microtubules, mitochondria, lysosomes, Golgi body, and centrioles. (Source: National Human Genome Research Institute. ► https://www.genome.gov/genetics-glossary/Organelle)

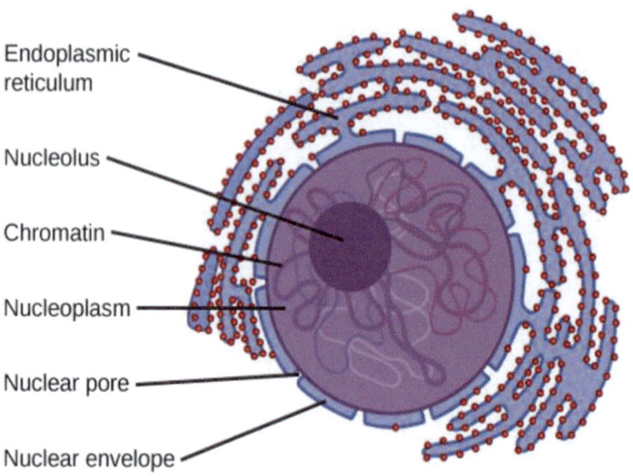

Fig. 1.4 Nucleus. Note intranuclear structures. The outermost boundary of the nucleus is the nuclear envelope. Notice that the nuclear envelope consists of two phospholipid bilayers (membranes)—an outer membrane and an inner membrane—in contrast to the plasma membrane, which consists of only one phospholipid bilayer. (*Source:* ► Concepts of Biology—1st Canadian Edition *by Charles Molnar and Jane Gair. It is licensed under a* ► Creative Commons Attribution 4.0 International License*). Molnar, C., & Gair, J. (2015). Concepts of Biology—1st Canadian Edition. BCcampus. Retrieved from* ► https://opentextbc.ca/biology/ *Chapter 3.3. Eukaryotic cells. Pp 95-112. All images*)

1.2.3.2 Chromatins

The mixture of DNA and protein that form cellular chromosomes is referred to as chromatin. DNA molecules in chromatins appear as granules or threads when a cell is non-dividing. When the cells divide, they look like short, rod-like, tightly coiled structures. These are called chromosomes.

1.2.3.3 Chromosomes

Human cells typically contain 46 chromosomes (except mature sex cells, which have 23 chromosomes). Chromosomes are structures found inside the nucleus of a cell. A chromosome is made up of proteins and DNA organised into genes. Each cell normally contains 23 pairs of chromosomes. The DNA molecules in chromosomes carry the master code for making all of a cell's enzymes and other proteins. Thus, they dictate both the structure and the function of the cells.

1.2.3.4 Nucleolus/Nucleoli

At the centre of the nucleus, one or more small non-membranous bodies called nucleolus/nucleoli are present. These are made up of ribonucleic acid (RNA) that helps make ribosomes. They perform protein synthesis.

1.2.3.5 Ribosomes

Ribosomes are intracellular structures made of RNA and protein and are sites of protein synthesis. Ribosomes have subunits composed of ribonucleic acid (RNA) (◘ Fig. 1.5). The RNA can be ribosomal RNA (rRNA), messenger RNA (mRNA), or transfer RNA (tRNA). Ribosomes are enzyme complexes responsible for protein synthesis. The ribosome reads the messenger RNA (mRNA) sequence and translates that genetic code into a string of specified amino acids, which grow into long chains to form proteins. When viewed through an electron microscope, ribosomes appear as clusters or single tiny dots floating freely in the cytoplasm (free ribosomes) or may be attached to the cytoplasmic side of the plasma membrane or the cytoplasmic side of the endoplasmic reticulum.

1.2.3.6 Mitochondria

Mitochondria are membrane-bound cell organelles that generate most of the chemical energy needed for the cell's biochemical reactions. Chemical energy produced by the mitochondria is stored in a small molecule called adenosine triphosphate (ATP). Mitochondria are oval-shaped, double-membrane organelles with ribosomes and DNA. They have two membranes: inner and outer (◘ Fig. 1.6). The inner layer possesses many folds called cristae. Embedded within the inner membrane is granular material called the matrix, which contains the main enzymes essential for producing adenosine triphosphate (ATP). They provide all the energy a cell needs to move, divide, contract, produce secretory products, and perform all other functions.

1.2.3.7 Centrosome

The centrosome is an organelle near the nucleus of a cell that contains centrioles (◘ Fig. 1.7). The centrosome is a cellular structure involved in the process of cell division. Before cell division, the centrosome duplicates, and then, as division begins, the two centrosomes move to opposite ends of the cell. A centriole is a small structure made of microtubules that exist as part of the centrosome.

1.2.3.8 Lysosomes

Lysosomes are membrane-enclosed organelles that pinch off from the Golgi apparatus (◘ Fig. 1.8). They contain chemicals (*enzymes*) that help degrade and recycle cellular waste through autophagy. They have an array of enzymes that break down all biological polymers—proteins, nucleic acids, carbohydrates, and lipids. They are also said to play a role in plasma membrane repair, bone resorption, and the immune response.

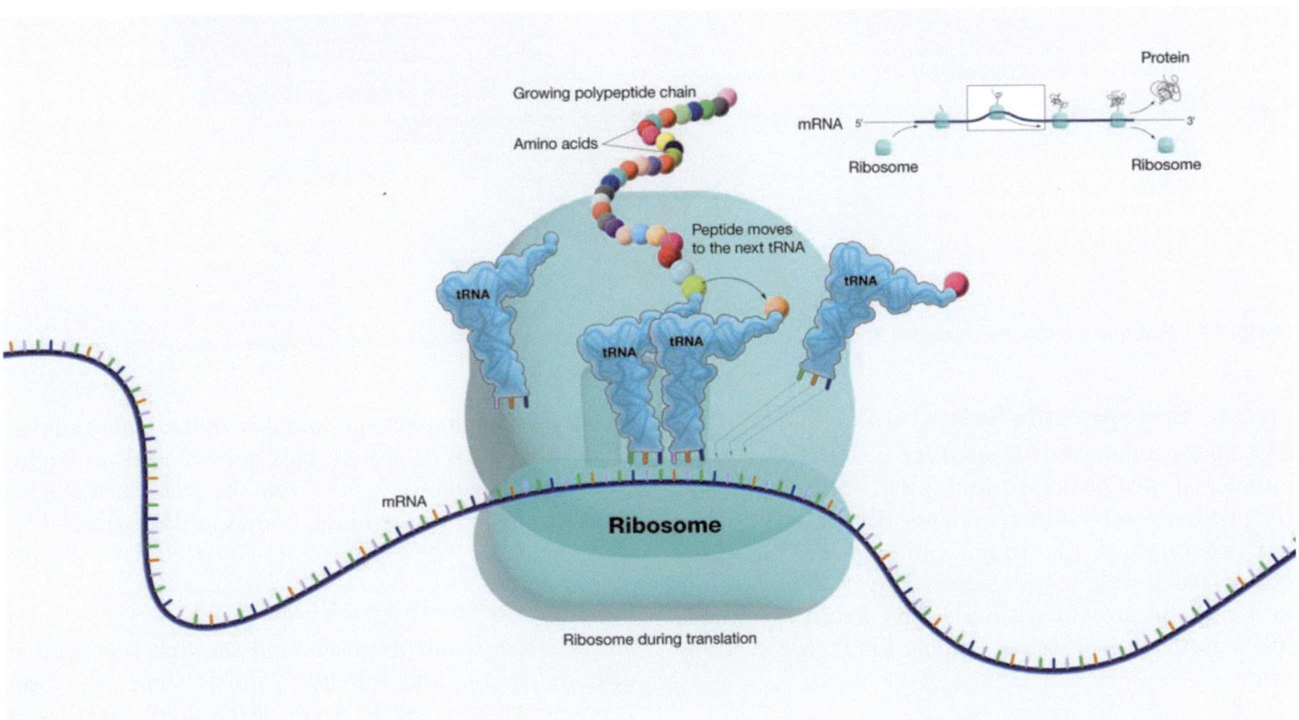

◘ **Fig. 1.5** Ribosome. (Source: National Human Genome Research Institute. ► https://www.genome.gov/genetics-glossary/Ribosome)

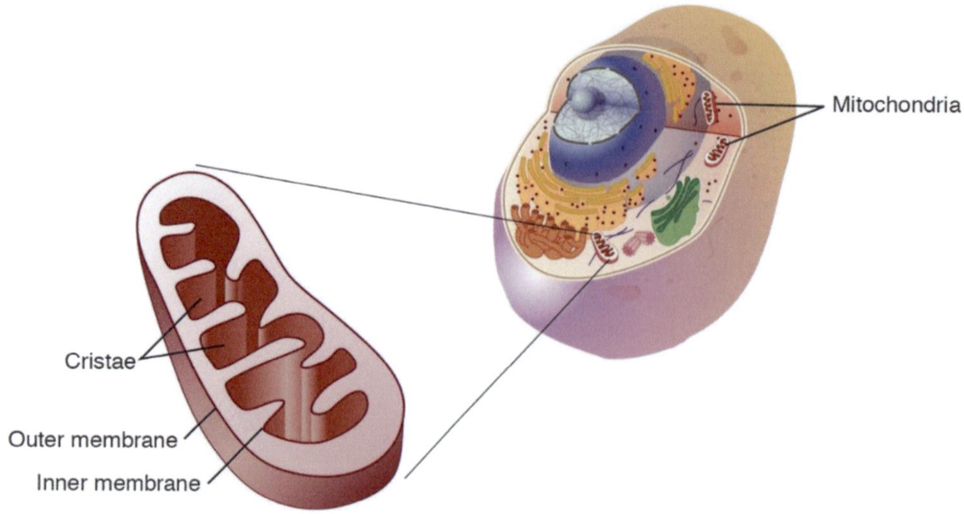

Fig. 1.6 Mitochondria. (Source: National Human Genome Research Institute. ► https://www.genome.gov/genetics-glossary/Mitochondria)

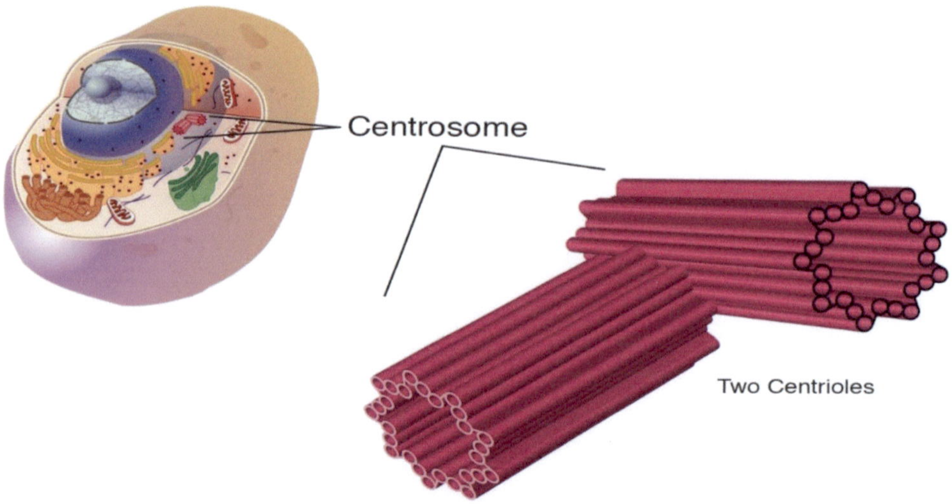

Fig. 1.7 Centrosome. (Source: National Human Genome Research Institute. ► https://www.genome.gov/genetics-glossary/Centrosome)

1.2.3.9 Endoplasmic Reticulum

The endoplasmic reticulum (ER) is a series of interconnected membranous tubules that collectively modify proteins and synthesise lipids (Fig. 1.9). There are two types of ER: rough and smooth. The rough endoplasmic reticulum is covered by many ribosomes and helps in protein synthesis. The smooth endoplasmic reticulum synthesises specific lipids and carbohydrates.

1.2.3.10 Golgi Apparatus (Golgi Body)

This is a complex of vesicles and folded membranes within the cytoplasm of most cells (Fig. 1.10), involved in secretion and intracellular transport. They modify, sort, tag, package, and distribute lipids and proteins. They help in protein biosynthesis and packaging protein molecules for export from the cell. The materials from the ER reach the Golgi bodies in the form of vesicles.

1.2.3.11 Vacuole and Vesicle

A vacuole is a membrane-bound sac that functions in cellular storage and transport and is somewhat more prominent than a vesicle. A vesicle is a small, membrane-bound sac that functions in cellular storage and transport; its membrane can fuse with the plasma membrane and the membranes of the endoplasmic reticulum and Golgi apparatus.

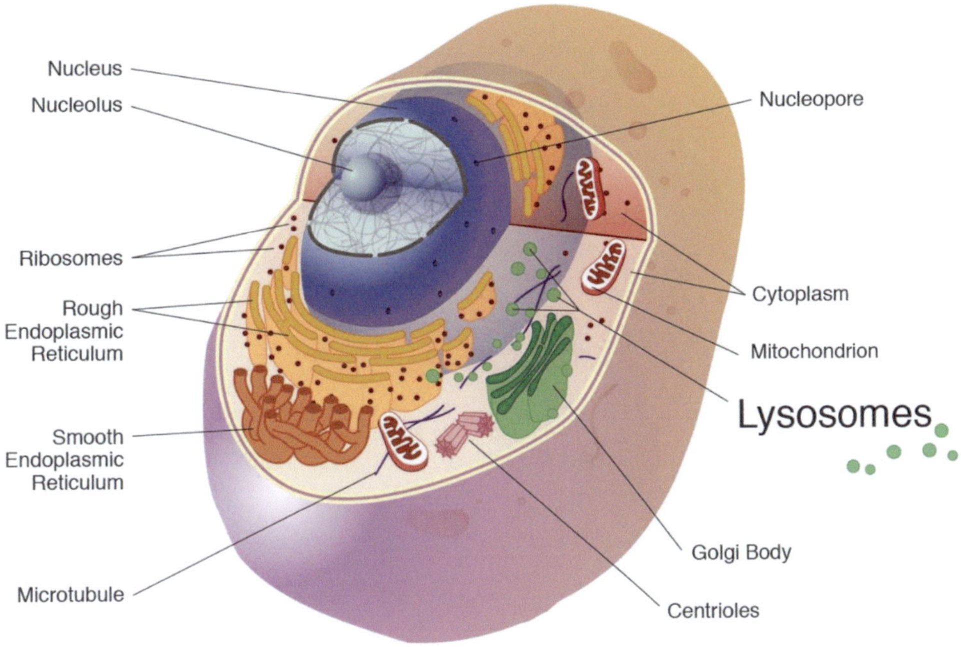

Fig. 1.8 Lysosome. (Source: National Human Genome Research Institute. ► https://www.genome.gov/genetics-glossary/Lysosome)

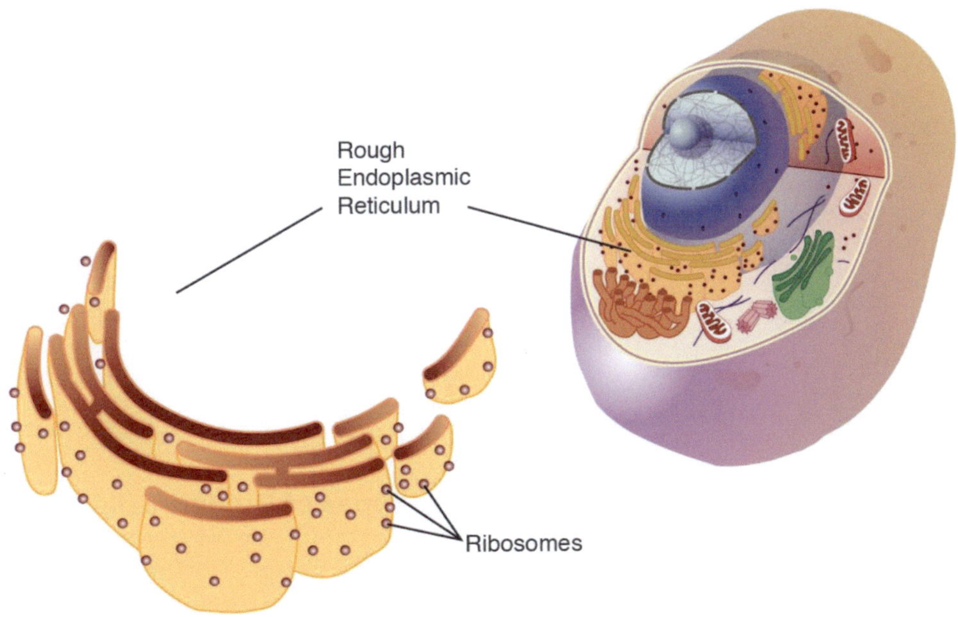

Fig. 1.9 Endoplasmic reticulum. (Source: National Human Genome Research Institute. ► https://www.genome.gov/genetics-glossary/Endoplasmic-Reticulum-rough)

1.2.3.12 Peroxisomes

Peroxisomes are tiny, round organelles enclosed by single membranes. They carry out oxidation reactions that break down fatty acids and amino acids. They also detoxify many poisons that may enter the body. Peroxisomes detoxify alcohol in liver cells. A by-product of these oxidation reactions is hydrogen peroxide, H_2O_2, which is contained within the peroxisomes to prevent the chemical from causing damage to cellular components outside of the organelle. Peroxisomal enzymes safely break down hydrogen peroxide into water and oxygen.

1

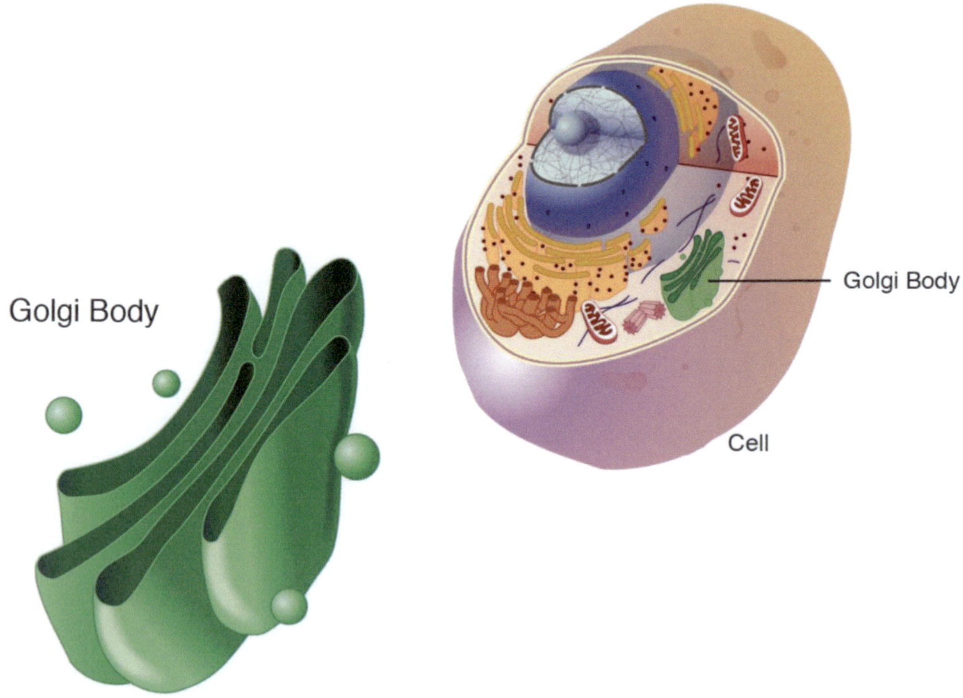

Fig. 1.10 Golgi body. (Source: National Human Genome Research Institute. ▶ https://www.genome.gov/genetics-glossary/golgi-body)

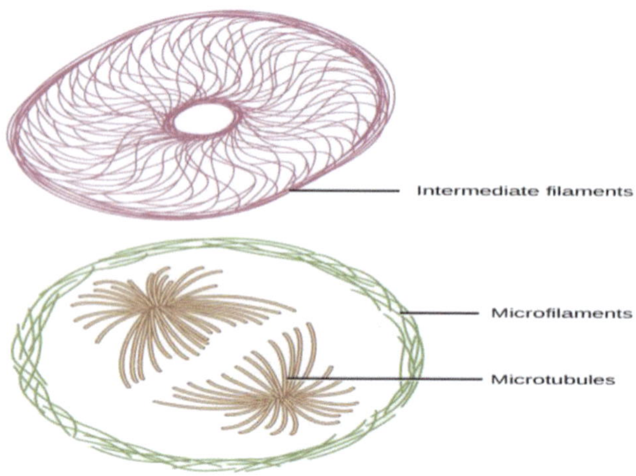

Fig. 1.11 Microfilaments, intermediate filaments, and microtubules compose a cell's cytoskeleton. (*Source:* ▶ Concepts of Biology—1st Canadian Edition *by Charles Molnar and Jane Gair. Licensed under a* ▶ Creative Commons Attribution 4.0 International License*). Molnar, C., & Gair, J. (2015). Concepts of Biology—1st Canadian Edition. BCcampus. Retrieved from* ▶ https://opentextbc.ca/biology/ *Chapter 3.3. Eukaryotic cells. Pp 95-112. All images*)

1.2.3.13 Cytoskeleton

The cytoskeleton is a network of fibres (Fig. 1.11). They can be divided into three types based on the composition of their protein subunits: (1) microfilaments, which are made up of actins; (2) microtubules, which are made up of tubulins; and (3) intermediate filaments, which are made up of a variety of subunits. The cytoskeleton maintains the cell's shape, secures organelles in specific positions, allows cytoplasm and vesicles to move within the cell, and enables unicellular organisms to move independently.

1.3 Types of Human Cells

The body is composed of many different types of cells, each with its own structure and function. Different tissues and cell types are shown in Table 1.2. A detailed description of cell types is provided in ▶ Chap. 2.

■ Table 1.2 Types of tissues and cells

Tissue	Cell type
Epidermis/oral mucosal epithelium	Keratinocytes Melanocytes Merkel cells Langerhans cells
Nerve cells	Neurons Neuroglial cells
Muscle cells	Skeletal Cardiac Smooth
Cartilage cells	Chondrocytes
Bone cells	Osteoblasts Osteoclasts Osteocytes
Blood vessels	Endothelial
Lining body cavities	Epithelial cells
Fat cells	Adipocytes (white and brown)
Fibrous cellular tissue	Fibroblasts
Red blood cells	Erythrocytes
White blood cells	Granulocytes (neutrophils, eosinophils, and basophils) Agranulocytes (monocytes and lymphocytes)
Platelets	Fragments of megakaryocytes
Sex cells	Spermatozoa Ova

1.4 Stem Cells

Stem cells are unspecialised cells of the human body. Two properties characterise stem cells: (1) the ability to self-renew and (2) the ability to differentiate into different types of cells. Stem cells exist in embryos (embryonic stem cells) and adults (adult stem cells).

Five types of stem cells exist: totipotent, pluripotent, multipotent, unipotent, and oligopotent stem cells.

1.4.1 Totipotent Stem Cells

Totipotent stem cells can divide and differentiate into cells of the whole organism. Totipotency has the highest differentiation potential. One example of a totipotent cell is a zygote, formed after a sperm fertilises an egg. Totipotent stem cells can differentiate into the three germ layers (endoderm, ectoderm, and mesoderm), germ cells (oocyte and sperm), and placental cells.

1.4.2 Pluripotent Stem Cells (PSCs)

Pluripotent stem cells form cells of all germ layers but not extraembryonic structures, such as the placenta. Embryonic stem cells (ESCs) are an example.

1.4.3 Multipotent Stem Cells

Multipotent stem cells have a narrower spectrum of differentiation than PSCs, but they can specialise in discrete cells of specific cell lineages. Somatic cells such as neural, bone marrow-derived, or haematopoietic stem cells (HSCs) fall into this category.

1.4.4 Unipotent Stem Cells

Unipotent stem cells are characterised by the narrowest differentiation capabilities and the unique property of dividing repeatedly. They can differentiate into a single type of cell. An example includes progenitor cells present during postnatal prostate development.

1.4.5 Oligopotent Stem Cells

Oligopotent stem cells usually consist of cells that reside in the tissue and have the ability to differentiate into cells of a specific tissue terminally. An example includes stem cells present on the mammalian ocular surface.

In embryos, foetuses, and adults, stem cells are found throughout the life cycle. Foetal and adult stem cells include umbilical cord stem cells, haematopoietic stem cells, and mesenchymal stem cells. The self-renewal and multi-lineage differentiation characteristics of stem cells make these cells uniquely suited for regenerative medicine, tissue repair, and gene therapy applications (■ Fig. 1.12).

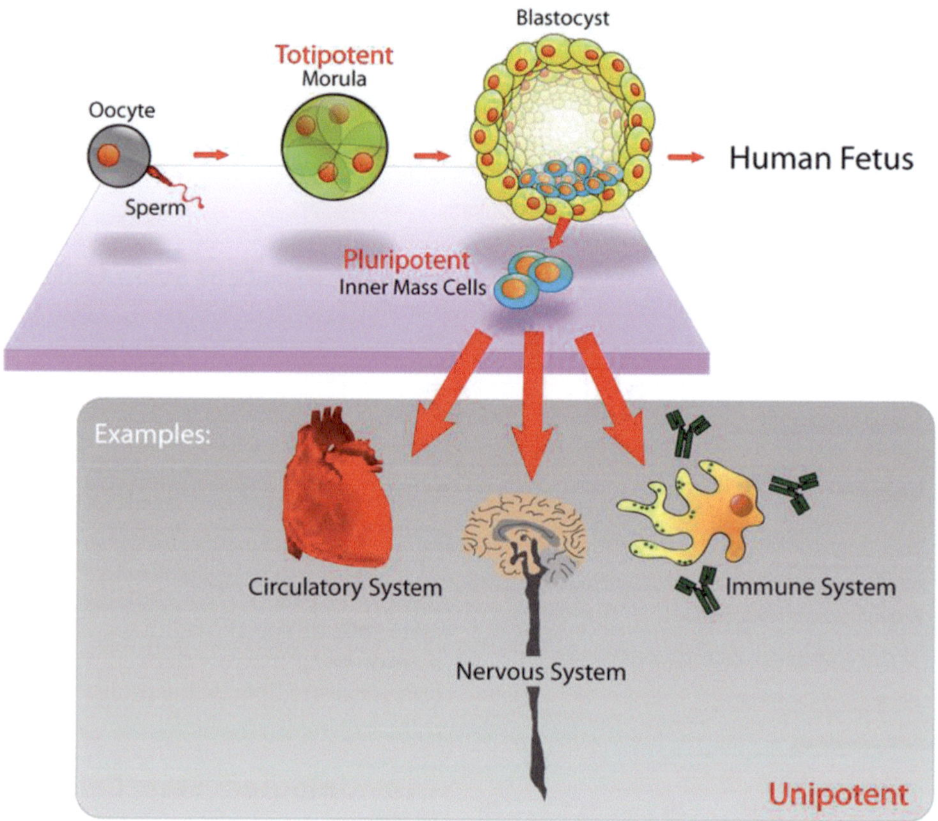

Fig. 1.12 Pluripotent: Embryonic stem cells are able to develop into any type of cell, excepting those of the placenta. Only embryonic stem cells of the morula are totipotent: able to develop into any type of cell, including those of the placenta. (Source: Wikipedia. ▸ Creative Commons ▸ Attribution-Share Alike 2.5 Generic license. ▸ https://en.wikipedia.org/wiki/Stem_cell)

1.5 Summary

Cells are the basic building blocks of all living things. A eukaryotic cell has a plasma membrane, cytoplasm, ribosomes, a true nucleus, and other membrane-bound organelles that allow for compartmentalisation of functions. The plasma membrane is a phospholipid bilayer embedded with proteins. The nucleus's nucleolus is the site of ribosome assembly. Ribosomes are either found in the cytoplasm or attached to the cytoplasmic side of the plasma membrane or endoplasmic reticulum. They perform protein synthesis. Mitochondria participate in cellular respiration; they are responsible for most of the cell's ATP. Peroxisomes hydrolyse fatty acids, amino acids, and some toxins. Vesicles and vacuoles are storage and transport compartments. Cells also have a centrosome and lysosomes. Stem cells are unspecialised cells of the human body. They can differentiate into any cell of an organism and have the ability to self-renew. There are two main types of stem cells: embryonic stem cells and adult stem cells.

Further Reading

Cell structure and function | Basic medical key 2016. https://basicmedicalkey.com/cell-structure-and-function-2/.

Chapter 3. Cell structure. In: Biology for Queensland: an Australian perspective unit 1 & 2. Oxford University Press; 2019.

Cell structure: SEER training. https://training.seer.cancer.gov/anatomy/cells_tissues_membranes/cells/structure.html.

Mitchell RN. The cell as a unit of health and disease. In: Mitchell RN, Kumar V, Abbas AK, Aster JC, editors. Pocket companion to Robbins and cotran pathologic basis of disease. 9th ed. Philadelphia: Elsevier; 2017. p. 3–36.

Molnar C, Gair J. Chapter 3.3. Eukaryotic cells. Concepts of biology—1st Canadian edition. BCcampus; 2015. pp. 95–112. https://opentextbc.ca/biology/.

Histology of Human Tissue Types

David F Wilson

Contents

S R Prabhu et al. (eds.), *Oral Histology and Oral Histopathology*, https://doi.org/10.1007/978-3-031-77481-2_2

2.1 Introduction

The interpretation of histological and histopathological images in an atlas depends upon an observer's fundamental knowledge and understanding of cell and tissue types. In the case of histopathology, an additional understanding of cell and tissue interactions in disease is important. In this chapter, a very abridged overview of normal cell and tissue types is presented to provide additional background to the sections of the book concerning oral histology and oral histopathology.

2.2 Embryologic Origin of Cell and Tissue Types

All tissues in the body derive from the three embryonic germ layers, namely the ectoderm, the mesoderm and the endoderm. These embryonic structures give rise to various types of epithelia along with other tissue components. The ectoderm gives rise to epithelial tissues such as the epidermis, the oral mucosal epithelium, tooth enamel and nerve tissue. The mesoderm gives rise to the soft and hard connective tissues and their various constituents, muscle, the haematopoietic system and the specialised epithelial cells called endothelial cells, which line blood and lymphatic vessels. The gastrointestinal tract and visceral organ epithelia derive from the endoderm.

2.3 Types of Epithelia

Epithelial tissues are widely distributed throughout the body. They form the covering of all external and internal body surfaces, are the major tissues in exocrine and endocrine glands and form the parenchyma of organs such as the liver and kidney. Specialised epithelia include myoepithelial cells that are found, for example, around salivary acini, neuroepithelial cells such as those found in the taste buds of the tongue and the previously mentioned endothelial cells lining blood vessels.

Surface epithelia cover and line all natural body surfaces. They provide a protective barrier against the external environment and are separated from underlying fibrous connective tissue by a basement membrane.

Surface epithelia, such as the epidermis and oral mucosal epithelium, may be non-keratinised, ortho-keratinised or para-keratinised (Fig. 2.1).

The two forms of keratin can be distinguished from one another at higher magnifications (Fig. 2.2) by examining the outermost epithelial layers. Orthokeratin is characterised by the presence of a zone of cells (the stratum granulosum) containing keratohyalin granules. Parakeratin does not have a granular zone but is histologically characterised by the presence of degenerate epithelial cell nuclei.

Various types of surface and lining epithelia are recognised and named largely depending upon the epithelial cell type present and their morphological arrangement. Examples include:

- Simple squamous epithelium.
- Simple cuboidal epithelium (Fig. 2.3).
- Simple columnar epithelium (Fig. 2.4).
- Stratified squamous epithelium (Fig. 2.5).
- Stratified cuboidal epithelium.
- Stratified columnar epithelium.
- Additionally, there are pseudostratified epithelia (Fig. 2.6) and transitional epithelia.

Glandular epithelium is found in many body organs and tissues. Glands may be exocrine (secretion via ducts onto a surface) or endocrine (secretion directly into the bloodstream) in type. For example, salivary glands (exo-

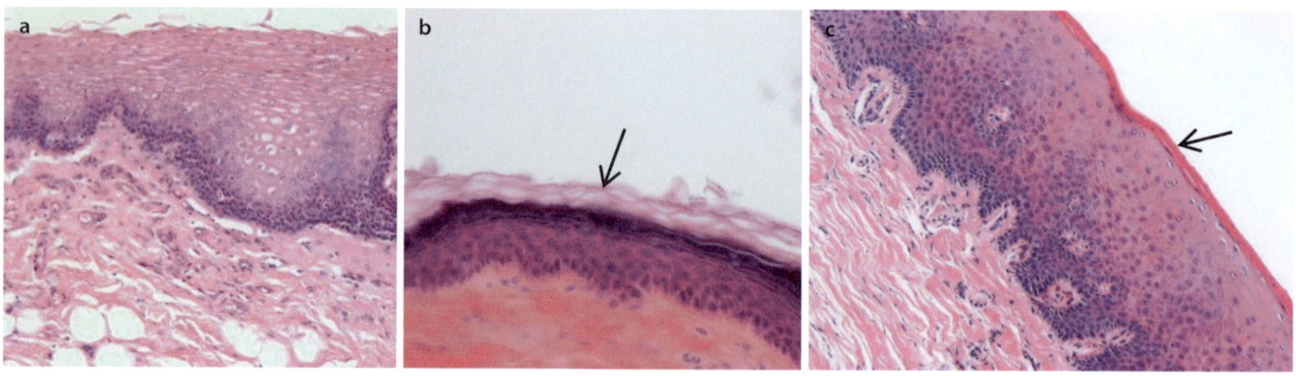

Fig. 2.1 Non-keratinised and keratinised lining epithelia. (**a**) Some lining epithelia, such as the buccal mucosa and floor of the mouth as well as sites such as the vagina and oesophagus, are non-keratinised. (**b** and **c**) The epidermis (**b**) is ortho-keratinised (arrow), while intra-oral sites such as the attached gingivae and the hard palate (**c**) exhibit parakeratosis indicated by the brightly eosinophilic surface layer of the epithelium (arrow)

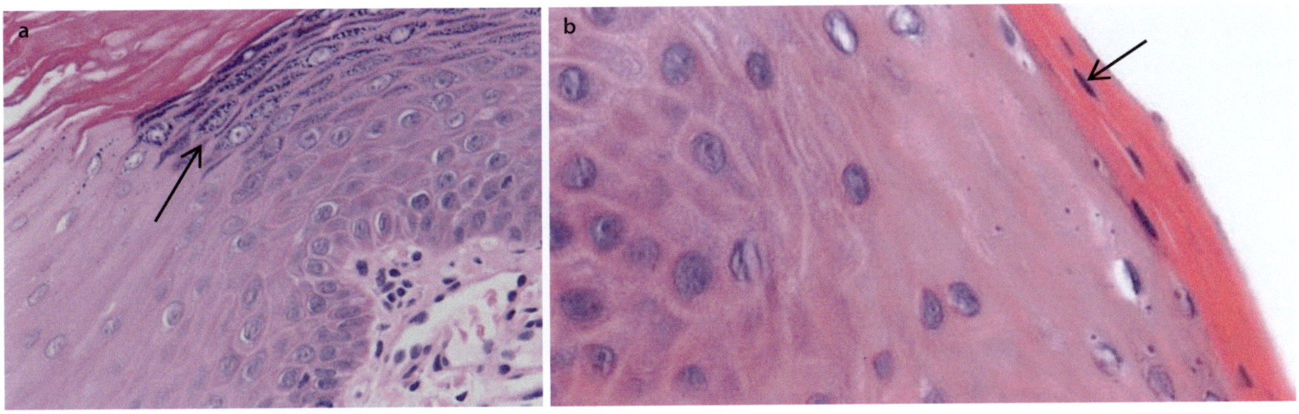

■ **Fig. 2.2** Orthokeratin (**a**) is characterised by a zone of intracellular keratohyalin granules (arrow). Parakeratin (**b**) is characterised by the presence of pyknotic epithelial cell nuclei (arrow) and the absence of a granular zone

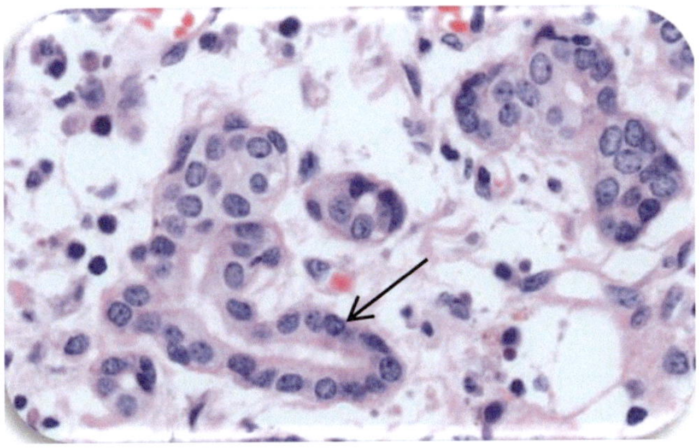

■ **Fig. 2.3** Simple cuboidal epithelium. Cuboidal epithelial cells (arrow) line an intercalated duct in a major salivary gland

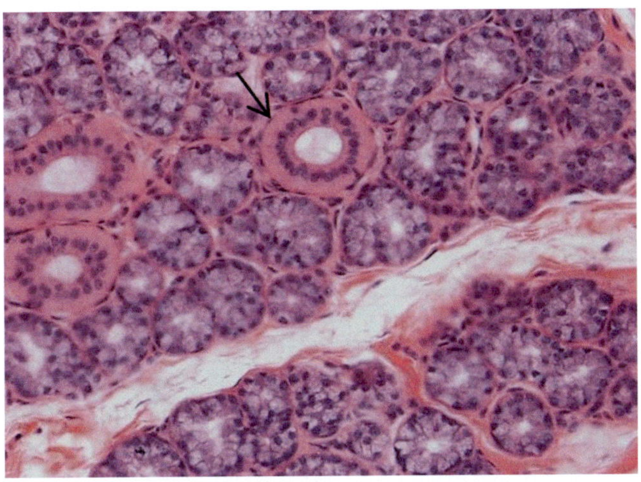

■ **Fig. 2.4** Columnar epithelium. A single layer of columnar epithelial cells (arrow) forms the lining of a striated duct in a salivary gland

crine) secrete saliva onto the oral mucosal surface; adrenal glands (endocrine) produce cortisol, androgenic hormones and adrenaline directly into the bloodstream.

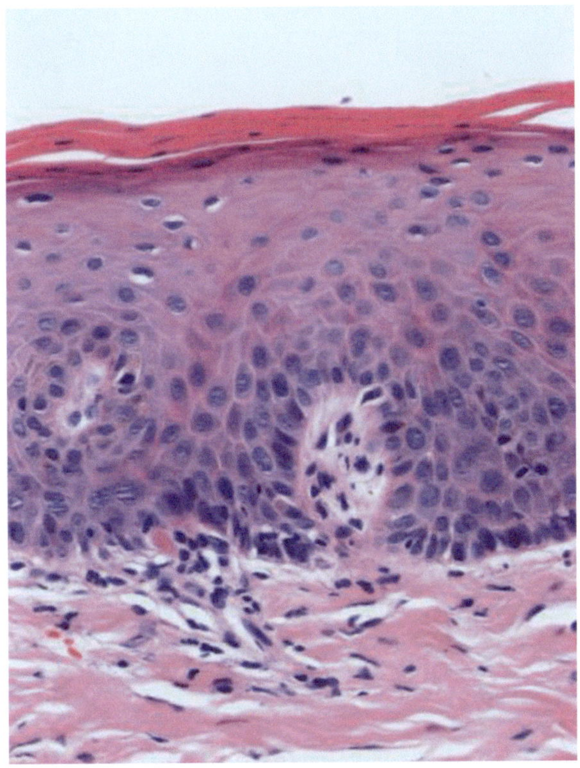

■ **Fig. 2.5** Stratified squamous epithelium. Oral mucosal epithelium is an example of stratified squamous epithelium. The descriptor 'squamous' refers to the flattened, outermost layers of epithelial cells

In the case of exocrine glands, both the secretory units of the glands and the ductal structures are epithelial. In the major and minor salivary glands, the secretory units (acini) (■ Fig. 2.7) are formed by discrete collections of epithelial cells that secrete their product into a central lumen, which is contiguous with a ductal system that carries saliva to the oral mucosal surface. The detailed structure of the salivary glands is presented in Sect. 20.10.

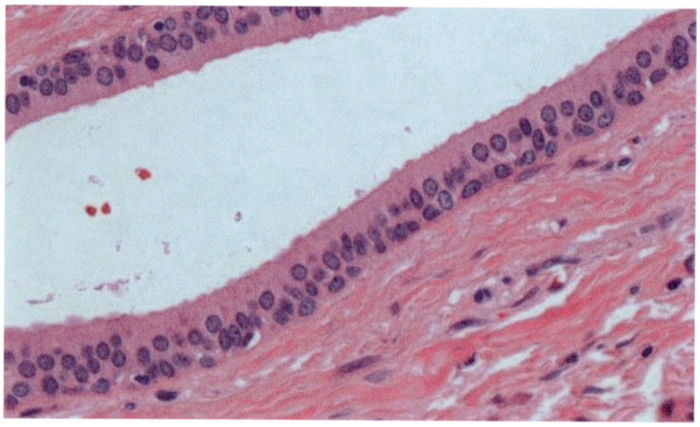

Fig. 2.6 Pseudostratified epithelium. An example of a pseudostratified columnar epithelium forming the lining of an excretory duct in a salivary gland

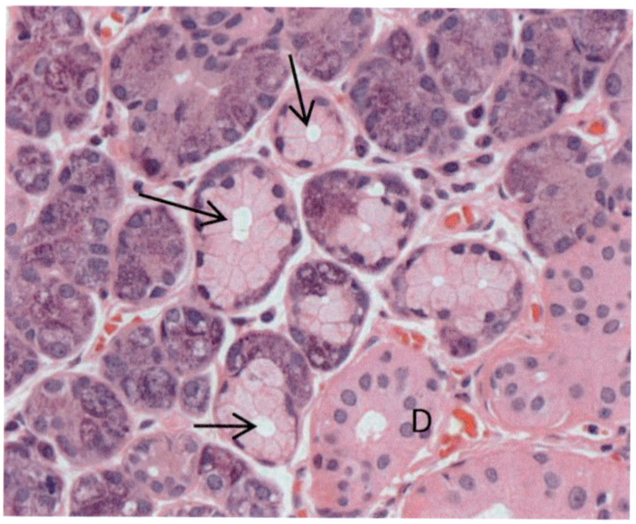

Fig. 2.7 Glandular epithelium. Photomicrograph of salivary gland tissue showing numerous discrete secretory units (acini). The lumens (arrows) of three acini are evident. Ductal structures (D) are also present

2.4 Basement Membrane (Basal Lamina)

Basement membrane, which is a specialised type of extracellular matrix, forms a thin, sheet-like structure in association with various tissues and cell types. Basement membranes are found in relation to:

- All lining epithelia
- The secretory units and ducts of glands, such as the salivary glands and kidney
- Fat cells, skeletal muscle fibres (cells) and peripheral nerve tissue, where they are associated with the Schwann cells that envelop axons
- The outer surface of capillaries and post-capillary venules and other blood and lymphatic vessels

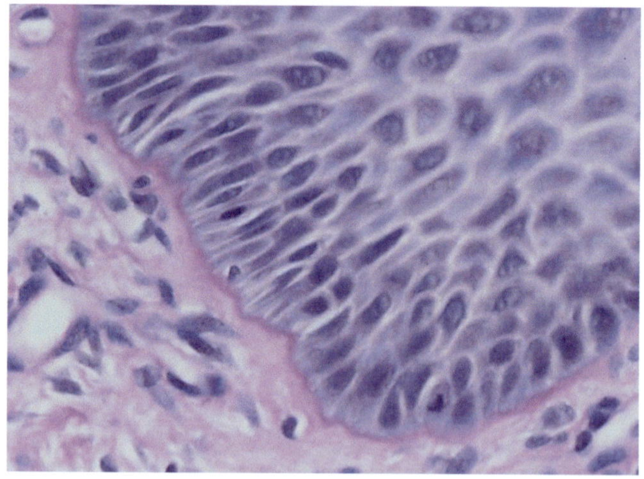

Fig. 2.8 The pink line at the base of the epithelium indicates a basement membrane providing a junction between the epithelium and the underlying connective tissue

Basement membranes have a well-established structure providing anchoring functions as well as a range of important biological functions, including signalling. In normal histological sections stained with haematoxylin and eosin (H&E), basement membranes are difficult to identify because of their dimensions and composition. The use of special stains such as Periodic acid - Schiff (PAS) used on light microscope sections (Fig. 2.8) can aid in the identification of basement membranes.

2.5 The Connective Tissues

The connective tissues are structural tissues that perform a variety of functions in the body and have a variety of appearances depending upon their function. The connective tissues occur either as soft connective tissue, specialised connective tissue or hard (calcified) connective tissue such as bone, pulp-dentine and the cementum of teeth. Examples of soft connective tissues are the various forms of fibrous connective tissue described below and the more specialised adipose tissue and blood. In addition, cartilage, tendons and ligaments are examples of soft connective tissues.

Fibrous connective tissues are composed of a variety of cell types embedded in a matrix of various types of collagens (predominantly type 1) and ground substances, which are collectively referred to as the extracellular matrix (ECM). These tissues also contain a range of blood and lymphatic vessels as well as peripheral nerve tissue. Soft fibrous connective tissues are usually classified as:

- Connective tissue proper (loose, dense regular and dense irregular)

- Elastic connective tissue
- Reticular connective tissue
- Mucous connective tissue (umbilical cord and dental papilla, which contain a high proportion of ground substance)

1. **Loose fibrous connective tissue proper** (◘ Fig. 2.9) is widely distributed in the body and is found, for example, subjacent to the lining epithelia of the mouth, the skin, the gastrointestinal system, and so on. It is also found in glands, where it forms a supportive framework for the epithelial components of the glands as well as well as the neurovascular supply. Loose fibrous connective tissue is also found in association with other tissues, such as muscle, adipose tissue, and peripheral nerves, where it provides a protective, supportive, and flexible matrix.
2. **Dense regular and dense irregular fibrous connective tissue** is found in relation to tendons and in tissues such as the dermis and the temporomandibular joint disc, respectively. In dense regular connective tissue, the fibroblasts are aligned along collagen bundles, whereas in dense irregular connective tissue, the fibroblasts are not aligned with the collagen bundles and collagen bundles themselves have an irregular arrangement
3. **Elastic fibrous connective tissue** is characterised by the presence of elastic fibres and is found in a variety of soft connective tissues such as the skin, some cartilage and the lungs. The elastic fibres consist of collections of microfibrils with varying orientations and provide the tissue involved with the ability to stretch and then recover and are prominent in, for example, arterial walls (◘ Fig. 2.10).
4. **Reticular connective tissue** contains very fine type 3 collagen fibres that form a delicate scaffolding (meshwork) of fibrous connective tissue containing small, terminal blood and lymphatic vessels and terminal nerve process in certain organs and tissues. Details are not easily seen in routine histological sections without the use of special stains. Reticular fibrous connective tissue occurs in sites such as the bone

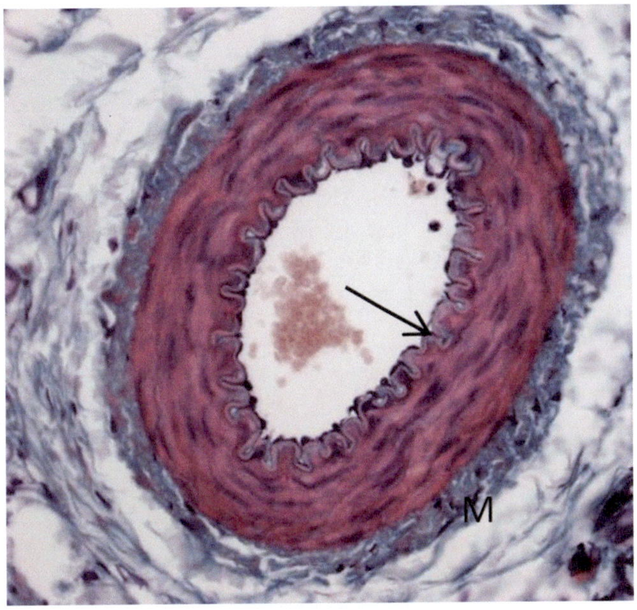

◘ **Fig. 2.10** A prominent elastin layer (arrow) is present, lining the luminal aspect of this artery. Smooth muscle (M) forms much of the remainder of the artery wall. These two components provide the vessel with the ability to expand and then recover during function. The folded character of the elastin layer in this micrograph is indicative of its ability to stretch when required

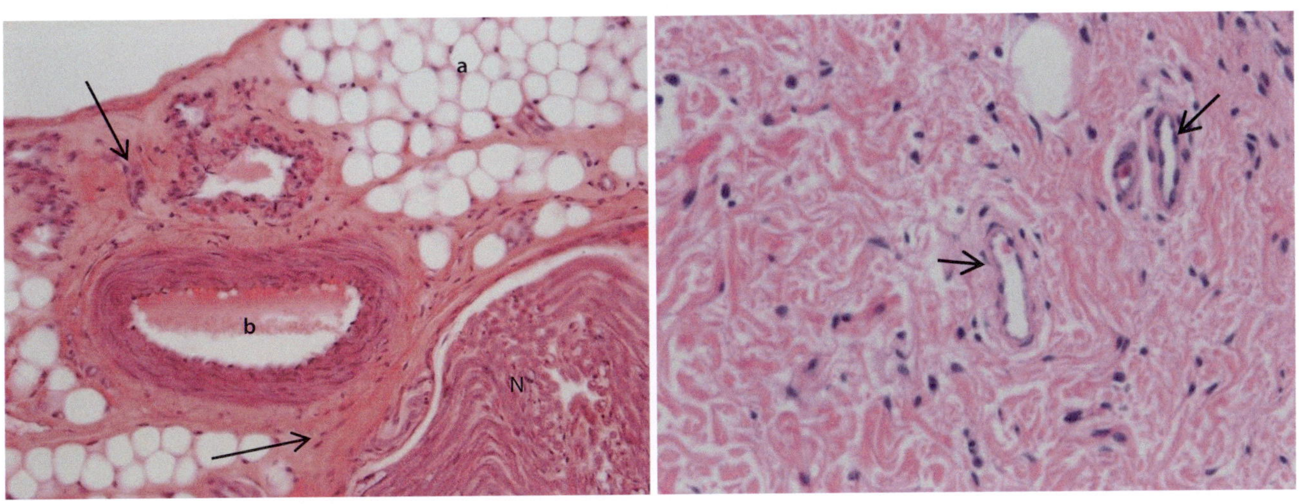

◘ **Fig. 2.9** Loose fibrous connective tissue proper. In the left-hand side (LHS) photomicrograph, fibrous connective tissue (arrows) provides a supporting matrix for other connective tissues such as adipose tissue (A), blood vessels (B) and peripheral nerve tissue (N). The micrograph on the right-hand side (RHS) shows eosinophilic (pink) loosely arranged collagen bundles in a pale background containing blood vessels (arrows) and a variety of cell nuclei representing different cell types, mostly fibroblasts marrow, liver, spleen and lymph nodes and in association with muscle and peripheral nerve fibres where the terms endomysium and endoneurium, respectively, are used to describe the reticular fibrous connective tissue and supporting loose fibrous connective tissue associated with these particular tissues.

5. **Cells of fibrous connective tissue**: Fibrous connective tissue contains a variety of cell types as well as cell types associated with blood and lymphatic vessels and peripheral nerves.

   The predominant fibrous connective tissue cell type is the fibroblast (◘ Fig. 2.11), which is responsible for the production of the fibrous (collagen and, where relevant, elastin) and non-fibrous components of the extracellular matrix (ECM). Fibroblasts are also responsible for ECM turnover and the rapid production of new ECM during wound healing. Inactive fibroblasts are referred to as fibrocytes, and a special type of contractile fibroblast called myofibroblasts is recognised. The latter cannot be differentiated from other fibroblasts in routine H- and E-stained sections and are important in the process of contraction observed in wound healing.

   An important but not easily seen cell in haematoxylin- and eosin-stained sections is the mast cell (◘ Fig. 2.12). Mast cells play significant roles in the normal maintenance of connective tissues and in immune-related processes. Mast cells are widely distributed in body tissues but, in particular, are found in mucosal and sub-mucosal connective tissues, usually adjacent to smaller blood vessels and near peripheral nerves. In histological sections, mast cells are seen as relatively large, well-delineated mononuclear cells, which may have a relatively eosinophilic cytoplasm. At high magnification, the cytoplasm shows the presence of large numbers of granules. These granules contain an extensive battery of bioactive molecules that have a variety of effects on cells

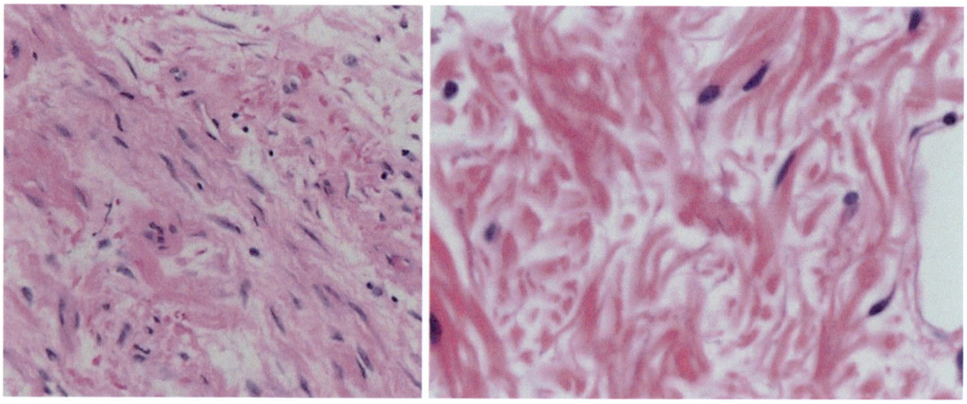

◘ **Fig. 2.11** Fibroblasts. Fibroblasts can be identified in light microscope sections by their basophilic and elongated nuclei, closely associated with the collagen of the ECM. Fibroblast cytoplasm is poorly delineated

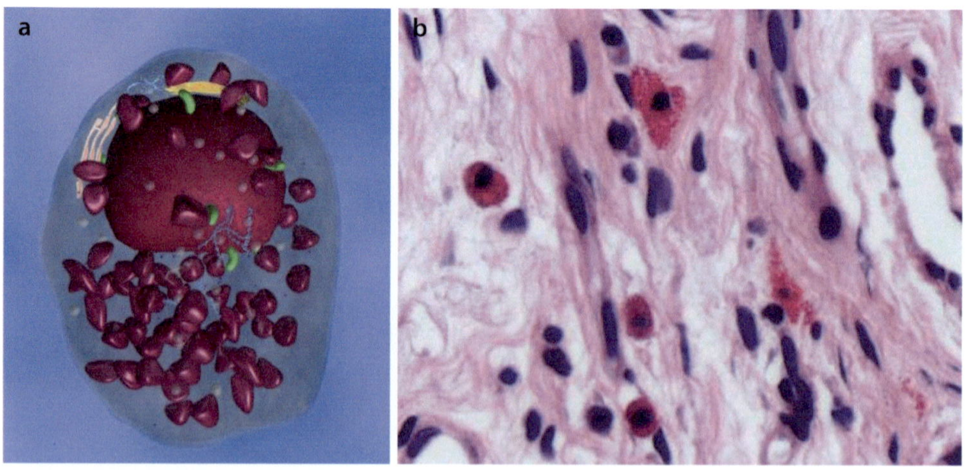

◘ **Fig. 2.12** (**a**) 3D graphic representation of a mast cell illustrating the presence of numerous cytoplasmic granules. (**b**) In this micrograph, mast cells present as mononuclear cells with brightly eosinophilic cytoplasm. This latter feature is not always evident in H&E-stained sections

and tissues. The full range of functions of mast cells is still not completely understood. Nevertheless, it is evident that they have important roles in body and tissue homeostasis, including important roles in some stages of inflammation and tissue repair, passive defence (passive immunity) and normal and type 1 hypersensitivity immunological reactions. Examples of the latter are allergies such as 'hay fever', asthma and anaphylaxis.

Other cells that are present in connective tissue include occasional lymphocytes and plasma cells, which are involved in immune surveillance and tissue macrophages, which in normal connective tissue are referred to as histiocytes. Tissue histiocytes have roles in relation to the phagocytosis of normal tissue and cell turnover products and in antigen processing. Other cell types seen in connective tissues are associated with vascular and lymphoid structures (e.g. smooth muscle in relation to the walls of larger blood vessels [see ◘ Fig. 2.9] and endothelial cells which line the lumen of blood and lymphatic vessels) and peripheral nerves, which contain Schwann cells as part of their structure.

6. **The calcified connective tissues** comprise the bone of the skeleton and the dental tissues dentine and cementum. Each of these is described in detail in relevant chapters in Part II, but a brief outline of bone histology is presented here to reinforce that bone is an example of connective tissue. When assessed macroscopically, a bone has a particular terminology applied when describing its morphology. For example, the terms cortical and cancellous bone are applied when describing the outermost bone layer and the innermost bone structure. Different terms are employed to describe histological bone types. The descriptors lamellar (Haversian) bone, woven (fibrous) bone and bundle bone are used in this context (◘ Figs. 2.13 and 2.14). Lamellar bone forms the adult human skeleton, while woven bone is involved in the embryogenesis of certain bones (e.g. the mandible) in bone healing and is also seen in bone pathologies. Bundle bone is found at the sites of tendon and ligamentous insertions on bones.
7. **Mature adipose tissue** is widely distributed in the human body and is categorised as specialised connective tissue. Fat tissue is the body's largest energy store—triglycerides—but also acts as a secretory and endocrine-like tissue. Fat comprises approximately 15–20% of body weight in males and 20–25% of body weight in females. Adipose cells are usually grouped into fat lobules (◘ Fig. 2.9) but can also be found scattered in tissue. Histologically, fat cells (◘ Fig. 2.15) are easily recognisable by their size and empty cytoplasm, the latter being due to loss of the lipid during tissue processing. Individual fat cells are embedded vascular loose fibrous connective tissue admixed with reticular connective tissue containing terminal vessels.

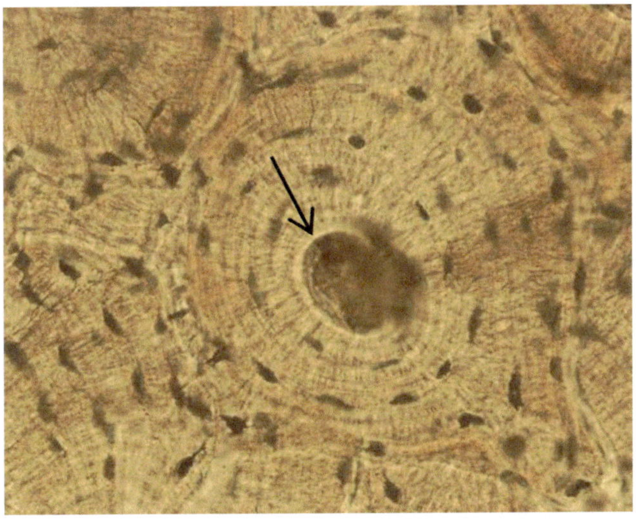

◘ **Fig. 2.13** Undecalcified section of bone illustrating lamellar bone showing an arrangement of circumferential lamellae arranged around a central Haversian canal (arrow). The Haversian canal supplies supporting connective tissue and blood supply to this form of bone

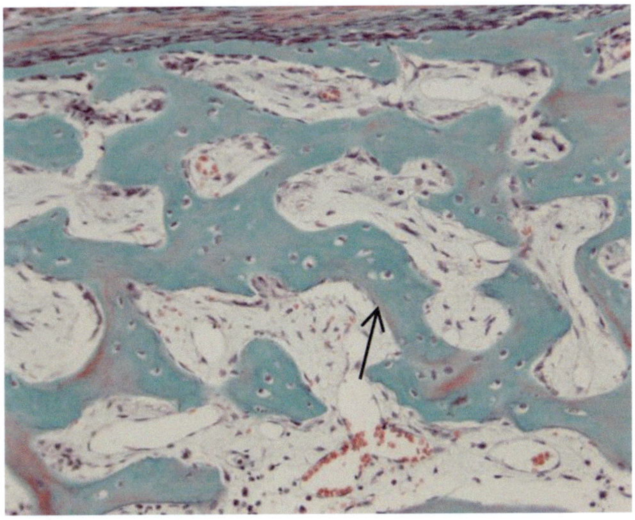

◘ **Fig. 2.14** Decalcified section of bone illustrating woven bone. The bone trabeculae (arrow) are devoid of a lamellar/Haversian pattern and are associated with a loose, vascular fibrous connective tissue stroma

8. **Cartilage** is a specialised connective tissue found in various sites in the body where it performs a variety of functions. Cartilage is a tough, resilient-flexible (compared to bone) tissue. It can cope with wear and tear (e.g. hyaline cartilage at the ends of long bones allows constant wearing/rubbing of one surface on

another without damage to the underlying bone). Three forms of cartilage are recognised:

- Hyaline cartilage
- Elastic cartilage
- Fibrocartilage

Hyaline cartilage has characteristic microscopic features (Fig. 2.16) and is found at various sites, including the articular surfaces of long bones, the epiphyseal plate (growth plate) of long bones and the ends of ribs (that joins ribs to the sternum), as well as forming the trachea, bronchi, larynx and the external nose. Hyaline cartilage has a specialised ECM made up principally of water, type 2 collagen and proteoglycans. The cells of cartilage are called chondroblasts (cells that differentiate into mature cartilage cells) and chondrocytes (cells that, along with the ECM, form the histologic structure of hyaline cartilage). Except for the articular surfaces of long bone and the epiphyseal plates, hyaline cartilage structures have a densely collagenous fibrous connective tissue perichondrium containing chondroblasts. Hyaline cartilage is avascular (absence of blood vessels), and cartilage cells receive nutritional supply by diffusion of nutrients through the ECM from the tissues (perichondrium) surrounding the cartilage. Articular hyaline cartilage receives nutrition from the synovial fluid in the joint spaces.

As the name suggests, elastic cartilage contains a prominent meshwork of elastin fibres as part of the ECM. Elastic cartilage is found in the external ear, the auditory canal and the larynx. The elastin component of the ECM provides flexibility to the body structures containing this form of cartilage. In haematoxylin- and eosin-stained histological sections, elastic cartilage closely resembles hyaline cartilage. Special stains are needed to identify the elastin in light microscope sections of elastic cartilage.

Fibrocartilage is a mixture of very densely collagenous fibrous connective tissue (type 1 collagen) containing areas of cartilage cells and small amounts of cartilage matrix. Sites where this form of cartilage is found include the intervertebral discs, the pubic symphysis, the discs of knee joints, parts of some ligaments and the articular surfaces of the temporomandibular joint. Readers are referred to ▶ Chap. 13 for details of the histological features of fibrocartilage applicable to the temporomandibular joint.

9. **Blood** is classified as a specialised connective tissue. Blood is made up of approximately 55% plasma and 45% cells. The functions of blood are many. These include oxygen and nutrient transport to the lungs and tissues, the ability to form blood clots, the carriage of inflammatory-immune cells and antibodies, the carriage of waste products to the kidneys and liver and contributing to the regulation of body temperature. Initial plasma is produced in the liver by

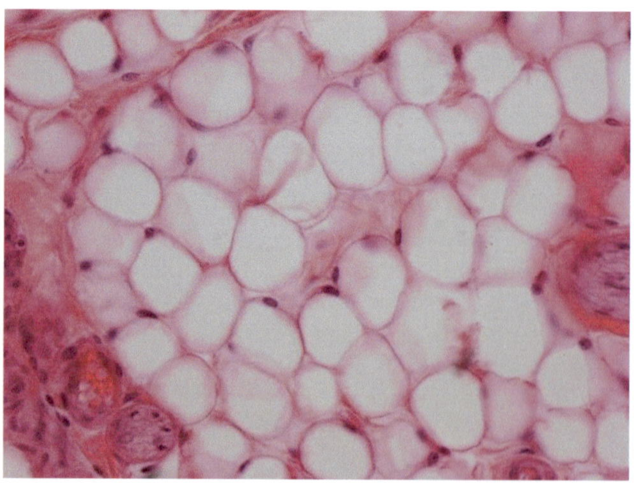

Fig. 2.15 In light microscope sections, mature fat cells are easily identified by their large size and clear cytoplasm

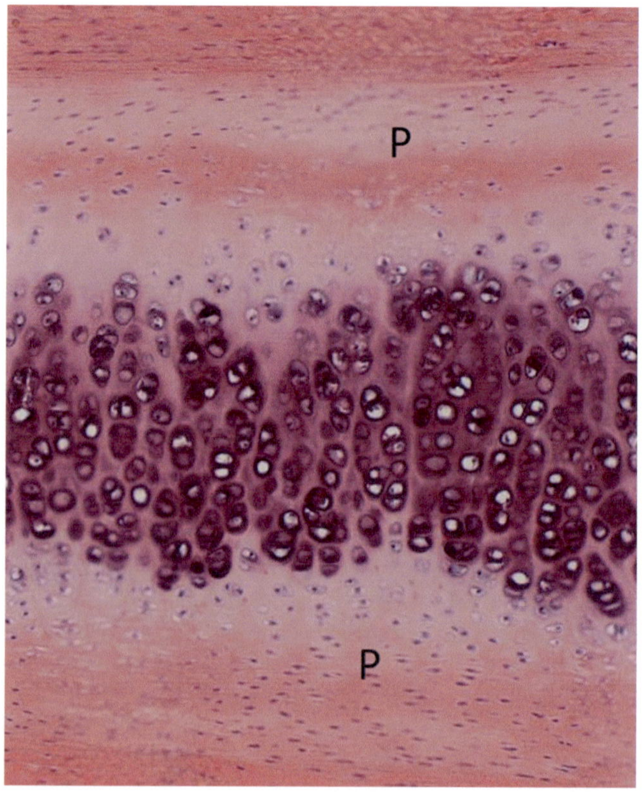

Fig. 2.16 Photomicrograph illustrating hyaline cartilage. The basophilic central zone in the micrograph comprises chondrocytes within lacunae and ECM. The surrounding perichondrium (P) consists of very dense fibrous connective tissue containing fibroblasts and chondroblasts

the reticuloendothelial cells. Other components are then added to produce whole plasma, which comprises water, proteins (e.g. albumin and antibodies), dissolved salts/ions, nutrients, hormones, cell and tissue waste products and gases.

The cellular compartment of blood is made up of the following:

- Erythrocytes (red blood cells) (about 45% of blood volume)
- Platelets (about 1% of blood volume)
- Leukocytes (white blood cells) (about 1% of blood volume)

The leukocyte population of cells consists of the following:

- Monocytes
- Lymphocytes (T and B types)
- Polymorphonuclear leukocytes

Immature mast cells and immature plasma cells (plasmablasts) may also be present in a blood smear.

The polymorphonuclear group of cells consists of the following:

- Neutrophils (polymorphonuclear neutrophils)
- Eosinophils
- Basophils

The various cells of blood develop from stem cells in the bone marrow—the process of haemopoiesis/lymphopoiesis (◘ Fig. 2.17). The lymphoid populations undergo further maturation in the thymus (T cells) and other lymphoid tissues, such as the lymph nodes and spleen, from where a variety of lymphoid cells can enter the blood or tissues.

Erythrocytes make up about 44% of the total blood cell count and are approximately 8 microns in diameter. They have a lifespan of about 120 days. Erythrocytes transport oxygen using haemoglobin and carbon dioxide. In haematoxylin- and eosin-stained sections, they can be seen as brightly eosinophilic cells lacking nuclei within blood vessels.

Platelets are very small anucleate cells about 2 microns in diameter which derive from megakaryocytes in the bone marrow. These cells live for 4–7 days and have a primary role in blood clotting. In addition, studies have shown that platelets also produce a range of bio-active agents (e.g. prostaglandins) and are involved in innate immunity and abnormal immune reactions. Individual platelets are not identifiable in light microscope sections.

Monocytes are bone marrow-derived cells that exist in the blood as monocytes and in normal connective tissues as histiocytes. In the various inflammatory states that can occur following injury (refer to ► Chap. 5), these cells are referred to as macrophages. Monocyte-derived cells also give rise to different types of multinucleate cells, such as osteoclasts and foreign body giant cells in tissues. In addition, specialised macrophage networks exist throughout the body in organs such as the lungs, liver (Kupffer cells), spleen, lymph nodes and brain (microglial cells) (◘ Fig. 2.18).

Lymphocytes are the effector cells of the immune system and play significant roles in both the maintenance of health and in human diseases, some of which can be due to abnormal immune system function. Furthermore, cells of the immune system are integral to inflammatory processes, especially chronic inflammatory processes (see ► Chap. 5). Some are involved in cancer cell surveillance. Lymphocytes are categorised as either:

- T-lymphocytes: Cells of this family are responsible for cell-mediated immunity.

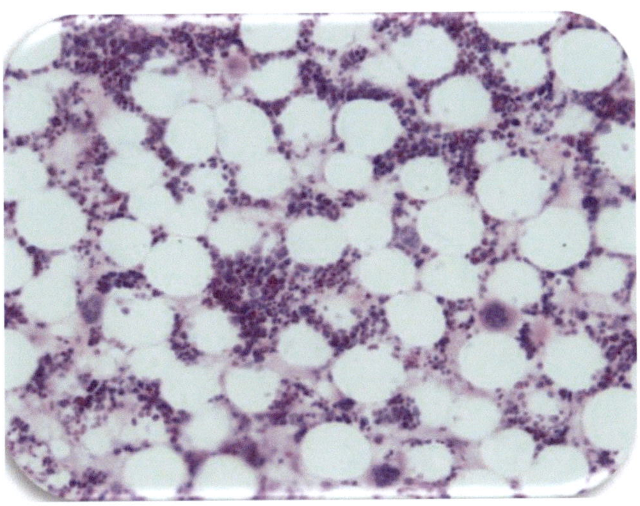

◘ **Fig. 2.17** Haemopoietic marrow contains the stem and precursor forms of the white blood cells

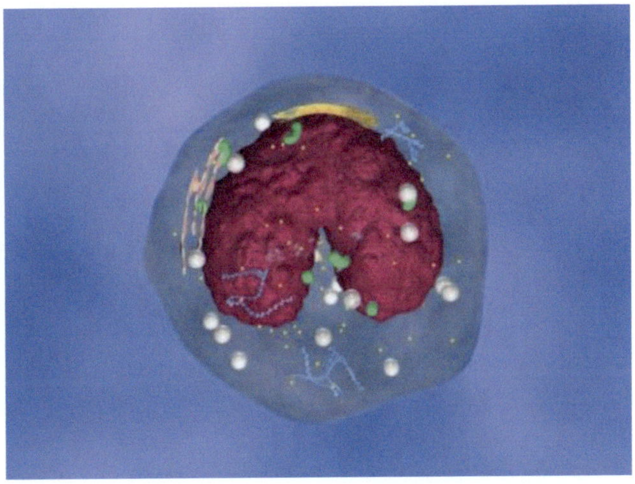

◘ **Fig. 2.18** 3D graphic representation of a blood monocyte. This cell type gives rise to a range of derived cell types

- B-lymphocytes: Cells of this family are responsible for antibody-mediated immunity.

Within these two broad groups, there are several subsets distinguished by cell surface markers (receptors) and by function. The principal T-lymphocyte subsets are as follows:

- T helper cells (T1 helper cells and T2 helper cells)
- T suppressor cells (often referred to as cytotoxic T cells)

The principal B-lymphocyte subsets are as follows:

- B cells (immature and memory types)
- Plasma cells (antibody-producing cells)

In addition to these cell types, an additional lymphocyte-like cell devoid of the usual T cell markers, called a natural killer cell, is recognised (◘ Fig. 2.19).

Although they are not normally found in circulating blood, mature, activated B-lymphocytes are called plasma cells. These cells are responsible for producing antibodies (immunoglobulins), which can exert their antigen-binding effects within circulating blood and in inflamed tissues. Microscopically, plasma cells can be identified as mononucleated cells with prominent, slightly basophilic cytoplasm. The prominence of the cytoplasm is due to the presence of prominent rough-surfaced endoplasmic reticulum involved in antibody production (◘ Fig. 2.20).

Polymorphonuclear leukocytes (polymorphs) are normal cellular constituents of blood. Their numbers vary depending upon the existence or otherwise of pathology in the body. Polymorphs in the circulation increase in numbers when there is inflammatory pathology in the body. All three cell types (◘ Fig. 2.21), but particularly neutrophils and eosinophils, leave the circulation and enter tissues at sites of inflammation, tissue damage or immunological injury (see ▶ Chap. 5). Each cell type is histologically characterised by a bi-lobed or tri-lobed nucleus with large numbers of cell-specific cytoplasmic granules.

The polymorphonuclear neutrophil is usually referred to as a 'neutrophil' or as a PMN. It is most commonly associated with acute inflammation (see ▶ Chap. 5), either de novo or as acute phase inflammation in pre-existing chronic inflammatory processes. Neutrophils are short-lived (a few days) first-line of defence cells. Their numbers in the circulation increase in cases of inflammatory pathology in the body. Neutrophils, like other inflammatory-immune cells, leave the circulating blood and enter tissues in response to a variety of molecular signals that are formed or released during cellular and tissue injury. Neutrophils contain large numbers of membrane-bound granules (previously called lysosomes). Three types of granules are now recognised: azuro-

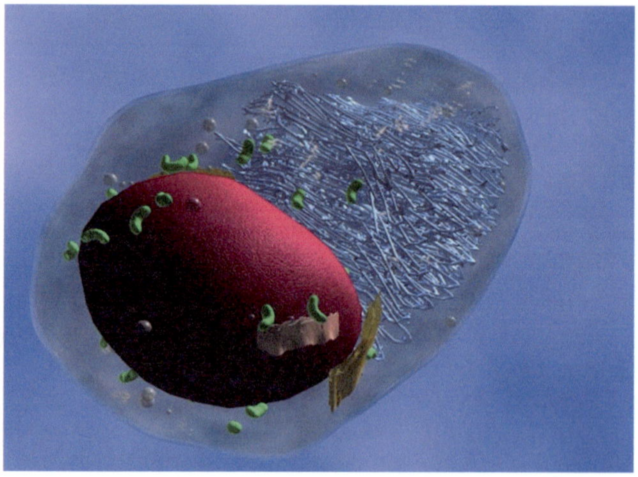

◘ **Fig. 2.20** 3D graphic representation of a plasma cell notable because of the presence of extensive rough-surfaced endoplasmic reticulum, which displaces the nucleus to one end of the cell. The microscopic features of plasma cells are detailed in ▶ Chap. 5

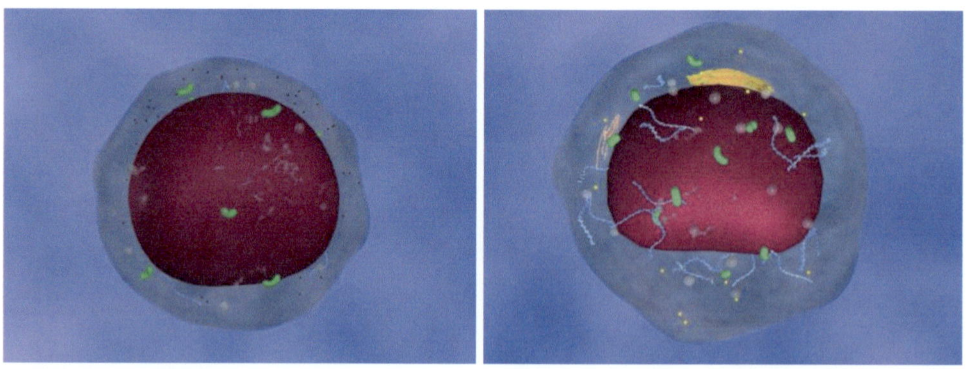

◘ **Fig. 2.19** 3D graphic representation of lymphocytes. Lymphocytes are classed as either T cells (LHS) or B cells (RHS). Unlike mature plasma cells, which have identifiable cellular features in tissue sections, lymphocytes are characterised by a basophilic, round nucleus and a paucity of cytoplasm

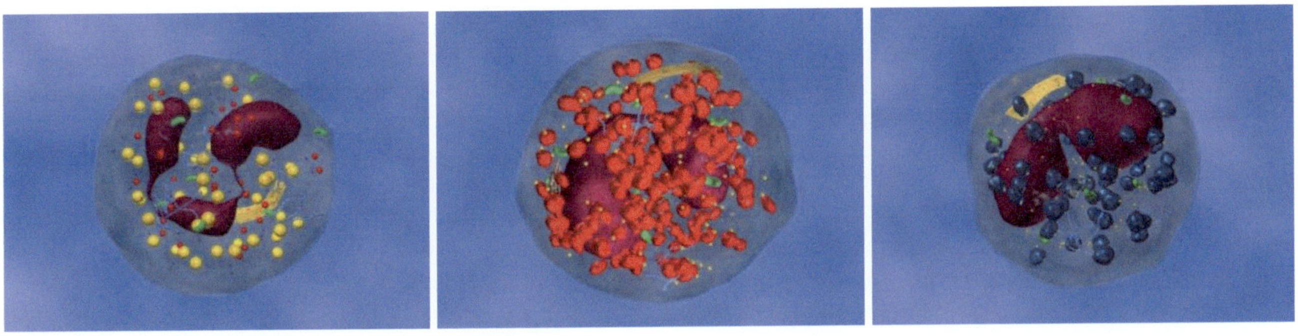

Fig. 2.21 3D graphic illustration of each of the polymorphonuclear leukocytes, namely, the neutrophil, the eosinophil and the basophil, respectively, showing their distinctive intracellular granules

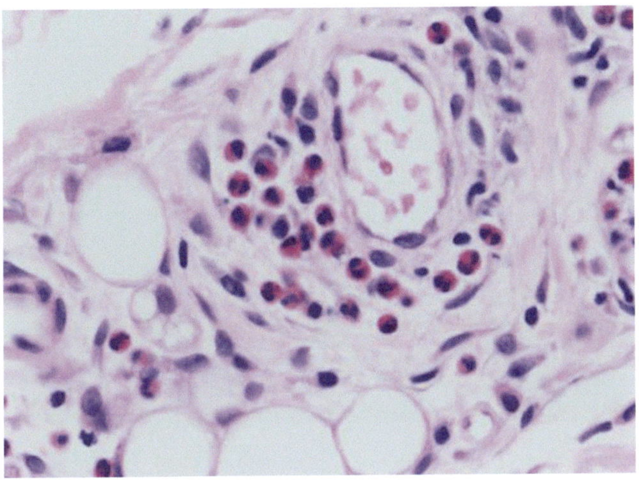

Fig. 2.22 Photomicrograph showing eosinophils with bi-lobed nuclei and intensely pink (eosinophilic) cytoplasm abutting a dilated capillary within loose fibrous connective tissue

phil granules, specific granules and small storage granules. The granules contain a variety of pre-formed enzymes, proteases and mediators capable of breaking down phagocytosed tissue, cellular debris and microorganisms. The granule contents are also capable of causing damage to normal tissue components if they escape the confines of the neutrophil. Additionally, some granule contents are involved in the regulation of processes such as inflammation.

Eosinophils are granule-containing polymorphonuclear leukocytes that occur in the circulation but which exist in much larger numbers in tissues, predominantly, mucosal and sub-mucosal tissues. While being capable of phagocytosis, eosinophils effect much of their activity outside the cell by releasing their granules and contents under the influence of a range of mediators. The granules stain intensely with eosin in haematoxylin- and eosin-stained sections (Fig. 2.22). Eosinophils have a range of activities and capabilities that occur when granules are released from the cytoplasm in response to a variety of stimuli. Historically, eosinophils have always been associated with defence against helminthic infections. However, it is now recognised that these cells also play roles in acute and chronic inflammation and, especially, in immune hypersensitivity reactions (allergies, systemic anaphylaxis, hives and asthma) where they interact with mast cells and basophils.

The basophil is the smallest of the polymorphonuclear leukocytes and circulates in the blood in small numbers. The basophil can be associated with inflammatory reactions but is very difficult to identify in H&E-stained sections. Basophils are most often functionally associated with mast cells in cases of type 1 hypersensitivity reactions (systemic and local anaphylactic-type reactions). Like mast cells, basophils have IgE-Fc fragment receptors on their surface. Interaction of antigen with the cell-bound IgE causes degranulation of the basophil and release of a wide range of predominantly pre-formed mediators, which, along with mediators derived from mast cells, contribute to allergic reactions such as asthma, anaphylaxis and the milder allergy 'hay fever'.

2.6 Muscle

Three types of muscle are recognised:
- Skeletal (striated muscle)
- Smooth muscle
- Cardiac muscle

Muscle as a tissue makes up about 50% of body mass and consists of specialised cells that contain contractile proteins (fibres). Stimulation of muscle cells causes these proteins to generate forces that cause movement. In skeletal muscle, the stimulation of cells is electrical and mediated by motor neurons that are under voluntary nervous control. In cardiac muscle, the stimulation of cells is also electrical, but it is generated within the cardiac muscle itself in highly specialised structures called 'nodes' that are made up of special types of cardiac muscle cells. These produce the contraction–relaxation cycle that is the 'heartbeat'. In smooth muscle, the stimulation causing the contraction of cells can be of different origins. For example, smooth muscle contraction and relaxation in the oesophagus is due to reflex impulses and signals from the autonomic system; smooth muscle contraction–relaxation in the uterus can be controlled by the sex hormones and the hormone oxytocin; smooth muscle contraction in blood vessels and the lungs can be controlled by cytokines (e.g. histamine and slow-reacting substances).

Depending upon the muscle type, the functions of muscle include the following:

- Movement of body parts of the musculoskeletal system—skeletal muscle
- Causing the pumping action of the heart—cardiac muscle
- Causing narrowing and then relaxation of arteries—smooth muscle
- Causing rhythmic movement—smooth muscle of the gastrointestinal system

1. **Skeletal muscle** consists of long individual muscle cells (called muscle fibres) arranged into discrete structures called fascicles. Many fascicles make up a single muscle (▫ Fig. 2.23). Each muscle is served by one nerve, one artery, and one or more veins. These become very highly branched to supply individual muscle cells (▫ Figs. 2.24 and 2.25).
2. **Smooth muscle** is found in the walls of hollow organs and structures in the body, for example, in arteries (▫ Fig. 2.9), arterioles and veins, the gastrointestinal tract, the bladder, the lungs and the uterus in females. Smooth muscle is also found in the eye, where it controls iris movements. Smooth muscle cells are considerably smaller than skeletal and cardiac muscle cells and are tightly arranged (▫ Fig. 2.26) in variously sized arrays depending upon the organ or tissue structure involved.
3. **Cardiac muscle** (▫ Fig. 2.27) is different from skeletal muscle in that:
   - The muscle cells are shorter (85–100 microns).
   - Each cell only contains one or, sometimes, two nuclei.

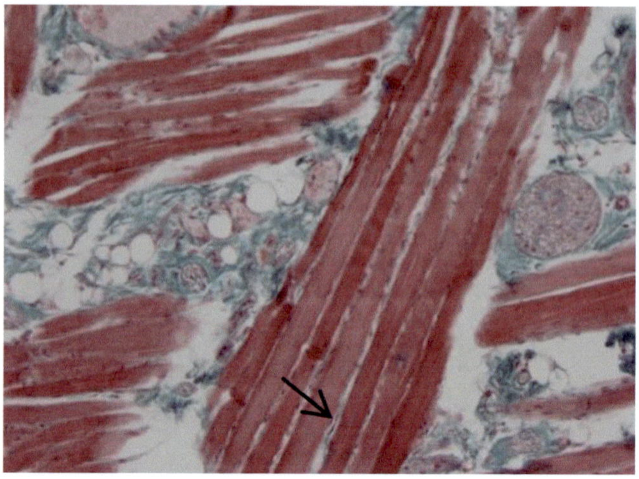

▫ **Fig. 2.24** Photomicrograph showing individual, elongated skeletal muscle cells, which can be seen in close proximity to each other. Each muscle fibre is surrounded by a basement membrane (not seen here) and a thin layer of delicate, reticular connective tissue that contains terminal blood vessels and terminal nerves. This layer is called the endomysium (arrow)

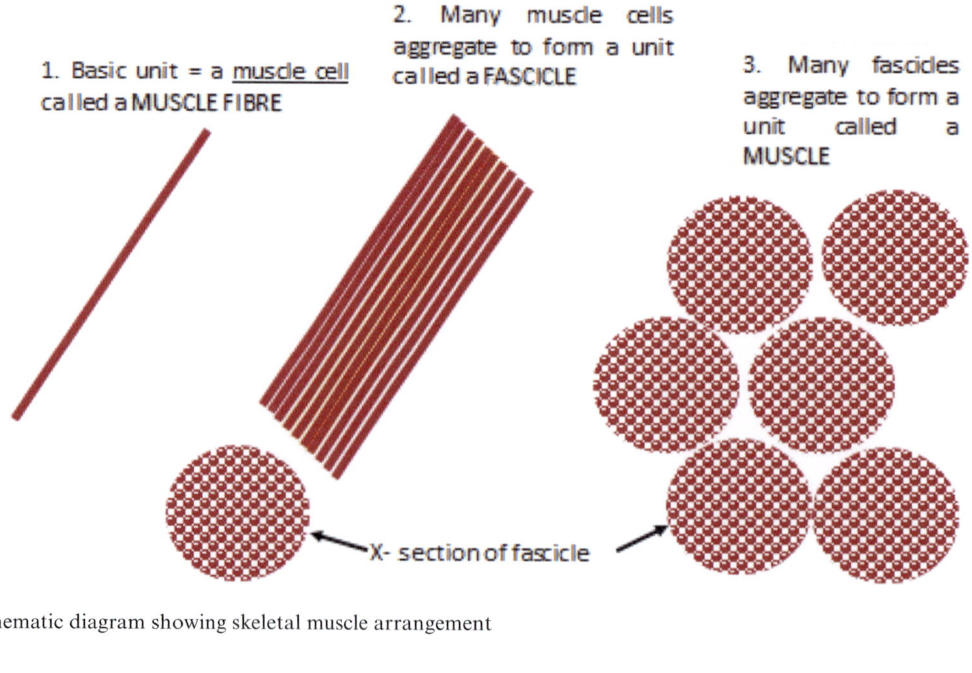

▫ **Fig. 2.23** Schematic diagram showing skeletal muscle arrangement

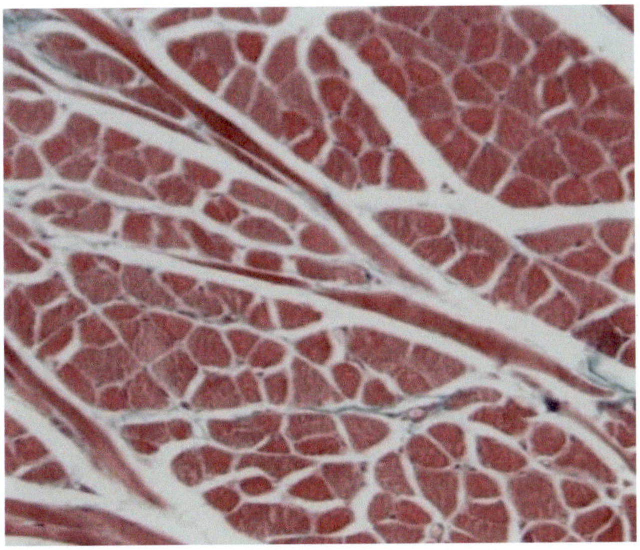

■ **Fig. 2.25** Photomicrograph of several skeletal muscle fascicles, each surrounded by a zone of supporting fibrous connective tissue called the perimysium. The perimysium is contiguous with the endomysium surrounding individual muscle cells, which in this micrograph are shown in cross section. Variable numbers of skeletal muscle fasciculi make up an individual muscle, which is enveloped in a prominent layer of tough fibrous connective tissue called the epimysium

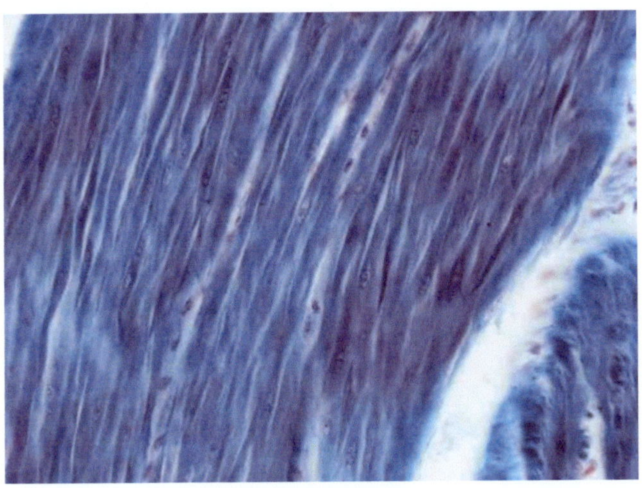

■ **Fig. 2.26** Smooth muscle. Photomicrograph showing a tightly packed, parallel array of smooth muscle cells. Individual cells are difficult to separate from one another. Purplish nuclear shapes indicate individual cells

- The muscle cells branch.
- Cardiac muscle cells and their branches link to one another by specialised intercellular junctions called intercalated discs.

Other differences include the facts that atrial cardiac muscle cells are smaller than ventricular cardiac muscle cells and cardiac muscle mitochondria occupy about 40% of cell volume compared to skeletal muscle cells, where mitochondrial volume is approximately 2%.

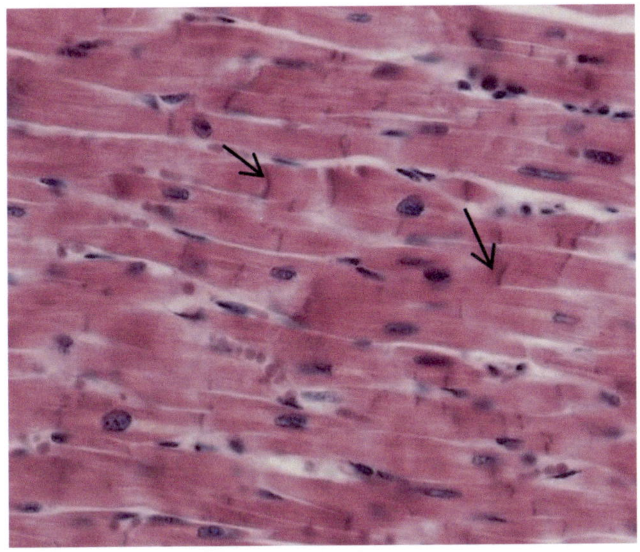

■ **Fig. 2.27** Histologically, cardiac muscle is seen to be made up of relatively short, closely packed and aligned cells. Intercalated discs reflecting cell-to-cell interconnections are indicated (arrows)

2.7 Peripheral Nerve Tissue

Peripheral nerve tissue observed in tissue sections can comprise somatic nerve branches and autonomic nerve tissue. The latter can include autonomic nerve branches as well as autonomic ganglion cell aggregates. Autonomic nerves are paired and arise from a chain of neurons containing ganglia alongside the spinal cord. The two major components of the autonomic system are the sympathetic and parasympathetic systems. The autonomic nervous system is a visceral efferent-only system (which sends motor impulses to the visceral organs). The somatic nervous system comprises the following:

- The cranial nerves: These are paired (12) and arise directly from the brain or brainstem and have ganglia outside the skull. Some are sensory-only nerves, others are motor nerves and a few are mixed nerves. These nerves mostly relate to the voluntary control of movement in the head and neck region.
- The spinal nerves: These are paired (31) and arise from the spinal cord and have their neurons in the sensory ganglia situated outside the spine. The motor neurons reside in the grey matter of the spinal cord. They control voluntary muscle movement and reflex responses.

Like skeletal muscle, peripheral nerves have a well-described structure. In summary, nerves consist of collections of nerve axons, the majority of which are enveloped by a myelin sheath produced by Schwann cells. Groups of axons are arranged into variously sized fascicles, which, in turn, make up a peripheral nerve. Other nerve components include connective tissue elements surrounding individual axons and fascicles and the whole nerve, each with a specific nomenclature (▫ Fig. 2.28) and blood vessels.

In routine tissue sections and because of their three-dimensional pathways, peripheral nerve branches are usually sectioned obliquely or in cross section rather than longitudinally such that only a portion of a nerve is microscopically observed. Furthermore, axons do not readily stain with H&E, and myelin is mostly lost during tissue processing because of its fatty composition (▫ Fig. 2.29).

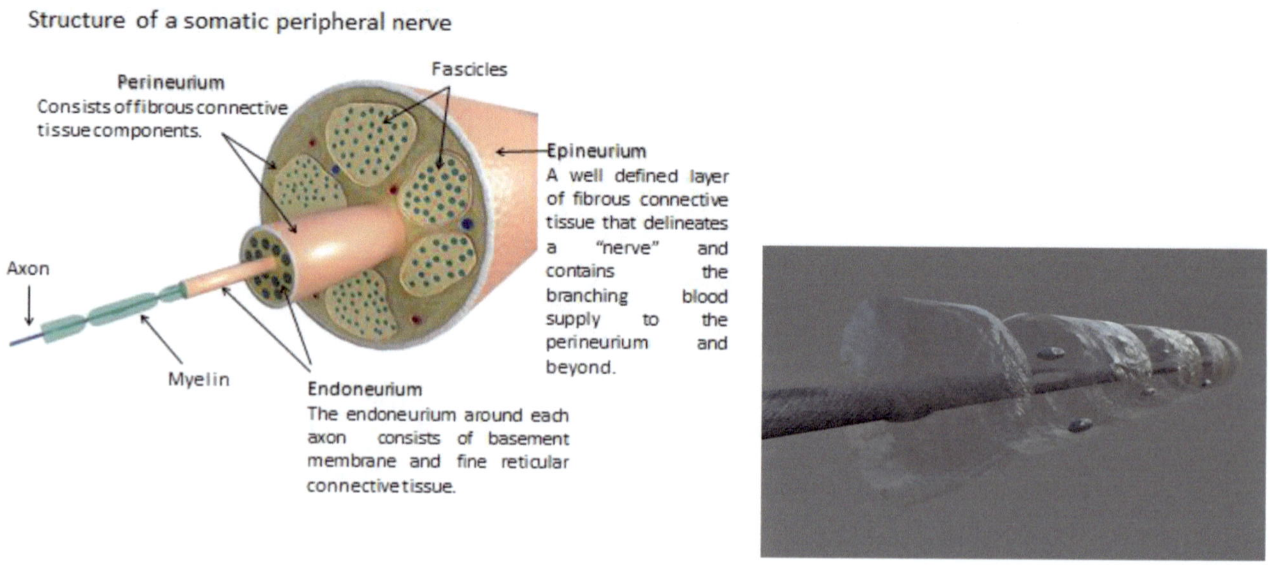

▫ **Fig. 2.28** 3D graphic diagrams illustrating the structure of a peripheral nerve. The fascicular structure can be observed in a larger nerve viewed in cross section but is not readily observed in the smaller branches of a nerve. A single myelinated axon within one fascicle making up the nerve in these diagrams is exaggerated in scale to illustrate the myelin. The interruptions in the myelin sheath seen in the diagrams are called the nodes of Ranvier

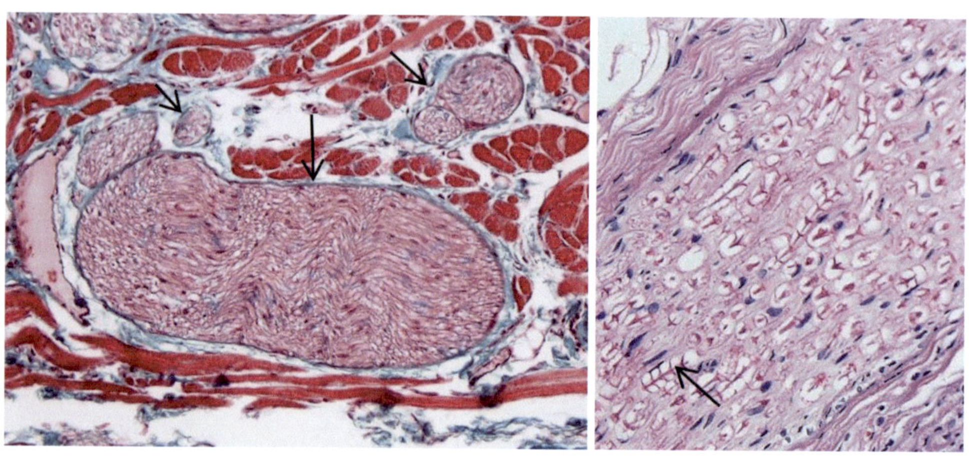

▫ **Fig. 2.29** Photomicrograph showing sectioned peripheral nerve branches. (LHS) Several nerve branches (arrows) of varying sizes sectioned obliquely or in cross section are evident. (RHS) A higher magnification view of a segment of a peripheral nerve branch shows small clear spaces where myelin has been lost during tissue processing, nodes of Ranvier (arrow) and longitudinally orientated cell nuclei. The latter comprise Schwann cells and fibroblasts. Other components such as collagen, reticular tissue and small blood vessels also make up nerve branches such as those seen here

2.8 Summary

The human body is made up of a diverse range of cell and tissue types, each characterised by particular microscopic features. Each cell and tissue type originates from one or more embryological layers in the early stages of embryogenesis. As embryogenesis progresses, the various cell and tissue types develop into their microscopically identifiable functional forms. Human tissues are classified as epithelial tissues, connective tissues and muscle and nerve tissues. Within each category, various sub-types are found, with their structural features reflecting their specific functions in the body.

Further Reading

Mescher AL. Junqueira's basic histology: text and atlas. 16th ed. 2021. isbn:9781260462982.

Young B, Woodford P, O'Dowd G. Wheater's functional histology: a text and colour atlas. 6th ed. 2013. isbn:9780702047473.

Histology of Cellular and Tissue Alterations

S R Prabhu

Contents

S R Prabhu et al. (eds.), *Oral Histology and Oral Histopathology*, https://doi.org/10.1007/978-3-031-77481-2_3

3.1 Introduction

If cells are placed under continuous stress, they can adapt. This process of cellular adaptation is a crucial mechanism that enables cells to maintain a steady state despite adverse conditions. These adaptations, characterised by reversible changes in the number, size, phenotype, metabolic activity, or functions in response to changes in their environment, play a significant role in disease. Understanding the two types of cellular adaptations, physiological and pathological, is key to comprehending the complex responses of cells to their environment. Physiological adaptations usually represent cellular responses to normal stimulation by hormones or endogenous chemical mediators, as evidenced in the enlargement of the uterus and breasts in pregnancy. Pathological adaptation represents responses to stress that allow cells to modulate their structure and function and thus escape injury. Distinct forms of pathological adaptations include cellular hypertrophy, hyperplasia, atrophy, metaplasia, and dysplasia. The term cellular dysplasia is frequently used in cellular pathology. It refers to abnormal cellular shape, size, and organisation changes and is usually not considered a true adaptation.

3.2 Hypertrophy

Hypertrophy is an increase in the size of cells, resulting in an increase in the size of the organ. In contrast, hyperplasia represents an increase in the size of the tissue due to an increase in the cell number (◘ Fig. 3.1). In hypertrophy, cells cannot divide as in the heart and striated muscles. Hypertrophy can be physiological or pathological and is caused either by increased functional demand or specific hormonal stimulation. A typical example is muscular hypertrophy in response to exercise. Exercise stimulates skeletal and cardiac muscle fibres to increase in diameter and accumulate more structural contractile proteins. Hypertrophy may compensate for injury when parenchymal cells are damaged or lost. For instance, following myocardial infarction, cardiac myocytes cannot divide to replace destroyed muscle fibres, but residual myocytes enlarge (hypertrophy) in an attempt to replace some of the functions of the lost myofibres. Benign masseteric hypertrophy is an example of facial muscle hypertrophy. This condition is idiopathic in most patients. Bruxism and habitual clenching may be a cause in some individuals. Literature often cites medication-induced gingival enlargement as gingival hypertrophy. However, medication-induced

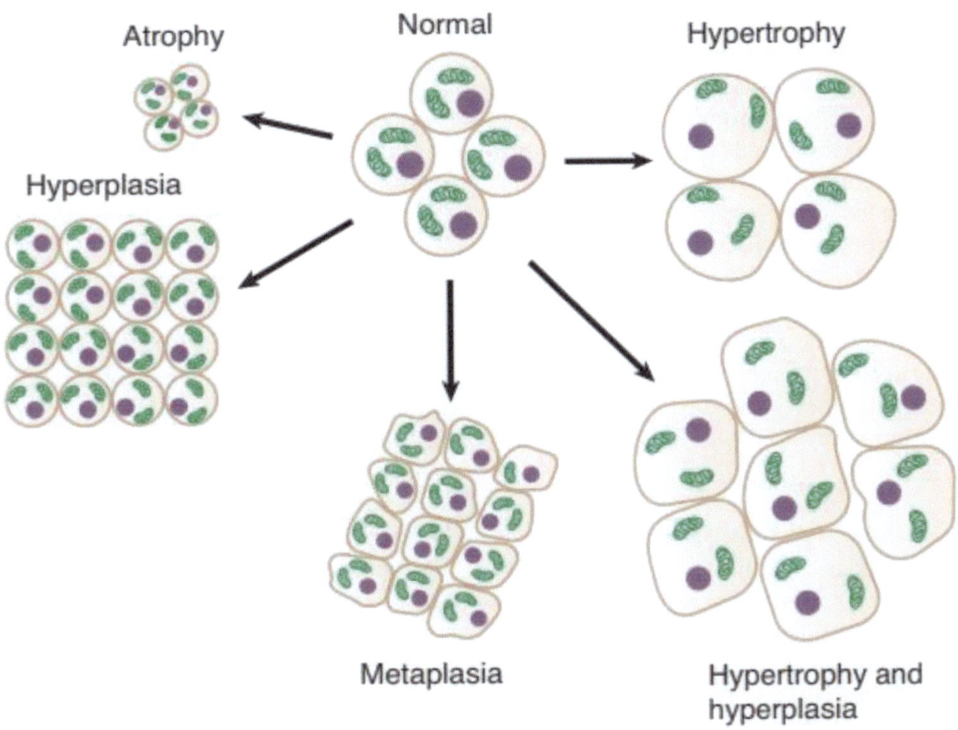

◘ **Fig. 3.1** Cellular adaptive changes to injury

gingival enlargement is characterised predominantly by the proliferation of fibroblasts and not purely by the increase in cellular size.

3

3.3 Hyperplasia

As defined above, hyperplasia refers to an increase in the number of cells (◘ Fig. 3.1) that increases the organ's size. This response can occur only in a cell population capable of cell division (mitosis). These are called labile cells. These include haematopoietic cells of the bone marrow, epithelial cells of the skin and mucosae of the mouth, intestine, vagina, and cervix, and ductal epithelia of exocrine glands, including those of the salivary glands, and epithelia of the uterus and the urinary tract. Cells in these tissues quickly undergo hyperplasia in response to hormonal stimulation, inflammation, or chronic physical trauma. The liver, kidney, and pancreas cells are stable cells with minimal replicative capacity in their normal state. However, these cells can proliferate in response to injury or loss of tissue mass. Hyperplasia differs from neoplastic cellular proliferation in that hyperplastic cells generally subside if the stimulus is removed.

3.3.1 Types of Hyperplasia

Hyperplasia can be physiological or pathological. Physiological hyperplasia is divided into two forms: compensatory and hormonal hyperplasia. Compensatory hyperplasia is cells' proliferation while maintaining their differentiated structure and function. The classic example of compensatory hyperplasia is hepatocyte regeneration in the injured liver. After partial hepatectomy, liver cells re-enter the cell cycle and replicate until the liver recovers its lost mass—hormonal hyperplasia results from excessive hormonal stimulation of target cells. The proliferation of glandular epithelium of the female breast at puberty and during pregnancy is an example of hormonal hyperplasia.

3.3.2 Some Causes and Examples of Hyperplasia

- **The increased physiological requirement**: This may result in hyperplasia, as seen in excessive menstrual bleeding (chronic blood loss). This causes hyperplasia of erythrocytic elements.
- **Hyperplasia due to immune responsiveness to many antigens**: Lymphoid hyperplasia, seen in enlarged tonsils and swollen lymph nodes in streptococcal pharyngitis, is an example of immune responsiveness to antigens.
- **Hyperplasia due to long-standing inflammation or chronic physical or chemical injury**: A hyperplastic response often accompanies the formation of calluses due to ill-fitting shoes.
- **Reactive hyperplastic lesions (RHLs)**: RHLs develop in response to chronic injury, simulating an exuberant tissue repair response. They represent some of the most common oral lesions, including traumatic (irritation) fibroma, inflammatory fibrous hyperplasia, oral pyogenic granuloma, pregnancy tumour, giant cell fibroma, peripheral ossifying fibroma, peripheral giant cell lesions, and epulis fissuratum (EF).
- **Increased levels of androgens**: Benign prostatic hyperplasia (BPH) is characterised by epithelial and stromal proliferation of the cellular elements of the prostate. Although the exact cause is not known, most experts consider increased levels of androgens (testosterone) and their metabolites to play a role in the development of BPH.
- **Chronic inflammation**: A pulp polyp (chronic hyperplastic pulpitis) seen in an open carious tooth is an example of hyperplasia of the inflamed pulp.
- **Human papillomavirus**: Multifocal epithelial hyperplasia (Heck's disease) is a wart-like growth in the mucous tissues of the mouth caused by certain subtypes of the human papillomavirus (HPV).
- **Medications**: Gingival hyperplasia (enlargement) is a well-known and common adverse reaction to several medications. Three major drugs are associated with gingival enlargement: calcium channel blockers, immune suppressants such as Cyclosporine A, and anti-epileptics such as Phenytoin.

3.4 Atrophy

Shrinkage of the size of cells by loss of cell substances is known as cellular atrophy (◘ Fig. 3.1). Atrophic cells may have diminished functions but are viable—atrophy results from decreased protein synthesis and increased protein degradation. Atrophic cells exhibit fewer mitochondria and endoplasmic reticulum. Autophagosomes take up damaged organelles where their digestion and lysis occur. Undigested residues remain in the cytoplasm as lipid-rich brown pigment imparting a brown colour to the atrophic organ (e.g. brown atrophy of the heart or the testis). Causes of atrophy may include decreased workload, as in immobilisation of a limb after a bone fracture (disuse atrophy), loss of innervation, diminished blood supply, inadequate nutrition, loss of endocrine stimulation, and ageing (senile atrophy).

3.4.1 Types and Examples of Atrophy

- Atrophy can be classified as physiological and pathological. The overall decrease in brain size over the years is an example of physiological atrophy. An atrophic brain shows narrow gyri, widened sulci, and dilated lateral ventricles. Bone and muscles in the elderly are atrophic, thin, and weak. The ovary, uterus, and breast undergo physiological atrophy after menopause.
- Pathological atrophy occurs as a result of inadequate nutrition and stimulation. Atrophic kidneys affected by atherosclerosis, atrophic leg muscles after spinal cord injury, and general cachexia due to malignant disease, HIV disease, or malnutrition are examples of pathological atrophy. Renewing physical activity of a disused limb, as in a fracture, may cause atrophy of the muscle cells to resume their usual size and function. Atrophy of the brain in Alzheimer's disease is due to extensive cell death. In this disease, the size of the brain cannot be restored.
- Atrophic glossitis is common in severe iron deficiency anaemia, vitamin B12 deficiency, and celiac disease. Acute atrophic candidiasis of the oral mucosa is usually associated with a bright red colour due to mucosal atrophy. Epithelium in oral lichen planus, oral lichenoid lesions, and sub-mucous fibrosis present as atrophy. A well-demarcated zone of epithelial atrophy, erythema, or ulceration characterises oral involvement of systemic lupus erythematosus. A detailed discussion of these conditions is beyond the scope of this chapter.

3.5 Metaplasia

Metaplasia is a reversible change in which one adult cell type replaces another (◘ Fig. 3.1). It is not known to occur during embryonic development. Generally, it results from persistent cellular trauma and is a protective mechanism. Metaplasia may be induced or accelerated by some abnormal stimulus, such as acid or base causing a change in pH, hormones, cigarette smoke, or alcohol, and a diet low in fruit, vegetable, and vitamin C and high in salt.

3.5.1 Examples of Metaplasia

- A typical example of metaplasia is the stratified squamous epithelial cells in the oesophagus becoming goblet cells when exposed to persistent acid reflux (Barrett's oesophagus).
- Another example is the ciliated columnar epithelium of bronchial mucosa changing into squamous epithelium when irritated by chronic cigarette smoke. After smoking cessation, the squamous epithelium may revert to the ciliated epithelium. If smoking is continued, the squamous metaplasia may progress to dysplasia (see below), showing disorderly arranged cells with cellular atypia. Initially, this change is reversible, but as the dysplasia becomes more severe, reversal becomes less likely, and there is a greater chance of progression to neoplasia.
- Metaplasia in radicular and dentigerous cysts: These cysts are lined by non-keratinising stratified squamous epithelium. Occasionally, the lining may microscopically exhibit metaplasia wherein goblet-like mucous cells, mixed with ciliated columnar cells, may replace stratified squamous epithelium.
- Metaplasia in denture-induced hyperplasia (epulis fissuratum): In this condition, distinct microscopic variations such as osseous and squamous metaplasia may occasionally be found.
- Necrotising sialometaplasia: This benign ulcerative lesion usually occurs at the posterior hard palate in the setting of trauma-induced ischemic necrosis (hypoxic injury) of minor salivary glands. Various contributing factors include cigarette smoking, bulimia, and trauma from local anaesthetic injections or dentures.

3.6 Cellular Dysplasia

Cellular dysplasia is linked to altered tissue architecture characterised by changes in cell size and shape, nuclear enlargement, cellular hyperchromatism, and disorderly arrangement of cells (◘ Fig. 3.2). It develops from sequential mutations in a proliferating cell population and is considered a pre-neoplastic (potentially malignant) disorder in several organs, such as the cervix, prostate, bladder, and mouth. In most cases, severe cellular dysplasia (intraepithelial carcinoma) leads to malignant transformation if not treated. Dysplasia of the uterine cervix is called cervical intraepithelial neoplasia (CIN). Cellular dysplasia can be observed in mucosal surfaces in response to chronic injury. Examples include chemical injury in the bronchi of cigarette smokers or viral injury in the setting of dysplasia of the uterine cervix. (Note: Often, terms such as fibrous, osseous, and cemental dysplasias are used in different clinical circumstances. These should not be confused with cellular dysplasia.)

3

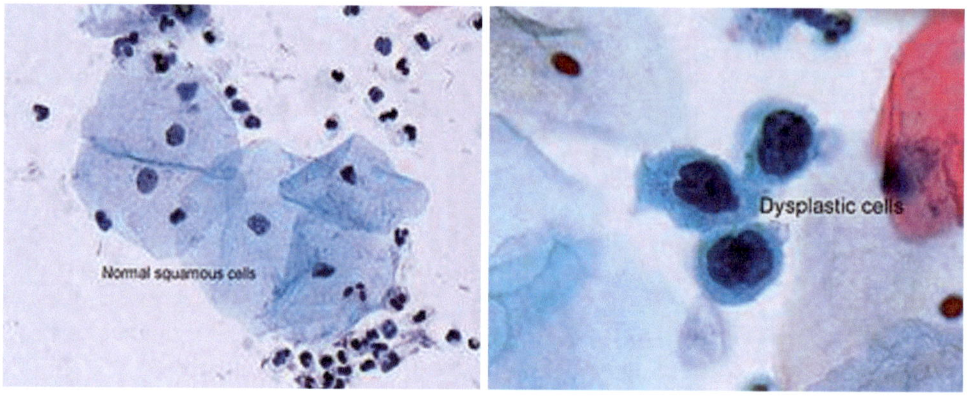

Fig. 3.2 Cellular dysplasia. Note the exfoliated normal squamous cells on the left and dysplastic cells with nuclear enlargement and cellular hyperchromatism on the right. (Wiki)

3.6.1 Examples of Dysplasia

Atypical endometrial hyperplasia, dysplastic bronchial mucosa in chronic cigarette smokers, and leukoplakia of the oral mucosa, vulva, or penis are some examples of dysplastic conditions. Oral lesions that may show cellular dysplasia include leukoplakia, erythroplakia, and chronic speckled white lesions. These and other dysplastic lesions are considered potentially malignant disorders (discussed in chapter….).

3.7 Cellular Degenerations

Non-lethal injury to a cell may cause cell degeneration (retrogressive change), manifested as some abnormality of biochemical function, a recognisable structural change, or a combined biochemical and structural abnormality. Degeneration is reversible but may progress to necrosis if the injury persists. Cellular degeneration includes hydropic degeneration, cellular fatty change, cloudy swelling, hyaline degeneration, mucoid (myxoid/myxomatous) degeneration, fibrinoid degeneration, and glycogen storage.

3.7.1 Hydropic Degeneration

Hydropic change means water accumulation within the cell's cytoplasm. Other synonyms are cloudy swelling because of the gross appearance of the affected organ and vacuolar degeneration because of cytoplasmic vacuolation. Hydropic swelling is an entirely reversible change upon removal of the injurious agent. Cellular swelling is the first manifestation of almost all forms of cell injury.

The common causes of hydropic degeneration include acute and sub-acute cell injury from various agents such as bacterial toxins, chemicals, poisons, burns, high fever, and intravenous administration of hypertonic glucose or saline. Hydropic change may be due to directly or indirectly acting chemical agents. These agents cause increased cell membrane injury. Some examples include cyanide poisoning, anti-neoplastic drugs, and tetrachloride. Some agents release highly toxic free radicals, causing lipid peroxidation and cell membrane damage with increased sodium and water influx, causing cellular swelling.

3.7.1.1 Examples of Hydropic Degeneration

- Injury to certain liver or kidney cells can cause hydropic degeneration. In the damaged organ (e.g. kidney), weight increases and it becomes swollen and pale in colour.
- Hydropic degeneration of the basal cells with scattered dyskeratotic keratinocytes (civatte, colloid, hyaline, or cytoid bodies) along the epithelial interface is common in lichen planus.
- Other oral disorders with microscopic evidence of hydropic degeneration of the basal epithelial cells include lupus erythematosus, oral lichenoid lesions, and oral graft lesions versus host reaction.

3.8 Cellular Fatty Change (Fatty Degeneration)

Fatty change (or older term fatty degeneration) is the accumulation of neutral fat within parenchymal cells. The term neutral fat is also taken as a synonym for triglycerides. Fatty change is widespread in the liver but may occur in other non-fatty tissues, such as the heart, skeletal muscle, and kidneys. The causes of fatty change in the liver include obesity, diabetes mellitus, alcoholism, starvation, protein-calorie malnutrition, chronic illnesses (e.g. tuberculosis), acute fatty liver in late pregnancy, hypoxia (due to anaemia or cardiac failure), use of hepatotoxins (e.g. carbon tetrachloride, chloroform, ether, aflatoxins, and other poisons), administration of methotrexate, steroids, halothane anaesthetic tetracycline, etc.

3.8.1 Examples of Fatty Change

Fattys change can occur in Reye's syndrome, polycystic ovary syndrome, chronic hepatitis B, chronic hepatitis C, and haemochromatosis. From the clinical point of view, fatty liver disease is paramount. It can be divided into two major types: non-alcoholic fatty liver disease (NAFLD) and alcohol-related fatty liver disease (AFLD).

- Non-alcoholic fatty liver disease (NAFLD) is a very common disorder. It refers to conditions where excess fat accumulates in the liver of people who drink little or no alcohol. Chronic liver disease is the most common cause, constituting a significant risk factor for progression to liver failure, cirrhosis, and hepatocellular carcinoma. A fatty heart is a typical finding in subjects with obesity and type 2 diabetes. Many cohort studies have shown an association between chronic kidney disease and NAFLD. A link between NAFLD and periodontitis through periodontal pathogens, inflammatory mediators, and oxidative stress has been reported.
- Alcoholic liver disease (ALD) can cause alcoholic ketoacidosis, liver fibrosis, liver cirrhosis, hypertension, cardiac myopathy, nutritional deficiencies, peripheral neuropathy, chronic pancreatitis, osteoporosis, and chronic parotid gland hypertrophy.

3.9 Cloudy Swelling (Cloudy Degeneration)

Cloudy swelling is a condition in which protein in cells forms minute visible droplets giving a cloudy appearance microscopically. This condition may occur in any inflamed tissue. This condition is also known as albuminous degeneration or parenchymatous degeneration. This change is usually reversible.

3.9.1 Examples of Cloudy Swelling

Parenchymatous organs such as the liver, kidneys, pancreas, or heart are commonly affected.

3.10 Hyaline Change

The word 'hyaline' means glassy (halos = glass). Hyalinisation is a common descriptive histologic term for the glassy, homogeneous, eosinophilic appearance of proteinaceous material in haematoxylin- and eosin-stained sections and does not refer to any specific substance. Hyaline change is seen in heterogeneous pathological conditions and may be intracellular or extracellular. Intracellular hyaline is mainly seen in epithelial cells.

3.10.1 Examples of Hyaline Change

- Zenker's degeneration in typhoid fever: Hyaline degeneration of the rectus abdominalis muscle occurs in this condition. The muscle loses its fibrillar staining and becomes glassy and hyaline.
- Mallory's hyaline represents aggregates of intermediate filaments in the hepatocytes in alcoholic liver cell injury.
- Nuclear or cytoplasmic hyaline inclusions are seen in some viral infections.
- Hyaline degeneration is frequently seen in multiple myeloma, plasmacytoma, and Helicobacter pylori infection; extracellular hyaline degeneration may occur in fibrous tissue in scars and some tumours due to the deposition of glycoproteins between collagen bundles.
- Russel bodies are seen in periapical granuloma and chronic inflammatory granuloma.
- Hyaline bodies, also called Rushton bodies, may be found in epithelial cells of the odontogenic cysts (radicular cysts and residual cysts) and tumours (ameloblastoma).

3.11 Mucoid Degeneration

Mucoid means mucus-like. The mucus is the secretory product of mucous glands and is a combination of proteins complex with mucopolysaccharides. Mucin, a glycoprotein, is its chief constituent. Mucin is usually produced by epithelial cells of mucous membranes, glands, and some connective tissues, such as ground substance in the umbilical cord. By convention, connective tissue mucin is termed myxoid.

3

3.11.1 Examples of Mucoid Degeneration

- Some examples of functional excess of epithelial mucin include catarrhal inflammation of the mucous membrane (e.g. respiratory tract, alimentary tract, and uterus), cystic fibrosis of the pancreas, mucin-secreting tumours (e.g. ovary, stomach, large bowel, etc.), and mucoid or myxoid change in some tumours such as myxomas, neurofibromas, fibroadenoma, and soft tissue sarcomas. This change is extracellular and seen in the connective tissue.
- A common microscopic feature is a mucoid substance in minor salivary gland mucoceles due to salivary duct obstruction. Other examples include pleomorphic adenomas of the parotid gland and oral focal mucinosis (OFM). OFM is a rare connective tissue disorder characterised by myxoid degeneration of sub-mucosal connective tissue.

3.12 Fibrinoid Degeneration

Fibrinoid degeneration is essentially extracellular. Two types of connective tissue degenerations occur: connective tissue fibrinoid and vascular fibrinoid. Connective tissue fibrinoid degeneration is formed by the breakdown of collagen fibres and the mucopolysaccharide ground substance between the fibres, resulting in a material with similar staining properties to fibrin.

3.12.1 Examples of Fibrinoid Degeneration

Connective tissue fibrinoid occurs in rheumatoid arthritis, and vascular fibrinoid is seen in conditions where vessel walls are damaged by the extravasation of fibrin into the wall's tissues.

3.13 Pathological Calcification

Pathological calcification refers to depositing calcium phosphates (CaP) or other calcific salts at sites that would not normally have become mineralised. Two distinct types of pathological calcification are recognised: dystrophic calcification and metastatic calcification.

- The deposition of calcium salts in dead or degenerated tissues with normal calcium metabolism and serum calcium levels characterises dystrophic calcification.
- Metastatic calcification occurs in apparently normal tissues and is associated with deranged calcium metabolism and hypercalcemia. Metastatic calcification deposition can be influenced by releasing excess calcium salts from bone, phosphate concentration, alkaline phosphatase activity, and viscera physicochemical conditions under alkalosis.

3.13.1 Examples of Pathological Calcification

- Some examples of extraskeletal pathological calcification include kidney and bladder stones, gall stones, chronic calculous prostatitis, testicular microliths, calcification in haemodialysis patients, atherosclerosis, scleroderma (systemic sclerosis), calcinosis cutis, calcific aortic stenosis, and tuberculous lesions in the lungs or lymph nodes. Metastatic calcification is commonly associated with hyperparathyroidism, sarcoidosis, and myeloma.
- Pulp stones and sub-mandibular salivary stones are examples of dystrophic calcification in the orofacial region.

3.14 Cellular Inclusions

Cells may accumulate abnormal amounts of intracellular substances in response to injury. These may be located in the cytoplasm, lysosomes, or the nucleus. These accumulations can broadly be grouped into lipids, proteins, glycogen, and pigments.

3.14.1 Abnormal Accumulation of Lipids

Abnormal accumulation of triglyceride depositions in the parenchymal cells of the liver are common. The kidney, heart, and other organs may also be affected. Fatty change is reversible; severe fatty change may cause cell death. Cholesterol depositions are due to excessive intake and defective catabolism. These accumulations may occur in macrophages (foam cells) and smooth muscle cells of blood vessels (atherosclerosis). In hyperlipidaemic syndromes, cholesterol-laden macrophages cause sub-epithelial connective tissue deposits on the skin or tendons. These are called xanthomas.

3.14.2 Abnormal Accumulation of Proteins

Abnormal accumulations of proteins are uncommon. These occur when proteins are presented to the cells in excess or the cells produce excessive amounts of proteins. In kidney disease (nephrotic syndrome, for example), when heavy protein leakage across the glomerular filter occurs, a large amount of protein is re-absorbed. This can cause pink hyaline protein cytoplasmic droplets in the renal tubular epithelium.

3.14.3 Abnormal Accumulation of Glycogen

Abnormalities of metabolism of either glucose or glycogen can cause excessive intracellular accumulation of glycogen. In poorly controlled diabetes mellitus, glycogen accumulates in the renal tubular epithelium, cardiac myocytes, and β-cells of the islets of Langerhans in the pancreas. Abnormal accumulation of glycogen also occurs in glycogen storage diseases. In these diseases, glycogen synthesis or breakdown is defective.

3.14.4 Accumulation of Pigments

Intracellular accumulation of pigments can occur from exogenous or endogenous sources. Carbon is the most common exogenous pigment from polluted air. Inhaled carbon can cause anthracosis in the lung parenchyma. Coal dust can cause pneumoconiosis in coal mine workers. Macrophages take up pigments from tattooing and persist until the cell's death. Endogenous pigments include melanin, haemosiderin, and lipofuscin.

3.14.4.1 Examples of Accumulation of Pigments

Melanin is the brown/black pigment normally present in the cytoplasm of cells in the basal layer of the epidermis, called melanocytes. The function of melanin is to block harmful ultraviolet (UV) rays from reaching the epidermal nuclei. It may accumulate in excessive quantities in benign or malignant melanocytic neoplasms. In inflammatory skin lesions, where the epidermis is damaged, melanin may be released from injured basal cells and taken up by dermal macrophages. This gives rise to post-inflammatory pigmentation of the skin. Excessive melanin pigmentation of the skin is a feature of certain diseases, such as Addison's disease (adrenal insufficiency) and neurofibromatosis. In Addison's disease, there is an increase in melanin production in the skin and mucous membranes due to the melanocyte-stimulating activity of high Adenocorticotropic hormone (ACTH) plasma levels.

3.14.4.2 Orofacial Examples

Oral pigmented lesions most commonly result from the implantation of exogenous materials or endogenous, excessive melanin deposition. A smoker's melanosis occurs due to long-term tobacco smoking. Polycyclic amines present in tobacco and free radicals produced by tobacco use stimulate oral melanocytes to produce melanin as a protective mechanism. The amalgam tattoo is one of the most common localised, exogenously derived pigmented oral mucosa lesions. This lesion is the result of iatrogenically embedded amalgam particles during dental procedures. Physiological pigmentation, or racial or ethnic pigmentation, is an increased production of endogenous melanin pigment by melanocytes in dark-skinned individuals. Other examples of endogenous oral pigmentation are oral melanotic macules, naevi, and perioral pigmentation in individuals with Peutz-Jeghers syndrome (an autosomal dominant disorder) and Laugier-Hunziker oral pigmentation. Occasionally, oral melanoma (a malignant neoplasm of melanocytes) has been reported to occur in the mouth.

Haemosiderin is a golden-yellow to brown pigment found in lysosomes within the cell cytoplasm. It comprises aggregates of partially degraded ferritin, protein-covered ferric oxide, and phosphate. Haemosiderin represents iron deposition and accumulates in tissues. For example, the haemoglobin is broken down in tissue haemorrhage, and haemosiderin is deposited in macrophages locally. This process occurs in many chronic inflammatory conditions. Excess of circulating iron can result in systemic haemosiderin accumulation as in primary haemochromatosis (an inherited disease), in which there is excessive absorption and widespread deposition of haemosiderin in the tissues, especially the liver, pancreas, heart, and skin. Other causes of systemic iron deposition include increased iron absorption from the intestine, haemolytic anaemia, and recurrent blood transfusions. The presence of iron in the tissues is termed haemosiderosis.

Oral examples: Haemosiderin deposition in tissues can occur in oral mucosa in chronic inflammatory conditions. One example is oral lichen planus, a chronic immunologically mediated mucocutaneous disorder. Haemosiderin deposition in tissues can also occur in haemorrhagic conditions.

Lipofuscin: It is a pigment derived from the oxidation of lipids, which accumulates with age, predominantly in the heart, liver, retina, and brain (so-called wear and tear pigment). It does not seem to damage cells and does not cause clinical problems.

3

Further Reading

Cunha SF, Melo DA, Braga CB, Vannucchi H, Cunha DF. Papillary atrophy of the tongue, and nutritional status of hospitalized alcoholics. An Bras Dermatol. 2012;87:84–9.

Damjanov I. Cell pathology. In: Damjanov I, editor. Pathology for the health professions. 4th ed. St. Louis: Elsevier; 2012. p. 1–20.

Giroux V, Rustogi AK. Metaplasia: tissue injury adaptation and a precursor to the dysplasia-cancer sequence. Nat Rev Cancer. 2017;17(10):594–604. https://doi.org/10.1038/nrc.2017.68.

Guggenheimer J, Close JM, Eghtesad B. Sialadenosis in patients with advanced liver disease. Head Neck Pathol. 2009;3:100–5.

Guzzardi MA, Iozzo P. Fatty heart, cardiac damage, and inflammation. Rev Diabet Stud. 2011;8(3):403–17. https://doi.org/10.1900/RDS.2011.8.403.

Han P, Sun D, Yang J. Interaction between periodontitis and liver diseases. Biomed Rep. 2016;5(3):267–76.

King TC. Chapter 1—Cell injury, cellular responses to injury, and cell death. In. Elsevier's integrated pathology. Mosby. 2007. pp. 1–20.

Miller MA, Zachary JF. Mechanisms and morphology of cellular injury, adaptation, and death. In: Pathologic basis of veterinary disease. 2017. pp. 2–43.e19. https://doi.org/10.1016/B978-0-323-35775-3.00001-1. Epub 2017 Feb 17. PMCID: PMC7171462.

Müller S. Oral lichenoid lesions: distinguishing the benign from the deadly. Mod Pathol. 2017;30:S54–67. https://doi.org/10.1038/modpathol.2016.121.

Pranay T, Kumar AS, Chhabra S. Civatte bodies: a diagnostic clue. Indian J Dermatol. 2013;58(4):327–9.

Ronen J, Shaheen S, Steinberg D, Justus KR. Acute fatty liver of pregnancy: a thorough examination of a harmful obstetrical syndrome and its counterparts. Cureus. 2018;10:e2164. https://doi.org/10.7759/cureus.2164. issn:2168-8184.

Senba M, Kawai K, Mori N. Pathogenesis of metastatic calcification and acute pancreatitis in adult T-cell leukemia under hypercalcemic state. Leuk Res Treatment. 2012;2012:128617. https://doi.org/10.1155/2012/128617. Epub 2011 Dec 1. PMID: 23198151; PMCID: PMC3504271.

Suzuki Y, Utsunomiya T, Morikawa M. A histochemical and Immunohistochemical study of mucous cyst-with special reference to mucoid substance and characteristics of inflammation. Int J Oral Med Sci. 2004;3(2):91–8.

Wallig MA, Janovitz EB. Morphologic manifestations of toxic cell injury. In: Hascheck and Rousseaux's handbook of pathology. 3rd ed. Elsevier; 2013. p. 77–104.

Weintraub JA, Lopez Mitnik G, Dye BA. Oral diseases associated with non-alcoholic fatty liver disease in the United States. J Dent Res. 2019;98(11):1219–26. https://doi.org/10.1177/0022034519866442. Atrophic glossitis, parotid gland enlargement, and sialadenitis may occur in alcohol-related liver disease.

Histology of Tissue Healing

S R Prabhu

Contents

S R Prabhu et al. (eds.), *Oral Histology and Oral Histopathology*, https://doi.org/10.1007/978-3-031-77481-2_4

4.1 Introduction

Tissue healing is an essential physiological process important for tissue homeostasis. Healing comprises two processes: regeneration and repair. Regeneration refers to the specific replacement of the tissue, such as the superficial epidermis of the skin or mucosal epithelium. In contrast, repair is a non-specific form of healing in which the wound heals by fibrosis and scar formation.

4.2 Regenerative Capacity of Cells

The body has three main types of cells depending upon their regenerative capacity: labile, permanent (non-dividing), and stable (quiescent).

4.2.1 Labile Cells

These cells are under continuous active division and replace the cells lost from the body. Examples of labile cells include the epidermis of the skin, the epithelia of the mucous membranes and ducts, and haemopoietic stem cells.

4.2.2 Stable Cells

The parenchymal cells of the most solid glandular organs are stable. Examples include the liver, kidneys, pancreas, mesenchymal cells such as fibroblasts, smooth muscle cells, endothelial cells, and lymphocytes. These cells normally exist in a non-dividing state but may enter the cell cycle in response to certain stimuli, such as cell injury. Regeneration following injury in the tissues that contain stable cells requires at least some healthy cells to undergo proliferation and regeneration. For example, when a part of the liver lobe is resected, the remaining liver cells proliferate at such a rate that the liver reaches a size similar to that before resection. While this process is commonly described as regeneration, it is more accurately viewed as compensatory growth.

4.2.3 Permanent Cells

These cells are unable to replicate in postnatal life. Nervous cells, also termed neurons, and skeletal muscle and cardiac cells are included in this group. Repair in these tissues always leaves permanent evidence (scar) of injury. For example, the heart cannot regenerate heart muscle after a heart attack (myocardial infarction), and lost cardiac muscle is replaced by scar tissue.

4.3 The Intrinsic Similarities and Differences Between Skin and the Oral Mucosa

When discussing the histological aspects of tissue healing, it is necessary to briefly discuss the intrinsic similarities and differences between skin and oral mucosa.

4.3.1 Epidermis and Epithelium

Healthy skin and oral mucosa share many features and intrinsic histological differences (◻ Fig. 4.1). Both tissues comprise stratified epithelia, consisting of keratinocytes, melanocytes, Merkel cells, and Langerhans cells with protective functions. The oral epithelium is generally thicker than the skin; the palate and buccal mucosa, for example, contain considerably more cell layers. A higher proliferation rate in the basal epithelial cell layer in the mucosa compared to the skin (20–30 versus 5–8 living cell layers, respectively) exists. The epidermis is entirely keratinised. The epithelium of the oral mucosa may be keratinised or non-keratinised, depending on the location. For example, the epithelium of the dorsum of the tongue, gingiva, and hard palate is keratinised, and the mucosa of the cheeks, lips, soft palate, and floor of the mouth is covered by non-keratinised epithelium.

4.3.2 Dermis and Lamina Propria

The stratified epithelium is supported by a sub-surface layer of connective tissues (dermis for skin and lamina propria for oral mucosa) that contains fibroblasts, macrophages, mast cells, blood vessels, and nerve endings embedded in the extracellular matrix (ECM) that provides the epithelium with structural support and nutrients needed for continuous renewal. In addition, more blood vessels are present in the oral mucosa than in the skin.

Dermis and lamina propria extracellular matrix (ECM) mainly consist of collagen type 1 and type 3 (both in a ratio of about 5:1). However, in non-keratinised oral epithelia (e.g. buccal mucosa and soft palate), the ECM has a looser structure and contains more elastin compared to skin, hard palate, or gin-

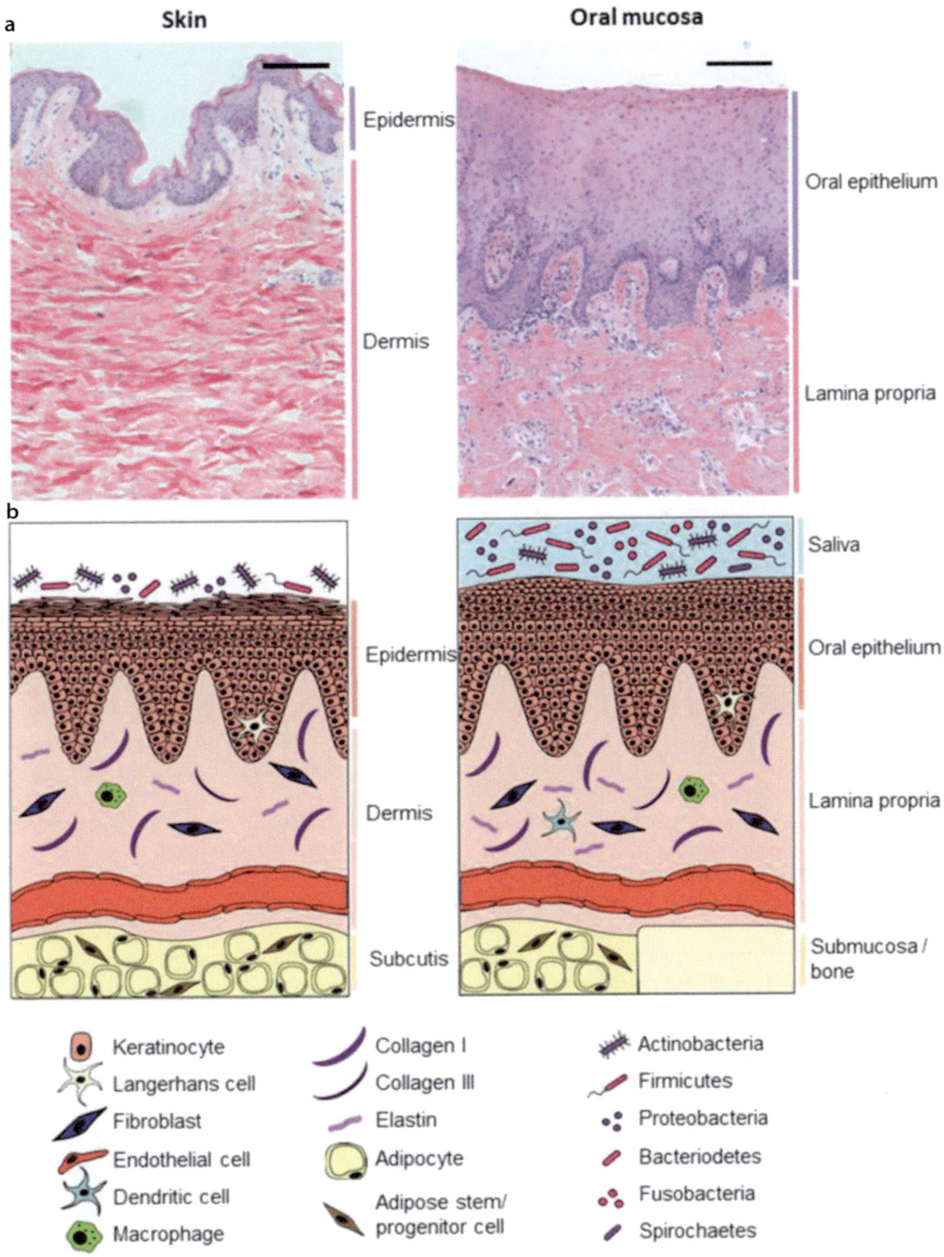

Fig. 4.1 Comparing healthy skin and oral mucosa. (**a**) Histological comparison between healthy skin (**left**) and gingiva (**right**) tissues. Haematoxylin and eosin staining of 5 µm paraffin-embedded tissue sections. Scale bar: 100 µm. (**b**) Graphical illustration comparing skin (**left**) and oral mucosa (**right**). (Source: Waasdorp M, Krom BP, Bikker FJ, van Zuijlen PPM, Niessen FB, Gibbs S. The Bigger Picture: Why Oral Mucosa Heals Better Than Skin. Biomolecules. 2021 Aug 6;11(8):1165. ► https://doi.org/10.3390/biom11081165. PMID: 34439831; PMCID: PMC8394648. Licensee MDPI, Basel, Switzerland. This open-access article is distributed under the terms and conditions of the Creative Commons Attribution (CC BY) license (► https://creativecommons.org/licenses/by/4.0/))

giva. In skin and buccal mucosa, the connective tissue layer is on top of an adipose tissue layer containing adipocytes, adipose stem, and progenitor cells. In contrast, the lamina propria of the hard palate and gingiva are attached directly to the bone via the mucoperiosteum.

4.4 Cellular Mechanisms in Cutaneous and Oral Mucosal Wound Healing

In the skin and oral mucosa, wound healing is a tightly regulated process that follows four partially overlapping phases: haemostasis, inflammation, prolifera-

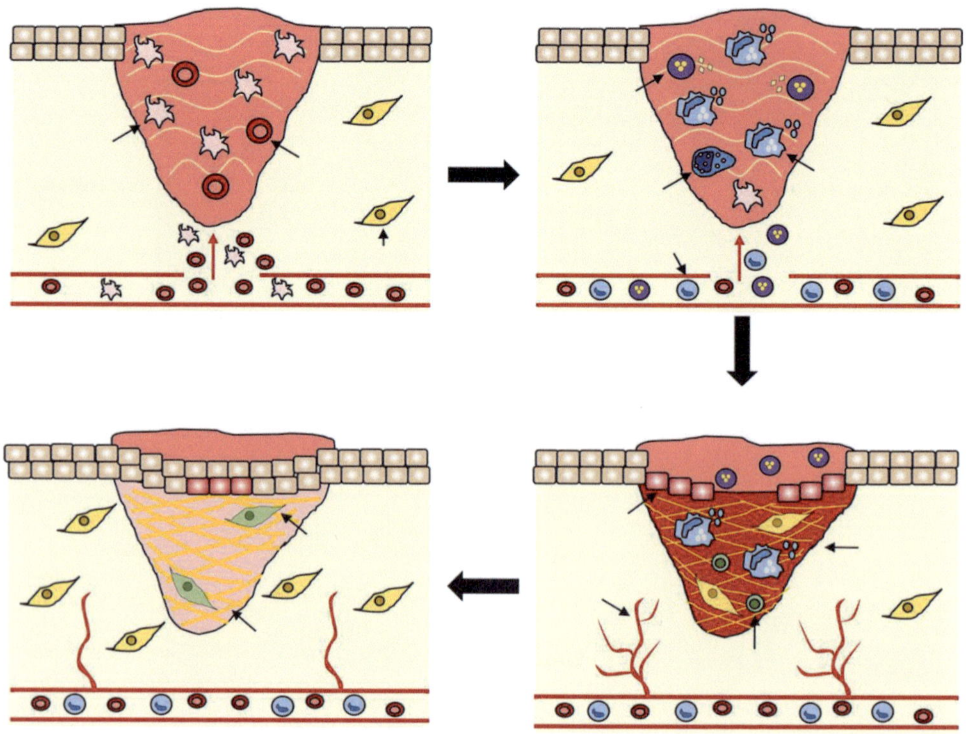

Fig. 4.2 The stages of wound repair and their major cellular components. Wound repair begins with haemostasis, where a platelet plug prevents blood loss, and a preliminary fibrin matrix is formed (Top left). Inflammation then ensues to remove debris and avoid infection, commencing with the neutrophil influx promoted by histamine release from mast cells. Monocytes arrive later and differentiate into tissue macrophages to clear remaining cell debris and neutrophils (Top right). During the proliferative phase, keratinocytes migrate to close the wound gap, blood vessels reform through angiogenesis, and fibroblasts replace the initial fibrin clot with granulation tissue (Bottom right). Macrophages and regulatory T cells (Tregs) are also vital for this stage of healing. Finally, fibroblasts remodel the deposited matrix further, blood vessels regress, and myofibroblasts cause overall wound contraction (Bottom left). (By Kind permission of Dr. H N Wilkinson, Centre for Atherothrombosis and Metabolic Disease, Hull York Medical School, The University of Hull, Hull HU6 7RX, United Kingdom Source: Wilkinson HN, Hardman MJ.) 2020 Wound healing: cellular mechanisms and pathological outcomes. Open Biol. 10: 200223. ► https://doi.org/10.1098/rsob.200223)

tion, and tissue remodelling, with each phase involving different cell types and (signalling) molecules (Fig. 4.2).

4.4.1 Haemostasis Phase

Immediately after an injury resulting in a wound, damaged blood vessels rapidly contract, and a blood clot forms, preventing further bleeding from vascular damage.

- Once a sufficient clot has formed, the coagulation process is switched off, preventing excessive thrombosis.
- At the same time, the injured vessel wall is repaired by smooth muscle cells and endothelial cells that proliferate in response to the released platelet-derived growth factor (PDGF).
- Endothelial progenitors are also recruited to aid this process as mature endothelial cells show limited proliferative capacity.

4.4.2 Inflammation Phase

- The inflammation phase of wound healing aims to remove debris from the injured site and prevent infection by pathogens. Innate inflammation evolved as the primary defence against pathogenic wound invasion.
- Within hours after wounding, in addition to neutrophils, monocytes, macrophages, mast cells, and T cells enter the wound bed in response to the chemokine gradients and drive the immune response against potential pathogenic invaders.
- After haemostasis, debris removal starts with resident cells via phagocytosis. Neutrophils are the first immune cells to enter the wounded area and play a crucial role in combatting microbial invasion via degranulation and phagocytosis. Neutrophils arrive early after injury and are recruited into the wound from damaged vessels.
- In addition to phagocytosing debris and killing microbial invaders by degranulation, neutrophils

secrete chemokines such as CCL2 and CCL3 to attract monocytes into the wounded area. Upon arrival, monocytes mature into macrophages, which contribute to the phagocytosis of debris and replace the neutrophil population, becoming the predominant immune cell type in the wounded area.
- In humans, it has been reported that 3 days after wounding, there is an influx of T cells in the oral mucosa, which resolves on day 6. The influx of T cells is delayed in the skin compared to the oral mucosa.
- Other less recognised immune cells in wound healing are mast cells. Mast cells have been shown to stimulate proliferation, angiogenesis, and ECM deposition and remodelling by releasing cytokines and growth factors.

Overall, the contribution of immune cells to wound healing appears to be prolonged in the skin compared to oral wound healing. This trend of faster resolution of the inflammation in the oral wound compared to skin was also reflected in the number of T cells and monocytes.

4.4.3 Proliferation Phase

The proliferation phase occurs hours or days after wounding.
- This healing phase is characterised by extensive activation of keratinocytes, fibroblasts, macrophages, and endothelial cells to orchestrate wound closure, matrix deposition, and angiogenesis.
- The highly vascularised and loosely organised granulation tissue rich in fibroblasts and endothelial cells provides the wound bed with structural support and nutrition.
- Meanwhile, epithelial cells re-epithelialise the wound bed in the proliferation, migration, and differentiation processes.
- Keratinocytes migrate laterally across the wound to reform the epidermal layer, and this process is termed re-epithelialisation.
- Stagnation of the blood flow in the wounded area leads to hypoxia and triggers the angiogenic response. Stimulation of endothelial cell proliferation and migration occurs, producing leaky vessels that provide the granulation tissue with nutrients and immune cells.
- Migration and proliferation of keratinocytes are key events in re-epithelialisation. Oral fibroblasts produce more hepatocyte growth factor (HGF) and keratinocyte growth factor (KGF), both known inducers of keratinocyte migration and proliferation compared to skin fibroblasts, which may explain the increased rate of re-epithelialisation of oral wounds compared to skin in vivo.
- While keratinocytes migrate and proliferate to restore the epithelial barrier, granulation tissue forms to replace the wounded dermis. Fibroblasts and endothelial cells start secreting fibronectin to create a dense fibrillary network that enables cell migration into the wound bed.
- When comparing skin and oral wounds, more fibroblasts are observed in the skin wound bed in vivo, suggesting that environmental factors rather than intrinsic differences between skin and oral fibroblasts determine cell migration and proliferation in vivo.

4.4.4 Remodelling Phase

- Once the wound is covered with a new epithelium and the host–microbial balance is restored, anti-inflammatory cytokines suppress inflammation.
- Macrophages switch from a pro-inflammatory (M1) to a pro-resolution (M2) phenotype and secrete growth factors, matrix metalloproteinases (MMPs), and tissue inhibitors of metalloproteinases (TIMPs) to stimulate (myo)fibroblast-mediated remodelling of the ECM. M1 macrophages are classically activated, typically by IFN-γ or lipopolysaccharide (LPS), and produce pro-inflammatory cytokines, phagocytise microbes, and initiate an immune response.

M1 macrophages produce nitric oxide (NO) or reactive oxygen intermediates (ROI) to protect against bacteria and viruses. M2 macrophages are alternatively activated by exposure to specific cytokines such as IL-4, IL-10, or IL-13. M2 macrophages will produce either polyamines to induce proliferation or proline to induce collagen production. These macrophages are associated with wound healing and tissue repair.

4.5 Types of Wound Healing in the Skin and Mucosa

Cutaneous and mucosal wound healing involves epithelial regeneration and connective tissue scar formation. Two categories of cutaneous or mucosal wound healing occur depending on the amount of tissue damage: healing by first intention and healing by second intention (◘ Fig. 4.3.)

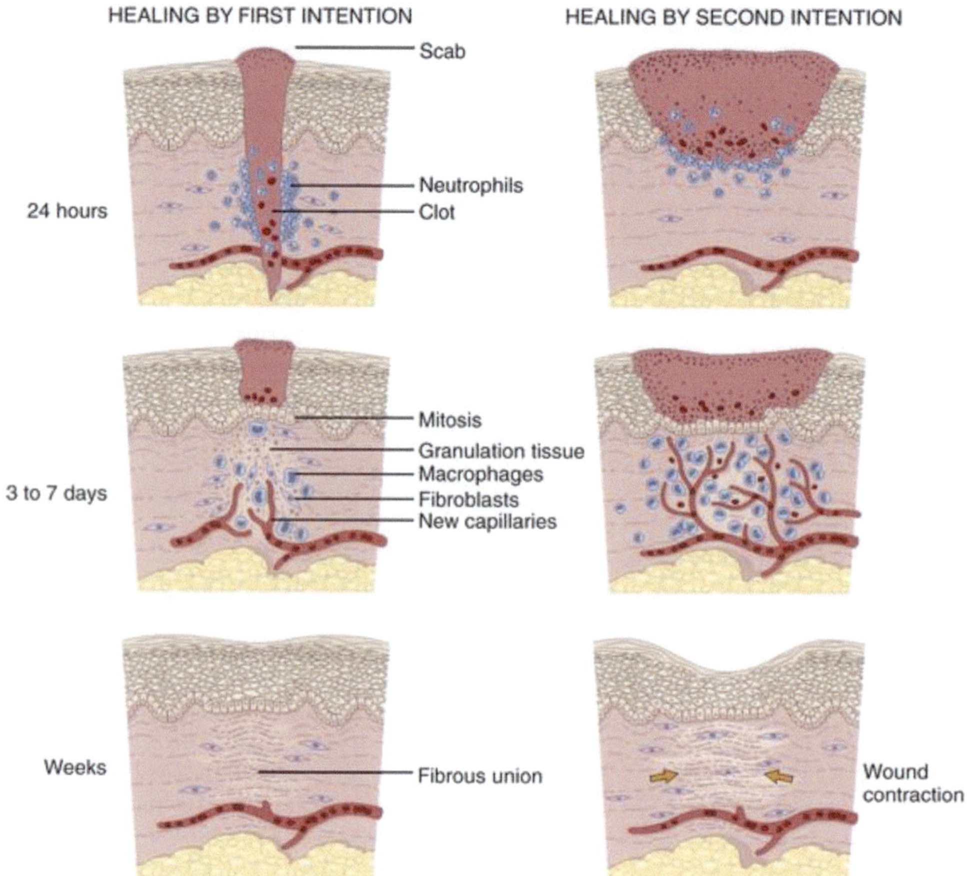

Fig. 4.3 Events in the skin and mucosal wound healing by first and second intentions (Source: By kind permission of Cao Xuan Cu)

4.5.1 Healing by First Intention (Primary Union)

A clean incision, such as a paper cut or sutured surgical wound, heals by the primary union or the first intention. In these types of injuries, the edges of wounds are approximated.

The first-intention healing process includes several events (Fig. 4.3).

- The narrow incisional space is filled with clotted blood containing fibrin and blood cells.
- This is followed by dehydration of the surface clot, resulting in a scab that covers the skin wound and seals it from the environment. The formation of a crusty scab is prevented under moist wound healing conditions, such as in the oral cavity.
- Within 24 h, neutrophils appear at the margins of the incision; these move towards the fibrin clot, and the basal cells at the cut edge of the epithelium show increased mitotic activity.
- Within 24–48 h, spurs of epithelial cells from the wound's edges migrate and grow along the cut margins of the wound (beneath the surface scab in the skin) to fuse in the midline, thus producing a continuous but thin epithelial layer.
- By day 3, neutrophils largely disappear and are replaced by macrophages, and granulation tissue invades the space created by the incision. Collagen fibres appear at the margins arranged vertically. Epithelial cell proliferation continues, and a thickened epidermal (epithelial) covering layer results.
- By day 5, the incisional space is filled with richly vascularised granulation tissue. Collagen fibrils begin to bridge the gap created by incision. The epidermis (epithelium in the mucosa) recovers its normal thickness, followed by the differentiation of epidermal (epithelial) cells and surface keratinisation.
- During the second week, collagen deposition and fibroblast proliferation continue, and oedema, leukocyte infiltration, and increased vascularity diminish.

- By the end of the first month, the scar is fully formed (skin) with connective tissue cells and devoid of inflammatory cells. The covering mucosal epithelium is normal in structure.

4.5.2 Healing by Second Intention (Secondary Intention)

The second type of wound healing process is known as healing by second or secondary intention. In this type of healing, there is an open wound with a more extensive loss of cells and tissue. Examples include inflammatory ulceration, abscess formation, and surface wounds that create significant defects (Fig. 4.3), which must be filled in the healing process.

- In the secondary intention of wound healing, the clot and scab are substantial at the surface of the skin wound, and the inflammatory cell infiltration is intense.
- Granulation tissue is abundant, growing from the margin to complete the repair.
- Wound contraction caused by myofibroblasts is a crucial feature. Regeneration of parenchymal cells cannot completely reconstitute the original architecture.

4.6 Healing of Palatal and Gingival Wounds

Healing of palatal and gingival wounds is typically characterised by without-scar tissue formation. This is due to the early onset of the inflammatory phase, decreased inflammatory mediators, fewer blood vessels, more cells originating from the bone marrow, rapid re-epithelialisation, and rapid fibroblast proliferation.

4.7 Healing of Dental Pulp Wounds

Dental pulp healing mainly relies on preserving the apical blood supply and surviving the damaged odontoblast layer. If the odontoblast layer is sufficiently intact, the odontoblasts can influence the formation of tubular or atubular reactionary (tertiary) dentin. Additionally, an opening of the pulp that causes only superficial dental pulp necrosis can provoke an inflammatory reaction that attracts pulpal stem cells or progenitor cells to the wound edge, where they differentiate into odontoblast-like cells that produce reparative dentin or osteodentin. However, persistent dental pulp inflammation can lead to necrosis.

4.8 Tooth Socket Healing

Like any other wound associated with tissue loss, the extraction socket heals by secondary intention. A well-defined, orderly sequence of biological events restores the continuity of the alveolar mucosa and bone following exodontia.

- Firstly, the socket fills with blood, which coagulates to produce a loosely adherent clot.
- Next, platelets within the clot retract, causing the gingival tissues to collapse into the clot-filled alveolus. The clot then stabilises by fibrin cross-linking within the first 24 h of the extraction.
- During the next 48 h, the clot is broken down by the fibrinolytic activity of the enzyme plasmin.
- After approximately 5 days, ingrowth of fibroblasts from the socket wall occurs, and angiogenesis results in the formation of capillaries, fixing the clot to the socket wall with granulation tissue. Fibroplasia (production of fibrous tissue) ensues, with the eradication of the fibrin by macrophages and replacement with granulation tissue. Gingival epithelium then proliferates and grows over the intact clot below the surface debris.
- Over the next 2 weeks, induced mesenchymal cells and osteoprogenitor cells in the residual periodontal ligament produce a variable amount of osteoid. This results in the formation of woven bone, which is then remodelled by subsequent osteoblastic and osteoclastic activity, resulting in the formation of mature lamellar bone.
- Gradually, the cortical bone of the empty socket (the radiographic lamina dura) is replaced, and the socket is filled by trabecular bone. Healing is complete at approximately 3 months post-extraction. This process is attributed to the abundant vascular supply of the alveolar process and accompanying periosteum, the responsiveness of the gingival epithelium, and the rapid turnover of periodontal connective tissue elements.

4.9 Healing of Jawbone Fracture

Jawbone fractures can heal by primary or secondary intention.

Primary intention

- Bone healing by primary intention can occur without callus formation.
- A good blood supply and an existing stable fixation without mobility of the bone fragments with a fracture gap of up to 1 mm are essential for healing by primary intention.

- Under these conditions, osteoblasts are activated within 1–3 days, and osteoid is established within a week.
- Bridging the gap with primary bone can take 4–6 weeks, depending on the gap distance. This primary bone contains large numbers of osteocytes and collagen fibres intertwined (woven bone) to create a spatial braid or plexus.
- The primary bone is replaced by mature secondary bone, characterised by a parallel collagen fibre arrangement. The concentric lamellae (lamellar bone) are better calcified, making the secondary bone stronger than the primary bone.

Bone healing by secondary intention (indirect bone healing) is characterised by callus formation.

- The indirect bone healing sequence can be summarised as follows: (1) inflammation and haematoma formation, (2) fragment stabilisation by periosteal and endosteal callus formation, (3) continuity restoration by membranous and endochondral bone formation, and (4) formation of osteons and Haversian canals and functional adaptation.
- After blood clot formation, osteocytes die on both sides of the fracture, and the bone matrix degrades. This is followed by the recovery phase, in which the dead cells, the thrombus, and the degraded bone matrix are cleaned up.
- The surrounding tissue prompts revascularisation, angiogenesis, and strong cell proliferation. The nature of the formed tissue is associated with fracture stability and tissue vascularisation. In cases of less stable fracture or poor vascularisation, a cartilaginous callus forms first, which is then converted to endochondral bone, followed by further transformation into the woven bone and conversion to the secondary (lamellar) bone as the stabilisation improves.
- When bone fragments show high mobility or a large gap, and in cases of periosteum damage, a connective tissue-like callus is formed that clinically appears as a pseudarthrosis in which the bone fragments opposite each other remain mobile.

4.10 Summary

In adult humans, optimal skin or mucosal wound healing involves several events, including rapid haemostasis, appropriate inflammation, mesenchymal cell differentiation, proliferation, migration to the wound site, angiogenesis, re-epithelialisation and synthesis, cross-linking, and alignment of collagen to provide strength to the healing tissue. Many cell types, including neutrophils, macrophages, lymphocytes, keratinocytes, fibroblasts, and endothelial cells, are involved in this process. Healing of tooth sockets comprises a wide range of processes, including coagulation and haemostasis, inflammation, proliferation, and modelling and remodelling, aiming to restore the lost architecture and functionality.

Further Reading

Chhabra S, Chhabra N, Kaur A, Gupta N. Wound healing concepts in clinical practice of OMFS. J Maxillofac Oral Surg. 2017;16(4):403–23. https://doi.org/10.1007/s12663-016-0880-z.

Delavary BM, van der Veer WM, van Egmond M, Niessen FB, Beelen RH. Macrophages in skin injury and repair. Immunobiology. 2011;216:753–62. https://doi.org/10.1016/j.imbio.2011.01.001.

Glim JE, Everts V, Niessen FB, Ulrich MM, Beelen RH. Extracellular matrix components of oral mucosa differ from the skin and resemble that of foetal skin. Arch Oral Biol. 2014;59:1048–55.

Kumar V, Abbas AK, Aster JC. Inflammation and repair. In: Kumar V, Abbas AK, Aster JC, editors. Robbins basic pathology. 10th ed. Philadelphia: Elsevier; 2018. p. 57–93.

Pastar I, Stojadinovic O, Yin NC, Ramirez H, Nusbaum AG, Sawaya A, Patel SB, Khalid L, Isseroff RR, Tomic-Canic M. Epithelialization in wound healing: a comprehensive review. Adv Wound Care. 2014;3:445–64. https://doi.org/10.1089/wound.2013.0473.

Politis C, Schoenaers J, Jacobs R, Agbaje JO. Wound healing problems in the mouth. Front Physiol. 2016;7:507. https://doi.org/10.3389/fphys.2016.00507. PMID: 27853435; PMCID: PMC5089986.

Reinke JM, Sorg H. Wound repair and regeneration. Eur Surg Res. 2012;49:35–43. https://doi.org/10.1159/000339613.

Ridiandries A, Tan JTM, Bursill CA. The role of chemokines in wound healing. Int J Mol Sci. 2018;19(10):3217. https://doi.org/10.3390/ijms19103217.

Rohani MG, Parks WC. Matrix remodelling by MMPs during wound repair. Matrix Biol. 2015;44–46:113–21. https://doi.org/10.1016/j.matbio.2015.03.002.

Rousselle P, Braye F, Dayan G. Reepithelialization of adult skin wounds: cellular mechanisms and therapeutic strategies. Adv Drug Deliv Rev. 2019a;146:344–65.

Rousselle P, Montmasson M, Garnier C. Extracellular matrix contribution to skin wound re-epithelialization. Matrix Biol. 2019b;75–76:12–26. https://doi.org/10.1016/j.matbio.2018.01.002.

Szpaderska AM, Zuckerman JD, DiPietro LA. Differential injury responses in oral mucosal and cutaneous wounds. J Dent Res. 2003;82:621–6. https://doi.org/10.1177/154405910308200810.

Szpaderska AM, Walsh CG, Steinberg MJ, DiPietro LA. Distinct patterns of angiogenesis in oral and skin wounds. J Dent Res. 2005a;84:309–14. https://doi.org/10.1177/154405910508400403.

Szpaderska AM, Walsh CG, Steinberg MJ, DiPietro LA. Distinct patterns of angiogenesis in oral and skin wounds. J Dent Res. 2005b;84:309–14.

Turabelidze A, Guo S, Chung AY, Chen L, Dai Y, Marucha PT, DiPietro LA. Intrinsic differences between oral and skin keratinocytes. PLoS One. 2014;9:e101480.

Waasdorp M, Krom BP, Bikker FJ, van Zuijlen PPM, Niessen FB, Gibbs S. The bigger picture: why oral mucosa heals better than skin. Biomolecules. 2021;11(8):1165. https://doi.org/10.3390/biom11081165.

Wilkinson HN, Hardman MJ. Wound healing: cellular mechanisms and pathological outcomes. Open Biol. 2020;10(9):200223. https://doi.org/10.1098/rsob.200223.

Winning TA, Townsend GC. Oral mucosal embryology, and histology. Clin Dermatol. 2000;18:499–511.

Histology of Types of Inflammation

David F Wilson

Contents

S R Prabhu et al. (eds.), *Oral Histology and Oral Histopathology*, https://doi.org/10.1007/978-3-031-77481-2_5

5

5.1 Introduction

Collectively, a significant number of pathological conditions affecting the teeth, oral soft tissues, salivary glands, and jawbones are characterised by the presence of inflammation. It is important, therefore, that students undertaking the study of oral histopathology have a good understanding of the light microscopic features of this process and an understanding of the dynamics of inflammatory processes. This chapter presents a brief overview of the histology of inflammation with a summary reference to underlying biological processes where relevant.

For histological diagnostic purposes, inflammation can be categorised as:

- Acute inflammation
- Chronic inflammation
- Granulomatous inflammation

Each of type of inflammation has relatively specific microscopic features, described in subsequent sections, allowing distinction between them. However, it should also be noted that there are aspects of commonality between each type when such features as the migration of inflammatory-immune cells to the site of injury, the interactions of chemical (inflammatory) mediators and chemokines with cells, the interactions of inflammatory cells themselves and processes such as phagocytosis are considered. For example, the cells that are seen microscopically in chronic inflammation have to reach the site of injury using the same mechanisms (transmigration from terminal blood vessels) as the predominant cell in acute inflammation. As another example, and as a generality, the chemical mediators operative in acute inflammation are also operative in chronic inflammation. Similarly, the process of phagocytosis which involves the removal of dead tissue, inflammatory debris and injurious agents by certain inflammatory cells is the same across each "type" of inflammation.

Histologically, a diagnosis of one or other forms of inflammation mainly rests on the identification of accumulations of one or more types of inflammatory-immune cells in an affected tissue. The inflammatory cell aggregations may be localised (focal) or more widely dispersed (diffuse). The terms acute inflammation, chronic inflammation or granulomatous inflammation are then applied depending upon the predominant cell types present along with, especially in the case of acute inflammation and granulomatous inflammation, the nature of changes observed in the affected tissue. The suffix "ïtis" denotes inflammation when used in diagnostic contexts such as gingivitis, pulpitis, periodontitis and so on.

In a general sense, inflammation is often referred to as a response to injury with that response having the ideal outcome of removing or otherwise eliminating the cause of that injury and allowing healing to be initiated. Inflammation can affect a localised area of an organ (e.g. an abscess in the skin) or a whole organ (for instance, hepatitis, pancreatitis or nephritis). Injuries may be exogenous as in the case of infective agents (bacteria or viruses), physical trauma (accidental or surgical trauma), thermal trauma, chemical trauma, electrical trauma or some forms of radiation. Tissue injury giving rise to inflammation can also be generated by endogenous abnormalities such as some of the immune hypersensitivities where abnormal immune cell functioning or abnormal antigen expression in tissue cells results in the recruitment of inflammatory-immune cells to tissues and the establishment of an identifiable inflammatory process. The mucocutaneous conditions such as lichen planus, mucous membrane pemphigoid and pemphigus vulgaris are examples of the latter. Failure to remove the causative agent in cases of inflammation results in the persistence of the process and can lead to tissue necrosis (abscess formation), particularly in the case of acute inflammation, and delayed healing in the case of chronic inflammatory conditions. Failure of an effective inflammatory process can be influenced by a range of factors, including the severity of the injury, the virulence of an infective agent and the presence of systemic factors that can influence the effectiveness of inflammatory-immune cells.

5.2 Acute Inflammation

Acute inflammation is usually the first-phase response to a tissue injury and, generally, is described as lasting from one to a few days before the cellular features of chronic inflammation predominate. However, if the injury is severe, acute inflammation can persist, leading to tissue destruction, cell necrosis and abscess formation. Acute inflammation can also arise in a pre-existing chronic inflammatory process. In the latter case, the inflammation is often described as "acute on chronic inflammation" or "subacute inflammation".

The initial histological hallmarks of acute inflammation are changes to the terminal vasculature and the presence of a variably intense polymorphonuclear leukocyte infiltrate, predominantly neutrophils (PMNs), in the affected tissue. However, in reality, it should be noted that when examining the histological features of acute inflammation, the microscopic field is almost invariably associated with the obvious presence of other inflammatory-immune cells, which can include macrophages, lymphocytes and plasma cells.

5.2.1 Vascular Changes

The vascular changes that occur in acute inflammation involve transient changes in regional arterioles and more marked and observable changes to the capillaries and post-capillary venules in the affected tissues, including the opening up of previously closed terminal vessels. The changes to the capillaries and post-capillary venules are dilation (◘ Fig. 5.1) and increased permeability and are initiated and maintained by a variety of chemical mediators. Permeability changes can also be due to direct microvasculature injury as a consequence of physical trauma, chemical injury or radiation. The chemical mediators involved in acute inflammation are derived from cells and plasma. Those derived from cells may exist as pre-formed mediators (e.g. histamine in mast cell granules and some molecules in PMN and macrophage granules). Others are synthesised by metabolic processes that occur in activated inflammatory cells and other cells (e.g. leukotrienes and prostaglandins). Some chemical mediators can have multiple roles (e.g. may act to cause vascular dilatation and also act as a chemokine [chemotactic agent]).

5.2.2 Permeability Changes

The permeability changes in the terminal blood vessels in acute inflammation allow both plasma constituents and cells to move to the extravascular tissue compartment. Both the plasma constituents, called inflammatory exudate, and inflammatory cells exit the blood vessels via widened intercellular junctions between the endothelial cells forming the walls of the vessels, with a smaller quantity of fluid also escaping by means of increased transcytosis across endothelial cells. Fluid inflammatory exudate consists of a number of plasma components including water, fibrinogen, albumin and antibodies. In the inflammatory field, the fibrinogen is converted to fibrin (◘ Fig. 5.2).

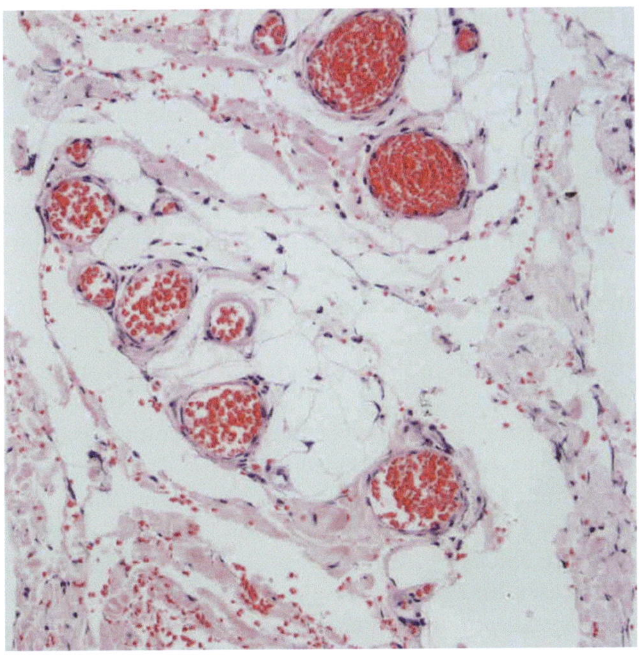

◘ **Fig. 5.1** Dilation of terminal capillaries and post-capillary venules is an initial histological feature of acute inflammation. Haemodynamic changes lead to a slowing of the blood-flow rate and the microscopic appearance of congestion of the erythrocytes within the vessels

5.2.3 Transmigration

The movement of inflammatory cells in acute and chronic inflammation from an intravascular to an extravascular location is a consequence of the cells initially marginating (adhering) on internal vessel walls (◘ Figs. 5.3 and 5.4) and then developing the ability to move (diapedesis and cell walking) along vessels walls (◘ Fig. 5.5) and exiting the vessels via the widened intercellular junctions. Once outside the vessels, the inflammatory cells move to the area of injury along a signalling gradient—the process of chemotaxis (◘ Fig. 5.6).

The rolling of leukocytes occurs because of weak adhesion molecule interactions with the endothelial cells, which then break. The expression of endothelial receptors is activated by inflammatory mediators such as interleukin-1 (IL-1) and tumour necrosis factor (TNF). The subsequent adhesion of leukocytes to the luminal endothelial cell walls occurs as a result of firm

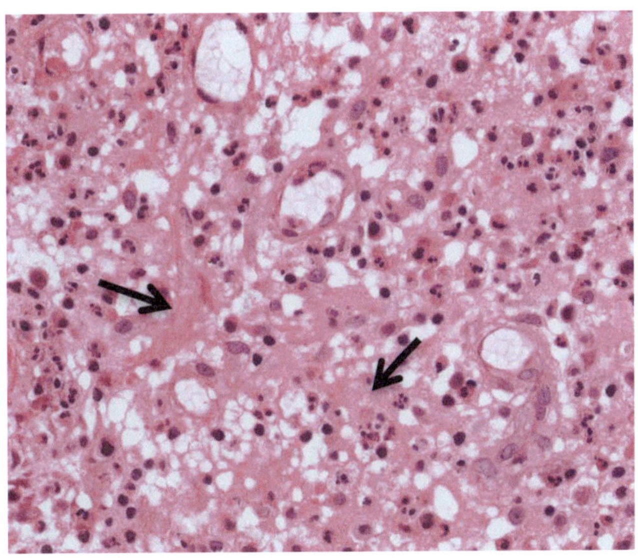

◘ **Fig. 5.2** Acute inflammation. The bubbly, eosinophilic material forming much of the background is the fluid inflammatory exudate made up of more visibly solid fibrin (arrows), derived from fibrinogen, and washed-out spaces where other fluid exudate components have been lost during tissue processing procedures

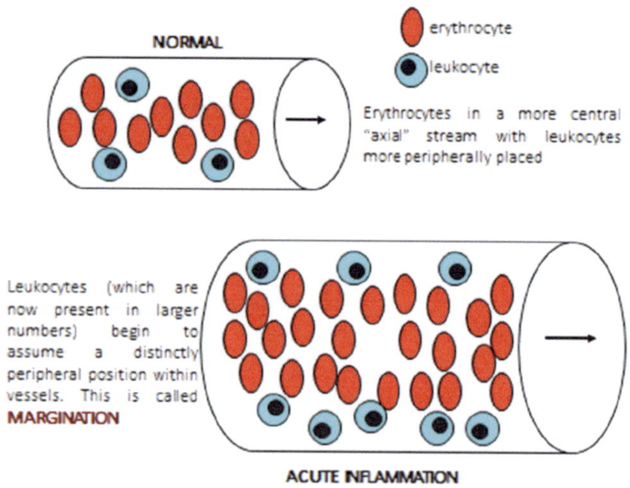

Fig. 5.3 One of the early changes seen in the microvasculature in acute inflammation is an increase in leukocyte numbers in the area of injury and their peripheral positioning within the vessels

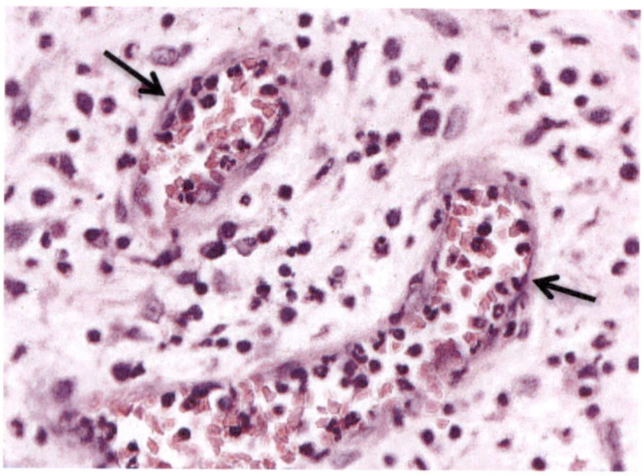

Fig. 5.4 Acute inflammation. In this photomicrograph, greater-than-normal white blood cell numbers are seen within the blood vessels (arrows), with some of these cells lining the internal vessel walls (marginating) prior to exiting the vessels

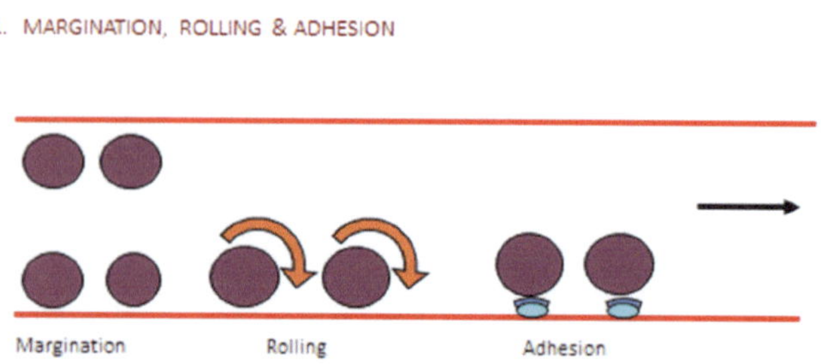

Fig. 5.5 Diagrammatic illustration of leukocyte margination, rolling and adhesion, which occurs on the luminal walls of the terminal blood vessels in the area of injury prior to cells leaving the vessels. These processes involve the binding of matching adhesion molecules on the endothelial cells and leukocytes. The expression of the receptors on the endothelial cells is initiated and modulated by some of the chemical mediators responsible for dilatation and permeability alterations

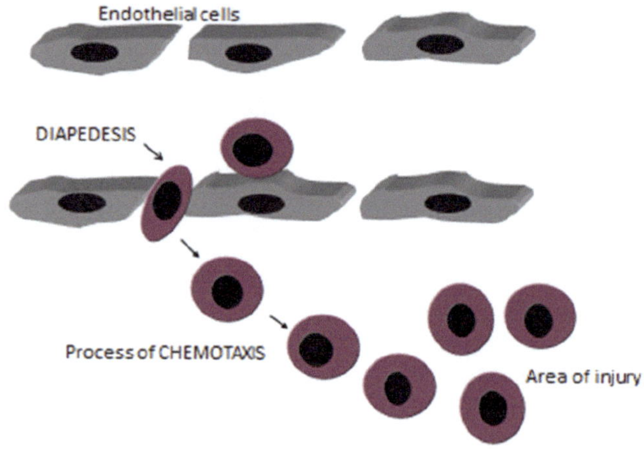

Fig. 5.6 Schematic diagram illustrating the movement (transmigration) of inflammatory cells from within terminal blood vessels to the extravascular compartment and their movement to the site of injury by the process of diapedesis

(high avidity) binding of adhesion molecules. Examples of adhesion molecules on endothelial cells include E-selectin, P-selectin, ICAM-1 (intercellular adhesion molecule-1) and VCAM-1 (vascular cell adhesion molecule-1). On leukocytes, L-selectin and integrins (there is a variety of these that interact with ICAM-1 and VCAM-1) are examples of adhesion molecules.

5.2.4 Neutrophil

The predominant cell type associated with acute inflammation is the polymorphonuclear neutrophil. Neutrophils are phagocytic cells that will ingest infectious agents in the circulation and in tissue and also tissue debris (extracellular matrix components and dead cells) in areas of injury. Neutrophils are short-lived (a few days) first-line of defence cells that are present as a normal component of blood. Their numbers in the circulation increase in cases of inflammatory pathology in the body. Neutrophils, like other inflammatory-immune cells, leave the circulation and enter tissues in response to a variety of molecular signals that are formed or released during cellular and tissue injury. Neutrophils contain large numbers of membrane-bound granules (previously called lysosomes) (Fig. 5.7). Three types of granules are recognised: azurophil granules, specific granules and small storage granules. The granules contain an extensive range of proteolytic enzymes and hydrolases and antibacterial agents such as lysozyme and myeloperoxidase involved in phagocytosis of cell and tissue debris and bacteria, respectively. Once they leave the circulating blood, neutrophils do not re-enter the circulation, and they undergo cell death in the inflamed area of tissue. As a consequence, extracellular release of the highly reactive granule contents from dead

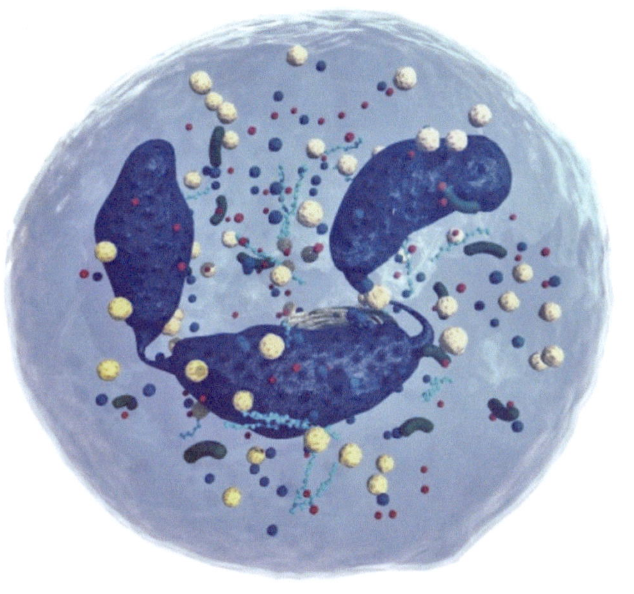

Fig. 5.7 The 3D graphic representation of a neutrophil showing a lobed nucleus and large numbers of cytoplasmic granules

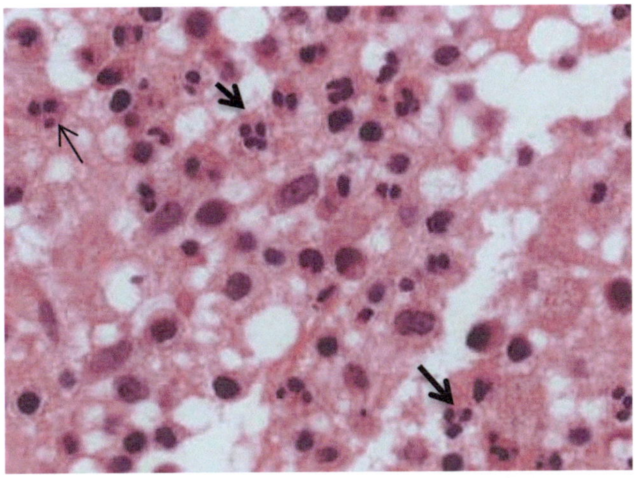

Fig. 5.8 Acute inflammation. In a histological section, neutrophils (arrows) can be recognised by their basophilic and apparently fragmented nuclei. Neutrophils are phagocytic cells with a short lifespan of one to a few days and, unlike longer-lived macrophages, cannot re-enter the circulation. Some of the cells in this micrograph are exhibiting signs of cell death and nuclear disintegration

and dying neutrophils can further damage normal tissue components and cause the persistence of inflammation as the granules escape the confines of the neutrophil. This negative outcome can contribute to the furtherance of the inflammatory process.

Other polymorphs (eosinophils and basophils), monocytes and circulating macrophages also exit (transmigrate) the terminal blood vessels in acute inflammation (and in chronic inflammatory processes). The eosinophils and basophils release a range of chemical mediators and enzymes from their granules that contribute to the inflammatory process. The monocytes become active macrophages in the extravascular environment. As previously mentioned, in the early phase of acute inflammation, neutrophils dominate the cellular exudate. Subsequently, macrophages become the major phagocytic cell component of the cellular exudate, with the microscopic field containing both cell types along with other cell types such as lymphocytes. In a microscopic acute inflammatory field, neutrophils can be recognised by their darkly staining (basophilic) and lobed nuclei (Fig. 5.8) but, with generally poorly delineated cytoplasm. Macrophages (Fig. 5.9) are mononuclear cells with a paler staining nucleus. The cell borders and cytoplasm of these cells can be difficult to identify in haematoxylin- and eosin-stained sections unless macrophages have been involved in phagocytosis (see later).

5.2.5 Necrosis

If the injury causing acute inflammation in an area of tissue is severe and persistent, the inflammatory process

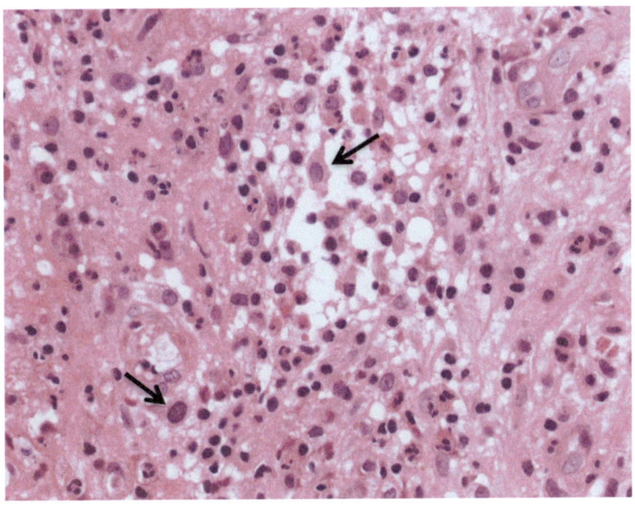

Fig. 5.9 Macrophages (arrows) in an inflammatory field are mononuclear cells with a round-to-ovoid, pale-staining nucleus. Lymphocytes characterised by their darkly staining nuclei and numerous pyknotic neutrophils are also evident in this photomicrograph

can lead to tissue necrosis and abscess formation with pus formation. Pus (Fig. 5.10) is a fluid collection of variable viscosity made up of tissue debris, dead and dying inflammatory cells and inflammatory exudate, and if the inflammatory process is due, for example, to a bacterial infection, evidence of the latter may be microscopically visible. The histological features of necrosis (Fig. 5.11) include an absence of viable tissue structures such as blood vessels and the accumulation of dead inflammatory and tissue cells. Dead and dying cells are characterised by their eosinophilic cytoplasm and

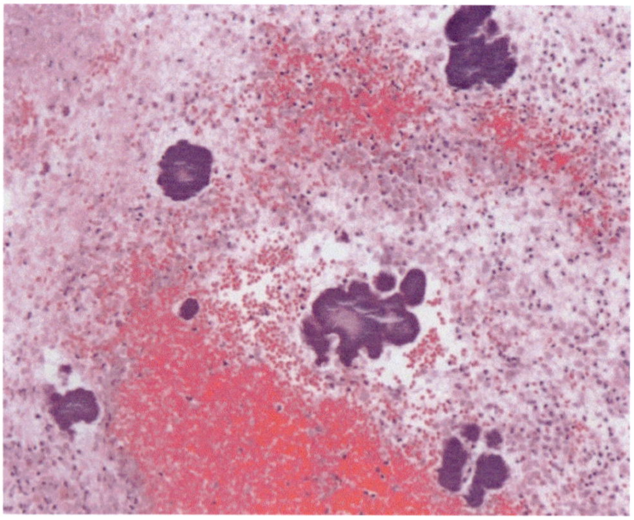

Fig. 5.10 In this photomicrograph, pus is seen to be made up of haemorrhagic, inflammatory fluid exudate containing large numbers of dead and dying inflammatory cells. In this particular instance, irregular, basophilic foci of bacteria are also evident

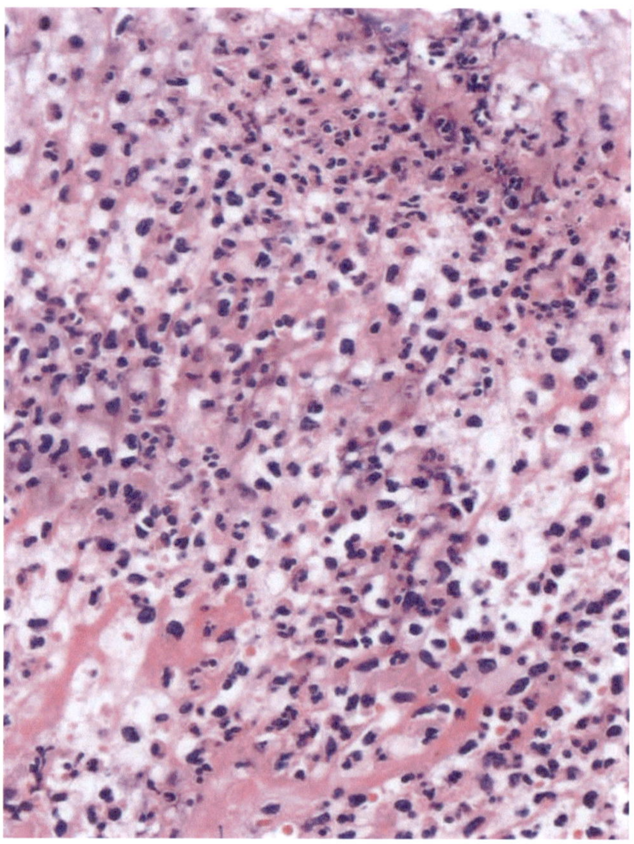

Fig. 5.11 Necrosis. Photomicrograph illustrating an absence of normal tissue structure and the accumulation of inflammatory cells, exhibiting the histological nuclear signs of cell death in a background of fibrinous inflammatory exudate

evidence of nuclear changes such as karyorrhexis (nuclear fragmentation), karyolysis (dissolution of the nucleus) or pyknosis (nuclear condensation).

5.3 Chronic Inflammation

Clinically, a chronic inflammatory disease is one that has been present for weeks, months or years. Histologically, chronic inflammation is characterised by the presence of chronic inflammatory cell populations, the relative absence of the prominent vascular changes seen in acute inflammation and, often, co-existing microscopic features of healing.

5.3.1 Cells of Chronic Inflammation

The family of chronic inflammatory cells comprises macrophages (Fig. 5.9), lymphocytes and plasma cells. Chronic inflammation is often the "second phase", but a more effective response to injury. This is because these cells are

- More capable of phagocytosis (macrophages)
- Capable of neutralising infectious agents (lymphocytes and plasma cells)
- More capable of removing tissue components damaged during inflammation (macrophages)
- More capable of triggering healing, mediated by growth-factor cytokines released from macrophages and lymphocytes

Microscopically, there is considerable variation as regards the chronic inflammatory cell types seen and their relative proportions in chronic inflammation. In some cases, a mixed chronic inflammatory cell population may be observed (Fig. 5.12) while other cases may be lymphocyte-predominant or plasma cell-predominant (Fig. 5.13).

Histological slides and photomicrographs present a relatively static picture of chronic inflammation. An appreciation of chronic inflammation is enhanced when the cellular dynamics of this process are understood. For example, in an inflammatory field, activated macrophages (Fig. 5.14) undertake a variety of functions related to phagocytosis of dead cells and other tissue components, the phagocytosis of bacteria and viruses, the recruitment of additional inflammatory cells such as lymphocytes to the area, the processing of antigens and the activation of cells involved in healing. The latter process is important in recruiting immune cells to the area and activating an immune system cascade of long-term

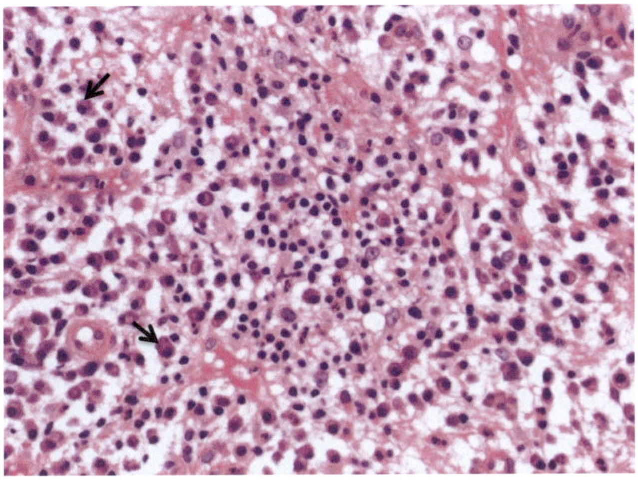

■ **Fig. 5.12** Chronic inflammation. Photomicrograph showing a mixed chronic inflammatory cell infiltrate with plasma cells (arrows) and lymphocytes characterised by small, round and darkly staining nuclei being evident in the central area of the micrograph

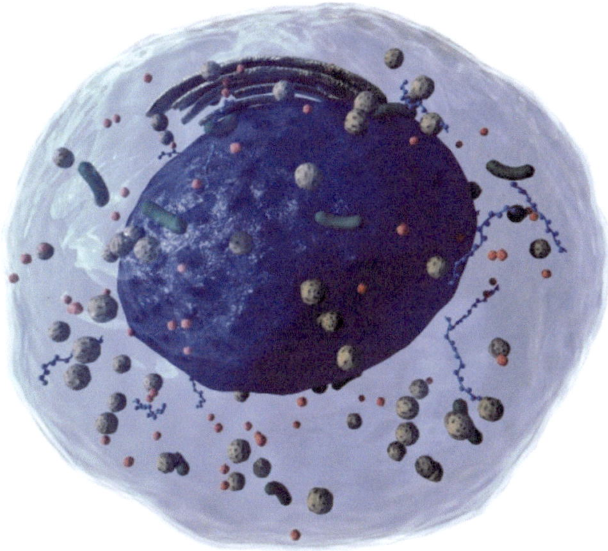

■ **Fig. 5.14** The 3D graphic representation of a macrophage. Activated macrophages are involved in a wide range of activities in acute and chronic inflammation. These roles include phagocytosis, antigen processing and presentation to cells of the lymphocyte family, cytokine synthesis, chemokine synthesis and growth-factor synthesis

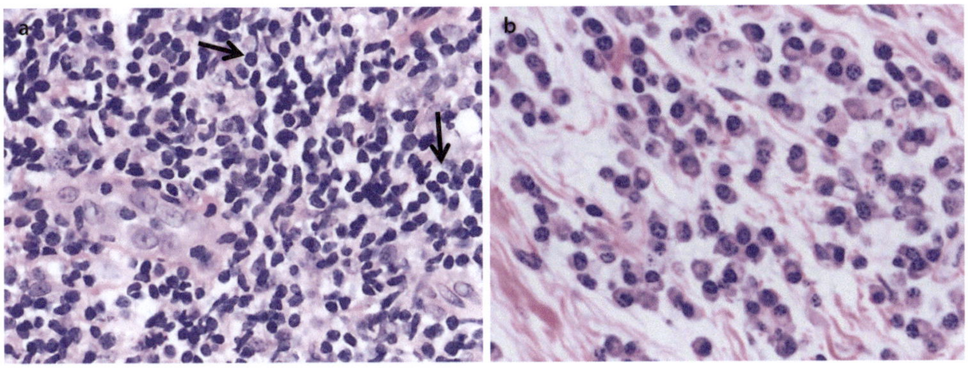

■ **Fig. 5.13** Chronic inflammation. (**a**) Photomicrograph showing a lymphocyte- (arrows) rich chronic inflammatory cell infiltrate. The lymphocytes are histologically identified by their darkly staining and rounded or, in some cases, distorted, due to artefact, nuclei with little or no cytoplasm being evident. (**b**) Photomicrograph illustrating plasma cell-rich chronic inflammatory infiltrate. The plasma cells have a rounded-to-ovoid shape with eccentrically placed nuclei and prominent, purplish cytoplasm. The latter reflects active antibody production by these B lymphocyte-derived cells

protective activity against, for example, the bacteria or viruses, which may have initially occurred in an area of inflammation. While the T lymphocyte subsets that occur in an inflammatory field cannot be specifically identified in haematoxylin- and eosin-stained sections, it is important to appreciate that these cell types can also be undertaking a variety of functions. For example, T1 helper cells release monocyte chemotactic factor and also interferon-y, which increases the phagocytic capability of macrophages. As another example, T2 (CD4+) helper cells interact with CD40+ B cells to produce antibody-producing plasma cells.

5.3.2 Phagocytosis

An important role of macrophages (and neutrophils) in inflammation is phagocytosis. Phagocytosis is a particular form of endocytosis, defined by the fact that the term phagocytosis describes the active taking into the cell and digestion (cell eating) of particulate material equal to or greater than 0.5 μm (microns) in size. In inflammatory fields, this can include dead and dying cells, cellular and tissue debris and organisms such as bacteria. In this section, the phenomenon of phagocytosis is exemplified by reference to the phagocytosis of a bacterium.

Phagocytosis of bacteria is carried out in a stepped fashion, beginning with the organisms being "coated" with an opsonising agent. Opsonising agents include a wide range of proteins such as complement fractions C1q, C3b and C4 and antibodies, and they allow phagocytic cells to attach to and then engulf their target. One well-researched opsonin is the complement fraction C3b activated from plasma during inflammation. Both neutrophils and macrophages possess C3b receptors on the cell membrane (◘ Fig. 5.15), and this allows them to attach to a bacterium opsonised with C3b (◘ Fig. 5.16). The bacterium is then engulfed and brought into the cell, where it is surrounded by a membrane to form a phagosome. The next stage involves the fusion of a lysosomal granule containing a battery of destructive enzymes with the phagosome and the release of those enzymes into the phagosome to form a phagolysosome, where the bacterium is digested and destroyed. Undigestable bacterial components form a residual body while other components are excreted from the phagocyte.

Phagocytosis of non-bacterial materials (◘ Fig. 5.17) having a dental context includes phagocytosis of dental root-filling materials seen in periapical granulomas and phagocytosis of amalgam in amalgam tattoos occurring in the oral mucosa. This phenomenon can also be seen microscopically in cases of haemosiderin pigmentation of the oral mucosa and in some pigmented lesions where there is pigmentary incontinence.

Histologically, inflammation is intimately associated with the healing of damaged tissues. Microscopic evidence of healing in inflammatory fields can be manifested by the presence of granulation tissue (◘ Fig. 5.18), immature fibrous connective tissue or fibrosis, the latter occurring in long-standing chronic inflammatory lesions. The topic of healing is detailed in ► Chap. 4.

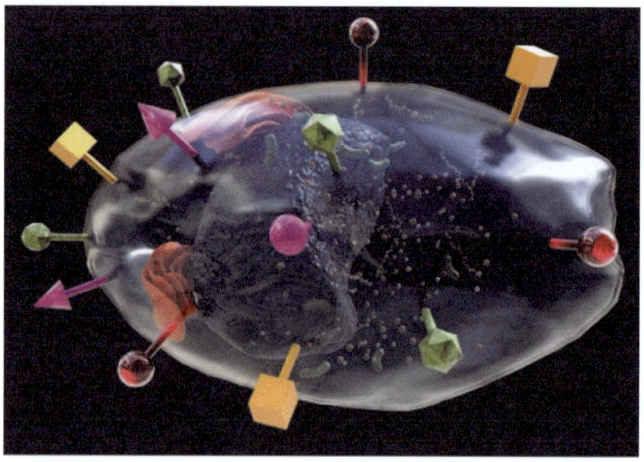

◘ **Fig. 5.15** The 3D graphic showing a variety of stylised receptors on a phagocytic cell. Receptor types include C3B and Fc receptors, both of which are important in bacterial phagocytosis in inflammation. The receptors allow a phagocyte to identify and attach to a target to be phagocytosed

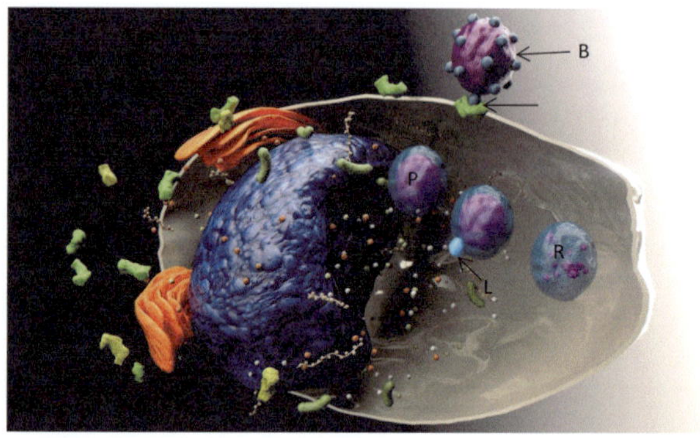

◘ **Fig. 5.16** The 3D graphic of a stylised cutaway macrophage illustrating the processes involved in phagocytosis of a bacterium. A C3b-opsonised bacterium (B arrow) is recognised by a C3b receptor (arrow) on the phagocytic cell and bound to the cell. Subsequently, the bacterium is taken into the cell and surrounded by a membrane to form a phagosome (P). A lysosomal granule (L arrow), containing destructive enzymes, then fuses with the phagosome and releases its contents into the phagosome to bring about the killing and lysis of the bacterium. Any undigestable bacterial components form a residual body (R)

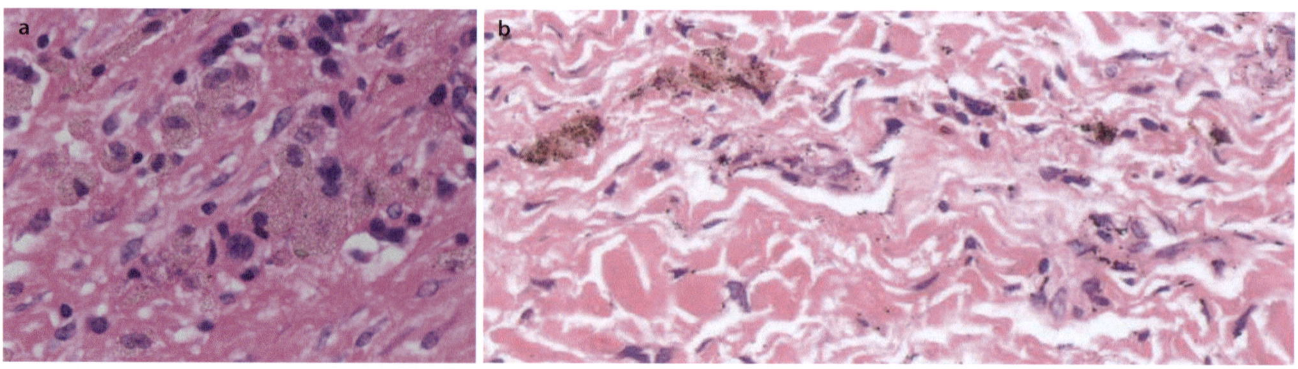

◘ **Fig. 5.17** (**a**) Photomicrograph from a periapical granuloma showing numerous macrophages containing brownish root-filling material. (**b**) Amalgam tattoo. Finely granular, brown material is seen within obscured phagocytic macrophages

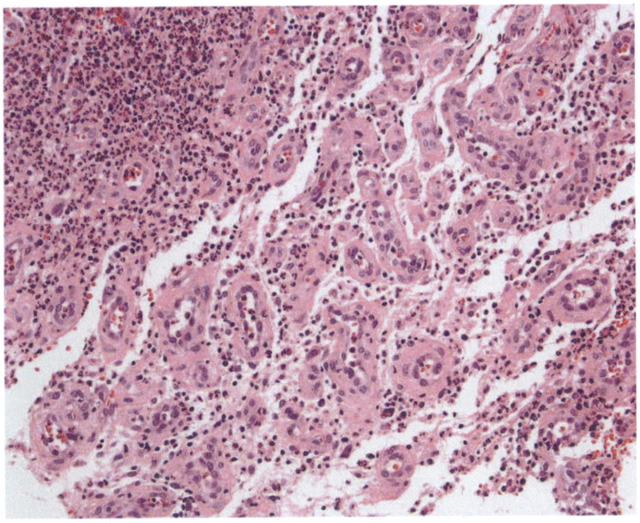

Fig. 5.18 Photomicrograph showing an area of granulation tissue within a markedly inflamed inflammatory background. The granulation tissue consists of newly formed capillaries and capillary buds with plump endothelial cells admixed with inflammatory cells

5.4 Chemical Mediators

A detailed discussion of chemical mediators is beyond the scope of this chapter. However, it is useful to have some understanding of these biologically active agents in order to appreciate the dynamics and complexity of events occurring in inflammation. The chemical mediators, some of which have already been referred to in the sections on acute and chronic inflammation, comprise a diverse group of rapidly generated and rapidly acting endogenous chemicals derived from cells and plasma. Mediators are involved in initiating and modulating the various processes that occur in the different types of inflammation and in other biological processes such as healing and allergies. Those derived from cells may exist as pre-formed mediators (e.g. histamine in mast cell granules and some molecules in neutrophil and macrophage granules) or as cytokines such as the interleukins and interferons. Others are synthesised by metabolic processes that occur in activated inflammatory cells and other cells (e.g. leukotrienes and prostaglandins produced from arachidonic acid, an essential fatty acid residing in the phospholipid layer of cell membranes). Some can have multiple roles (e.g. may act to cause vascular dilatation and also act as a chemokine [chemotactic agent]). Plasma-derived mediators include the complement system and its fractions and bradykinin. The complement system consists of a group of plasma proteins that can be activated by a variety of means including immunoglobulins. In the context of inflammation, there are various ways in which the complement system can act. As an example, the complement system generates activated complement proteins that bind to injury-causing agents such as bacteria, opsonising (coating) them and enabling engulfment by neutrophils and macrophages, which carry receptors for complement (see also section on phagocytosis). Other small fragments such as C3a and C5a act as chemical mediators to recruit and activate neutrophils and macrophages at the site of injury by, for example, inducing arachidonic acid metabolism and the production of additional chemical mediators such as the prostaglandins and leukotrienes. An additional method in which complement fractions can act is by direct damage to bacterial cell walls. Examples of chemical mediators, their source and their actions are presented in Table 5.1.

Table 5.1 The chemical mediators, their sources and their actions occurring in inflammatory processes

Mediators	Sources	Roles
Histamine	Mast cells, basophils	Vasodilation, vascular permeability, modulation of some adhesion molecules
Serotonin	Platelets	Vascular permeability
Bradykinin	Plasma	Vascular permeability, causing pain
Complement fraction C3a	Plasma	Vascular permeability
Complement fraction C5a	Plasma	Vascular permeability, chemotaxis, leukocyte activation
Complement fraction C3b	Plasma	Opsonising agent
Leukotriene B4	Leukocytes	Chemotaxis, leukocyte activation
Leukotrienes C4, D4 and E4	Leukocytes, mast cells	Vascular permeability, some also cause bronchoconstriction and vasoconstriction
Prostaglandin PGI2	Inflammatory cells, endothelial cells, platelets	Vasodilation, anti-platelet aggregation
Prostaglandin PGE2	Inflammatory cells, endothelial cells, platelets	Vasodilation, smooth muscle relaxation
Platelet-activating factor (PAF)	Leukocytes, mast cells	Vascular dilation, chemokine, platelet aggregation
IL-1 and TNF	Macrophages, lymphocytes	Chemotaxis, immune cell modulation, modulation of adhesion molecule expression
Interleukin-6 (IL-6)	Macrophages and T cells	Proliferation of B cells
Interferon-gamma (IFN-gamma)	T cells and natural killer cells	Activation of macrophages to increase their bactericidal activity and promote antigen presentation

5.5 Granulomatous Inflammation

Two forms of granulomatous inflammation are recognised:

- Immune-mediated granulomatous inflammation
- Foreign body granulomatous inflammation

However, nowadays, the term "granulomatous inflammation" is generally reserved to describe immune-mediated granulomatous inflammation. Immune-mediated granulomatous inflammation is a complex pathological process associated with a range of human diseases, including tuberculosis, tertiary syphilis, Crohn's disease, sarcoidosis and the rare condition of oro-facial granulomatosis. This form of inflammation develops and continues in affected tissues because of the persistence of the injurious agent and the resulting and complex interactions of the immune system and its cells. In some cases, such as tuberculosis, the injury (mycobacterium) associated with the granulomatous condition is known. In other diseases, including Crohn's disease and sarcoidosis, the nature of the injury is unknown.

5.5.1 Immune-Mediated Granulomatous Inflammation

In light microscope sections, immune-mediated granulomatous inflammation is a distinctive pattern of chronic inflammation in which the predominant cell type is an activated macrophage with a modified epithelial cell-like appearance. The modified macrophage is called an epi-

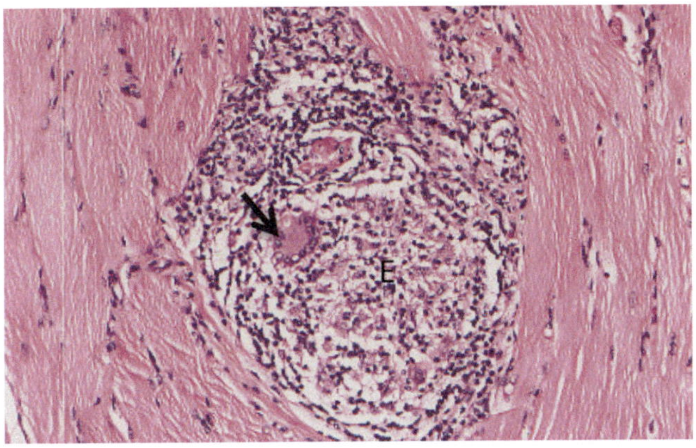

Fig. 5.19 Immune-mediated granulomatous inflammation. A well-delineated granuloma within the skeletal muscle is evident. A focus of eosinophilic epithelioid cells (E) surrounded by darkly staining lymphocytes can be seen. A multinucleate giant cell (arrow) is also evident, but these cells are not a feature of some conditions classified as immune-mediated granulomatous disease

thelioid cell. The diagnostic feature of granulomatous inflammation is the presence of discrete epithelioid granulomas, often within a background of generalised chronic inflammation. Granulomas can be caseating and associated with necrosis, as in tuberculosis, or non-caseating, as is the case in conditions such as sarcoidosis and Crohn's disease. These are collections of epithelioid cells usually associated with immune cells such as lymphocytes (Fig. 5.19). Multinucleate giant cells may or may not be present in the granulomas.

5.5.2 Foreign Body Granulomatous Inflammation

Foreign body granulomatous inflammation (Foreign body reaction) describes the condition where persistent chronic inflammation occurs due to the persistence of exogenous foreign material—usually solid—within the tissue. Histologically, a foreign body reaction is usually characterised by features of normal chronic inflammation admixed with immature fibrous connective tissue and granulation tissue and the presence of multinucleated giant cells (Fig. 5.20) closely associated with the foreign material. Examples of materials that can elicit a multinucleate giant response when introduced to tissues include silica, talc powder (intravenous drug users), suture materials, plant materials, keratin and some endodontic materials.

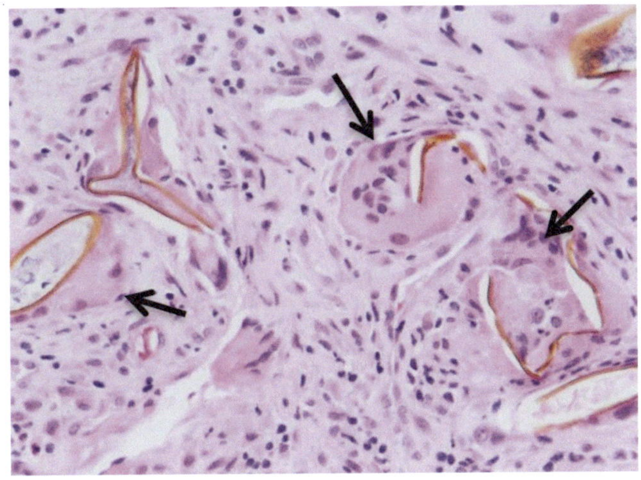

Fig. 5.20 Foreign body reaction. Irregularly shaped fragments of yellow-brown foreign material in chronically inflamed, immature fibrous connective tissue are evident. Variously sized and shaped multinucleated giant cells (arrows) are seen associated with the foreign material, which in this particular case is a plant-origin component of a proprietary product, sometimes used as part of the treatment of dry sockets

5.6 Summary

Inflammation is a response to injury, with that response having the ideal outcome of removing or otherwise eliminating the cause of that injury and allowing healing to be initiated. Inflammation can affect a localised area of an organ (e.g. an abscess in the skin) or a whole organ (for instance, hepatitis). Injuries may be exogenous as in the case of infective agents (bacteria or viruses), physical trauma (accidental or surgical trauma), thermal trauma, chemical trauma, electrical trauma or some forms of radiation. Tissue injury giving rise to inflammation can also be generated by endogenous abnormalities such as some of the immune hypersensitivities. For histological diagnostic purposes, inflammation can be categorised as acute inflammation, chronic inflammation and granulomatous inflammation. Each type of inflammation has relatively specific microscopic features, allowing distinction between them. A diagnosis of one or other form of inflammation mainly rests on the identification of accumulations of one or more types of inflammatory-immune cells in an affected tissue and in the case of acute inflammation, changes in the terminal microvasculature. However, there are aspects of commonality between each type when such features as the migration of inflammatory-immune cells to the site of injury, the interactions of chemical (inflammatory) mediators and chemokines with cells, the interactions of inflammatory cells themselves and processes such as phagocytosis are considered.

Further Reading

Herrington S. Cell injury, inflammation and repair. In: Herrington S, editor. Muir's textbook of pathology. Boca Raton: CRC Press; 2014. p. 41–7.

Kumar V, Abbas AK, Aster JC. Chapter 3. Inflammation and repair. In: Robbin's basic pathology. 10th ed. Philadelphia: Elsevier; 2018. p. 57–93.

Nunes AC. Introductory chapter: overview of the cellular and molecular basis of inflammatory process. In: Nunes AC, editor. Translational studies on inflammation [internet]. London: IntechOpen; 2020 [cited 2022 Aug 06]. https://www.intechopen.com/chapters/68815. https://doi.org/10.5772/intechopen.88967.

Prabhu SR. Inflammation: an overview. In: Prabhu SR. Textbook of general pathology for dental students. Springer. 2023. pp. 41–47.

Histology of Odontogenesis: An Overview

S R Prabhu

Contents

S R Prabhu et al. (eds.), *Oral Histology and Oral Histopathology*, https://doi.org/10.1007/978-3-031-77481-2_6

6.1 Introduction

Odontogenesis refers to the process of tooth formation, eruption and integration with its surrounding tissues. It encompasses primary and permanent dentition development. Odontogenesis involves the intra-oral molecular embryological process in which teeth are formed from specialised embryonic cells until their root formation and eruption are completed. Genetically complex processes regulate initial dental histological organisation, histodifferentiation, morphodifferentiation, spatial tooth arrangement, amelogenesis, dentinogenesis, cementogenesis, periodontal ligament formation and tooth eruption. A cascade of gene expression occurs to direct cells along the appropriate differentiation pathways. Signalling pathways involved in this cascade include (1) bone morphogenetic protein (BMP), (2) fibroblast growth factor (FGf), (3) sonic hedgehog (Shh), (4) Wingless-related integration site (Wnt) and (5) ectodysplasin A (EDA). Determining specific tooth types at their correct positions in the jaws is called patterning of the dentition.

6

The first morphological sign of tooth formation is a thickening of the oral epithelium, which later forms a dental lamina. The dental lamina gives rise to epithelial tooth buds with surrounding condensed mesenchyme. The tooth development is divided into three stages: bud, cap and bell (Fig. 6.1). The bud and cap stages are the

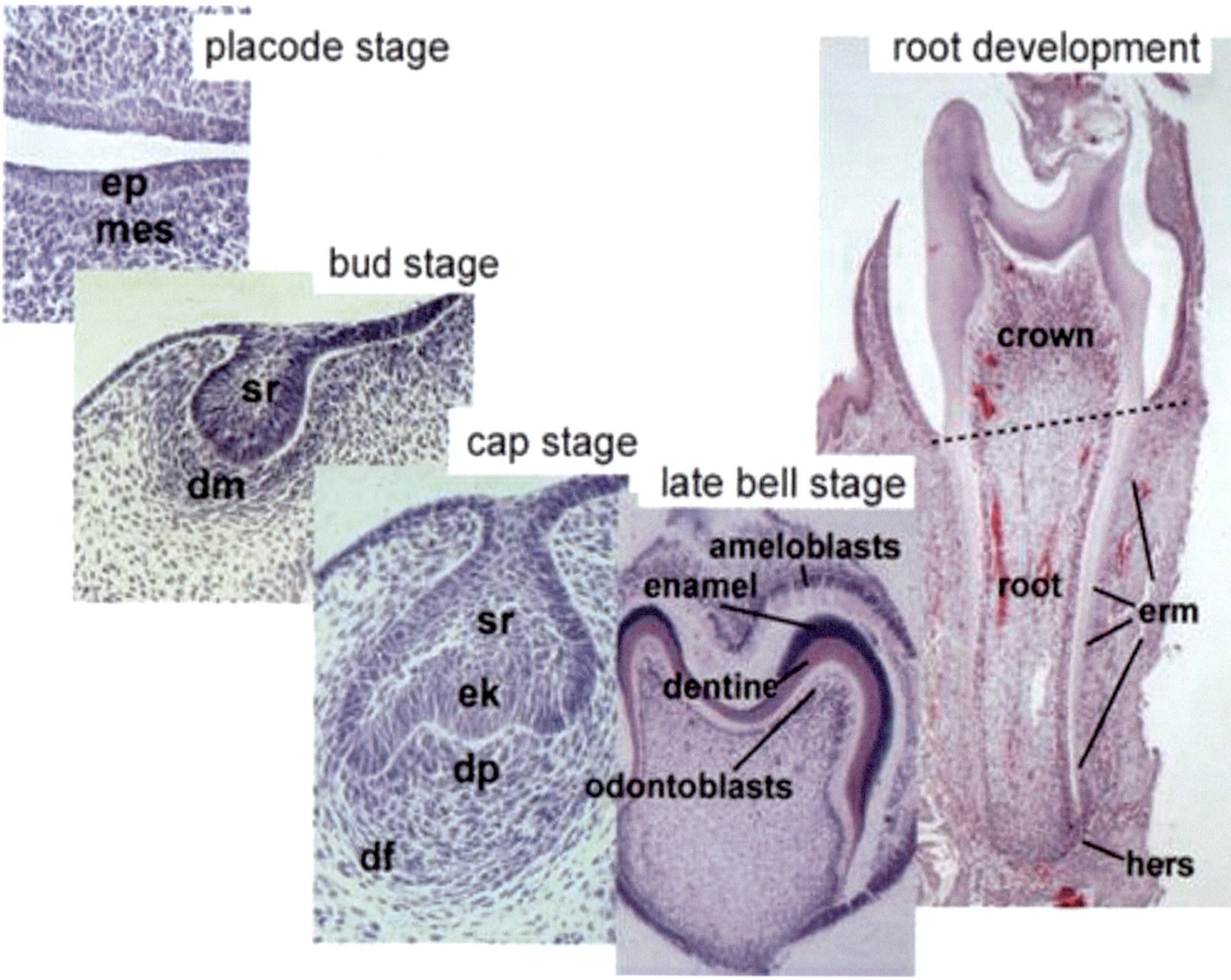

Fig. 6.1 Histology of important stages of tooth development. Note that all early development is directed at creating the crown, and only then root formation is initiated. Ameloblasts differentiate from the epithelium and odontoblasts from the mesenchyme, and they deposit the matrices of enamel and dentine, respectively. Ameloblasts and enamel are missing on the root, which is covered by the softer dentin and cementum. *ep* epithelium, *mes* mesenchyme, *sr* stellate reticulum, *dm* dental mesenchyme, *dp* dental papilla, *df* dental follicle, *ek* enamel knot, *erm* epithelial cell rests of Malassez, *hers* Hertwig's epithelial root sheath. (Source: Thesleff, I. and Tummers, M., Tooth organogenesis and regeneration (January 31, 2009), StemBook, ed. The Stem Cell Research Community, StemBook. ► https://doi.org/10.3824/stembook.1.37.1; ► http://www.stembook.org. CC BY 3.0)

first and second stages of tooth development. During the early bell stage, the enamel organ resembles a bell. In the late bell stage, the tooth germ increases in size, and the hard tissues of the teeth start forming. For a detailed description of odontogenesis, the reader is referred to standard textbooks on the subject. This chapter focuses on the histological features of odontogenesis. A detailed description of amelogenesis, dentinogenesis, cementogenesis and periodontal ligament is presented elsewhere in the book.

6.2 Initiation of Odontogenesis

The timing of tooth development is different for different teeth. Most teeth develop during intrauterine life. Deciduous ▶ central incisors are the first to develop, followed by the ▶ first molars, lateral incisors and canines. The mandibular central incisor is the first to initiate its development, and the maxillary central incisor starts its development slightly afterwards. The development of the first permanent molar commences in the fourth month of intrauterine life. The second molar is initiated in the first year and the third molar in the fourth or fifth years after birth.

Most of the connective tissue cells underlying the primitive oral epithelium are neural crest (ectomesenchyme) in origin. Tooth development initiates with a thickening of the oral epithelium, which exhibits odontogenic inductive potential and can induce the initiation of tooth development when recombined with non-odontogenic neural crest-derived mesenchyme. The neural crest is a pluripotent cell population derived from the lateral ridges of the neural plate during early embryogenesis. Cranial neural crest-derived ectomesenchyme contributes to the formation of condensed dental mesenchyme at the initial bud stage and, subsequently, to the formation of the dental papilla and follicle in the developing tooth germ.

The initiation of odontogenesis starts from the primitive oral epithelium (oral ectoderm) that lines the primary oral cavity ("stomodeum"). Tooth development initiates with a thickening of the oral epithelium. This is called a primary epithelial band (PEB), followed by localised thickenings or placodes (◘ Fig. 6.1) forming within the primary epithelial bands. Certain areas of basal cells of the epithelium proliferate more rapidly than the adjacent cells. These are roughly horseshoe-shaped and correspond in position to the future dental arches of the upper and lower jaws. This initial change occurs when the embryo is about 6 weeks old.

6.3 Formation of Dental and Vestibular Laminae

Around the seventh week of intrauterine life, the PEB grows deeper into the mesenchyme. Two divisions quickly occur, forming an inner (lingual) process called the dental lamina and an outer (buccal) process called the vestibular lamina. The dental lamina connects the developing tooth bud to the epithelium of the oral cavity and serves as the primordium for the ectodermal portion of the deciduous teeth. The successors of deciduous teeth develop from a lingual extension of the free end of the dental lamina. The lingual extension of the dental lamina is called the successional lamina. The basement membrane separates the epithelium of the dental lamina from the underlying mesenchyme.

The vestibular lamina (also called the lip furrow band) proliferates within the mesenchyme and leads to the formation of the vestibule. The cells of the vestibular lamina rapidly enlarge and then degenerate. This results in the formation of a cleft that becomes the vestibule between the cheek/lip and the tooth-bearing areas.

6.4 Crown Formation: Stages of Morphogenesis

Based on the shapes of the epithelial part of the enamel organ, the developmental history of teeth is divided into three morphologic stages, namely the bud, cap and bell. These stages are descriptive of the morphology of the developing tooth germ and do not describe the functional changes that occur during development.

6.4.1 Bud Stage

Corresponding to the future positions of the deciduous teeth in the dental arch, dental lamina thickens from the free edge into small, ten rounded swellings (◘ Fig. 6.2). This is the bud stage of tooth development. The swellings are the tooth buds of the deciduous teeth and are primordia of the epithelial part of enamel organs responsible for enamel formation. In the bud stage, low columnar cells are peripherally located, and polygonal cells are located centrally. At this stage, increased mitotic activity occurs in cells of the tooth bud and ectomesenchyme. The ectomesenchymal cells immediately subjacent to the tooth bud are packed closely beneath and around the epithelial bud. This results in increased cellular density, called condensation of ectomesenchyme.

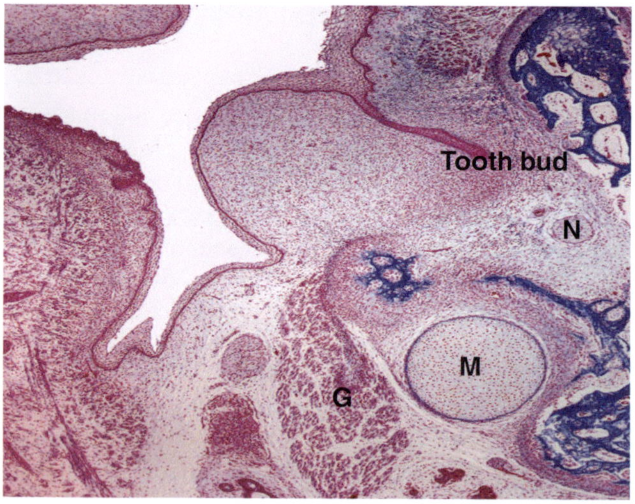

Fig. 6.2 Bud stage of tooth development in the mandible. This section is taken from a human foetus and is displaying a cross section of parts of the developing mandible and its surrounding tissues. The mandibular bone is under development, and a tooth bud is seen among the spicules of bone. A cross section of Meckle's cartilage (M) and the inferior alveolar nerve (N) are seen, and glandular parenchyma is seen inferiorly (G) and medially to Meckle's cartilage. (Source: ► https://www.anatomicum.com/files/images/modified/fullsize/34.jpg. Courtesy of Dr. Mathias Nordvi)

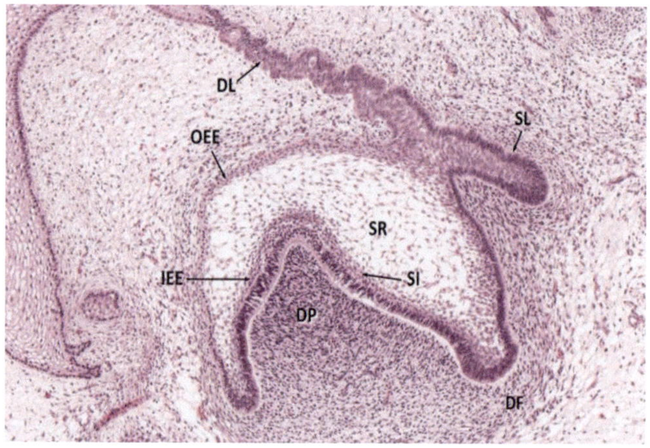

Fig. 6.3 Haematoxylin and eosin-stained histology section shows a developing tooth in the "cap" stage. The inner and outer enamel epithelia (IEE and OEE) are present and separated by the stellate reticulum (SR) and stratum intermedium (SI). The dental lamina (DL) is still present, and the successional lamina (SL) can be seen to the right of the image. The dental papilla, composed of mesenchymal cells, is surrounded by the IEE, and the dental follicle (DF) surrounds the developing tooth structure. (Source: Takata, T., Miyauchi, M., Ogawa, I., Mighell, A. (2018). Odontogenic Pathology. In: Farah, C., Balasubramaniam, R., McCullough, M. (eds) Contemporary Oral Medicine. (Springer.com). ► https://doi.org/10.1007/978-3-319-28100-1_22-1

This becomes the dental papilla, which is responsible for the formation of dental pulp. The condensed ectomesenchyme surrounding the entire tooth bud and dental papilla becomes a dental sac (also known as dental follicle) responsible for forming the periodontal ligament at later stages of tooth development.

6.4.2 Cap Stage

The transition from bud to cap stage indicates the onset of morphologic differences between tooth germs that give rise to different types of teeth. The tooth bud transforms into a cap by differential proliferation and infolding of the odontogenic epithelium. The epithelial bud continues to proliferate and grow unequally in its different parts. This leads to a shallow invagination on its deep surface, giving it the shape of a cap (Fig. 6.3). The peripheral cells of the "cap" later form the outer and inner enamel epithelium. This structure is called the enamel organ. The enamel organ, dental papilla and dental sac (follicle) constitute the tooth germ. The cells in the centre of the enamel organ synthesise and secrete glycosaminoglycans into the extracellular space between the epithelial cells. Glycosaminoglycans are hydrophilic and draw water into this space and force central cells of the enamel organ apart from each other. Because these cells retain connections with each other through their desmosomal contacts, they become star shaped. Now, the centre of the enamel organ is termed the stellate reticulum.

At the late cap stage, further folding of the enamel organ establishes future cusp shapes as the teeth enter the bell stage. During the bell stage, specific cell populations differentiate before hard tissue formation.

6.4.3 Bell Stage

Cell growth in the enamel organ leads to the next stage of tooth development, the bell stage. This stage of tooth development is characterised by the enamel organ growing into a bell shape as its undersurface deepens and covers the dental papilla (Fig. 6.4). Both the enamel organ and the dental papilla remain encapsulated by a mesenchymal tissue called a dental sac (dental follicle).

In the bell stage, two important events occur: histodifferentiation and morphodifferentiation. A high degree of histodifferentiation is achieved in the early bell stage. Histodifferentiation refers to the differentiation of cells of the enamel organ into four distinct cell groups based on their morphology and function. These include outer enamel epithelium (OEE), inner enamel epithelium (IEE), stellate reticulum and stratum intermedium. Morphodifferentiation refers to the morphogenesis of the enamel organ via the folding of the IEE layer into a

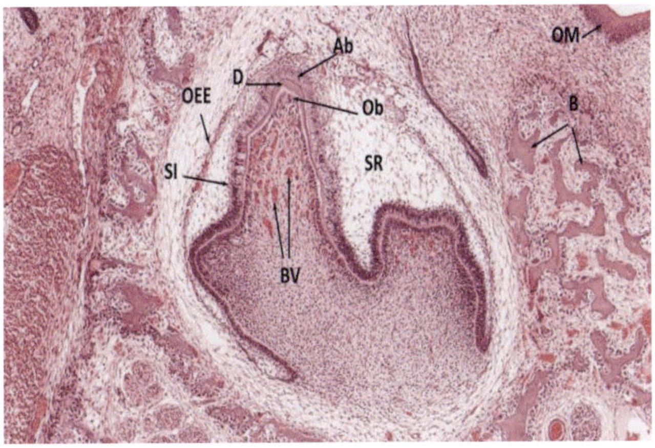

Fig. 6.4 Haematoxylin and eosin-stained histology section shows a developing tooth at the "bell" stage. Dentin (D) can be seen (in its greatest quantity at this stage at the future cusp tip) being laid down by odontoblasts (Ob). Ameloblasts (Ab) are also present. The stellate reticulum is still present (SR) as are parts of the stratum intermedium (SI). The pulp is more developed at this stage too, and blood vessels (BV) are infiltrating it. The outer enamel epithelium (OEE) can be seen and will soon fuse with the stratum intermedium (SI) to become the reduced enamel epithelium. Bone (B) can be seen forming around the developing tooth, and the oral mucosa (OM) is visible at the top right corner of the image. Source: Takata, T., Miyauchi, M., Ogawa, I., Mighell, A. (2018). Odontogenic Pathology. In: Farah, C., Balasubramaniam, R., McCullough, M. (eds) Contemporary Oral Medicine. Springer, Cham. ► https://doi.org/10.1007/978-3-319-28100-1_22-1

three-dimensional structure that resembles the future tooth crown. By the start of the bell stage, the shape of the tooth has already been decided.

- **Outer enamel epithelium (OEE)**: The OEE cells are cuboidal epithelial cells on the outer surface of the enamel organ (Fig. 6.4). This structure has high mitotic activity. It is avascular; it derives its nutrition from the capillary loops in the mesenchyme of the dental sac surrounding the enamel organ.
- **Inner enamel epithelium**: This comprises a single layer of columnar epithelial cells on the enamel organ's undersurface and adjacent to the dental papilla (Fig. 6.4). Before amelogenesis, these cells differentiate into tall columnar cells (ameloblasts). These cells exert an organising influence on the underlying mesenchymal cells of the dental papilla, which later become odontoblasts (Fig. 6.4). At the late bell stage, cells of the IEE of the enamel organ stop dividing. They elongate and rapidly induce adjacent neural crest-derived cells of the dental papilla to differentiate into odontoblasts. Odontoblasts first appear at the sites of the future cusp tips. They are responsible for the secretion of the dentin matrix as they differentiate along the length of the dental papilla adjacent to the internal enamel epithelium. The formation of predentine precedes dentine formation. This first layer signals the overlying inner enamel epithelial cells to differentiate into ameloblasts and begin secreting the enamel matrix. The odontoblasts migrate in an apical direction and lay down coronal dentine, while ameloblasts migrate in a coronal direction and deposit enamel of the tooth crown.
- **Stellate reticulum**: Stellate reticulum cells are star-shaped cells situated in the centre of the enamel organ (Fig. 6.4). These cells synthesise and secrete glycosaminoglycan into the inter-cellular space, which draws water into the inter-cellular space. Intercellular water separates the cells apart, while intercellular adhesions remain through desmosomes, resulting in a star-shaped appearance of the stellate reticulum cells. The stellate reticulum has a cushion-like consistency, offering support and protection to the enamel-forming cells.
- **Stratum intermedium**: In the bell stage, some epithelial cells between the inner enamel epithelium and the stellate reticulum differentiate into two or three stratified layers of cells called the stratum intermedium (Fig. 6.4). These cells are situated over the IEE and are connected to the cells of the stellate reticulum and inner enamel epithelium by desmosomes. Stratum intermedium cells show the high activity of the enzyme alkaline phosphatase and act, together with the IEE cells, as a single functional unit in enamel formation.
- **Cervical loop:** The OEE and the IEE are continuous, and their junction forms the bell's rim, termed the cervical loop. Cells of the cervical loop continue to proliferate and play crucial roles in root formation (Fig. 6.5).

Two other significant events occur during the bell stage: the dental lamina joins the tooth germ to the oral epithelium fragments, eventually separating the developing tooth from the oral epithelium, and the inner enamel epithelium completes its folding, providing evidence to recognise the shape of the future crown pattern of the tooth—the folding results from intrinsic growth caused by differential rates of mitotic division within the inner enamel epithelium. The cessation of mitotic division within cells of the inner enamel epithelium determines the shape of a tooth.

- **Transitory structures**:

  The enamel knot, enamel cord, and enamel niche are transitory structures seen in the enamel organ during the early bell stage of tooth development. Of these,

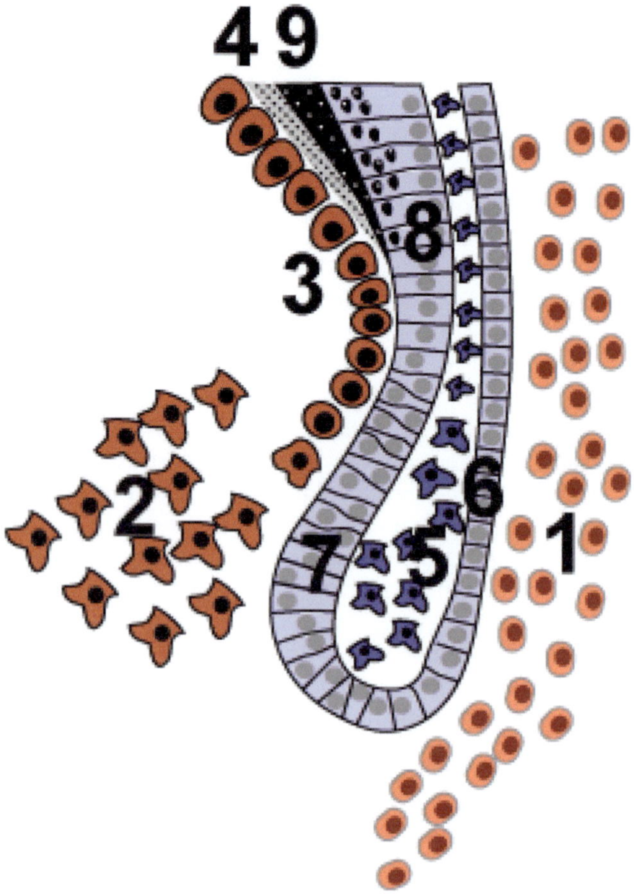

Fig. 6.5 Schematic diagram of the cervical loop area: (1) dental follicle cells, (2) dental mesenchyme, (3) odontoblasts, (4) dentine, (5) stellate reticulum, (6) outer enamel epithelium, (7) inner enamel epithelium, (8) ameloblasts, (9) enamel. (Source: ► https://en.wikipedia.org/wiki/Cervical_loop#/media/File:Cervical-loop.png. Image credit: M. Tummers 2004. Creative Commons Attribution-ShareAlike License 4.0)

the enamel knot is the most significant in functional development. Recent studies suggest it may represent an important signalling centre during tooth development (e.g. bone morphogenetic proteins [BMP-2 and BMP-7]). Enamel knot is seen as densely packed cells in the advanced cap stage, the molar tooth germ shows a single primary enamel knot that induces the formation of secondary enamel knots at the tips of the future cusps and, thereby regulates crown patterning. Depending on the plane of histological sections, cells extending from the enamel knot across the stellate reticulum to the outer enamel epithelium may be seen. This structure is the enamel cord. The narrow, ectomesenchyme-filled space between the dental ledge and an enamel organ is called enamel niche.

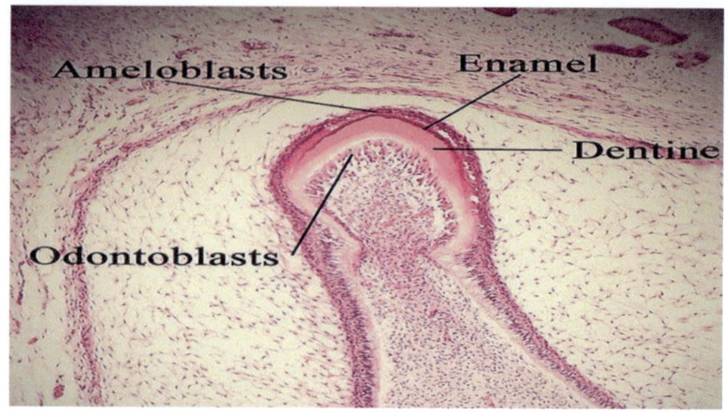

Fig. 6.6 Histology of developing tooth with enamel, dentine, ameloblasts and odontoblasts labelled. The tooth bud is in the maturation/crown stage. Human tooth development. (Source: Wikipedia. ► https://en.wikipedia.org/wiki/Human_tooth_development. CC-BY-SA licence)

6.4.4 Advanced Bell Stage: Hard Tissue Formation of the Crown

Until the crown assumes its final shape during the early bell stage, all cells of the inner enamel epithelium continually divide. After that, until the tooth crown attains its full size, only cells at the cervical margin of the enamel organ divide. At the sites of the future cusp tips, a layer of dentin will first appear, mitotic activity ceases and the short columnar cells of the inner enamel epithelium elongate and become taller. These cells also show reverse polarity, with their nuclei aligned adjacent to the stratum facing the dental papilla. At the same time, the undifferentiated ectomesenchymal cells of the dental papilla increase rapidly in size and, ultimately, differentiate into dentin-forming cells called odontoblasts (Fig. 6.6). An organising influence from the cells of the inner enamel epithelium initiates the differentiation of odontoblasts from the undifferentiated ectomesenchyme of the dental papilla. The odontoblasts begin to elaborate the organic matrix of dentine, resulting in their movement towards the centre of the dental papilla, leaving behind the cytoplasmic extension around which the dentine is formed. This gives a tubular structure to the dentine.

During the advanced bell stage, dentin formation occurs first as a layer along the future dentinoenamel junction in the region of future cusps. This process proceeds pulpally and apically. Immediately after that, ameloblasts (differentiated from IEE cells) lay down the first layer of the enamel matrix over the dentin in the future incisal and cuspal areas (Fig. 6.6). This process pro-

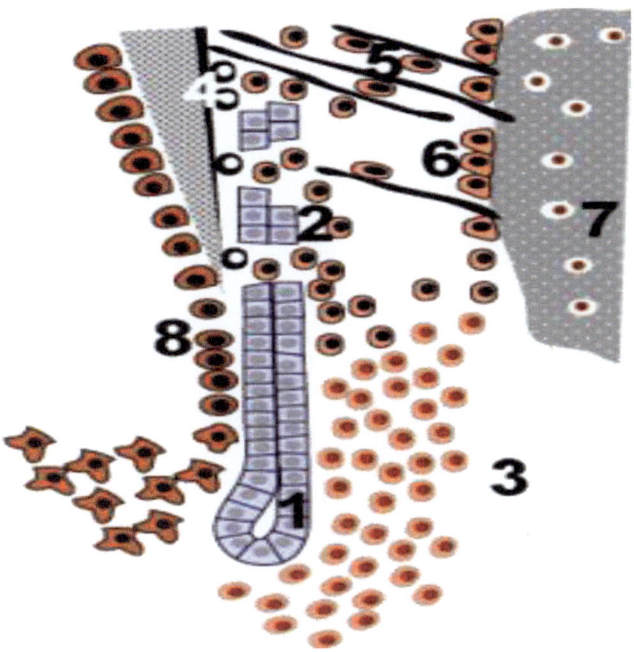

Fig. 6.7 Schematic representation of the HERS, epithelial rests of Malassez (ERM) and associated cells. The HERS (1), epithelial rests of Malassez (2), dental follicle (3), cementoblasts (4), periodontal ligament (5), osteoblasts (6), bone (7), odontoblasts (8). (Source: Wikipedia. ► https://en.wikipedia.org/wiki/Epithelial_cell_rests_of_Malassez. CC-BY-SA licence) (Credit. M Tummers)

ceeds coronally and cervically in all directions. The growth of cervical loop cells (formed by the OEE and IEE cells) into the deeper tissues creates Hertwig's epithelial root sheath (HERS) (Fig. 6.7), which determines the outline, number, length, shape and size of the future roots.

The molars of the permanent dentition have no deciduous predecessors. When the jaws have grown long enough, the dental lamina burrows posteriorly beneath the lining epithelium of the oral mucosa into the ectomesenchyme. This backward extension successively gives off epithelial outgrowths that, together with the associated ectomesenchymal response, form the tooth germs of the first, second and third molars.

6.5 Root Formation

Development of the tooth root starts following crown formation. At the late bell stage of tooth development, when amelogenesis and dentinogenesis are well advanced, the double-layered Hertwig's epithelial root sheath (HERS) extends around the dental papilla (future dental pulp) and between the dental papilla and dental follicle, leaving only the basal portion of the dental papilla not enclosed. The rim of the HERS at this stage is called the epithelial diaphragm. Once the epithelial diaphragm has formed, the root dentine and cementum formation process begin. This structure encloses the primary apical foramen; the cells of the HERS initiate the differentiation of odontoblasts from the ectomesenchymal cells at the periphery of the dental papilla that faces the root sheath. These odontoblasts form a dentine matrix for a single-rooted tooth. The spatial position of the root sheath relative to the bone at the base of the tooth crypt remains relatively constant. Elongation of the root occurs in a vertical direction mainly because of the relative movement of the tooth crown towards the mucosa. Only approximately two-thirds of the tooth root is formed at tooth emergence. It may take up to 3 years for the root apex to close. HERS also participates in determining the number of tooth roots. As the process of root formation is in progress, the HERS (now called the epithelial diaphragm) develops tongue-shaped epithelial protrusions that join horizontally to form a bridge called the furcation, where the root becomes divided, constituting the base of the pulp cavity; after the formation of the furcation, root development in multi-rooted teeth is driven by the apical growth of the HERS, in the same way as in single-rooted teeth. Thus, the growth of the HERS in different orientations contributes to the formation of multi-rooted teeth, including two-rooted lower molars and three-rooted upper molars.

6.5.1 Formation of Root Dentine Cementum and Periodontal Ligament

Tooth root development occurs through the reciprocal interactions between Hertwig's epithelial root sheath (HERS), the underlying dentine surface and the surrounding mesenchyme. Hertwig's epithelial root sheath is involved in the induction of odontoblast differentiation and subsequent dentin deposition during root formation via epithelial–mesenchymal interactions. Changes follow the induction of root dentine formation in both the composition and morphology of the HERS cells. The cuboidal cells become more flattened, and perforations appear in the outer epithelial layer of HERS. Following this, the basal lamina of the inner epithelial layer disintegrates. This change makes the epithelial bilayer of HERS perforated via localised (focal) apoptosis (physiological cell death), forming a mesh-like structure of epithelial cells surrounding the tooth root. This mesh-like structure facilitates the continuous interaction among epithelial cells and their collective interaction with the neural crest-derived mesenchyme, as well as contact between dental follicle cells and newly formed dentine. Epithelial rests of Malassez (ERM) cells persist within a mesenchymal matrix during postnatal life.

After they initiate contact with dentine, cells in the dental follicle differentiate into cementoblasts, which produce cementum-specific extracellular matrix proteins, including collagen fibres. Cells of HERS eventually either undergo apoptosis, get incorporated into the mineralised matrix of the cementum or migrate to the developing periodontal ligament to form the epithelial rests (◘ Fig. 6.8) of Malassez (ERM). In the apical

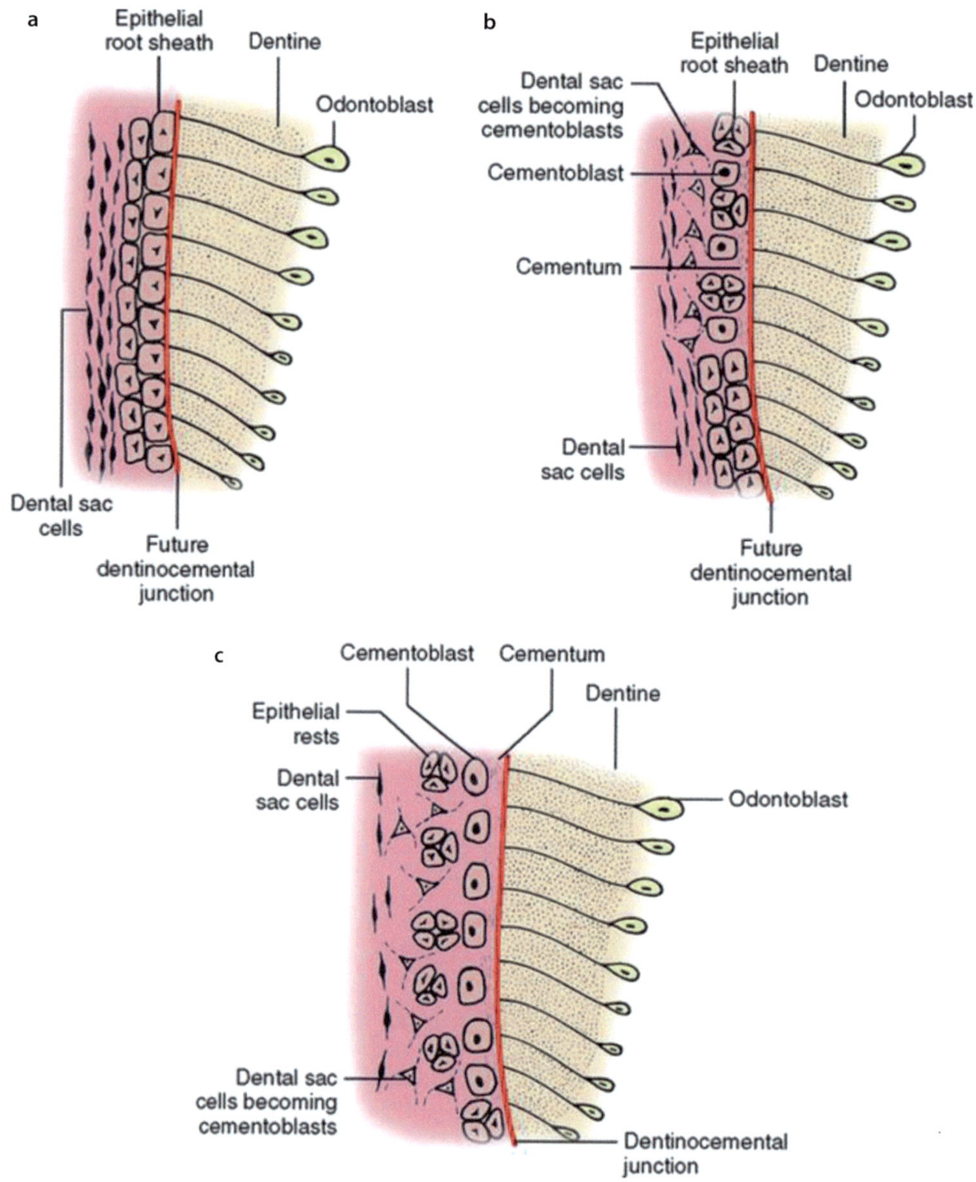

◘ **Fig. 6.8** Root formation. (**a**) The epithelial root sheath separates dentine from the dental sac cells. (**b**) The epithelial root sheath breaks up, and the dental sac cells become cementoblasts. (**c**) The epithelial root sheath moves away from dentine, and the dentinocemental junction is formed. (Root Formation and Attachment Apparatus. Chapter 21. Pocket Dentistry Courtesy of Dr. Cau Xuan Cu. Clinicalpub@gmail.com)

region of the root, cementoblasts remain embedded in the matrix, giving rise to the cellular cementum. By contrast, the rest of the root is covered by acellular cementum. The formation and degeneration of the HERS are essential for the development of periodontal ligament (PDL), which starts with the migration of dental follicle cells in contact with the HERS in between the root and alveolar bone, coinciding with the beginning of the perforation of HERS. During the migration of dental follicle cells, several cytoplasmic processes project from the leading edges of cells and begin secreting collagen fibres. Initially, these collagen fibres are disorganised but become arranged in a structured manner as development progresses.

6.6 The Role of Growth and Transcription Factors in Tooth Development

The mouse tooth has long been a model organ for studying developmental biology, such as epithelial–mesenchymal inductive interactions, differentiation and pattern formation. The human tooth development shares significant similarities to that of the mouse in the early process, including the lamina, the bud and the cap stages.

Tooth development is regulated by epithelial–mesenchymal interactions, which are mediated by signalling pathways including hedgehog (Hh), Wnt, fibroblast growth factor (FGF), transforming growth factor beta (Tgfβ), bone morphogenic protein (BMP), and ectodysplasin (EDA).

- One of the essential genes regulating placode formation is the transcription factor *p63*, expressed throughout the surface ectoderm.
- Around embryonic day 11.5 (E11.5), multiple genes encoding growth factors are expressed in the thickened dental epithelium. They include FGF8, FGF9, BMP2, BMP4, BMP7, Shh, Wnt10a and Wnt10b. These epithelial signalling molecules are responsible for the induction of gene expression, including msh homeobox 1 gene (MSX1), MSX2, LEF1, distal-less homeobox 1 gene (DLX1), DLX2, Patched (PTC), glioma-associated oncogene homolog (GLI1) and Syndecan-1 in the adjacent dental mesenchyme.
- At the bud stage, in response to the epithelial inductive signals, the dental mesenchyme begins to express genes encoding signalling molecules, including BMP4, FGF3, activin-βA and Wnt5a.
- A unique set of signalling molecules, including Shh, BMP2, BMP4, BMP7, FGF4 and FGF9, are expressed in the enamel knot. Therefore, the enamel knot is a signalling centre to control the patterning of the tooth cusps.
- Bone morphogenic protein (Bmp), transforming growth factor beta (Tgfβ), sonic hedgehog (Shh), muscle segment homeobox 2 (MSX2) and Distal-Less Homeobox 2 (DLX2) are expressed in HERS cells.
- Mesenchyme adjacent to the HERS also shows expression of Nuclear Factor I-C (NFIC) protein, fibroblast growth factor (FGF), transforming growth factor beta (TGFβ), bone morphogenic protein (BMP) and Wingless-integrated (Wnt) protein.

6.7 Determination of Position, Number and Types of Teeth

From the experimental data, the signals for controlling the position and the number of tooth germs along the oral surface appear to originate from the oral epithelium. FGF-8 seems to have a role in determining the positions where the tooth germs will form. The PAX9 gene is one of the earliest mesenchymal genes defining tooth germs' localisation. PAX9 gene expression co-localises with the exact sites where tooth germs appear. Signalling molecules often regulate the expression of transcription factors. Determination of tooth types is a process called patterning of dentition. This process involves the expression of various genes.

Two hypothetical theories have been proposed for dentition patterning to explain how these different shapes (incisiform, caniniform and molariform) are determined. These are called field theory and clone theory.

Genes responsible for the determination of tooth type include varying gene expressions (DLX1&2, BARX-1 and MSX1&2) in different regions of the dental arch and by specifically programmed ectomesenchyme (◘ Fig. 6.9a and b).

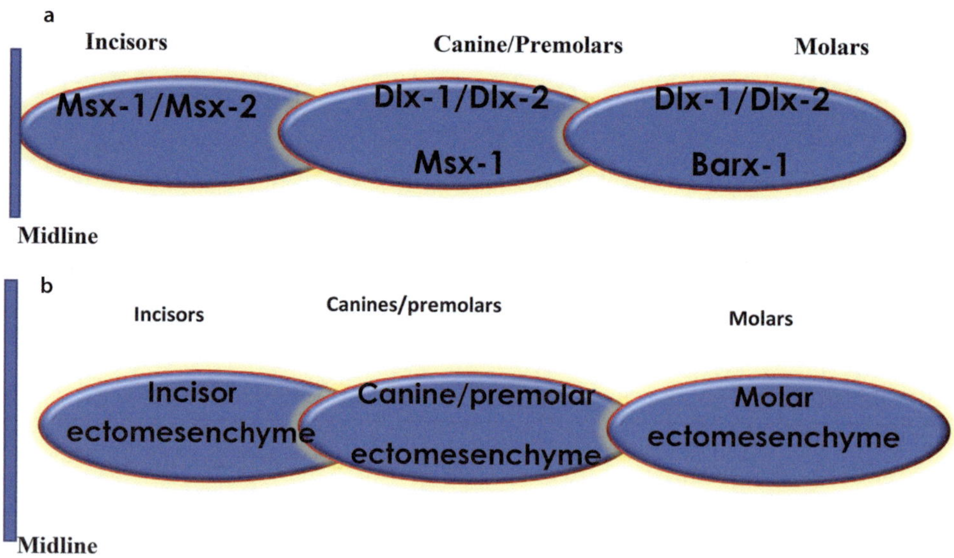

Fig. 6.9 (**a**) The field theory. This suggests that varying gene expressions in different arch regions determine tooth type. (Courtesy of Professor D F Wilson, Adelaide). (**b**) The clone theory. This suggests that tooth type is determined by specifically programmed dental ectomesenchyme. (Courtesy of Professor D F Wilson, Adelaide)

6.8 Formation of the Permanent Teeth

The initiation of successional permanent teeth occurs between week 20 in utero and 10 months after birth and the permanent molars between week 20 in utero for the first molars and 5 years of age for the third molars. The permanent dentition also arises from the dental lamina. The tooth germs that give rise to the permanent incisors, canines and premolars form because of further proliferative activity within the dental lamina at its deepest part. This increased proliferative activity leads to the formation of another tooth bud on the lingual aspect of the deciduous tooth germ, which remains dormant for some time. The permanent molars, on the other hand, have no deciduous predecessors. When the jaws have grown sufficiently for some time, beneath the lining epithelium of the oral mucosa, the dental lamina burrows backwards into the ectomesenchyme. This backward extension of dental lamina successively gives off epithelial outgrowths. These outgrowths, together with the response of the associated ectomesenchyme, form the tooth germs of the permanent first, second and third molars.

6.9 Vascular and Nerve Supply During the Early Stages of Tooth Development

During the cap stage, clusters of blood vessels are found forming branches around the tooth germ in the dental follicle and entering the dental papilla. During the bell stage, their number increases at the beginning of the deposition of the matrix. In the dental follicle, adjacent to the enamel epithelium, vessels are concentrated. The enamel organ is avascular.

During the bud-to-cap stage, nerve fibres are seen approaching the tooth bud, targeting the dental follicle. A rich plexus of nerves forms around the tooth germ in the dental follicle. Nerve fibres penetrate the dental papilla (pulp) as dentinogenesis begins. Histochemical studies show that autonomic nerve fibres are absent. The initial innervation of the developing teeth is concerned with the sensory innervation of the future periodontal ligament and pulp. Nerve fibres do not enter the enamel organ.

6.10 Tooth Eruption

Soon after the formation of the root is initiated, the tooth begins to erupt in an axial direction until it assumes its final position in the mouth with its occlusal surface in the occlusal plane. The crown of the tooth escapes from its bony crypt and passes through the lining mucosa of the oral cavity. At the beginning of the eruptive movement, a layer consisting of ameloblasts and remnants of the other three layers of the enamel organ are present, covering the tooth crown. Ameloblasts and adjacent cells of this layer are collectively called reduced enamel epithelium. The bone overlying the erupting tooth is soon resorbed, and the crown escapes through the mucosal connective tissue, broken down before the erupting tooth. The reduced enamel epithelium and the oral epithelium fuse and form a solid layer of epithelial cells over the crown of the tooth. The central cells in this mass degenerate, through which the crown of the tooth erupts. Epithelial cells of the oral epithelium and the reduced enamel epithelium form the dentogingival junction.

6.11 Summary

Odontogenesis, or tooth development, is the process of tooth formation, eruption and integration with its surrounding tissues. It encompasses the primary and the permanent dentition development. Teeth develop from ectoderm and mesoderm; the enamel develops from the ectoderm of the oral cavity, whereas other tissues develop from the associated mesenchyme. Development involves three stages. Early in the sixth week of intrauterine life, dental laminae appear as U-shaped thickenings of the oral epithelium. This is called the bud stage. The localised proliferation of cells in the dental laminae occurs, forming round or oval swellings, the tooth buds, which grow into the mesenchyme. Each jaw has ten tooth buds, one for each deciduous tooth. In the tenth week of intrauterine life, tooth buds for the permanent teeth develop from deeper continuations of the dental lamina lying on the lingual side of the deciduous buds. The permanent molars with no deciduous predecessors develop as buds from backward extensions of the dental laminae. Tooth buds for the permanent teeth appear at different ages during the foetal period, except for the second and third permanent molars, which occur after birth at about 4 months and 5 years, respectively. The deeper surface of each ectodermal tooth bud becomes invaginated by mesenchyme called the dental papilla, which is responsible for the formation of future dentine and dental pulp. This stage is called the cap stage. The cap-shaped covering over the dental papilla is called an enamel organ, which will produce the future tooth enamel. The outer cellular layer of the enamel organ is called the outer enamel epithelium, and the inner lining of the "cap"-like structure is called the inner enamel epithelium. The cellular region between the above two layers is called the stellate reticulum. As the enamel organ and dental papilla form, the surrounding mesenchyme condenses to form the dental sac, which later forms the cementum and periodontal ligament. As the invagination of the enamel organ continues, the developing tooth structure assumes a bell shape, and this stage is called the bell stage. The mesenchymal cells in the dental papilla, adjacent to the inner enamel epithelium, differentiate into odontoblasts, which produce and deposit predentine adjacent to the inner enamel epithelium. Predentine later calcifies to form dentine. As the dentine thickens, the odontoblasts regress towards the centre of the dental papilla, but odontoblastic processes remain embedded in the dentine. These processes are called Tomes' processes. Cells of the inner enamel epithelium near the dentine form ameloblasts. These cells produce enamel over the dentine layer to form the tooth crown. As the amount of enamel increases, the ameloblasts regress. Enamel and dentine form the crown through this process, beginning at the cusp or tip of the tooth and progressing to the future root. The inner and outer enamel epithelia come together in the cervical region of the tooth and form an epithelial fold, called the epithelial root sheath. This sheath grows into the mesenchyme and begins the formation of the root. The odontoblasts near the sheath form the dentine, continuous with that of the crown. As the dentine increases, the pulp cavity (pulp chamber) gets smaller and narrower, forming a root canal. Blood vessels and nerves enter the root. The inner cells of the dental sac form cement-forming cells called cementoblasts. Cementum is deposited over the root dentine, and it meets the enamel at the cervical region of the tooth. As teeth develop, the jaws ossify, and the outer cells of the dental sac also become active in bone formation. Each tooth root is surrounded by bone and is held in its bony socket or alveolus by the periodontal ligament.

Further Reading

Berkowitz BKB, Holland GR, Moxham BJ. Early tooth development. In: Oral anatomy, histology and embryology, 5th ed. Elsevier; 2018. pp. 350–368.

Daniel Diego J. Development of teeth. In: Essentials of oral histology and embryology—A clinical approach. 5th ed. 2019. pp. 59–74.

Kumar GS. Development and growth of teeth. In: Orban's oral histology and embryology, 14th ed. Reed Elsevier India. 2015. pp. 22–38.

Nanci A. Development of the teeth and its supporting tissues. In: TenCate's oral histology-development, structure and function, 9th ed. 2018. pp. 68–86.

Takata T, Miyauchi M, Ogawa I, Mighell A. Odontogenic pathology. In: Farah C, Balasubramaniam R, McCullough M, editors. Contemporary oral medicine. Cham: Springer; 2018. https://doi.org/10.1007/978-3-319-28100-1_22-1.

Histology of Enamel and Amelogenesis

S R Prabhu

Contents

S R Prabhu et al. (eds.), *Oral Histology and Oral Histopathology*, https://doi.org/10.1007/978-3-031-77481-2_7

7.1 Introduction

Tooth enamel, dentine, and cementum are calcified structures. Enamel covers the crown of the tooth. The enamel composed of approximately 96% inorganic apatite crystals and 4% organic material and water, and it is a highly mineralized and hardest tissue in the body. The organic component of enamel is the protein enamelin found between and on the crystals, which aids enamel permeability. This is similar to the protein keratin found in the skin.

This chapter briefly describes the physical and chemical properties and histological features of enamel and amelogenesis. The chapter on Odontogenesis (▶ Chap. 6) provides an overview of the developmental aspects of all tooth tissues.

7.2 Physical Properties

7.2.1 Colour

The colour of enamel varies from yellow to shades of grey depending on the transparency of the enamel. The more transparent the enamel, the more yellowish enamel appears, showing the colour of the underlying dentine. Conversely, the enamel may show shades of blue at the incisive edges, where dentine is absent.

7.2.2 Thickness

Enamel is thickest at the incisive edges and cusp tips. At the cervical margins, it is thin, forming a fine knife edge.

- Deciduous teeth: cusp tips and incisal edges—1.3 mm, lateral surfaces—less than 1 mm, cervical margin—feather edge.
- Permanent teeth: cusp tips and incisal edges—2.5 mm, lateral surfaces—1.3/1.5 mm, cervical margin—feather edge.

7.2.3 Density

The density of enamel decreases from the surface of the enamel to the dentinoenamel junction (DEJ) and from incisive edges to the cervical margin.

7.2.4 Hardness

The hardness of enamel is greatest at incisive margins and decreases steadily towards the cervical margins. It drops considerably at the DEJ.

7.2.5 Permeability

Enamel can act as a semi-permeable membrane for some radioactive tracers. It permits complete or partial passage of molecules like c-labelled iodine.

7.2.6 Elasticity

The enamel has a high modulus of elasticity, the average being 19×10^6 pounds per square inch. The average value for breaking stress is 11,000 pounds per square inch.

7.2.7 Refractive Index

Enamel is birefringent with a high refractive index.

7.3 Chemical Properties

7.3.1 Inorganic Content

The inorganic content of enamel is 96–97% of its weight. The remainder is formed by organic content and water. The inorganic component is calcium phosphate in the form of crystalline hydroxyapatite ($Ca_{10}(PO_4)_6(OH)_2$. The primary mineral hydroxyapatite (HA) has a typical apatite lattice structure as ($A_{10}(BO_4)_6C_2$), where A, B, and C are defined by Ca, PO_4, and OH, respectively. Pure HA contains 39.68% by weight calcium and 18% by weight phosphorus, resulting in a Ca/P mole ratio of 1.67. Other trace elements in enamel are aluminium, barium, copper, molybdenum, strontium, sulphur, and tin.

7.3.2 Organic Content

The organic matrix of enamel consists of enzymes such as serine proteases, metalloproteinases, phosphatases, and traces of other proteins. These proteins include amelogenin, proline-rich non-amelogenin, enamelin, tuftelin, and amelin. Enamel proteins consist of 1–2% of the total composition. These proteins are located mainly at the enamel rod interface. The proteins play a role in the modulation of the stress in enamel and contribute to the elastic and viscoelastic behaviour.

7.3.3 Water

Water is present in the enamel between crystals (hydroxyapatite), rods and surrounding the rods.

7.4 Histology of Mature Enamel

Enamel is difficult to study in conventional decalcified sections because of its high inorganic content. Enamel crystals dissolved during decalcification. Therefore, the best method to study enamel structure is using thin undecalcified ground sections with a light microscope utilising transmitted light (◘ Fig. 7.1). This technique is time-consuming, and details are limited by the thickness of the sections. One of the best ways to study and understand the enamel structure is by examining enamel with a scanning electron microscope (SEM). It offers a three-dimensional picture of the enamel and thus helps in its better understanding at a large magnification range (2–3× to thousands of times). The transmission electron microscopy (TEM) technique has enormous resolution and magnification capability, which provides details at the individual crystal and subcellular levels.

7.4.1 Enamel Rods

The enamel is composed of enamel prisms or rods, rod sheaths, and cementing interprismatic substances. The basic structural unit of enamel is the enamel 'rod' or prism' formed by ameloblasts during amelogenesis. Enamel rods extend from the dentinoenamel junction (DEJ) to the tooth's surface. Enamel rods appear as cylinders in cross-section, and interlocking enamel rods are deposited in an approximate keyhole shape (◘ Fig. 7.2). Each enamel rod has three parts: head (broadest part), neck, and tail. Each rod is filled with crystals. Those in the head follow the long axis of the rod, and those in the tail lie in the cross axis to the head. Each rod interdigitates with its neighbour, the head of one rod nestling against the necks of the rods to its left and right (◘ Fig. 7.3). The surface of each rod is known as the rod sheath (prism sheath), and the centre is the core. Rod sheaths contain more enamel protein than other regions. Interrod regions exist between the enamel rods and have different crystallite orientations and a higher organic content than the enamel rods. In some areas, enamel rods show an undulating course in certain areas of the cusps, where they become twisted.

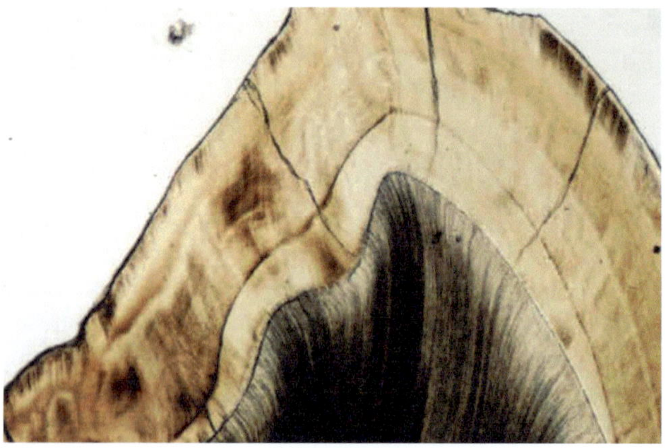

◘ **Fig. 7.1** Light microscopy. Undecalcified ground section of a tooth crown. At this magnification, the enamel appears as a structureless, yellow-brown tissue overlying dentine in which the tubule pattern is discernible. A dark line within the enamel is a prominent stria of Retzius, possibly representing a neonatal line, and is seen to encompass the coronal dentine cusp. The three dark lines extending through the enamel are cracks produced during section preparation. (Courtesy of Professor David F Wilson, Adelaide, Australia)

Enamel rods do not run horizontally from the amelodentinal junction to the anatomical enamel surface except for a zone close to the cementoenamel junction where a few layers of rods may run horizontally or even apically. At the sides of teeth, enamel rods extend from the amelodentinal junction and are orientated cuspally. In cuspal regions and incisally, enamel rods are arranged in a complex spiral-based pattern that greatly strengthens the enamel. Enamel in these regions is often referred to as gnarled enamel.

7.4.2 Incremental Lines

Two types of incremental lines in enamel are recognised. These are cross striations and the striae of Retzius. Both are described as being reflections of the incremental growth of enamel and enamel rods as enamel formation moves from the amelodentinal junction to the anatomical tooth surface. In ground sections, cross striations appear as closely apposed dark and light bands across individual enamel rods. Cross striations generally represent a daily, incremental pattern of enamel formation of about 4 microns. The striae of Retzius, also seen in ground sections, are similarly considered to be a reflection of the rhythmic pattern of enamel formation, but with a periodicity of several days (approximately one week). In ground sections, the striae of Retzius appear as dark lines of variable thickness and intensity. At the sides of the teeth, striae run from the amelodentinal junction obliquely to the anatomical enamel surface (◘ Fig. 7.4). Striae at the sides of teeth intersect the actual anatomical surface in the perikymata (◘ Fig. 7.5). In cuspal regions, the striae envelop the dentine (see ◘ Fig. 7.1). When a ground section of a tooth crown is viewed microscopically in cross-section, incremental lines appear as concentric growth rings. Deciduous and some permanent teeth in which the enamel is only partially formed before birth may, in ground sections, show an accentuated stria of Retzius due to the sudden envi-

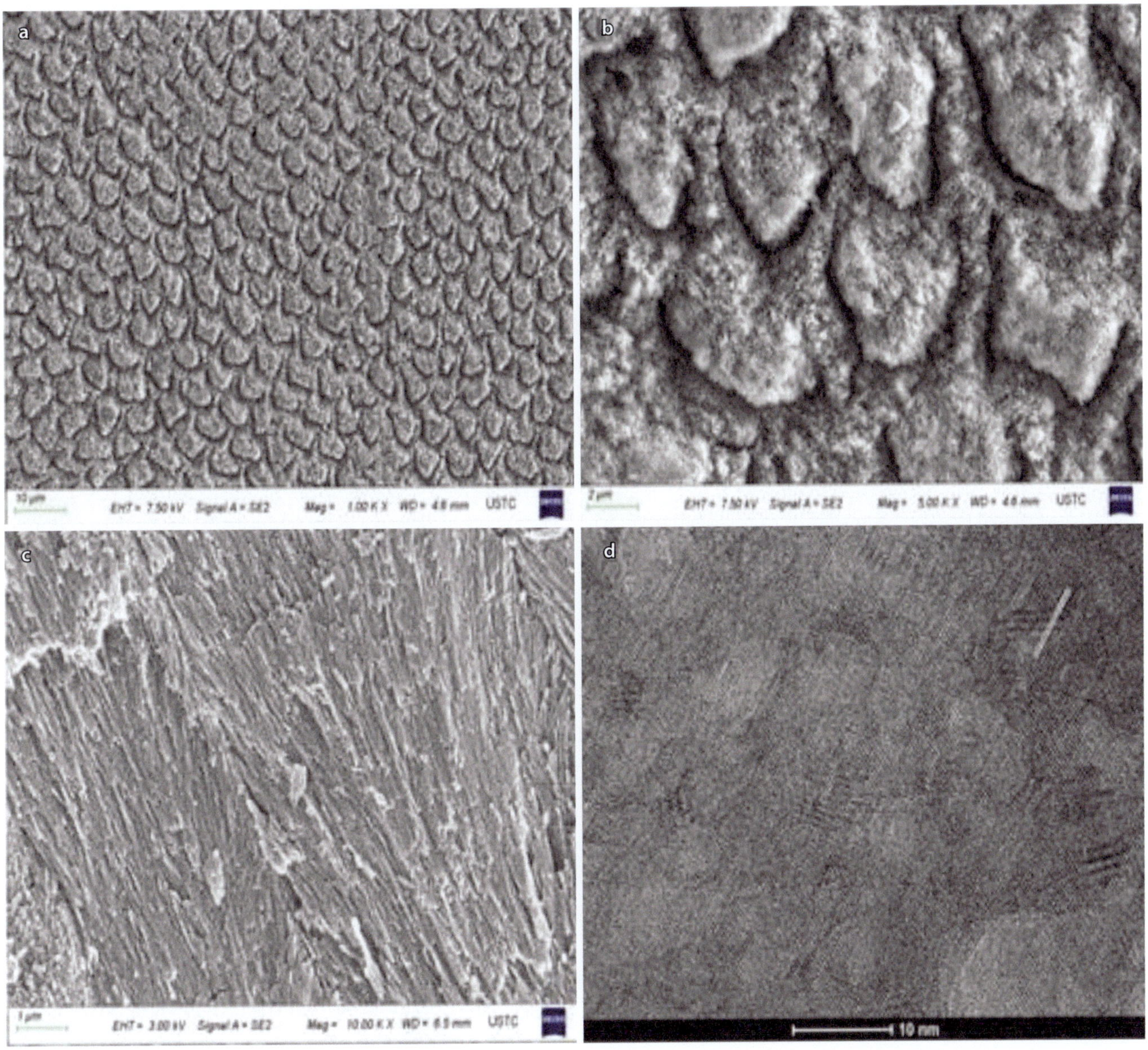

Fig. 7.2 Scanning electron microscope (SEM) micrograph of acid-etched enamel shows highly ordered crystallites assembled into enamel prisms (**a–c**). (**a**) Enamel prisms; (**b**) the magnified micrograph of (**a**); (**c**) parallelly oriented crystals assembling into prisms; (**d**) the high-resolution transmission electron micrograph (HRTEM) of enamel crystals (d-spacing = 0.093 nm). (Source: Zhang, Y. Y., Li, Q. L., & Wong, H. M. (2021). Cell-Free Biomimetic Mineralization Strategies to Regenerate the Enamel Microstructure. *Crystals* **2021**, *11*(11), 1385. ▶ https://doi.org/10.3390/cryst11111385 (MDPI Open Access))

ronmental and nutritional change at birth. This is known as the neonatal line (Fig. 7.1). The neonatal line separates prenatal enamel from postnatal enamel.

7.4.3 Hunter-Schreger Bands

A longitudinally sectioned tooth may show an alternating series of dark and light bands in the enamel in a ground section examined in reflected light (Fig. 7.6). These are called Hunter-Schreger bands. These are most easily seen on the lateral surfaces of permanent teeth and reflect the fact that enamel rods are arranged into groups of rods, which, in the inner two-thirds of the enamel, bend such that each group of rods is out of phase with its neighbours. In a ground section, this will produce the histological picture of groups of rods being sectioned in different orientations, as shown in Fig. 7.6. Hunter-Schreger bands are an optical phenomenon produced by the refraction of light due to this particular internal structure of the enamel.

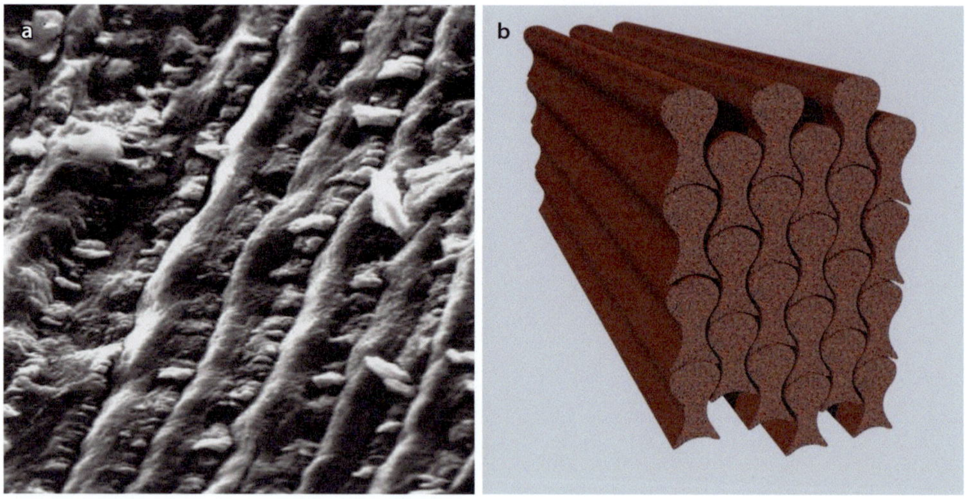

■ **Fig. 7.3** Scanning electron micrograph of artificially fractured adult enamel. Parts of several enamel rods exhibiting a rounded contour, each separated by a layer of fractured enamel material, are evident (**a**). The rounded profiles represent the 'head' region of rods while the fractured zones are the 'inter-rod' (neck-tail) components of adjacent enamel rods. Interpretation of the micrograph can be made easier by reference to the schematic 3D diagram (**b**). (Courtesy of Professor David F Wilson, Adelaide, Australia)

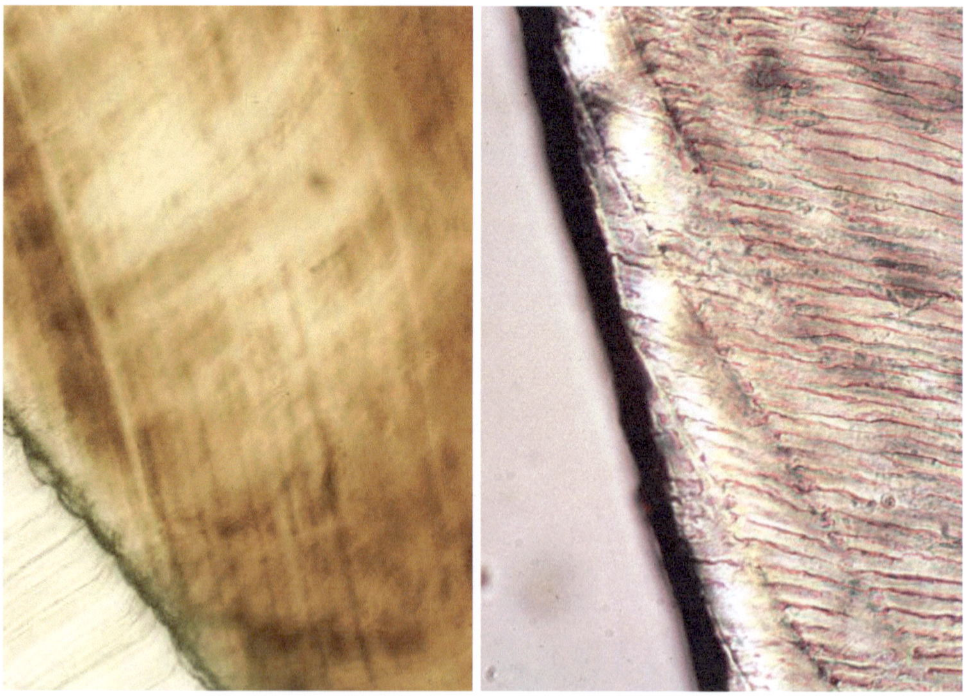

■ **Fig. 7.4** Ground sections from the side of a tooth showing variably prominent striae of Retzius in the enamel. The lines reach the enamel surface at an oblique angle at the sides of teeth (RHS), but in the coronal region, they are seen to encompass the dentine (■ Fig. 7.1). (Courtesy of Professor David F Wilson, Adelaide, Australia)

7.4.4 Enamel Lamellae

Enamel lamellae are thin, longitudinally oriented linear defects arranged radially in the enamel. They are hypomineralised structures that extend from the tooth surface, reaching a considerable distance backwards into the enamel, usually beyond the DEJ (■ Fig. 7.7). They are found more in the cervical half of the crowns and are more numerous in the interdental area than buccally or lingually.

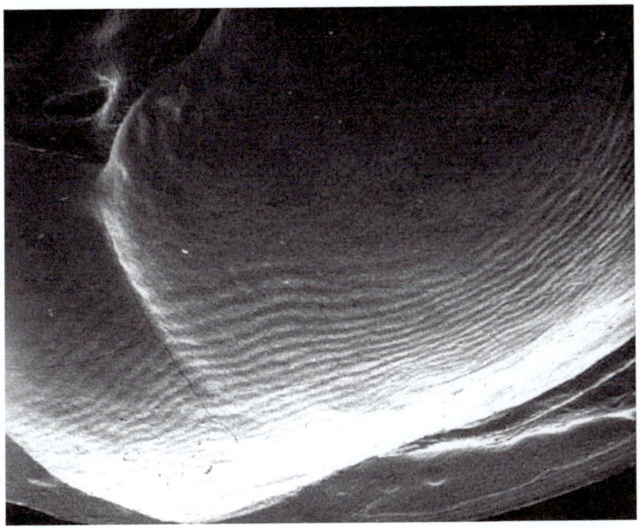

Fig. 7.5 Scanning electron micrograph of a permanent molar showing bands of perikymata at the sides of the tooth. (Courtesy of Professor David F Wilson, Adelaide, Australia)

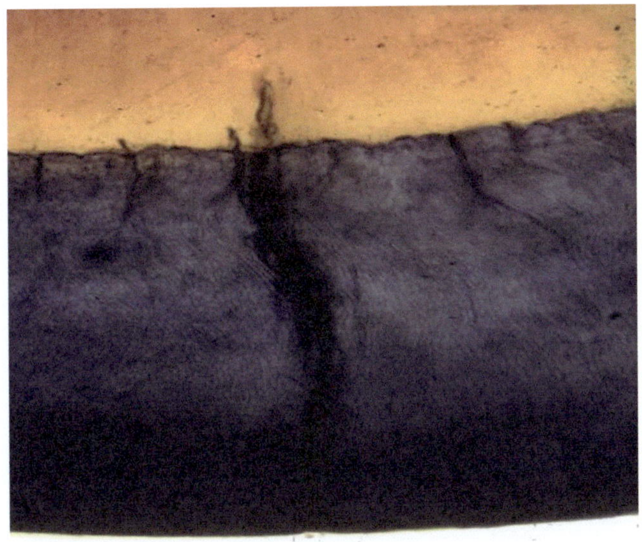

Fig. 7.7 Ground section of a tooth showing a dark lamella extending from within the dentine through the enamel to the anatomical tooth surface. (Courtesy of Professor David F Wilson, Adelaide, Australia)

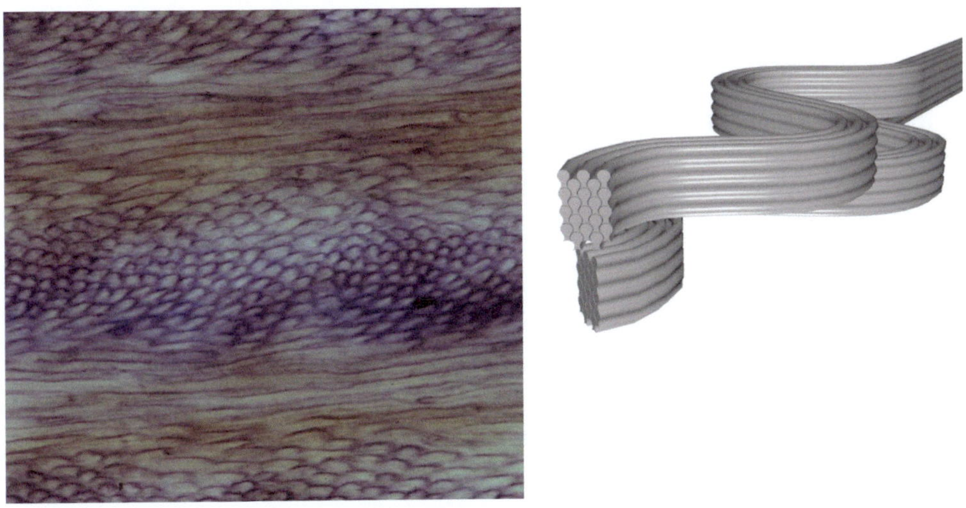

Fig. 7.6 Ground section of a permanent tooth showing Hunter-Schreger bands in the inner two-thirds of enamel where adjacent groups of rods have been cut in different orientations relative to the plain of section. Enamel rods run straight to the anatomical surface in the outer third of the enamel at the sides of teeth. The 3D schematic diagram indicates the bending of groups of enamel rods in the inner two-thirds of the enamel as they travel from the amelodentinal junction towards the enamel surface. (Courtesy of Professor David F Wilson, Adelaide, Australia)

7.4.5 Enamel Tufts

Enamel tufts are hypomineralised areas of tooth enamel which can be best viewed in transverse sections. They project from the dentinoenamel junction (DEJ) and reach a short distance in the enamel, where they appear to be branched ~~as~~ like tufts of grass (Fig. 7.7).

7.4.6 Enamel Spindles

Enamel spindles are seen at the DEJ and extend into the enamel. During the early appositional phase of odontogenesis, odontoblastic processes are situated between the cells of the inner enamel epithelium of the enamel organ before the differentiation of secretory ameloblasts. Often, they terminate as rounded or pointed

7

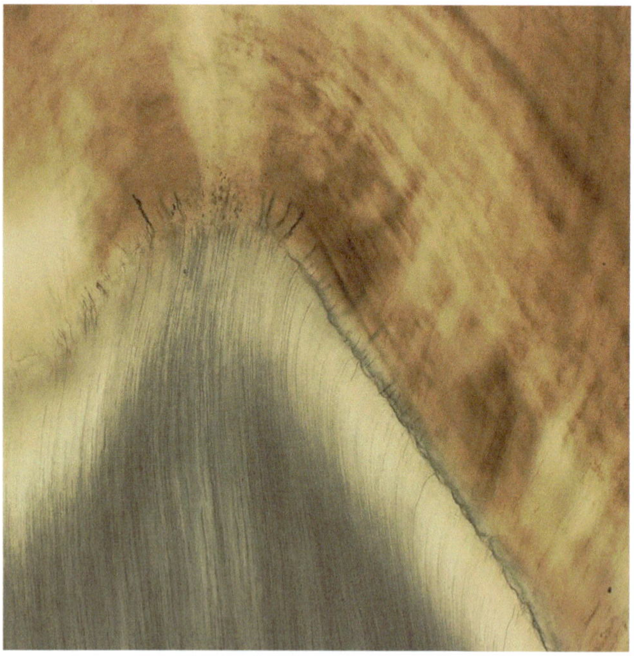

Fig. 7.8 The ground section of a tooth shows short, dark structures called spindles extending from the dentine for a short distance into the enamel. (Courtesy of Professor David F Wilson, Adelaide, Australia)

spindle-shaped processes in the enamel at the DEJ, running right angles to the dentine surface (Fig. 7.8). Enamel spindles appear dark under transmitted light. These living odontoblastic processes possibly contribute to sensitivity at the DEJ.

7.4.7 Amelodentinal Junction (Dentinoenamel Junction)

In the ground sections of the tooth, the amelodentinal junction (ADJ) (also known as dentinoenamel junction—DEJ) appears as a scalloped line. The DEJ is a complex structure that unites two dissimilar calcified tissues and prevents the development of cracks from enamel into the dentine. The DEJ is scalloped with convexities directed towards the dentin and concavities towards the enamel. The arrangement of ameloblasts during amelogenesis is responsible for the concave (pitted) appearance of the ADJ. The irregular shape of the ADJ strengthens the adhesion between the enamel and dentine.

7.4.8 Gnarled Enamel

Enamel forming the cusp of a tooth is characterised by twisting, intertwining groups of enamel rods (Fig. 7.9) called gnarled enamel. Gnarled enamel resists shearing forces.

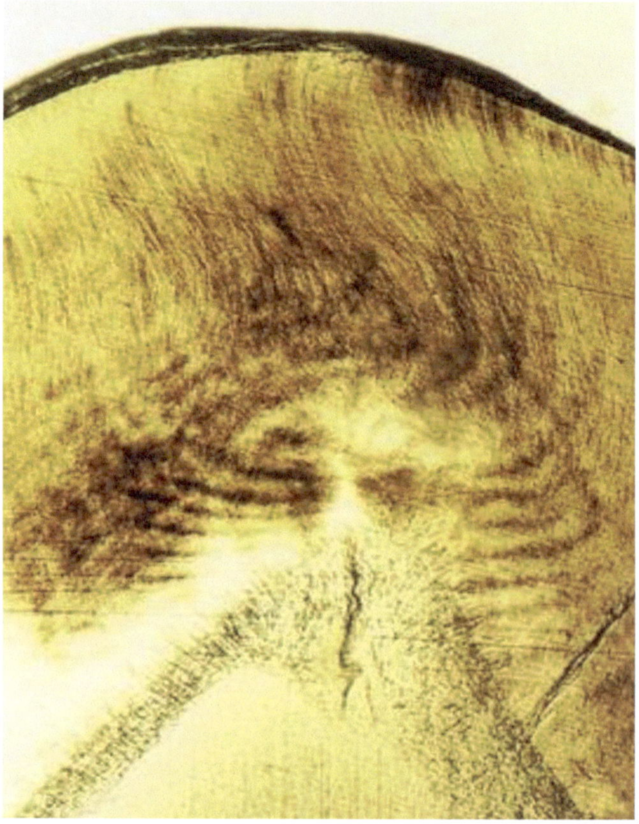

Fig. 7.9 Gnarled enamel showing twisted intertwining groups of enamel rods. (Courtesy of Dr. Cao Xuan Cu. Source: clinicalpub@gmail.com. Pocket Dentistry)

7.4.9 Surface Enamel and Primary Enamel Cuticle (Nasmyth's Membrane)

The surface layer of enamel is harder and less soluble and contains five to ten times more fluoride than the subsurface enamel. The enamel cuticle, a delicate membrane called Nasmyth's membrane, or primary enamel cuticle, covers the entire crown of newly erupted teeth. Forces of mastication soon remove this cuticle. The cuticle is the secretory product of ameloblasts when enamel formation is completed. At the anatomical surface, a very thin, prismless enamel zone occurs on all deciduous teeth and 70% of permanent teeth. This is common on the lateral and cervical areas of enamel. The prismless (rodless) enamel at the sides of teeth in permanent teeth is associated with perikymata (Fig. 7.10). This area is more heavily mineralised than the rest of the enamel.

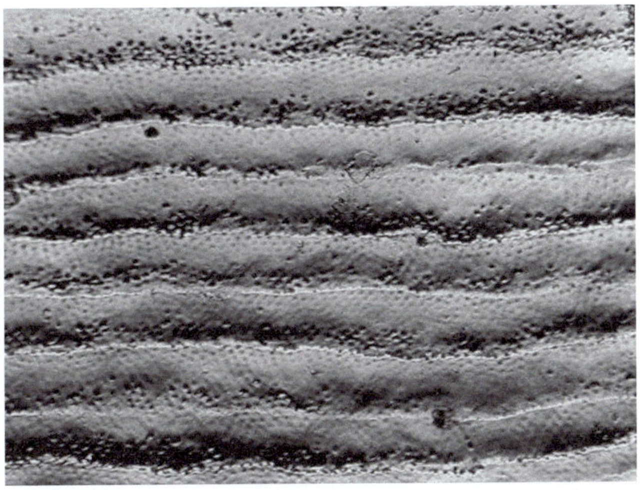

Fig. 7.10 Pale zones of prismless (rodless) enamel devoid of Tome's process impressions separated by zones where enamel rods reach the anatomical surface in the perikymata. (Courtesy of Professor David F Wilson, Adelaide, Australia)

7.5 Age Changes in Enamel

Loss of enamel on the occlusal surfaces due to wear (attrition) is a prominent age-related change in the structure of enamel. Another notable age-related change is a marked decrease in the permeability of enamel. Change in the colour of teeth is a common feature in aged individuals. Teeth become darker, which may be associated with the changes in the underlying dentine seen through progressively thinning layers of translucent enamel.

7.6 Histology of Amelogenesis

The tooth enamel is fully formed before the eruption of the tooth. Enamel is produced by cells derived from the ectoderm. Amelogenesis starts at the bell stage of tooth development (see ▶ Chap. 6). At this stage, ectodermal cells invaginate to produce two layers of simple cuboidal cells called the Inner Enamel Epithelium (IEE) and Outer Enamel Epithelium (OEE). The borderline between the IEE and the underlying connective tissue of the dental papilla subsequently becomes the dentine-enamel junction (DEJ). Other epithelial cells between the IEE and OEE include the stratum intermedium and stellate reticulum cells. These four groups of cells collectively form the enamel organ. Ameloblasts are responsible for laying down enamel matrix. Their differentiation from preameloblasts (whose origin is from inner enamel epithelium) is the result of signalling from the ectomesenchymal cells of the dental papilla. At the free end of the enamel organ, the IEE and OEE layers are continuous to form a cervical loop.

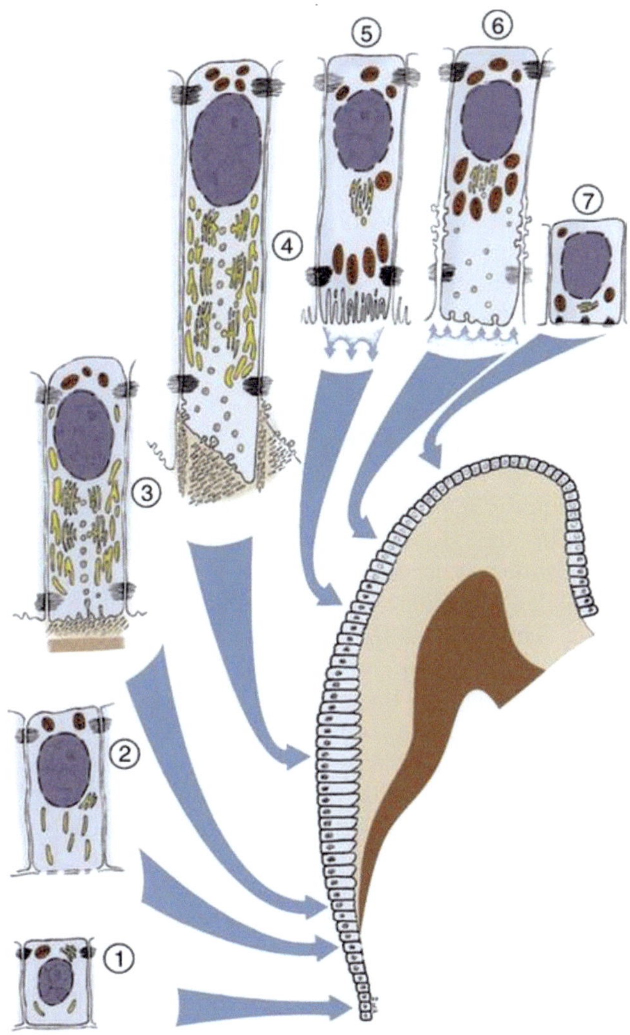

Fig. 7.11 Schematic representation of the various functional stages in the life cycle of ameloblasts as would occur in a human tooth. (1) Morphogenetic stage; (2) histodifferentiation stage; (3) initial secretory stage (no Tomes' process); (4) secretory stage (Tomes' process); (5) ruffle-ended ameloblast of the maturative stage; (6) smooth-ended ameloblast of the maturative stage; (7) protective stage. (Source: Pocket Dentistry. 7: Enamel: Composition, Formation, and Structure. Courtesy of Dr. Cao Xun Cu. Clinicalpub@gmil.com. Pocket Dentistry)

The enamel organ cells undergo numerous morphological changes at the beginning, during, and at the end of the maturation stage of amelogenesis. Amelogenesis is generally subdivided into several functional phases. The IEE cells undergo six functional stages in their lifespan. These are (1) morphogenic, (2) organising, (3) formative, (4) maturative, (5) protective, and (6) desmolytic (Fig. 7.11).

7.6.1 Morphogenic Stage

This stage determines the DEJ and tooth crown shapes. The enamel organ grows around a cluster of neural crest-derived mesenchymal cells (dental papilla), with a basement membrane separating the two. The adjacent pulpal layer is a cell-free zone containing cytoplasmic processes of the superficial cells of the dental pulp. Soon, the basement membrane disappears, and hemidesmosome attachments are lost, allowing IEE cells (preameloblasts) more mobility.

7.6.2 Organising Stage

This stage is characterised by the changes in the appearance of the IEE cells due to their differentiation. Differentiation occurs when the cuboidal IEE cells next to the dental papillae elongate and become columnar in shape. The nuclei of IEE cells move to the apical side of the cell (polarisation), while organelles needed for secretion accumulate on the basal side. These are considered preameloblasts. The cell-free zone between the IEE and the dental papilla disappears, resulting in epithelial cells coming into close contact with the dental papilla cells, which differentiate into dentine-forming cells (odontoblasts). During the final stages of the organising stage, dentine formation (dentinogenesis) begins. The appearance of the first dentine layer (predentine) formed by odontoblasts is essential for enamel formation. This occurs first at the cusp tips and progresses to the cervical regions of a tooth. Differentiation from preameloblasts (originating from the inner enamel epithelium) to ameloblasts is the result of signalling from the ectomesenchymal cells of the dental papilla. Initially, the preameloblasts will differentiate into presecretory ameloblasts and then into secretory ameloblasts, which lay down the tooth enamel. In this stage, the ameloblasts become longer; the nucleus migrates towards the proximal end and the Golgi apparatus and centrioles migrate towards the distal end. This change is referred to as the 'Reversal of Polarity'. At this stage, the nutrition for the ameloblasts is cut off from the dental papilla and is now derived from the capillaries of the dental sac (dental follicle). This nutritional source change is called the 'reversal of nutrition'.

7.6.3 Formative Stage

The first dentin (predentin) layer forms before ameloblasts enter their formative stage. Predentin is composed primarily of collagen but also contains non-collagenous proteins. During the enamel matrix formation, ameloblasts do not change the length and arrangements seen in the organising stage.

7.6.4 Maturative Stage

After the thickness of the enamel matrix has been formed in the occlusal or incisal area, enamel maturation (mineralisation) occurs. The ameloblasts are slightly smaller during enamel maturation and closely attached to the enamel matrix. The stratum intermedium cells lose their cuboidal shape and assume a spindle shape. Ameloblasts show cytoplasmic vacuoles containing material resembling an enamel matrix.

7.6.5 Protective Stage

When the enamel has been fully formed and calcified, the outer enamel epithelium and nonfunctional ameloblast layer cells fuse to form a stratified layer of cells called reduced enamel epithelium (REE). This layer covers the enamel of the crown of the tooth. Its function is to protect the enamel from contacting the connective tissues of the surrounding dental sac and prevent cementum formation until the tooth erupts.

7.6.6 Desmolytic Stage

The reduced enamel epithelium (REE) induces atrophy of the connective tissue, separating it from the oral epithelium and leading to tooth eruption. REE releases proteolytic enzymes, which cause the breakdown of collagen fibres. As the tooth approaches oral epithelium, both epithelium and REE proliferate and fuse with each other, forming an epithelial plug. This eventually degenerates to form a pathway for eruption.

7.7 Summary

Dental enamel is the hardest and most mineralised tissue, composed of approximately 96% inorganic apatite crystals and 4% organic material and water. About 96% of the enamel is calcium, phosphate, and water (as OH) of a form known as hydroxyapatite ($Ca_{10}(PO_4)_6.2OH$). The basic unit of enamel is called an enamel rod (enamel prism). This develops from a protein matrix in which amelogenin is the predominant component. The enamel matrix proteins are eventually and completely degraded and removed by proteinases to form mineral-enriched tooth enamel. Other microscopic enamel structures consist of incremental lines (Hunter-Schreger bands), enamel tufts, spindles, lamellae, and gnarled enamel. The process of enamel formation is referred to as amelogenesis. Enamel development is regulated by cells of the enamel organ called ameloblasts. These heavily polarised cells lay down a proteinaceous matrix that serves as a template for crystal growth. Enamel matrix proteins are secreted by ameloblasts into the enamel space and are later degraded and proteolytically removed, also by ameloblasts. Amelogenesis is considered to have three stages. The first stage is known as the presecretory stage (inductive stage), the second is the secretory stage, and the third is known as the maturation stage. Ameloblast differentiation from inner enamel epithelium (IEE) is initiated during the inductive stage. Proteins and an organic matrix form a partially mineralised enamel in the secretory stage. The maturation stage completes enamel mineralisation.

Further Reading

Berkovitz BKB, Holland GR, Moxam BJ. Enamel. In: Berkovitz BKB, Holland GR, Moxam BJ, editors. Oral anatomy histology and embryology. 5th ed. Edinburgh: Elsevier; 2018. p. 123–43.

Desai D. Chapter 4. Enamel. In: Kumar GS, editor. Orban's oral histology and embryology, 14th ed. Elsevier. pp. 40–71.

Diekwisch TG, Berman BJ, Anderton X, et al. Membranes, minerals, and proteins of developing vertebrae enamel. Microsc Res Tech. 2002;59(5):373–95.

Farci F, Soni A. Histology, tooth. [Updated 2022 Jul 4]. In: StatPearls [Internet]. Treasure Island: StatPearls Publishing; 2023. https://www.ncbi.nlm.nih.gov/books/NBK572055/.

Nanci A. Chapter 7. Enamel: composition, formation, and structure. In: TenCate's oral histology. 9th ed. St. Louis: Elsevier; 2018. p. 118–56.

Rao N. Histology of enamel. In: Prabhu SR, editor. Textbook of oral and maxillofacial anatomy and embryology. Oxford: Oxford University Press; 2006. p. 198–206.

Histology of Dentine and Dentinogenesis

Sandhya Tamgadge and Avinash Tamgadge

Contents

S R Prabhu et al. (eds.), *Oral Histology and Oral Histopathology*, https://doi.org/10.1007/978-3-031-77481-2_8

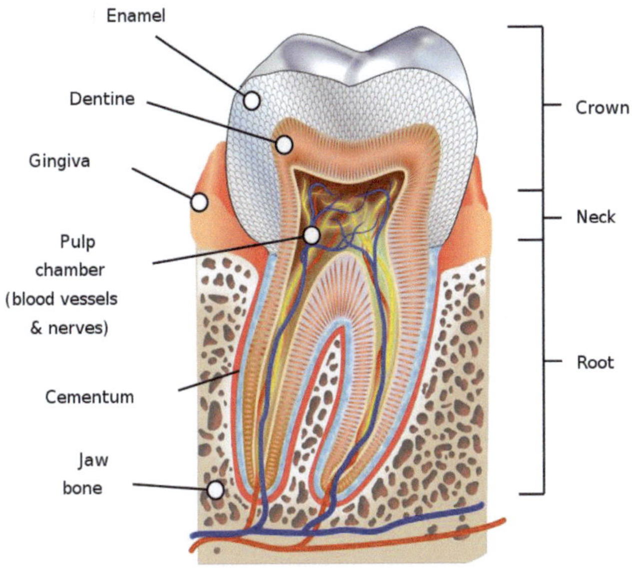

Fig. 8.1 Diagram of a human molar showing the enamel, dentine, cementum, pulp, and the surrounding tissues. (Source: "Human tooth diagram-en. svg from Wikimedia Commons by K. D. Schroeder, CC-BY-SA 4.0"CC BY-SA 4.0)

8.1 Introduction

Dentine is the mineralised and highly sensitive tissue that constitutes the major bulk of the tooth. Dentine is present as an enclosed cylindrical wall around the central core of soft pulp tissue. Dentine is present in the crown and the root and opens at the root tip through a single foramen at the apex and, sometimes, through accessory canals. Dentine is deposited by specialised cells called odontoblasts. They cover the entire pulpal surface of the dentinal wall (Fig. 8.1).

8.2 Physical Properties of Dentine

- Dentine is yellowish in contrast to the enamel. It is less hard than enamel but slightly stronger than bone or cementum.
- Dentine is more radiolucent than enamel. It is resilient, and this allows it to bear masticatory forces without damaging the brittle overlying enamel.

8.3 Chemical Properties

- Dentine is a collagen-based mineralised tissue consisting of inorganic apatite crystallites embedded in an organic extracellular matrix.
- The inorganic portion comprises 70% mineralised components (calcium hydroxyapatite crystals), 20% organic components, and 10% water by weight (50% inorganic, 30% organic, and 20% water by volume).
- Dentine is less mineralised than enamel but more mineralised than bone or cementum.

8.3.1 Inorganic Component

- Calcium hydroxyapatite crystals in dentine are smaller in size as compared to enamel.
- The major inorganic components of dentine include calcium, phosphorus, carbonate, sodium, and magnesium.
- The crystallites also contain trace elements, including fluoride.

8.3.2 Organic Matrix

- The organic matrix of dentine comprises collagenous and non-collagenous proteins. The collagenous matrix comprises 90% of collagen, mainly type 1 and small amounts of types 3 and 5 collagens. A few other non-collagenous matrix proteins and lipids are also found in the organic matrix.
- Non-collagenous components include proteoglycans (such as decorin, biglycan, fibromodulin, lumican, osteoadherin, and versican), several glycoproteins such as osteocalcin, osteonectin, and the small integrin-binding ligand N-linked glycoprotein (SIBLING) proteins (i.e. osteopontin, bone sialoprotein, dentine matrix protein 1, dentine sialophosphoprotein, and matrix extracellular phosphoglycoprotein), and some serum proteins.
- Small amounts of several growth factors (insulin growth factor 2 [IGF-2], bone morphogenetic protein 2 [BMP-2], and transforming growth factor [TGF]-beta) are also identified in dentine.
- The organic component of the dentine matrix also contains small amounts of enzymes such as collagenase (MMP-1) and tissue metalloproteinases (TMPs).
- The nature of the dentine organic matrix components results in greater compressive strength, higher tensile strength, and higher flexural strength than enamel.

8.4 Histology of Dentine

Dentine can be examined by optical microscopy (undecalcified and decalcified sections), transmission electron microscopy (TEM), and scanning electron microscopy (SEM).

- Dentine is a dense calcified tissue that constitutes the major bulk of the tooth. It is avascular and highly sensitive.
- The dentine matrix is secreted by specialised cells called odontoblasts. Cell bodies are within the pulp, but their processes extend within the dentinal tubules.

8.4.1 Dentinal Tubules

- Dentinal tubules are cylindrical canals running from the pulp to the dentinoenamel junction (DEJ) in the crown and the cemento-dentinal junction (CEJ) in the root.
- All tubules are arranged circumferentially and radially around the pulp chamber, perpendicular to the tooth's longitudinal axis.
- Anatomical variations of both the number and size of dentinal tubules from the crown to the apex of the root canal exist. For example, the number of tubules near the pulpal surface of the dentine varies between 50,000 and 60,000/mm^2. The ratio between the number of tubules per unit area on the pulpal and outer surfaces of the dentine is about 4:1.
- The dentinal tubules follow a gently curved path with a slight 'S' (sigmoid course) in shape (Fig. 8.2a and b) as tubules are slightly longer than the dentine thickness. These curvatures, called primary curvatures, begin at the pulpal surface. The first convexity is directed towards the apex of the tooth. Tubules are straighter in the incisal ridges, cusps, and root areas. Branches of the dentinal tubules near the outer surface are referred to as terminal branches. These are Y-shaped (Fig. 8.3a). Regular secondary curvatures are also present throughout the entire length of the tubules.
- The dentinal tubules display a tapered lumen of 1 µm in diameter in the mid-portion of dentine, reaching a diameter of 2.5 µm near the pulp.
- The tubules have lateral branches (Fig. 8.4), called canaliculi or microtubules, which originate more or less at right angles along their circumference.
- The dentinoenamel junction (DEJ), also known as the amelodentinal junction (ADJ), is a scalloped structure with convexities towards dentine and concavities towards enamel (Fig. 8.4). Scalloped structures of the DEJ contain micro-scallops and collagen type 1 fibrils. The DEJ is less mineralised than either enamel or the primary dentine.
- A few odontoblastic processes cross the dentinoenamel junction and enter the enamel for a few millimetres. These are known as enamel spindles (Fig. 8.4).

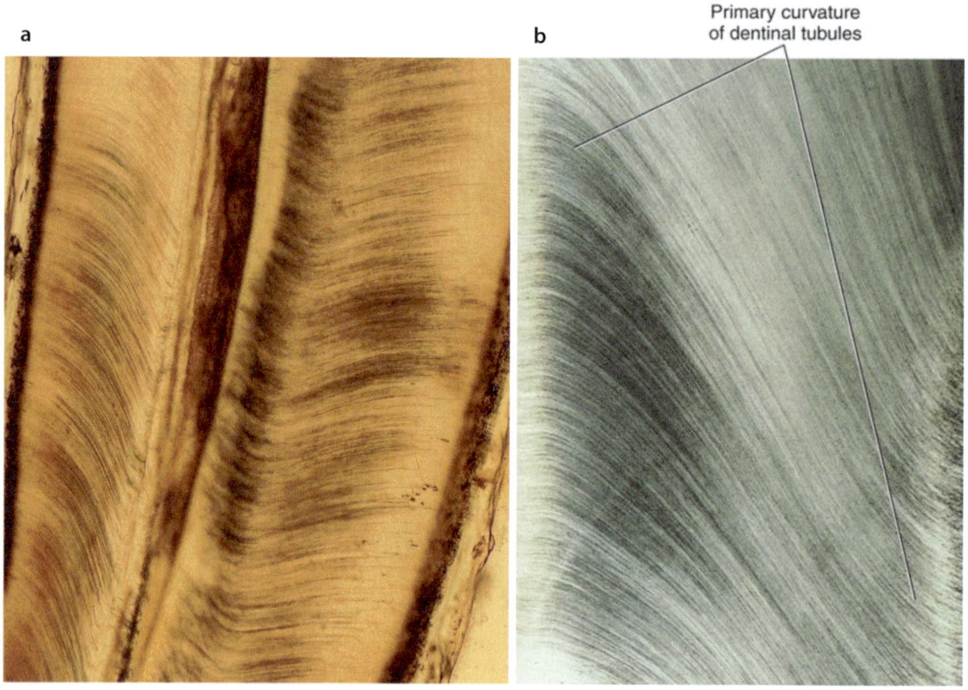

Fig. 8.2 (**a** and **b**) Dentinal tubules. The undecalcified (ground) section of dentine shows dentinal tubules with gentle 'S'-shaped primary curvature. (Image B. Source: Chapter 13. Dentine and Pulp. Pocket Dentistry. Courtesy of James McIntosh, PhD, Assistant Professor Emeritus, Department of Biomedical Sciences, Baylor College of Dentistry, Dallas, TX)

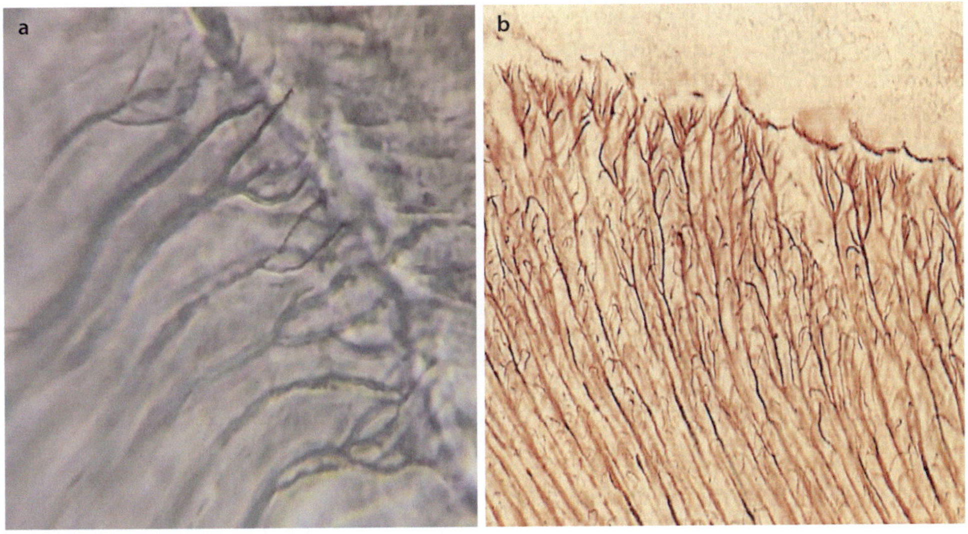

Fig. 8.3 (**a** and **b**) Dentinal tubules. Y-shaped terminal branches (**a**) and lateral branching of dentinal tubules close to the dentinoenamel junction (**b**). (Image Source: Berkovitz BKB, Holland GR, Moxham BJ: Oral anatomy, histology, and embryology, ed 4, Edinburgh, 2010, Mosby.) Ground section showing dentinal tubules and their lateral branching close to the dentinoenamel junction (DEJ) (Courtesy of Professor David F Wilson, Adelaide, Australia)

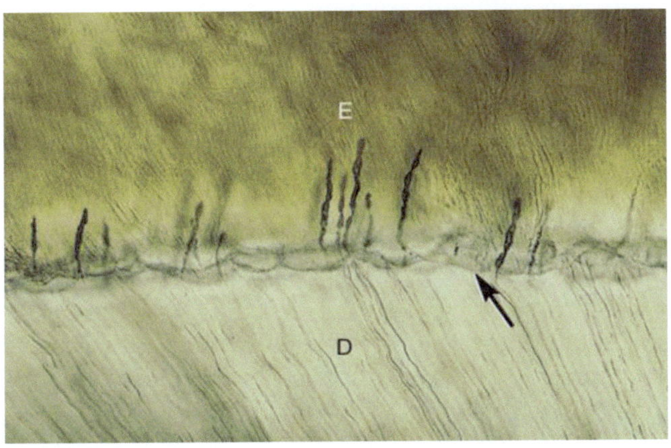

Fig. 8.4 Dentinoenamel junction (DEJ), enamel, and dentine. (Source: Pocket Dentistry. Chapter 1. Lee W. Boushell and John R. Sturdevant.) Microscopic view of scalloped dentinoenamel junction (DEJ) (arrow). E is enamel and D is dentine. (From Bath Balogh M, Fehrenbach MJ: Illustrated dental embryology, histology, and anatomy, ed 3, Saunders, 2011, St. Louis. Courtesy James McIntosh, PhD, Assistant Professor Emeritus, Department of Biomedical Sciences, Baylor College of Dentistry, Dallas, TX)

8.4.2 Contents of Dentinal Tubules

8.4.2.1 Odontoblast Processes

Odontoblast processes (also called Tomes' fibres) are extensions of odontoblasts.

- The odontoblast processes contain vesicles, microtubules, and intermediate filaments.
- The main organelles associated with protein synthesis (e.g. rough endoplasmic reticulum Golgi material) are present in the odontoblast cell body but do not extend into the process.
- A thin, proteinaceous membrane (lamina limitans) is located lining the wall of the dentinal tubule, which consists mostly of glycosaminoglycans (GAGs).

8.4.2.2 Dentinal Fluid

Dentinal tubules are filled with dentinal fluid.

- The fluid content of the dentine tubules varies by depth, with superficial dentine containing the lowest fluid content and dentine closest to the pulp containing more fluid.
- Dentinal fluid has a similar composition as plasma or interstitial fluid.
- Fluid from terminal pulpal blood vessels flow through the fenestrations in the vessels.
- Once this fluid leaves the capillary, it penetrates through the odontoblast and, then, the predentine layer, where it may be combined with the secretory products of the odontoblast.
- The increased pulpal pressure of dentinal fluid tends to clean the tubule and hinder bacteria from entering the pulp.

8.4.2.3 Sensory Nerve Terminals

Sensory nerve axons may be seen adjacent to the odontoblast processes. Nerve receptors play an important role in dentine sensitivity.

- Sensory nerve terminals are limited mainly to the dentine of the crown beneath the cusps, where they may be found in 50–80% of the tubules and project up to 200 μm from the pulp.

- Few tubules are innervated in the mid-coronal dentinal regions, and fewer than 5% are innervated in the cervical and root dentine.
- The axon is narrower than the odontoblast process and often contains mitochondria.
- No specialised contact exists between the nerve and the odontoblast process.

8.5 Predentine

Predentine is the newly formed dentine before calcification and maturation. It is the innermost layer of dentine located adjacent to the pulp.

- Predentine is usually thicker, where active dentinogenesis occurs. Its presence is necessary for maintaining the integrity of the dentine.
- Predentine contains types 1, 3, and 5 collagens.
- Predentine can be easily identified as a band of dentine's newly formed organic matrix in decalcified sections (◘ Fig. 8.5). It gradually converts into mineralised dentine as various non-collagenous matrix proteins are incorporated at the mineralisation front.
- Predentine can be 10–40 μm in width, depending on its rate of deposition. The thickness of predentine remains constant because the amount that calcifies is replaced by adding a new unmineralised matrix.

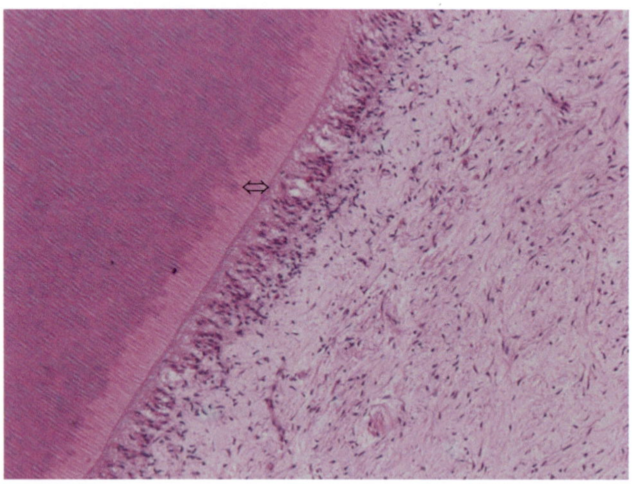

◘ **Fig. 8.5** Dentine (decalcified section stained with H&E). Pale hypo-calcified area in the dentine is predentine (two-way arrow). Primary dentine is the bulk of dentine (blue arrowhead) (Courtesy of Professor David F Wilson, Adelaide, Australia)

8.6 Primary Dentine (Circumpulpal Dentine)

The bulk of the dentine that surrounds the pulp is primary dentine (◘ Fig. 8.5), which is also known as circumpulpal dentine.

- Primary dentine is formed before tooth eruption during tooth development.
- Primary dentine may be 6–8 mm thick in the crown and a little thinner in the roots.
- The outer layer of the primary dentine that is closest to the enamel is known as the mantle dentine.
- Primary dentine is formed by the newly differentiated odontoblasts.
- Primary dentine includes intertubular and peritubular dentine (see later).

8.7 Secondary Dentine

Secondary dentine forms after the completion of root formation and tooth eruption.

- When contacts between antagonistic cusps are established, the formation of secondary dentine starts and continues throughout life. This is also known as reactive dentine.
- Secondary dentine represents a much slower deposition.
- The continuous formation of secondary dentine leads to an uneven reduction in pulp chamber dimensions.
- Apart from the decreasing number of dentinal tubules, there is no structural or chemical difference between primary and secondary dentine.
- The histological differentiation between secondary and primary dentine is based on a shift in tubule direction between the two layers (◘ Fig. 8.6).

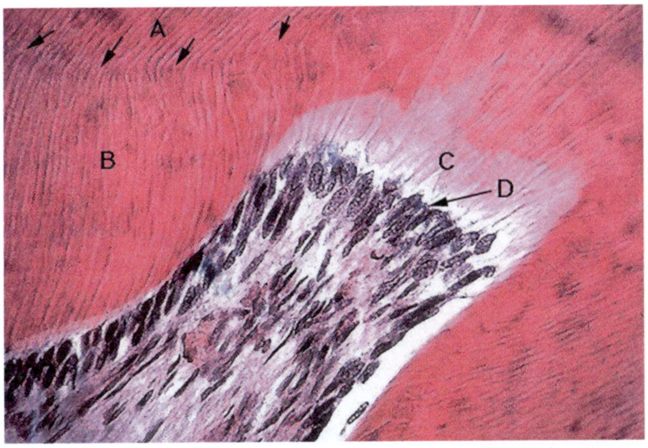

Fig. 8.6 The decalcified section of a tooth stained with H&E shows primary dentine (**A**), secondary dentine (**B**), predentine space (**C**), and odontoblasts (**D**). The boundary between primary dentine and secondary dentine is also evident (arrows). (Source: University of Kentucky Digital Lab. ► https://www.uky.edu/~brmacp/oralhist/module5/lab/imgshtml/image32.htm)

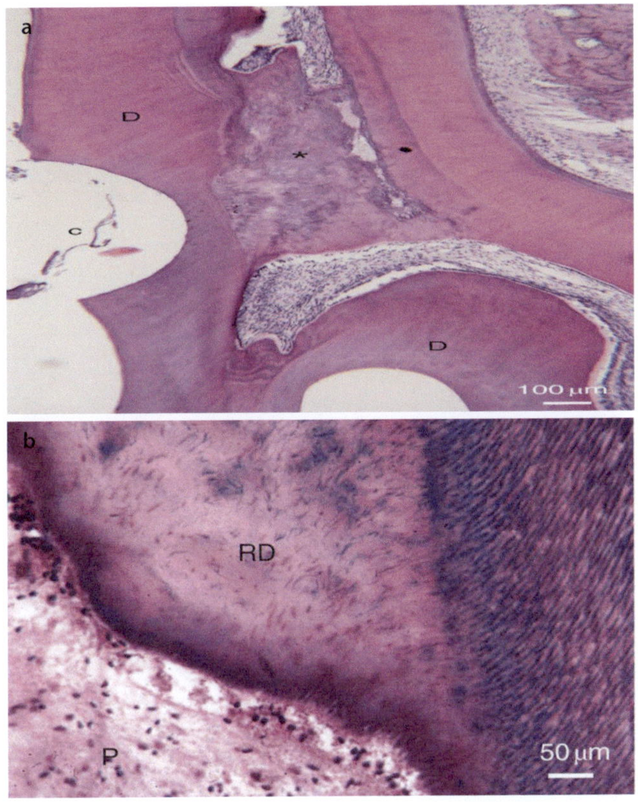

Fig. 8.7 (Figure a) Ninety days after a pulp exposure and filling of the cavity with a dental cement, reparative dentine (*) partially occludes the exposed mesial root pulp. Dentine (D). (Figure b) Reactionary osteodentine (RD), stains as a pink/violet structure. Pulp, (P). (*Source:* Pocket Dentistry Chapter 5. Dentine, Pulp and Tooth pain). Michel Goldberg. Biomédicale des Saints Pères, Université Paris Descartes, INSERM UMR-S 1124. With a contribution by Bradley K. Formaker, Ph.D., University of Connecticut School of Dental Medicine, Farmington, CT)

8.8 Tertiary Dentine (Reactionary/Reparative Dentine)

Tertiary dentine (or reactionary/reparative dentine) forms in response to various stimuli, such as attrition, caries, or a dental procedure.

- Unlike primary or secondary dentine, which is formed by all odontoblasts along the entire pulp–dentine border, tertiary dentine is produced only by odontoblasts directly subjected to the stimulus.
- The architecture and amount of tertiary dentine depend on the strength and duration of the stimulus.

Tertiary dentine is subdivided into reactionary or reparative dentine.

8.8.1 Reactionary Dentine

The reactionary dentine is deposited by pre-existing odontoblasts in situations where odontoblasts become hyper-plastic and deposit excess dentinal tissue in response to an external stimulus. This is a protective mechanism.

8.8.2 Reparative Dentine

When the stimuli are more significant and if the odontoblasts have been disrupted, dentine is formed by newly differentiated odontoblast-like cells. This is called 'reparative dentine' (Fig. 8.7a). Reparative dentine may have tubules continuous with those of the secondary dentine but are scant and irregularly formed.

8.8.3 Osteodentine

The rapidly formed tertiary dentine sometimes contains entrapped odontoblasts and few tubules, thereby significantly resembling bone. This is called osteodentine (Fig. 8.7b).

8.9 Sclerotic Dentine

Sclerotic dentine (physiologic sclerotic dentine and translucent dentine) is characterised by the accumulation of mineral deposits within the lumen of the dentinal tubules.

- When mineral deposits affect several adjacent tubules together, the dentine becomes glassy in appearance and becomes translucent (Fig. 8.8).

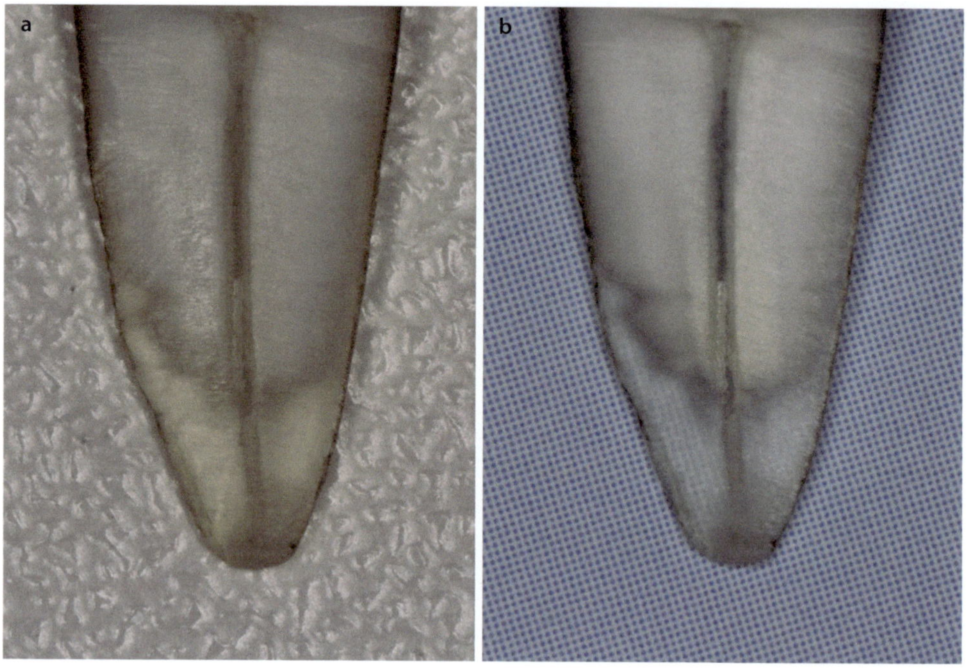

Fig. 8.8 (**a** and **b**) The distribution of physiologic sclerotic dentine on the vertical root section (serrated line). (Source: F. Kabartai, T. Hoffmann, C. Hannig. The physiologic sclerotic dentine: A literature-based hypothesis. Medical Hypotheses. Volume 85, Issue 6, December 2015, Pages 887-890). PMID: 26404871. ▶ https://doi.org/10.1016/j.mehy.2015.09.016. With permission from Elsevier)

- Sclerotic dentine is located more at the mesial and distal areas of the roots than at the buccal or lingual areas.
- The sclerotic root dentine increases with age, proceeding from the apex towards the crown.

8.10 Mantle Dentine

Mantle dentine is a variant of primary dentine. It is so named because it forms a layer or mantle over the rest of the dentine, representing the first deposition of dentine.

- Mantle dentine interdigitates with enamel at the scalloped dentinoenamel junction peripherally and extends centrally towards the pulp in the zone of interglobular dentine (Fig. 8.9).
- The mantle dentine layer width varies between 20 and 150 μm.
- Mantle dentine comprises large collagen fibres, some of which are 0.1–0.2 μm in diameter, in contrast to the primary dentinal–collagen matrix, which is 50–200 nanometres (nm).
- Mantle dentine is slightly less mineralised and contains fewer defects than circumpulpal dentine.

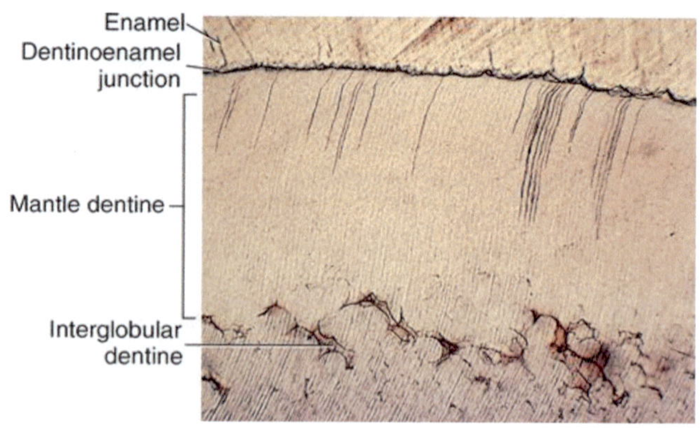

Fig. 8.9 The undecalcified (ground) section of dentine shows mantle dentine occupying the area bounded by dentinoenamel junction above and interglobular dentine below. (Pocket dentistry. Chapter 8. Dentine. With permission)

8.11 Intertubular Dentine (ITD)

Intertubular dentine (ITD) composed of calcified matrix dispersed between the dentine tubules (◘ Fig. 8.10). Type 1 collagen (50–200 nm in diameter) is the major protein of intertubular dentine.

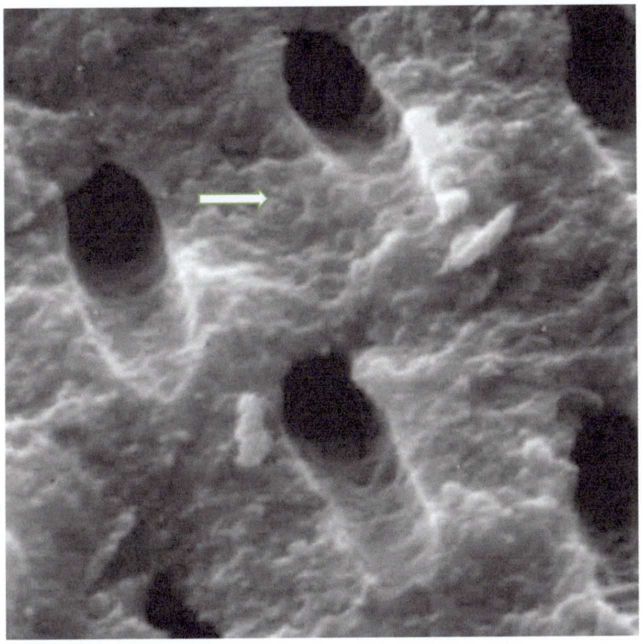

◘ **Fig. 8.10** Intertubular dentine. In cross section, dentinal tubules are approximately round in shape. The calcified matrix between tubules is referred to as the intertubular dentine (white arrow) (Courtesy of Professor David F Wilson, Adelaide, Australia)

8.12 Peritubular Dentine (PTD)

The dentine that encircles dentinal tubules is peritubular dentine (◘ Fig. 8.11). Peritubular dentine is highly mineralised and usually devoid of collagen fibrils.

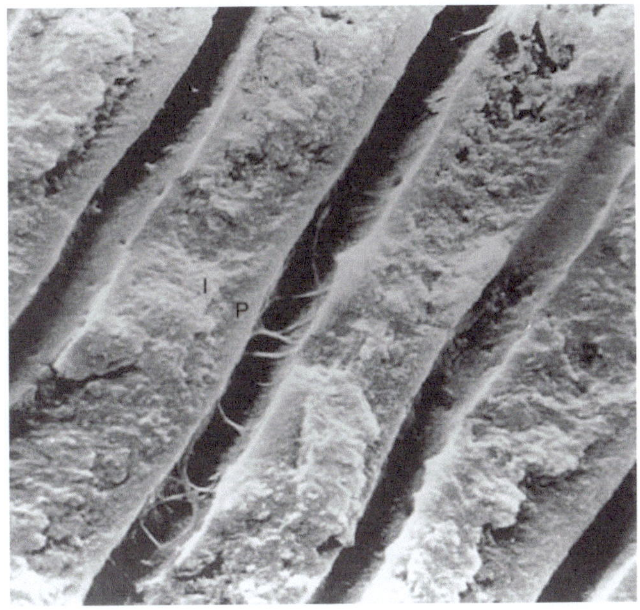

◘ **Fig. 8.11** Peritubular dentine (P) is more mineralised than intertubular dentine (I). (From Brännström M: Dentine and pulp in restorative dentistry, London, 1982, Wolfe Medical.) Source: Lee W. Boushell and John R. Sturdevant. Chapter 1. Clinical Significance of Dental Anatomy, Histology, Physiology, and Occlusion. Pocket Dentistry: with permission)

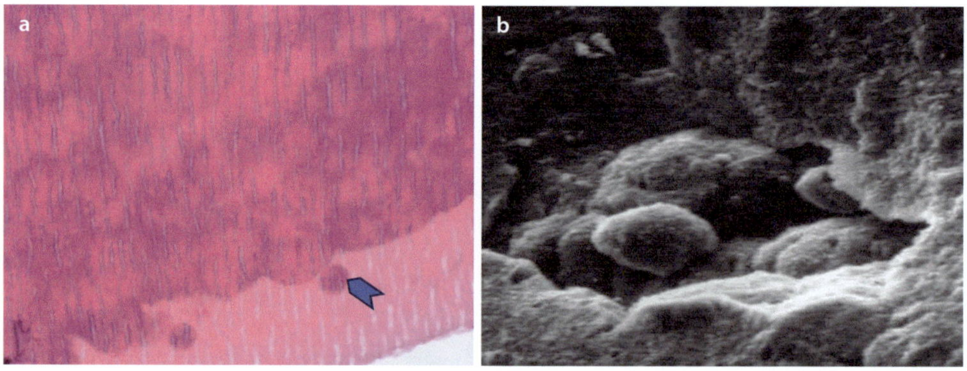

Fig. 8.12 (**a** and **b**) The junction between the calcified dentine and the predentine is seen to be irregular. This reflects the globular calcification (blue arrow) pattern that occurs in dentine. The calcifying globules are called calcospherites (Courtesy of Professor David F Wilson, Adelaide, Australia)

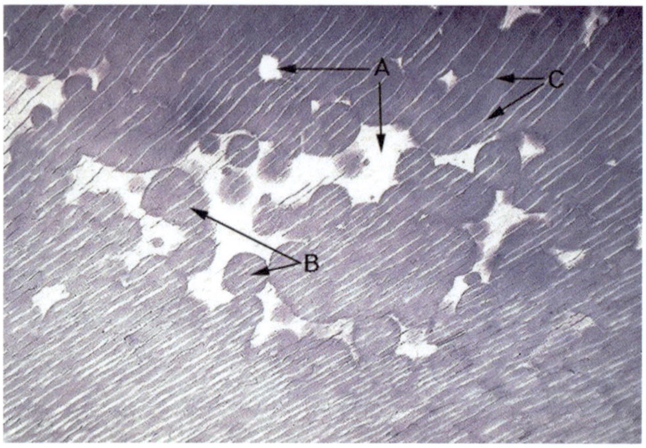

Fig. 8.13 Photomicrograph shows interglobular dentine (**A**), globular dentine (**B**), and dentinal tubules (**C**). (Source: University of Kentucky. Digital Lab. (with permission) ▶ https://www.uky.edu/~brmacp/oralhist/module5/lab/imgshtml/image24.htm)

8.13 Interglobular Dentine (IGD)

Most of the minerals in dentine are deposited as globules (calcospherites), which fuse to form a uniform calcified structure (Fig. 8.12a, b). In some areas in the crown, the fusion may be incomplete. This results in hypo-mineralised 'spaces' between the calcospherites, with the 'spaces' referred to as interglobular dentine (Fig. 8.13).

8.14 Tomes' Granular Layer

Tomes' granular layer represents a relatively hypo-mineralised zone in the root adjacent to the circumferential cemento-dentinal junction (CDJ).

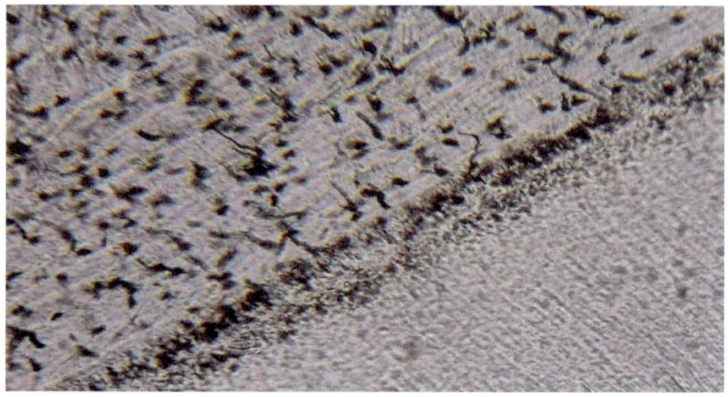

Fig. 8.14 Tomes' granular layer in dentine just below the DEJ. The tissue above the DEJ is the cellular cementum of the root

- Due to the tapering morphology of the root and gradually decreasing dentinal wall thickness, there is difficulty in the placement of the entire length of dentinal tubules, which leads to crowding, looping, and intertwining of terminal branches of dentinal tubules near the cemental surface.
- Current understanding is that dentinal tubules in these areas branch more profusely and loop back on themselves, forming air spaces, which, in ground sections, appear as dark granular areas (Fig. 8.14). The other theory of forming a granular layer refers to the incomplete fusion of calcospherites in the root dentine.

8.15 Lines Associated with the Curvatures of Dentinal Tubules

Dentine-forming cells secrete matrix in consistent rhythmic phases, resulting in the formation of successive microscopic growth lines inside tooth crowns and roots.

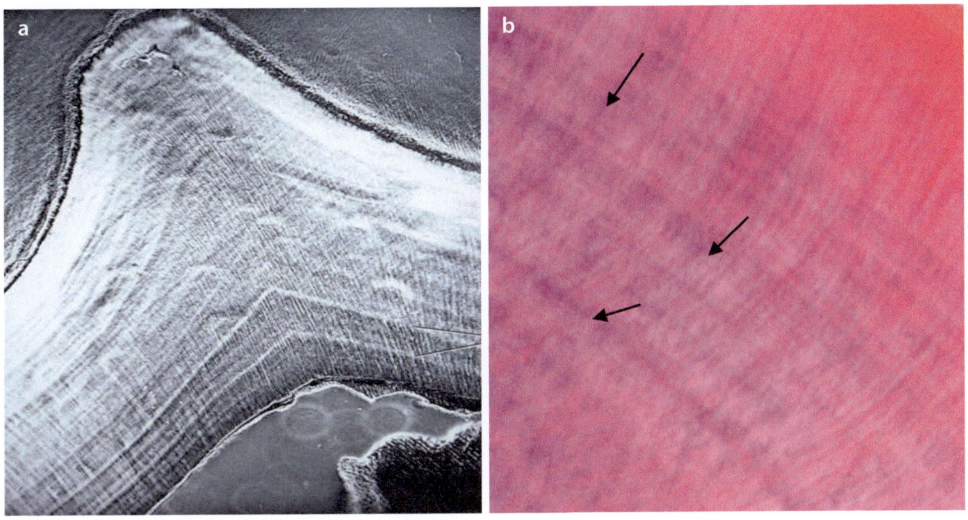

▣ **Fig. 8.15** (**a** and **b**) Incremental lines of von Ebner in dentine (**a**) and (**b**). Decalcified section of dentine showing incremental lines (Arrows) (Courtesy of Professor David F Wilson, Adelaide, Australia)

These are called incremental lines. A variety of lines perpendicular to the dentinal tubules can be seen when sections of dentine are viewed using different techniques.

8.15.1 Incremental Lines of von Ebner

Also called imbrication lines, these lines appear as fine lines or striations in dentine (▣ Fig. 8.15a and b). In cross sections, they are at right angles to dentinal tubules and represent rhythmic, recurrent daily deposition of dentine.

- The distance between the lines corresponds to the daily rate of deposition, which in crown varies from 4 to 8 μm and becomes decreasingly less as root formation progresses.

8.15.2 Contour Lines of Owen

These are hypo-calcified and accentuated incremental lines (▣ Fig. 8.16). They reflect a major interruption in the deposition of dentine due to a metabolic disruption during odontogenesis.

8.15.3 Schreger Lines

Lines associated with the sigmoid primary curvature of dentinal tubules known as Schreger lines are occasionally visible in horizontal sections as broad concentric bands in the circumpulpal dentine.

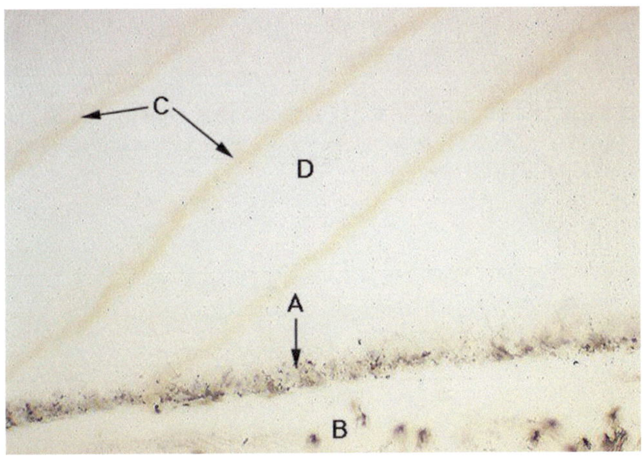

▣ **Fig. 8.16** Contour lines of Owen. Distinctly different coloured lines (C) that traverse the dentine (D) are contour lines of Owen. Tomes' granular layer (A) and dentine (D) are other structures seen in the ground section. (Source: Source: University of Kentucky. Digital Lab. (With permission). ▸ https://www.uky.edu/~brmacp/oralhist/module5/lab/imgshtml/image29.htm)

8.15.4 Neonatal Line

This line separates the prenatal and postnatal dentine, mostly found in deciduous and first permanent molars (▣ Fig. 8.17). This line is the result of incomplete calcification due to metabolic disturbances at the time of birth. It indicates abrupt changes in environment and nutrition faced by newborns.

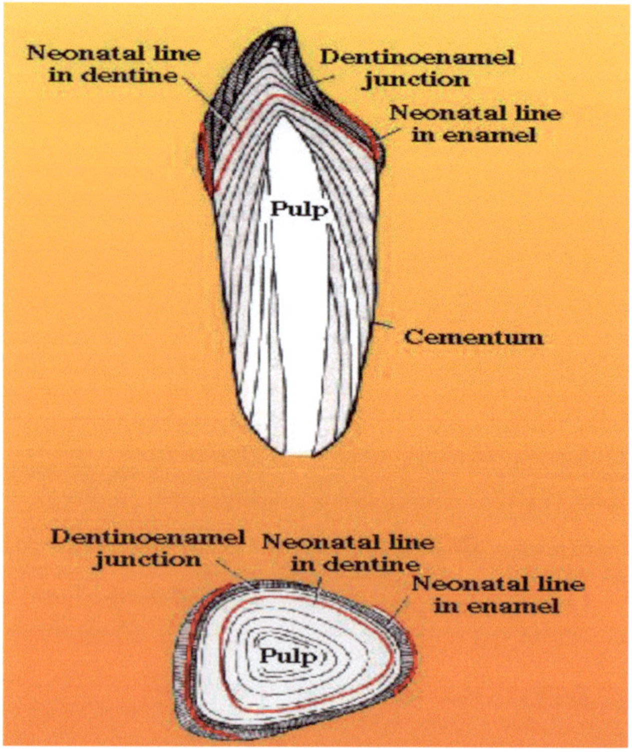

Fig. 8.17 The diagram shows neonatal lines (red) in dentine and enamel. (Source: ► http://www.ostia-antica.org/dahp/cd1/html/cap3_3.htm) (with permission)

8.16 Dead Tracts

The literal meaning of dead tracts is dead or empty dentinal tubules (tracks or tunnels). When odontoblastic processes disintegrate in response to various injuries (such as dental caries and attrition), the tubules appear empty in dried ground sections. These air-filled tubules,s when observed under the light microscope, appear darker in transmitted light (Fig. 8.18).

- Dead tracts are often found in the area of narrow pulpal horns because of the crowding of odontoblasts.
- The body protects this empty, open-ended tubule by forming reparative dentine and sealing the damage at the pulpal ends. In the ground sections, such groups of tubules appear black in transmitted and white in reflected light.
- Dead tracts are possibly the initial step in forming sclerotic dentine.

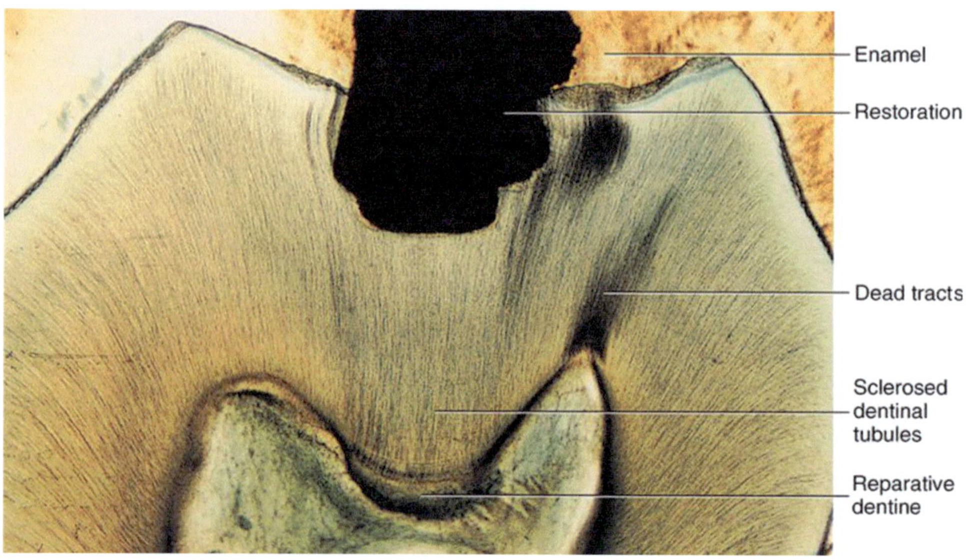

Fig. 8.18 Black dead tracts (open tubules) underlie a black (dense) restoration that appears associated with sclerosed dentinal tubules. Tubules lie adjacent to the reparative dentine, which is seen on the roof of the pulp chamber. Each of these tubules probably resulted from stimulation from the overlying restoration. (Source: Pocket Dentistry . Chapter 8. Dentine.) ► https://pocketdentistry.com/8-dentin/ (With permission)

8.17 Innervation of Dentine and Theories of Dentine Sensitivity

Dentine hypersensitivity is defined as a short, sharp pain arising from exposed dentine in response to various mechanical and chemical stimuli. As compared to soft tissues which are richly innervated, dentine is avascular and without any stromal component to transmit nerve impulses to the brain, generated due to external stimuli. Following are the proposed pathways of dentine sensitivity towards the brain.

Dentine is sensitive to external stimuli. Dentine sensitivity is attributed to intratubular nerves, the odontoblastic processes, or fluid movement in the dentinal tubules.

Three main theories of pain conduction through dentine have been proposed:

8.17.1 Direct Neural Stimulation Theory

Dentinal tubules contain nerves in the predentine accompanying odontoblastic processes, predominantly in the region of pulp horns. The direct neural stimulation theory states that nerves present in the dentine get directly stimulated. The nerves in the dentinal tubules do not extend throughout the dentine. Because of this, topical application of anaesthetics does not abolish sensitivity. Hence, this theory is not popular.

8.17.2 Transduction Theory

This theory presumes that the odontoblast processes are first excited by the stimulus, and the impulse is then transmitted to the nerve endings in the deeper dentine. This theory is also not popular since neurotransmitter vesicles are absent in the odontoblast processes to facilitate the synapse or synaptic specialisation.

8.17.3 Hydrodynamic Theory

This theory proposes that mechanical or osmotic forces applied to the extremity of the dentinal tubules would be transmitted to the sensory transduction apparatus via fluid displacement, either in or out of the tubules.

- Hydrodynamic theory describes that various stimuli such as heat, cold, removal of moisture by air blast, and mechanical or osmotic pressure affect dentinal fluid movement inside the dentinal tubules.
- Fluid movement, either inwards or outwards, stimulates the pain mechanism in the tubules by mechanical disturbance of the nerves closely associated with the odontoblasts and their processes. Thus, these nerve endings may act as mechanoreceptors when affected by the mechanical displacement of the tubular fluid (◻ Fig. 8.19). This is the most popular theory.

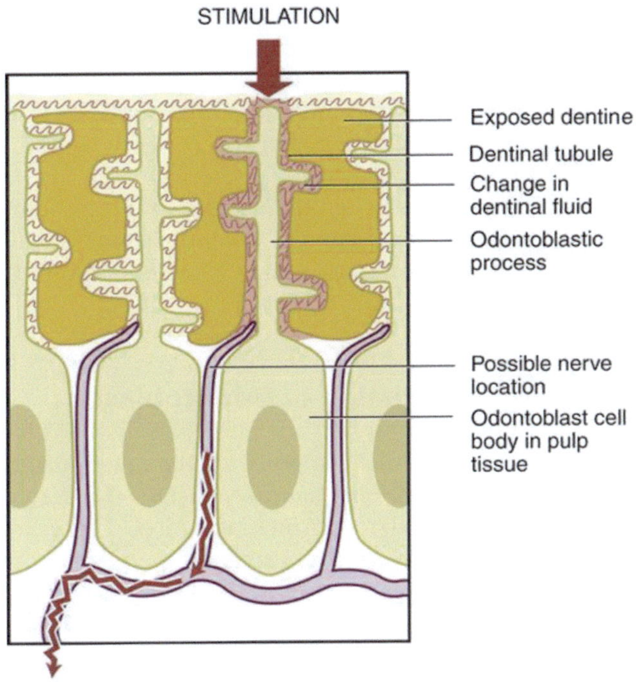

◻ **Fig. 8.19** Possible mechanism involved in the hydrodynamic theory of dentinal hypersensitivity. Stimulation of the exposed dentinal tubules (such as with cold water) causes changes in the dentinal fluid, which is then transmitted to the nerves associated with the odontoblast cell bodies in the pulp tissue. (Source: Dentine and Pulp. Chapter 13. Pocket Dentistry) ▶ https://pocketdentistry.com/13-dentin-and-pulp/ (with permission)

8.18 Histology of Dentinogenesis

Dentinogenesis refers to dentine formation. Dentine formation begins when the tooth germ has reached the bell stage of development. It starts at the cuspal edges and incisal surfaces of the teeth and proceeds towards the root.

- Ectomesenchymal cells of the dental papilla (future pulp) are involved in dentine formation after an inductive influence occurs, which is derived from the inner enamel epithelium (IEE).
- Inductive influence initiates dentinogenesis involving molecular signalling pathways. Dentine formation is a continuous process.

- Odontoblasts synthesise the primary dentine during odontogenesis but also secondary dentine during the life of the tooth and tertiary dentine when the tooth is challenged by pathological stimulations such as caries, attrition, and abrasion.

Dentine formation can be subdivided into three important stages: (1) differentiation of odontoblasts, (2) deposition of the organic matrix, and (3) mineralisation of organic matrix.

8.18.1 Differentiation of Odontoblasts

- The enamel organ is composed of the outer enamel epithelium (OEE), inner enamel epithelium (IEE), stellate reticulum, and stratum intermedium (◘ Fig. 8.20). The inner and outer enamel epithelia meet at the rim of the enamel organ and form the cervical loop. The dental papilla's ectomesenchymal cells (derived from the neural crest) surround the enamel organ.
- The cells bordering the dental papilla are called inner enamel epithelium (IEE). These are short columnar cells characterised by high glycogen content.
- Odontoblast differentiation is regulated by reciprocal molecular interactions between the cells of the IEE and dental papilla.

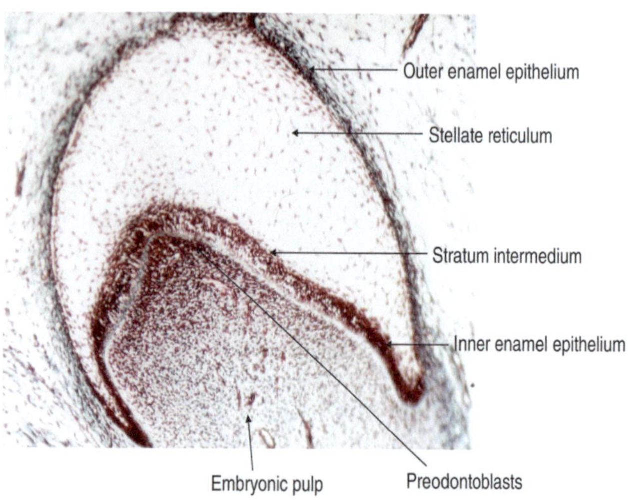

◘ **Fig. 8.20** Light micrograph of a tooth germ at the bell stage. The enamel organ comprises four layers: the outer enamel epithelium, the stellate reticulum, the stratum intermedium, and the inner enamel epithelium. A basement membrane separates the inner enamel epithelium from the pre-odontoblasts at the tip of the pulp horn. These cells line the periphery of the embryonic pulp. (Michel Goldberg. Biomédicale des Saints Pères, Université Paris Descartes, INSERM UMR-S 1124. With a contribution by Bradley K. Formaker, Ph.D., University of Connecticut School of Dental Medicine, Farmington, CT. Chapter 5. Dentine, Pulp and Tooth Pain. Pocket Dentistry with permission)

- Odontoblasts synthesise the components of the predentine (type 1 collagen, glycoproteins, and other non-collagenous proteins) and are responsible for its mineralisation.
- Cells of the dental papilla differentiate into odontoblasts only after cells of the IEE elongate and exhibit reverse polarity.
- The ectomesenchymal cells of the dental papilla adjoining the acellular zone now rapidly enlarge and elongate first to become pre-odontoblasts and, soon thereafter, to become odontoblasts. The cytoplasm of these cells increases in volume to contain increasing amounts of protein-synthesising organelles.
- Odontoblasts exhibit highly ordered rough endoplasmic reticulum (RER), a prominent Golgi apparatus, secretory granules, and numerous mitochondria. Odontoblasts are also rich in RNA and contain one or more prominent nucleoli in their nuclei.
- The acellular zone between the dental papilla and the inner enamel epithelium gradually disappears as the odontoblasts differentiate and increase in size and occupy this zone.

8.18.2 Deposition of Organic Matrix

- Approximately 90% of the organic matrix is type 1 collagen; the remaining 10% of the matrix includes glycoproteins and non-collagenous proteins (NCPs). NCPs comprise glycoproteins/sialoproteins, proteoglycans, phosphoproteins, and growth factors.
- The dentine matrix that forms before the initiation of mineralisation is known as predentine (◘ Fig. 8.21).
- The odontoblasts synthesise mainly type 1 collagen. A small amount of type 5 collagen is also found in the extracellular matrix.
- In addition to proteoglycans and collagen, the odontoblasts also secrete dentine sialoprotein and phosphophoryn, a highly phosphorylated phosphoprotein involved in extracellular mineralisation. Odontoblasts have also been found to secrete the enzymes acid phosphatase and alkaline phosphatase.
- The extracellular matrix molecules are also involved in the odontoblast differentiation process via receptors. Fibronectin interacts with plasma membrane proteins, including one receptor of 165-kDa. The 165-kDa receptor and the fibronectin accumulate at the apical pole of polarising odontoblasts.
- Various growth factors and their receptors have been shown to be present at the enamel organ–dental papilla interface during tooth development and have

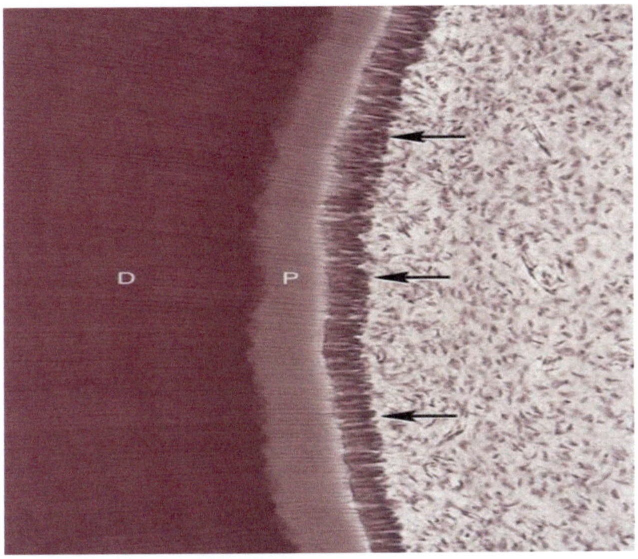

Fig. 8.21 Microscopic view of odontoblasts (arrows) producing predentine (P) that will mature into dentine (D). (Source: Chapter 13. Dentine and Pulp. Courtesy of James McIntosh, PhD, Assistant Professor Emeritus, Department of Biomedical Sciences, Baylor College of Dentistry, Dallas, TX. Pocket dentistry. (With permission))

been implicated in odontoblast differentiation. These include growth hormone (GH), IGF-1, transforming growth factors (TGF) β1, -2, and -3 , and bone morphogenetic proteins (BMP)-2, -4, and -6.

8.18.3 Mineralisation of the Organic Matrix

- The first layer of dentine is unmineralised. Mineralisation begins and proceeds after a certain width of the dentine matrix is laid down.
- Mineralisation of predentine begins at the dentinoenamel junction during tooth development and progresses towards the pulp of the tooth.
- Odontoblasts can take up and store calcium and actively transport calcium ions to the mineralisation site via active transport through the cell.
- Deposition of calcium occurs onto a template formed by type 1 collagen, and mineral crystal deposition occurs at the gap zone within the collagen fibrils.
- A pool of chondroitin sulphate (CS), decorin, and biglycan is secreted at the mineralisation front and is transported intra-cellularly along the odontoblast process.
- Another important glycoprotein in directing mineralisation is dentine phosphoprotein (DPP). This has a high affinity for calcium and hydroxyapatite surfaces.
- Matrix vesicles are required for the mineralisation of mantle dentine. After mantle dentine has been synthesised and secreted, odontoblast differentiation is complete.
- Dentine is mineralised in the presence of matrix vesicles which are hydroxyapatite-containing membrane-enclosed vesicles secreted by odontoblasts. These are believed to serve as nucleation centres for the mineralisation of dentine. One of the key proteins involved in the mineralisation process is dentine phosphoprotein secreted by odontoblasts.

8.19 Summary

Dentine is the mineralised tissue that constitutes the major bulk of the tooth and is present as an enclosed cylindrical wall around the central core of soft pulp tissue. Dentine comprises cylindrical canals called dentinal tubules running from the pulp to the dentinoenamel junction (DEJ) in the crown and the cemento-dentinal junction (CEJ) in the root. The dentine matrix is secreted by specialised cells in the pulp called odontoblasts. Extensions of odontoblasts called odontoblast processes are found in the dentinal tubules, usually about one-quarter of the total length of the tubule. Dentinal tubules are also filled with dentinal fluid, and sensory nerve terminals may be seen adjacent to the odontoblast processes.

The newly formed dentine before calcification and maturation is called predentine. It is the innermost layer of dentine located adjacent to the pulp. The bulk of the dentine that surrounds the pulp is primary dentine, which is also known as circumpulpal dentine. Mantle dentine is the variant of primary dentine. Dentine formed after the completion of root formation and tooth eruption is termed secondary dentine. Dentine that forms in response to various stimuli, such as attrition, caries, or a dental procedure, is called tertiary dentine. Sclerotic dentine (physiologic sclerotic dentine and translucent dentine) is characterised by the accumulation of mineral deposits within the lumen of the dentinal tubules. The collagen matrix dispersed between the dentine tubules is intertubular dentine (ITD). Most of the mineral in dentine is deposited as globules (calcospherites), which fuse to form a uniform calcified structure. Hypo-mineralised spaces sometimes present between the globules are termed interglobular dentine. The hypo-mineralised zone in the root adjacent to the circumferential cemento-dentinal junction (CDJ) is called Tomes' granular layer. The disintegration of odontogenic processes can occur due to trauma, such as restorations. This may result in empty dentinal tubules. These are called dead tracts.

Dentine-forming cells secrete matrix in consistent rhythmic phases, resulting in the formation of successive microscopic growth lines inside tooth crowns and roots. These are called incremental lines. Two types of lines exist: incremental lines of von Ebner and contour lines of Owen. The line that separates the prenatal and postnatal dentine is called the neonatal line.

Dentine is sensitive to external stimuli. Dentine sensitivity is variously attributed to intratubular nerves, the odontoblastic processes, or fluid movement in the dentinal tubules (hydrodynamic theory).

Dentinogenesis refers to dentine formation. Dentine formation begins when the tooth germ has reached the bell stage of development. Dentine formation can be subdivided into three important stages, namely differentiation of odontoblasts, deposition of the organic matrix, and mineralisation of the organic matrix.

Further Reading

Avery JK. Oral development and histology. In: Oral development and histology. 3rd ed. New York: Theime; 1988. p. 298–332.

Coffey CT, Ingram MJ, Bjorndal AM. Analysis of human dentinal fluid. Oral Surg Oral Med Oral Pathol. 1970;30(6):835–7.

Couve E, Osorio R, Schmachtenberg O. The amazing odontoblast: activity, autophagy, and aging. J Dent Res. 2013;92(9):765–72. https://doi.org/10.1016/j.mehy.2013.05.015.

Goldberg M, Kulkarni AB, Young M, Boskey A. Dentin: structure, composition and mineralisation. Front Biosci (Elite Ed). 2011a;3(2):711–35.

Goldberg M, Kulkarni AB, Young M, Boskey A. Dentin: structure, composition and mineralization. Front Biosci (Elite Ed). 2011b;3(2):711–35. https://doi.org/10.2741/e281. PMID: 21196346; PMCID: PMC3360947.

Kabartai F, Hoffmann T, Hannig C. The physiologic sclerotic dentin: a literature-based hypothesis. Med Hypotheses [Internet]. 2015;85(6):887–890. https://doi.org/10.1016/j.mehy.2015.09.016. http://www.ncbi.nlm.nih.gov/pubmed/21197505.

Kinney JH, Marshall SJ, Marshall GW. The mechanical properties of human dentin: a critical review and re-evaluation of the dental literature. Crit Rev Oral Biol Med. 2003;14(1):13–29.

Kumar GS. Orban's oral histology and embryology. 13th ed. New Delhi: Elsevier; 2010.

Leonora J, Tieche JM, Steinman RR. The effect of dietary factors on intradentinal dye penetration in the rat. Arch Oral Biol. 1992;37(9):733–41.

Liu XX, Tenenbaum HC, Wilder RS, Quock R, Hewlett ER, Ren YF. Pathogenesis, diagnosis and management of dentin hypersensitivity: an evidence-based overview for dental practitioners. BMC Oral Health. 2020;20(1):1–10.

Nanci A. Ten Cate' s oral histology development, structure, and function. Elsevier. 2018. p. 824.

Okiji T. Odontoblasts: Specialized hard-tissue-forming cells in the dentin-pulp complex. Congenit Anom (Kyoto). 2021;56(4):144–53.

Özok AR, Wu MK, Ten Cate JM, Wesselink PR. Effect of dentinal fluid composition on dentin demineralization in vitro. J Dent Res. 2004;83(11):849–53.

Slootweg PJ. Dental pathology—A practical introduction. Berlin: Springer; 2007. 1–80 p.

Tjäderhane L. Dentin basic structure, composition, and function. In: Versiani M, Basrani B, Sousa-Neto M, editors. The root canal anatomy in permanent dentition. Cham: Springer; 2019. https://doi.org/10.1007/978-3-319-73444-6_2.

Vennat E, Bogicevic C, Fleureau JM, Degrange M. Demineralized dentin 3D porosity and pore size distribution using mercury porosimetry. Dent Mater. 2009;25(6):729–35.

Vennat E, Wang W, Genthial R, David B, Dursun E, Gourrier A. Mesoscale porosity at the dentin-enamel junction could affect the biomechanical properties of teeth. Acta Biomater. 2017;51:418–32.

Histology of Cementum and Cementogenesis

Kshipra Deshpande

Contents

S R Prabhu et al. (eds.), *Oral Histology and Oral Histopathology*, https://doi.org/10.1007/978-3-031-77481-2_9

9.1 Introduction

Cementum is a hard, avascular connective tissue covering the tooth root. It furnishes an attachment medium for collagen fibres that bind the tooth to the surrounding structures. Due to its intermediary position, forming the interface between root dentine and periodontal ligament, cementum is a component of the tooth itself but belongs functionally to the dental attachment apparatus, that is, the periodontium. Dental cementum is unique in various aspects; it is avascular and not innervated, does not undergo continuous remodelling like bone, but continues to grow in thickness throughout life, thus helping to maintain the tooth in its functional position in the dental occlusion.

9.2 Physical Properties

9

- Cementum is pale yellow in colour and can be distinguished from enamel by its lack of lustre and darker hue, softer than dentine, more permeable than dentine, and its thickness varies in different teeth and in the same tooth in different regions.
- Cementum is thinnest at the cementoenamel junction (20–50 μm) and thickest towards the apex (150–200 μm).

9.3 Chemical Composition

- By volume, cementum contains 45% inorganic material, 33% organic material, and 22% water; on a wet weight basis, it contains 65% inorganic material, 23% organic material, and 12% water. The inorganic material consists mainly of calcium and phosphate in the form of hydroxyapatite and trace elements in varying amounts. Cementum has the highest fluoride content of all the mineralised tissues.
- The organic material of cementum consists primarily of type I collagen (90%) type III collagen (5%) and non-collagenous proteins.
- Non-collagenous proteins play important roles in matrix deposition, initiation, and control of mineralisation and matrix remodelling. They consist of bone sialoprotein (BSP), osteopontin, tenascin, fibronectin, and osteocalcin.
- Cementum is rich in proteoglycans. These include chondroitin sulphate, heparan sulphate, hyaluronate, keratan sulphates–fibromodulin and lumican, versican, biglycan, and osteoadherin. Cementum also contains growth factors. These include TGF-β, various BMPs, FGF, IGF, EGF, and PDGF. A cementum-derived growth factor is seen exclusively in cementum.

9.4 Cementum-Associated Cells: Cementoblasts and Cementocytes

Cementoblasts are derived initially from the dental follicle. The main organic matrix of cementum, i.e. collagen and protein polysaccharides, is synthesised by cementoblasts. The collagen fibrils produced by the cementoblasts form a fibrous fringe perpendicular to the periodontal space at the superficial surface. These cells retreat and intermingle with the fibroblasts of the periodontal ligament.

Cementoblasts can be inducted from periodontal ligament (PDL) stem cells throughout life, as evidenced by physiological areas of cemental repair. Cementoblasts' cellular turnover is slower than that of osteoblasts. Furthermore, it appears that cementoblasts can alter their rate of cementum deposition.

Cementocytes are spider-like cells entrapped in the cemental matrix (Fig. 9.1). The cementocytes lie in lacunae, and their process extends through channels called canaliculi, which are directed towards the PDL, and cementocytes communicate with each other through these canaliculi. The central cell mass appears round or oval, and the diameter ranges from 8 to 15 μm. The cytoplasm is palely basophilic, and the nucleus is centrally located. The number of cementocytes depends on the rate of formation of cellular cementum. The more rapidly the cementum is laid, the greater the number of cementocytes seen.

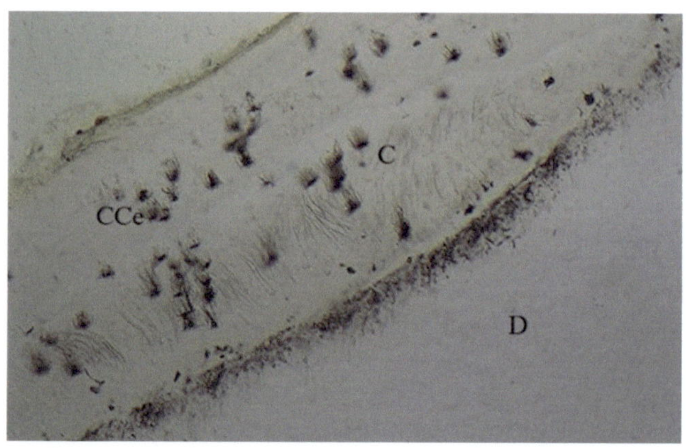

Fig. 9.1 Cellular cementum (ground section). *C* cementum. *D* dentine. *CCe* spider-like structures are cementocytes lacunae and canaliculi, which in a living tooth would be occupied by cementocytes and their cytoplasmic extensions

9.5 Classification and Structure of Cementum

Cementum can be classified into three different types based on the presence or absence of cells, the nature or types of organic fibres, or a combination of both. The three main types are cellular intrinsic fibre cementum (CIFC), acellular extrinsic fibre cementum (AEFC), and mixed stratified cementum, which exhibits cellular and acellular cementum lines.

9.5.1 Cellular Cementum (◘ Figs. 9.1, 9.2)

Cellular cementum contains cells known as cementocytes. It is found mainly in the apical third and furcation areas. Three main subtypes of cellular cementum are recognised.

- Cellular intrinsic fibre cementum (CIFC)
- Cellular mixed fibre cementum
- Cellular mixed stratified cementum

9.5.1.1 Cellular Intrinsic Fibre Cementum (CIFC)

Cellular intrinsic fibre cementum (CIFC) mainly occupies the middle and apical third. Cementocytes are present in lacunae and show canaliculi. Cementoblasts forming this type of cementum are derived from the dental follicle. Non-collagenous proteins and proteoglycans are present in the cemental matrix. Both cellular and acellular cementum are separated by incremental lines into layers, which indicate periodic formation. These incremental cementum lines are more mineralised than enamel and dentine due to less collagen and more ground substance. As cellular cementum is rapidly formed, the incremental lines are placed further apart than in AEFC.

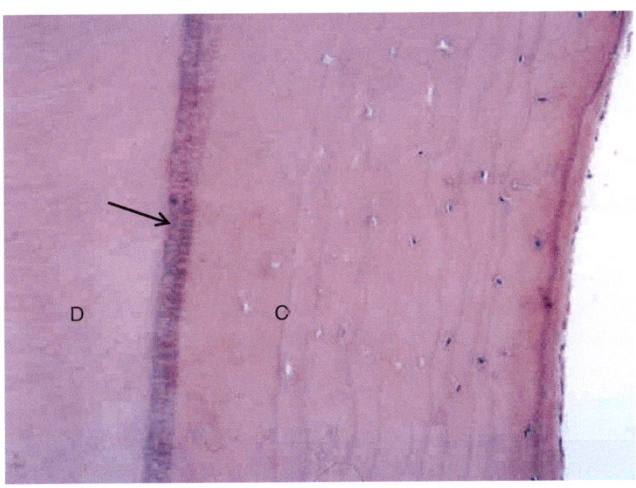

◘ **Fig. 9.2** Decalcified specimen showing cellular cementum (C) abutting primary (acellular) cementum (arrow). *D* dentine. Lacunae, some of which contain cementoblast nuclei, are evident, as are incremental lines. A layer of cementoblasts abutting a thin, pale layer of cementoid is seen on the outer cementum surface. As described in the text, cellular cementum can be made up of cementum subtypes (Courtesy of Professor David Wilson, Adelaide, Australia)

9.5.1.2 Cellular Mixed Fibre Cementum (CMFC)

The cellular mixed fibre cementum (CMFC) is a variant formed at a faster rate with less mineralised fibres. The collagen fibres of CMFC are derived from the periodontal ligament fibroblasts and the cementoblasts. These intrinsic and extrinsic fibres form an intricate pattern running between each other at almost right angles and different orientations. However, the number of intrinsic fibres is comparatively less than the extrinsic fibres. The fibre bundles originating from the fibroblasts are ovoid or round, 5–7 μm in diameter, and the fibres originating from the cementoblasts are much more delicate and smaller, measuring 1–2 μm in diameter.

9.5.1.3 Cellular Mixed Stratified Cementum (CMSC)

In this type of cementum, the cellular intrinsic fibre cementum alternates with acellular extrinsic fibre cementum. It is formed by cementoblasts and fibroblasts. It appears primarily on the apical third of the root and furcation areas. The thickness varies from 100 to 1000 μm. The cells incorporated into cellular cementum (cementocytes) are like osteocytes. They are best viewed in mineralised ground sections (◘ Fig. 9.1a). At the light microscopic level, lacunae in the deeper layers of cementum appear to be empty, suggesting the complete degeneration of cementocytes located in these areas.

Intrinsic fibres are produced by cementoblasts. They are smaller and usually oriented parallel to the surface. Extrinsic fibres (Sharpy's fibres) are produced by the periodontal ligament (PDL) fibroblasts. They are larger bundles oriented perpendicularly to the surface of the cementum.

9.5.2 Acellular Cementum

Acellular cementum is devoid of cells. It is continuously and slowly produced throughout life. It appears as a relatively thin, amorphous layer overlying the dentine in sections (◘ Fig. 9.3).

Acellular extrinsic fibre cementum (AEFC) (◘ Fig. 9.4) is termed primary cementum as it forms first. AEFC extends from the cervical margin to the apical third of the root. It is the only type of cementum seen in single-rooted teeth. AEFC is formed by cementoblasts derived from Hertwig's epithelial root sheath (HERS) and periodontal ligament fibroblasts. Cementocytes are absent in AEFC. Extrinsic (Sharpey's) fibres, which form the bulk of the acellular cementum, are mineralised except for their inner cores. Non-collagenous proteins fill the space between the extrinsic fibres. This type of cementum is formed slowly and regularly. Therefore, the incremental lines (lines of Salter) run parallel to the surface and closer together. Cementoid is not seen in this type of cementum. The main function of AEFC is anchorage, especially in single-rooted teeth.

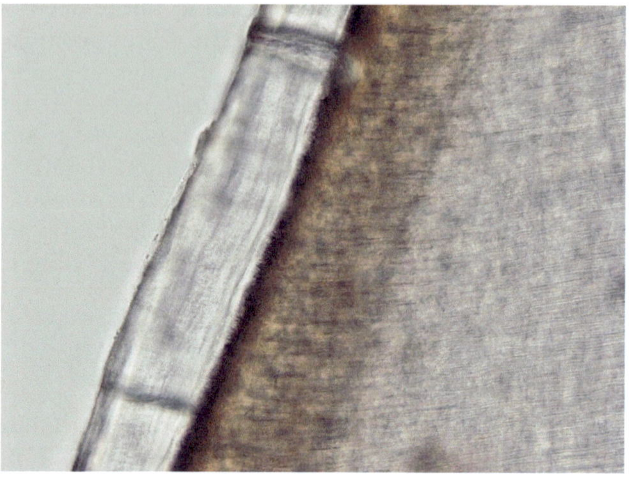

◘ **Fig. 9.3** The undecalcified section of cementum shows acellular cementum with incremental lines of salter and the overlying dentine. (Courtesy of Professor David Wilson, Adelaide, Australia)

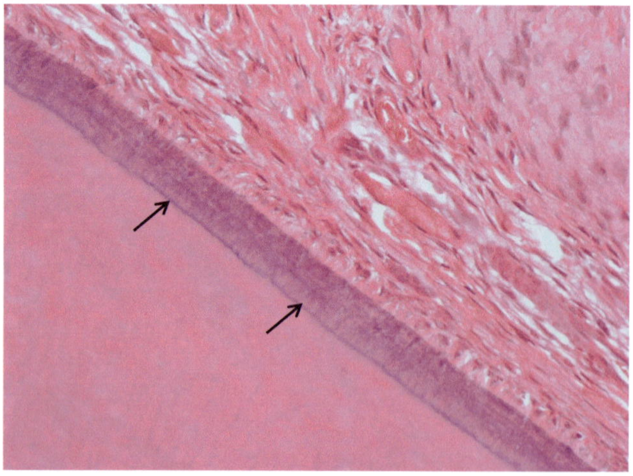

◘ **Fig. 9.4** Decalcified section showing acellular cementum (arrows) (Courtesy of Professor David Wilson, Adelaide, Australia)

9.5.3 Other Varieties of Cementum

9.5.3.1 Acellular fibrillar cementum (AFC)

AFC consists of a mineralised matrix containing neither collagen fibres nor cementocytes. AFC is found to be isolated patches or as the most cervical part of AEFC on enamel just coronal to the cementoenamel junction (CEJ). Its composition of non-collagenous proteins is very similar to that of AEFC. AFC is formed when there is a premature loss of reduced enamel epithelium (REE) protecting the newly formed enamel at the cervical margin of the tooth.

9.5.3.2 Intermediate cementum

The term 'intermediate cementum' indicates a narrow zone containing cellular elements between dentine and cellular mixed stratified cementum (CMSC). Sometimes, dentine is separated from cementum by a zone known as the intermediate cementum layer, which does not exhibit characteristic features of either dentine or cementum. As it appears hyaline (structureless), it is also known as the hyaline layer. This layer is predominately seen in the apical two-thirds of molars and premolars and rarely observed in incisors or deciduous teeth. The probable function might be to seal the sensitive root dentine.

9.6 Cementodentinal Junction (CDJ)

The terminal apical area of the cementum where it joins the internal root dentine is called the cementodentinal junction (CDJ). CDJ is smooth in permanent teeth and scalloped in deciduous teeth. CDJ is a wide zone containing large quantities of collagen associated with glycosaminoglycans like chondroitin sulphate and dermatan sulphate, resulting in increased water content, contributing to stiffness. This reduction in its mechanical property helps it to redistribute occlusal loads to the alveolar bone. The cemental fibres intermingle with the dentinal fibres at the CDJ more in cellular cementum than in acellular cementum, aiding in cementum attachment to the dentine. The width of CDJ is 2–3 μm and remains relatively stable.

9.7 Cementoenamel Junction (CEJ)

The cementoenamel junction (CEJ) is where cementum and enamel unite at the cervical region of the tooth. Three main types of junctions are recognised.

9.7.1 Gap Junction

In about 10% of the teeth, enamel and cementum do not meet. This occurs when enamel epithelium in the cervical portion of the root is delayed in its separation from dentine. In such cases, there is no cementoenamel junction. Instead, the zone of the root is devoid of cementum (◘ Fig. 9.5).

9.7.2 Edge-to-Edge Junction

In approximately 30% of all teeth, cementum meets the cervical end of enamel in a relatively sharp line (◘ Fig. 9.6)

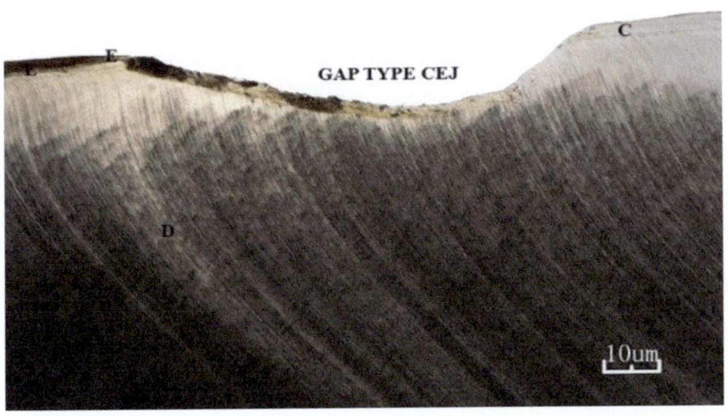

◘ **Fig. 9.5** Cementoenamel junction: Gap type (ground section). *C* cementum, *E* enamel. The main bulk of the tooth is dentine

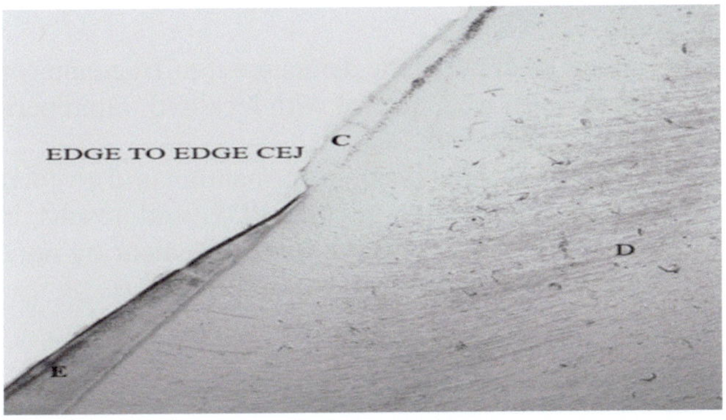

◘ **Fig. 9.6** Cementoenamel junction: Edge-to-edge type (ground section).. *C* cementum, *E* enamel, and *D* dentine

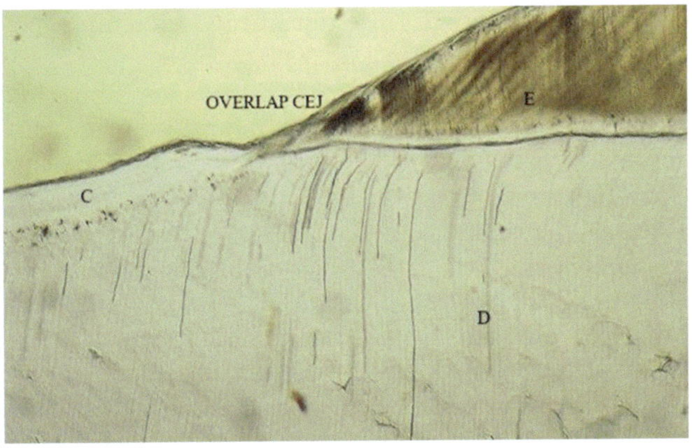

◘ **Fig. 9.7** Cementoenamel junction: Overlap type (ground section).. *C* cementum, *E* enamel, *D* dentine

9.7.3 Overlap Junction

In approximately 60% of the teeth, the cementum overlaps the cervical end of the enamel for a short distance. This occurs when the enamel epithelium degenerates at its cervical termination, permitting connective tissue to come in direct contact with the enamel surface. (◘ Fig. 9.7)

Recent studies have shown the presence of the fourth type of CE junction: the enamel overlapping the cementum. In deciduous teeth, the enamel and cementum meeting edge-to-edge is the most common type, followed by the cementum overlapping the enamel.

9.8 Functions of Cementum

Anchorage: The primary function of cementum is to provide a medium for attaching collagen fibres that bind the tooth to the alveolar bone. Collagen fibres of the periodontal ligament cannot merge into dentine; cementum is necessary for connective tissue attachment.

Adaptation: Cementum establishes the functional adaptation of teeth to masticatory and other forces. Deposition of cementum in an apical area can compensate for loss of tooth substance from occlusal wear. The continuous deposition of cementum is of considerable functional importance. As the most superficial layer of cementum ages, a new layer of cementum must be deposited to keep the attachment apparatus intact.

Repair: Cementum is the major reparative tissue for root surfaces. Root damage, such as fractures and resorptions, can be repaired by depositing new cementum. The cementum formed during repair resembles cellular cementum because it forms faster.

Hypercementosis: Hypercementosis is an abnormal thickening of cementum. It may be diffuse or circumscribed. It may affect all teeth of the dentition, be confined to a single tooth, or even affect only parts of one tooth. Hypercementosis may be due to teeth exposed to great stress, chronic periapical inflammation, nonfunctioning teeth, sequela of injuries to the cementum, advanced age, and neoplastic and non-neoplastic diseases such as Paget's disease, benign cementoblastoma, florid cemento-osseous dysplasia, acromegaly, calcinosis, and some forms of arthritis.

9.9 Cementogenesis

9.9.1 Formation

The process of formation of cementum is known as cementogenesis. In a forming tooth, at the advancing root edge, Hertwig's epithelial root sheath (HERS), which is derived from the extension of inner enamel epithelium (IEE) and outer enamel epithelium (OEE), releases enamel proteins. HERS sends an inductive message to the ectomesenchymal cells of the dental papilla (pulp). These ectomesenchymal cells now differentiate into odontoblasts and produce a layer of predentine along the inner aspect of HERS. Once dentine formation is underway, breaks occur in HERS. Therefore, the inner layer of the dental follicle (dental sac) meets predentine. Cells of the dental follicle now differentiate into cementoblasts, which are the main cells responsible for cementum formation. Cementoblasts synthesise an organic matrix, which is uncalcified.

9.9.1.1 Formation of Cellular Cementum

It is deposited over acellular cementum and is less mineralised than acellular cementum. Cementoblasts, derived from the dental follicles, secrete the collagen fibres and ground substances, forming the intrinsic fibres of the cellular cementum. Cementum growth is a rhythmic process, and as a new layer of cementoid is formed, the older matrix calcifies. This results in the entrapment of cementoblasts in their matrix, resulting in the formation of cellular cementum.

9.9.1.2 Formation of the Acellular Cementum

It is preceded by mineralisation of the first layer of dentine. It is associated with the secretion of cementum-related proteins such as bone sialoproteins (BSP), osteopontin, and fibrillar collagen. Cementoblasts derived from HERS meet dentine and lay down ground substances and collagen fibrils, forming acellular cementum. Connective tissue fibres from PDL pass into the cementum and attach the tooth to the surrounding bone. These are called Sharpey's fibres. These are extrinsic fibres of the acellular cementum.

In permanent teeth, this acellular extrinsic fibre cementum is formed after the tooth has erupted when two-thirds of the root has formed. Before this, the acellular cementum lining the root is the acellular intrinsic fibre cementum.

Incremental lines seen during cementogenesis are called lines of Salter. They occur during periods of rest and activity and are closer in acellular cementum, which is formed slowly.

9.10 Mineralisation

This begins in the depth of the precementum. Fine hydroxyapatite crystals are deposited, first between and then within the collagen fibrils, by a process identical to bone tissue mineralisation. The width of the precementum layer is about 3–5 µm. Establishing the appropriate condition for crystallisation and growth of the individual crystals in cementum is slow and extends over several months.

9.11 Developmental Anomalies of Cementum

Developmental anomalies of cementum are common. These include:

- Concrescence: Concrescence of teeth is a form of fusion which occurs after root formation has been completed. In this condition, teeth are united by cementum only.
- Cementicles: Small, globular masses of cementum found in the apical, middle third, and furcation of roots.
- Cemental tears: It is the detachment of fragments of cementum. It is associated with localised, rapid periodontal breakdown.
- Ankylosis: It is the fusion of cementum and alveolar bone by obliteration of the PDL and results in resorption of the root and its replacement by bone tissue. It is an uncommon condition.

9.12 Clinical Considerations

- Tooth movement: Cementum is more resistant to resorption than bone, and it is for this reason that orthodontic tooth movement is possible.

- Trauma or excessive occlusal forces can cause cementum to resorb. The damage is usually repaired after the cessation of trauma, either by forming acellular or cellular cementum.
- Transverse fractures of the root due to trauma may heal by the formation of a new cementum.
- In periodontal pockets, dental plaque and its by-products can cause numerous alterations in the physical, chemical, and structural characteristics of cementum.
- Cemental caries can be seen on exposed surfaces of cementum associated with gingival recession of older individuals.
- In forensic dentistry, counting the cemental incremental lines is helpful for the determination of the age of an individual.

9.13 Summary

Cementum is bone-like mineralised tissue lining the dentine of the root, which functions both to protect the root and as an attachment surface used to anchor the periodontal ligament to the tooth. It forms the periodontal apparatus of the tooth along with the periodontal ligament, alveolar bone, and gingiva. It is formed by cementoblasts. It is composed of 45–50% inorganic hydroxyapatite and 50–55% organic material and water. Cementum is classified based on the presence or absence of cells as cellular or acellular cementum. Based on the presence of fibres, cementum is further classified as cellular intrinsic fibre cementum and acellular extrinsic fibre cementum. Other varieties of cementum are also described. Anchorage, adaptation, and repair are the major functions of cementum.

Acknowledgements The author sincerely thanks Professor David Wilson (Adelaide) and the Department of Oral Pathology and Microbiology, Govt: Dental College and Hospital Nagpur and Mumbai for the Photomicrographs of Histology of Cementum.

Further Reading

Foster BL. Methods for studying tooth root cementum by light microscopy. Int J Oral Sci. 2012;4:119–28.

Gonçalves PF, Antonio E, Antonio S, Sallum W, Zaffalon M, et al. Dental cementum reviewed: development, structure, composition, regeneration and potential functions. Braz J Oral Sci. 2005;4(12)

Kumar GS. Cementum. In: Orban's oral histology and embryology. 14th ed. Elsevier; 2015. p. 116–34.

Nancy A, editor. Periodontium. In: Ten Cate's oral histology. 9th ed. p. 445–72.

Peeran SW, Ramalingam K, Thiruneervannan R. Cementum. In: Peeran SW, Ramalingam K, editors. Essentials of periodontics & oral implantology. 1st ed; 2021. p. 1–17.

Shafer HL. Developmental disturbances of oral and paraoral structures. In: Rajendran R, Sivapathasundharam B, editors. Shafer's textbook of oral pathology. 7th ed. p. 184–210.

Suchetha A, Aparna Suraj N, Sapna N, Darshan B, Apoorva S, Bhat D. Cementum in disease - Review. Int J Curr Adv Res. 2021;10(01(C)):23688–92.

Yamamoto T, Hasegawa T, Yamamoto T, Hongo H, Amizuka N. Histology of human cementum: Its structure, function, and development. Jpn Dent Sci Rev. 2016;52:63–74.

Histology of the Dental Pulp

S R Prabhu

Contents

S R Prabhu et al. (eds.), *Oral Histology and Oral Histopathology*, https://doi.org/10.1007/978-3-031-77481-2_10

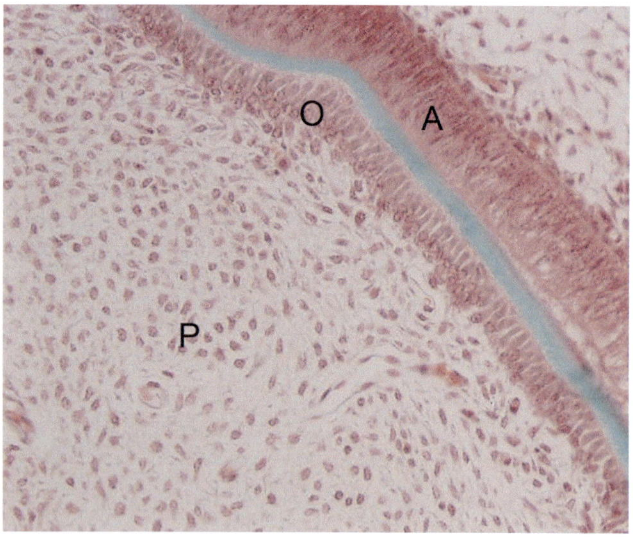

Fig. 10.1 During tooth formation, odontoblasts (O) differentiate from the dental papilla (P). In this micrograph, the odontoblasts have already laid down a thin layer of dentine matrix (green) that abuts differentiating ameloblasts (A). (Courtesy Professor David F Wilson, Adelaide, Australia)

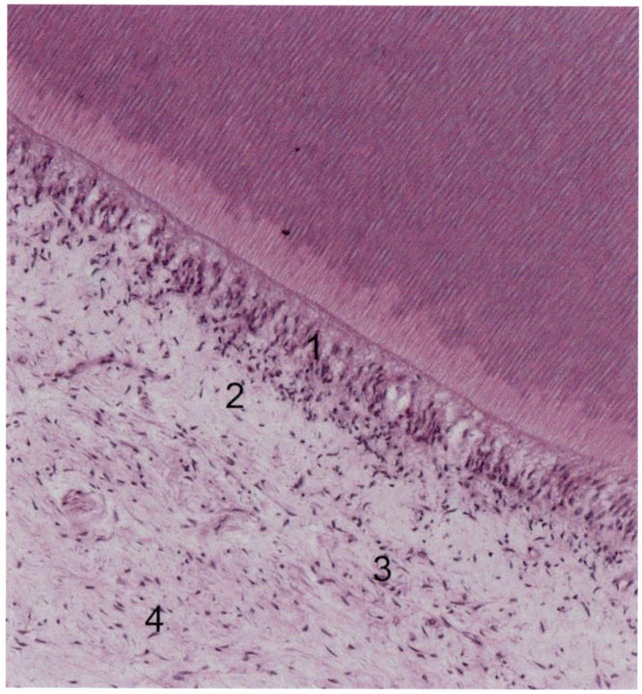

Fig. 10.2 Photomicrograph illustrating the four zones of the dental pulp: the odontoblastic zone (1), the cell-free zone of Weil (2), the cell-rich zone (3), and the zone consisting of blood vessels and nerves (4). (Courtesy Professor David F Wilson, Adelaide, Australia)

10.1 Introduction

The dental pulp is a soft connective tissue found in the pulp chamber of the crown and root canals. The root canal opens into the periodontium via the apical foramen, through which blood vessels and nerves of the dental pulp enter and leave. This establishes a form of communication between the pulp and surrounding periodontal tissue.

The dental pulp is derived from the dental papilla during odontogenesis (Fig. 10.1) and is responsible for dentine formation (see ▶ Chap. 6). Pulp also forms secondary dentine throughout life and, when confronted by mild stimuli such as caries or trauma, produces tertiary dentine. By either weight or volume, 75–80% of dental pulp is water.

10.2 Histology

The dental pulp consists of cells, an extracellular matrix of fibres, and a ground substance. The cellular components of the dental pulp include odontoblasts, fibroblasts, undifferentiated mesenchymal cells, and defence cells. The extracellular matrix acts as a scaffold to stabilise the pulp's structure. Fibrous components of the pulp include collagen fibres. Types 1 and 3 collagen fibres are predominant, and types 5 and 6 are in small amounts. The bulk of the dental pulp in the centre consists of blood vessels and nerves surrounded by the fibroblasts and intercellular matrix. The non-fibrous type 4 collagen is in the basement of blood vessels in the pulp. The ground substance forms the environment that surrounds both cells and fibres of the pulp. It is rich in proteoglycans, glycoproteins, and water.

Histologically, the dental pulp has four distinct zones: (1) The odontoblastic zone at the periphery of the pulp; (2) the cell-free zone of Weil, beneath the odontoblastic zone, which is prominently seen in the coronal pulp; (3) the cell-rich zone, which is in the coronal pulp adjacent to the cell-free zone; and (4) the core of the pulp consisting of blood vessels and nerves (Fig. 10.2).

10.3 Cellular Components of Pulp Tissue

10.3.1 Odontoblasts

Odontoblasts are responsible for the formation of dentine. They are terminally differentiated cells lining the periphery of the pulp and cannot divide. They are columnar in the coronal portion of the pulp (Fig. 10.3) and cuboidal in the root canals. A terminally differentiated odontoblast is a polarised columnar cell showing a

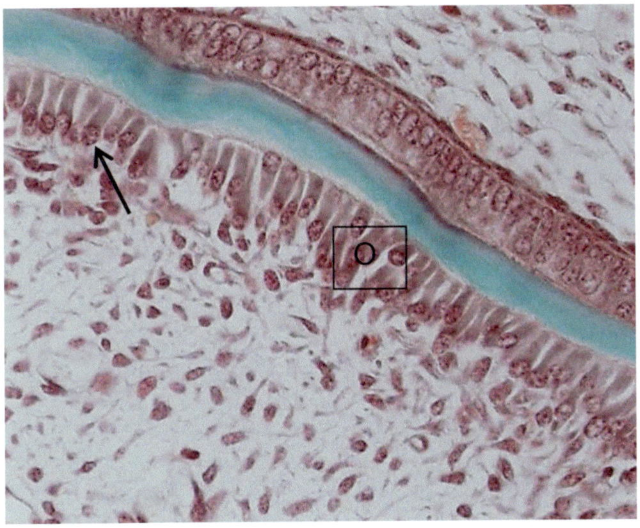

■ **Fig. 10.3** Odontoblasts (O) are tall, columnar cells (arrow) with a basally situated nucleus. (Courtesy Professor David F Wilson, Adelaide, Australia)

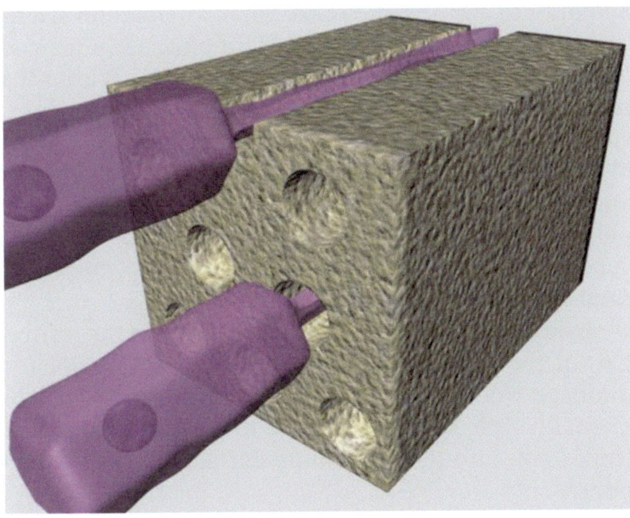

■ **Fig. 10.4** Schematic diagram illustrating odontoblast processes within dentine tubules. (Courtesy Professor David F Wilson, Adelaide, Australia)

long process or extension called the odontoblastic process. This extends within a dentinal tubule. The number of odontoblasts corresponds to the number of dentinal tubules. Odontoblasts also show smaller processes linking them to adjacent odontoblasts. A characteristic of odontoblasts is cytoplasmic extensions called odontoblast processes (■ Fig. 10.4) that initially extend into the dentine to the dentinoenamel junction. These processes are longer in the crown, whereas they are shorter in the root canals. During dentine formation, dentine forms around odontoblastic processes, and as the odon-

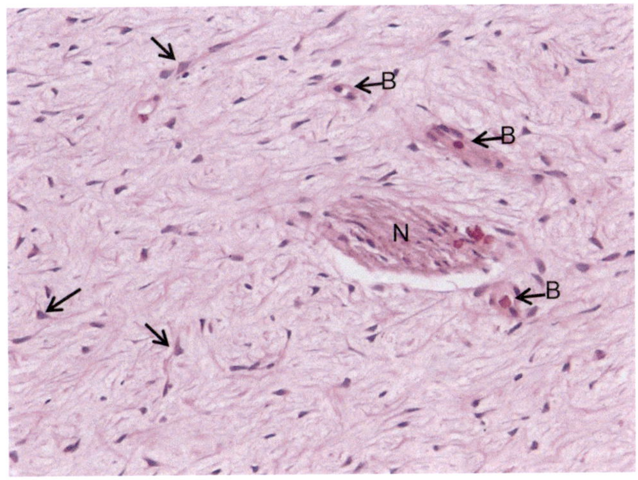

■ **Fig. 10.5** Photomicrograph of the cell population in the pulp proper. Fibroblasts (arrows) are identifiable, but other cell types, exclusive of inflammatory cells, as described below, are generally very difficult to identify in routine haematoxylin- and eosin-stained sections. Nerve tissue (N) and small blood vessels (B arrow) are also seen in this micrograph. (Courtesy Professor David F Wilson, Adelaide, Australia)

toblasts move towards the pulp, these processes lengthen and the dentine thickness increases. As teeth age, the process of intratubular dentine formation occurs, resulting in the gradual retraction of odontoblastic processes towards the pulp.

An active odontoblast has a large nucleus in its basal part and a Golgi apparatus in its apical part. In the cell body, mitochondria and rough-surface endoplasmic reticulum are scattered. During development, members of the transforming growth factor (TGF)-beta family control the synthetic activity of odontoblasts. Odontoblasts can produce pro-inflammatory mediators such as lipopolysaccharides and cytokines (interleukin-8) in response to bacterial toxins. They also act as sensory receptors by passing information from the outer dentine to nerve fibres in the periphery of the pulp. Some types of junctional complexes exist between adjacent odontoblasts: desmosomes (adhering junctions), gap junctions, and tight junctions. Desmosomes maintain positional relationships between odontoblasts; gap junctions participate in the intercellular communication and passage of small molecules, and tight junctions constitute predentine–pulp barrier and permeability.

10.3.2 Fibroblasts

Fibroblasts are the most abundant cell type in the pulp (■ Fig. 10.5). They form a loose network of cells linked by adherence type and gap junctions. Fibroblasts produce extracellular collagen fibres and ground substance for the pulp tissue. They have a stellate (star-shaped) shape and extensive processes. In young pulp tissue, fibroblasts show a centrally located large oval nucleus and cytoplasm containing intra-cellular Golgi apparatus, rough-surface endoplasmic reticulum, and mitochondria. In the ageing pulp, fibroblasts are smaller and spindle-shaped, with few organelles. In inflammatory conditions, fibroblasts can secrete angiogenic factors such as fibroblast growth factor 2 (FGF-2) and vascular endothelial growth factor (VEGF) to promote healing.

10.3.3 Undifferentiated Mesenchymal Cells

Undifferentiated mesenchymal cells (stem cells) are abundant in young pulp tissue. They are polyhedral in shape and larger than fibroblasts, with peripheral processes and prominent nuclei. They are predominantly found in the cell-rich zone along the blood vessels. When needed, they can differentiate into odontoblasts, fibroblasts, or macrophages.

10.3.4 Defence Cells

Defence cells in pulp tissue include T lymphocytes, macrophages, dendritic cells, mast cells, and plasma cells. Lymphocytes are present in small numbers; they increase when the pulp is inflamed due to toxins or trauma. Macrophages are involved in eliminating dead cells and other tissue components. Dendritic cells capture foreign antigens and present them to lymphocytes. Dendritic cells are closely associated with vascular and neural elements. In inflammatory conditions, other blood-derived cellular elements appear in the pulp, including neutrophils, eosinophils, basophils, plasma cells, and mast cells.

10.4 Fibres

Fibres in pulp tissue are principally type 1 and type 3 collagen fibres, which exist in the extracellular matrix surrounding the cells. Collagen is predominantly produced by pulpal fibroblasts. Type 4 collagen is non-fibrous and found in the basement membrane of the blood vessels in the pulp. A small amount of types 5 and 6 collagen fibres are also present in the pulp. Type 1 collagen is also produced by odontoblasts because this type of collagen is found in dentine, which is the product of odontoblasts.

10.5 Ground Substance

Ground substance is a gel-like intercellular substance. It supports the cells and acts as the transport medium for nutrients from the vasculature to the cells and metabolites from the cells to the vasculature. Ground substance is composed of glycosaminoglycans (GAGs), proteoglycans, and water. Four types of GAGs (chondroitin sulphate, dermatan sulphate, heparan sulphate, and hyaluronic acid) exist in the pulp. These are hydrophilic molecules that swell when hydrated, forming a gel that fills the extracellular space. Proteoglycans are functionally diverse molecules formed by the attachment of GAGs to a protein core.

10.6 Vasculature and Lymphatic Supply

The dental pulp is richly vascularised. Its blood supply is derived from the superior and inferior alveolar arteries and drained by the same veins. Small arteries and arterioles enter the pulp via the apical foramina, accompanied by sensory and sympathetic nerve bundles. Within the root canals, they send branches to the periphery. Capillaries are present between and below the odontoblastic cell layers and between the odontoblastic layer and predentine. Veins and venules are also present in the pulp, and venous–venous anastomosis and arteriole–venous anastomosis occur. The terminal network of capillaries is present in the coronal pulp tissue.

Lymphatic vessels are more abundant in the central part of the pulp than in the peripheral part. Lymphatic drainage from the anterior teeth drains into the submental lymph nodes, and those draining the posterior teeth drain into the submandibular and cervical lymph nodes.

10.7 Nerves of the Dental Pulp

The dental pulp is innervated. Nerve bundles run centrally in the pulp of the root (◘ Fig. 10.6). These follow the blood vessels closely. Some fibres from the central bundle in the root travel to the periphery. Coronal pulp is heavily innervated where it ends in the odontoblastic or sub-odontoblastic regions. The plexus of nerves beneath the odontoblastic region is known as the plexus of Raschkow, which becomes evident after the tooth has erupted. Branches from this plexus pass into the odontoblastic layer, between the odontoblastic layer and pre-

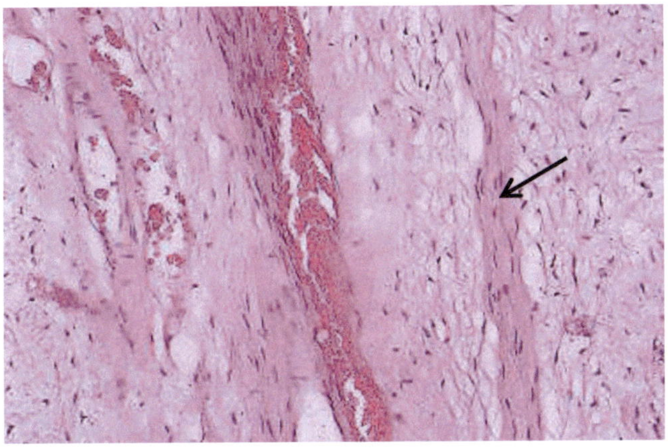

◘ **Fig. 10.6** Larger nerve branches (arrow) and blood vessels are seen in the tooth root canal. These branch into smaller structures as the dentine is approached. (Courtesy Professor David F Wilson, Adelaide, Australia)

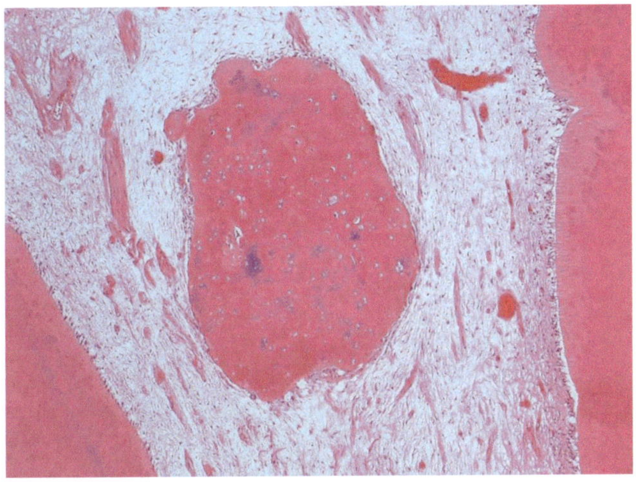

◘ **Fig. 10.7** Photomicrograph showing a discrete pulp stone within the soft tissue of the pulp. (Courtesy Professor David F Wilson, Adelaide, Australia)

dentine, accompany odontoblastic processes, and end up in the dentinal tubules. Nerve fibre types in the pulp include afferent nociceptors and autonomic fibres.

Afferent nociceptors carry the sensation of sharp pain centrally. Afferent nociceptors include three classes: thermal nociceptors, mechanical nociceptors, and polymodal nociceptors. Thermal nociceptors are activated by extremes of temperature, mechanical nociceptors by intense pressure applied to the pulp tissue, and polymodal nociceptors by high-intensity mechanical, chemical, or thermal stimuli. The cell bodies of nociceptor neurons are found in the trigeminal ganglion.

Autonomic fibres are sympathetic efferents supplying smooth muscles of arterioles. They mediate the vasoconstrictive effect. The vaso-dilation in the pulp is caused by axon reflexes involving afferent nerves.

10.8 Age Changes in the Dental Pulp

As age advances, dental pulp shrinks in size because of continuous deposition of secondary dentine at a slow rate. Pulp is less vascular and more fibrous. The neural innervation is reduced, and mineralised deposits (pulp stones) are often seen in older pulps (◘ Fig. 10.7). Large pulp stones can be detected on radiographs.

10.9 Summary

The dental pulp is the soft connective tissue that occupies the central cavity of the tooth. It consists of fibroblasts, odontoblasts, undifferentiated mesenchymal cells (stem cells), and defence cells embedded in a collagenous and ground substance matrix. The fibrous component comprises a combination of collagen types 1 and 3. The ground substance comprises a non-fibrous matrix consisting of glycosaminoglycans and glycoproteins. Odontoblasts form dentine, whereas fibroblasts form loose fibrous connective tissue. Undifferentiated mesenchymal cells are multi-potent and, when needed, can differentiate into fibroblasts, odontoblasts, or macrophages. Defence cells include lymphocytes, macrophages, and antigen-presenting dendritic cells. Dental pulp has a rich blood and nerve supply. Age changes in the dental pulp result in more fibrous and less vascular tissue and pulp calcifications.

Further Reading

Avery J, Chiego DJ Jr. Dental pulp. In: Avery J, Chiego DJ Jr, editors. Essentials of oral histology and embryology—A clinical approach, 3rd ed. Mosby; 2006. pp. 121–136.

Berkovitz BKB, Holland GR, Moxham BJ. Dental pulp. In: Berkovitz BKB, Holland GR, Moxham BJ, editors. 5th ed. Elsevier; 2018. pp. 176–194.

Joseph B. Histology of the dental pulp. In: Prabhu SR, editor. Textbook of oral and maxillofacial anatomy, histology and embryology. Oxford: Oxford University Press; 2006. p. 223–6.

Kumar GS. Pulp. In. Kumar GS, editor. Orban's oral histology and embryology, 12th ed. Elsevier; 2008. pp. 109–136.

Histology of the Periodontal and Gingival Fibres

G. S. Deepak Pateel and Ooi Der Jiun

Contents

S R Prabhu et al. (eds.), *Oral Histology and Oral Histopathology*, https://doi.org/10.1007/978-3-031-77481-2_11

11.1 Introduction

The teeth in the oral cavity are structurally and functionally anchored to the jawbone through the facilitation of a group of tissues called the periodontium. The periodontium comprises cementum, periodontal ligament (periodontal membrane and alveolo-dental ligament), alveolar bone, and gingiva. The periodontal ligament can be defined as an 'Investing and supporting connective tissue structure by which a tooth and tooth root is anchored within its alveolus; it consists of bands of collagen fibres connecting tooth cementum to both gingival tissue and alveolar bone and the cementum of adjacent teeth'. The aligned fibrous network is responsible for the firm anchorage of the tooth to the bone, provides mechanical stability, and protects the underlying tissues through the absorption of forces. The histology of the periodontal ligament plays an essential role in understanding this crucial functional role of the periodontal ligament (PDL).

11.2 Development and Organisation of Periodontal Ligament

PDL formation occurs synchronously with root, cementum, and alveolar bone formation and tooth eruption. Periodontal ligament formation can be briefly explained under three headings: (1) differentiation of PDL-forming cells, (2) formation of Sharpey's fibres, and (3) establishment of continuous-anchoring fibrous bands.

11.2.1 Differentiation of PDL-Forming Cells

Development of the periodontal ligament begins after the formation of the crown of the tooth. With the completion of crown formation, the outer and inner enamel epithelia proliferate at the cervical ends of the tooth germ to form a cervical loop. Root formation begins with the activation and proliferation of the cervical loop. The activated portion will now be referred to as Hertwig's epithelial root sheath (HERS), and the bent terminal end portion of the HERS will be referred to as the epithelial diaphragm. HERS plays a vital role in the formation of root and periodontal ligaments. They stimulate the peripheral cells of the dental papilla (DP), adjacent to them, to differentiate as odontoblasts and form root dentin on the medial aspect, similar to coronal dentin formation (◘ Fig. 11.1a). At the same time, the outer aspect of the HERS, the dental follicle (DF), is stimulated and gets differentiated into dental follicle inner (DFI), middle (DFM), and outer (DFO) cells. These cells differentiate into cementoblasts, fibroblasts, and osteoblasts, forming the cementum, periodontal ligament, and alveolar bone, respectively (◘ Fig. 11.1a, b).

11.2.2 Formation of Sharpey's Fibres

Activated DFM cells differentiate into fibroblasts and produce collagen fibres, which insert into the simultaneously forming cementum on one side and alveolar bone on the other side. The fibres anchored to the cementum and bone are called Sharpey's fibres. The formation of Sharpey's fibres starts at the tooth side first (◘ Fig. 11.2a). The formation of cementum involves the deposition of a matrix perpendicular to the orientation of cementum fibres on the newly formed root dentin. The deposited matrix becomes mineralised, leaving small spicules of collagen fibres unmineralised and protruding into the PDL space. The fibres of the periodontal ligament then become attached to these areas to form Sharpey's fibres. On the bone side, the PDL fibres attach to the bone matrix during the remodelling phase rather than in the newly formed matrix (◘ Fig. 11.2b).

11.2.3 Establishment of Continuous-Anchoring Fibrous Bands

The formation of PDL undergoes a continuous process of degradation and regeneration, which facilitates and is required during the eruption of teeth. The periodontal ligament structure gets organised when occlusal contact is established. During the initial phases of occlusal contact, the PDL fibres from the cementum and alveolar bone become thicker and meet each other. However, the central zone remains distinguishable (◘ Fig. 11.3a). As the occlusion is established, the fibres become thicker and more densely packed, resulting in fully mature and continuous-anchoring PDL fibre bundles (◘ Fig. 11.3b and 11.4). These developments begin with the dentogingival and transeptal fibres, which are near the cervical region. The development continues further in the downward direction, from the cervical region of the root towards the alveolar bone until the apex of the tooth with the PDL fibre arrangement. The entire process is analogous to the formation of root formation.

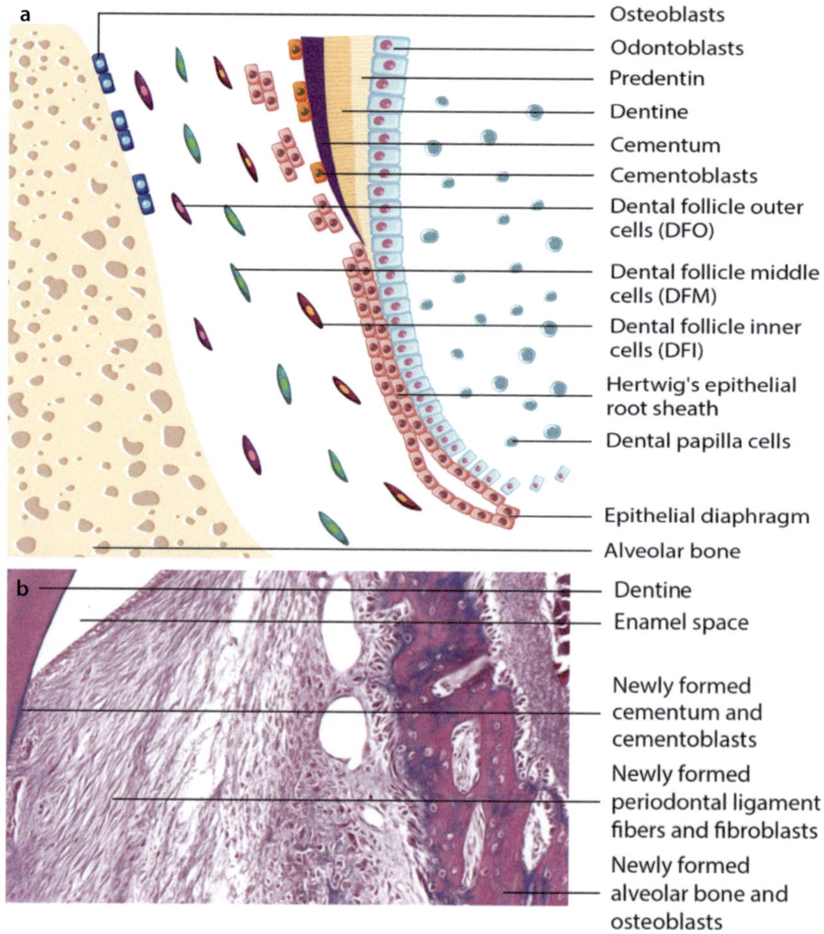

Fig. 11.1 **a** Schematic representation of differentiation of cells during the formation of periodontal ligament. **b** Histological features of the early periodontal ligament formation

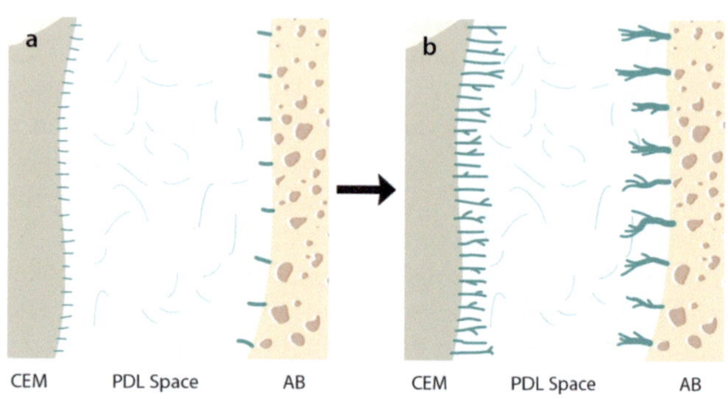

Fig. 11.2 Schematic representation of the formation of PDL fibres. CEM is cementum, PDL is periodontal ligament, and AB is alveolar bone

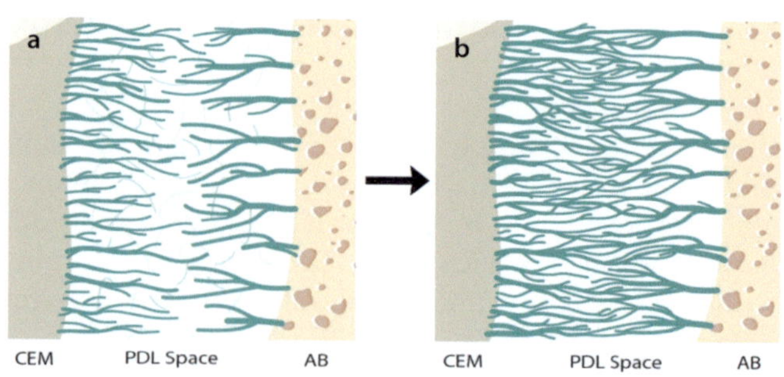

Fig. 11.3 Schematic representation of establishment of PDL fibres. CEM is cementum, PDL is periodontal ligament, and AB is alveolar bone

11.3 Structure of the Periodontal Ligament

The PDL is primarily composed of two components: the fibres and cells. The fibres are predominantly composed of type I collagen fibres. Types 3 and 12 are also present, especially during the remodelling and organisation of PDL fibres, respectively. Small amounts of types 5 and 6 are also reported to be associated with PDL.

Type 1 collagen is found in close aggregates of approximately 5 μm-diameter bundles, which are referred to as principal fibres. Several distinct groups of periodontal fibres are established at specific locations of the PDL and are referred to as the principal group of periodontal ligament fibres (▶ Fig. 6.4).

The principal fibres of periodontal ligament are composed of five types: (1) alveolar crest fibres, (2) horizontal fibres, (3) oblique fibres, (4) apical fibres, and (5) interradicular fibres (◻ Fig. 11.5).

11.3.1 Alveolar Crest Fibres

The alveolar crest fibres are oriented obliquely and extend from the cementum below the cemento-enamel junction to the crest of the alveolar process (◻ Fig. 11.6).

Function: These fibres resist occlusal forces, which can be either intrusive or extrusive forces applied to the tooth. They may also resist lateral tilting forces.

11.3.2 Horizontal Fibres

The horizontal fibres located apical to the alveolar crest are oriented almost horizontally and extend from the cementum to the alveolar bone. They are commonly found underneath the crest of the alveolar bone until the middle third of the root (◻ Fig. 11.7). These fibres resist lateral displacement of the tooth.

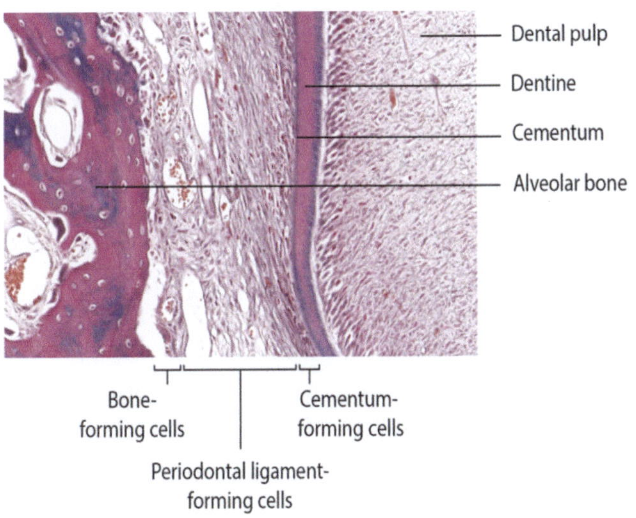

◻ **Fig. 11.4** Histology section of root development of tooth showing the establishment of PDL fibres

11.3.3 Oblique Fibres

Oblique fibres are located apically to horizontal fibres and extend to the apical third of the tooth. They constitute the most numerous fibres of the PDL. They run from the alveolar bone in a diagonal apical direction towards the cementum (◻ Fig. 11.8). These fibres resist intrusive forces subjected to the tooth during mastication.

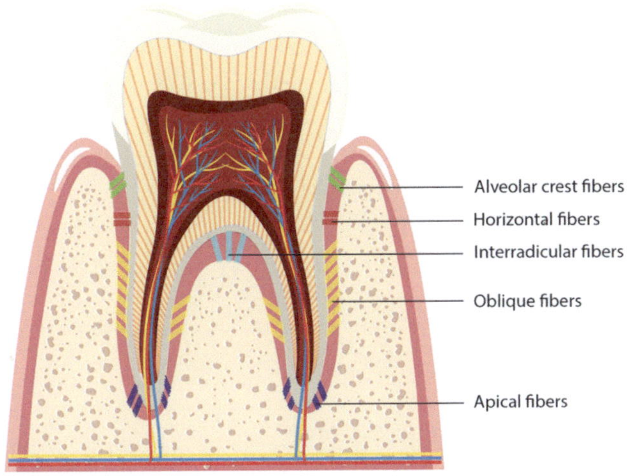

◻ **Fig. 11.5** Schematic representation of the principal fibres of PDL

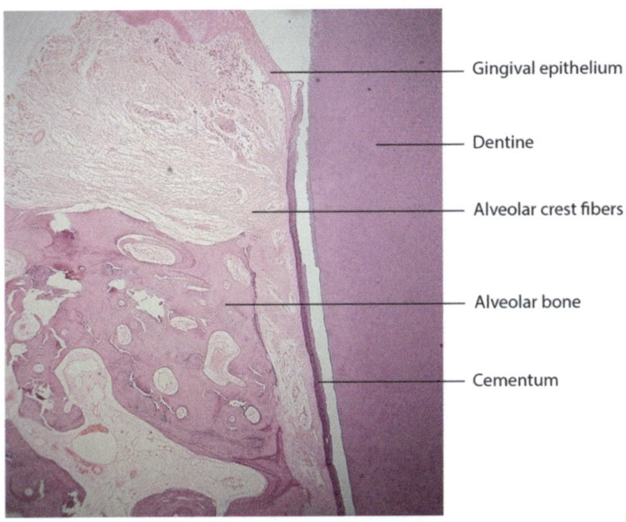

◻ **Fig. 11.6** Principal periodontal fibres. Histological section of tooth showing alveolar crest fibres of the PDL. (*Please note that the gap between dentin and cementum is an artefact*)

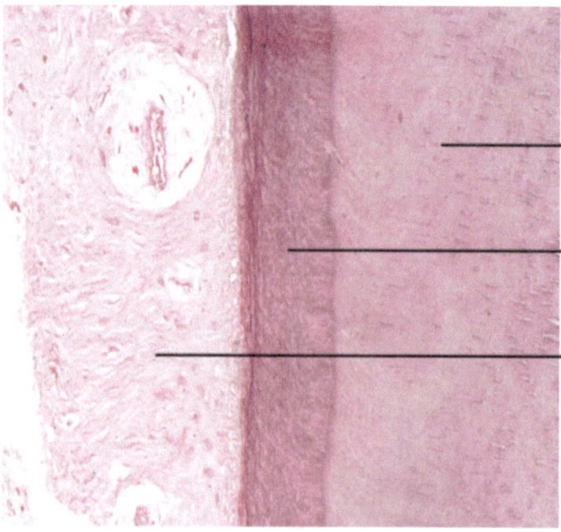

Fig. 11.7 Principal periodontal fibres. Histological section of tooth showing horizontal fibres of the PDL

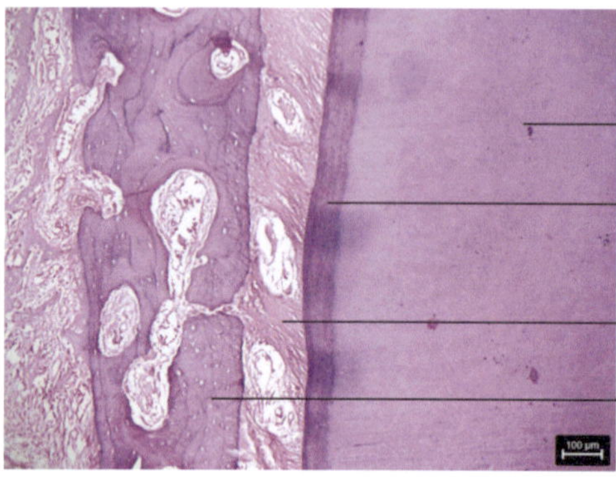

Fig. 11.8 Principal periodontal fibres. A histological section of a tooth shows oblique fibres of the PDL. (Reproduced with permission of Dr. Pooja Kamath, DY Patil University School of Dentistry, Navi-Mumbai, India)

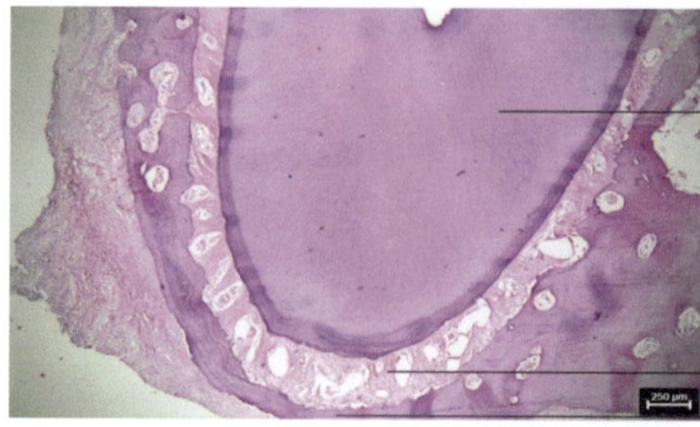

Fig. 11.9 Principal periodontal fibres. Histological section of tooth showing apical fibres of the PDL. (Reproduced with permission of Dr. Pooja Kamath DY Patil University School of Dentistry, Navi-Mumbai. India)

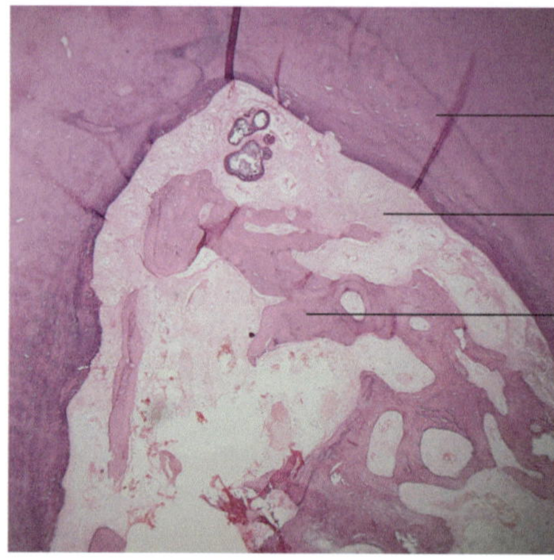

Fig. 11.10 Principal periodontal fibres. A histological section of a tooth shows interradicular fibres of the PDL. (Reproduced with permission of Dr. Harshvardhan S. Jois, India)

11.3.4 Apical Fibres

The apical fibres are located at the base of the socket and radiate from the cementum to the fundus of the alveolar bone (Fig. 11.9). These fibres prevent the tooth from being displaced in the occlusal or incisal direction, tipping, and damage to the nerves and blood vessels at the apical area of the tooth.

11.3.5 Interradicular Fibres

Interradicular fibres in the multi-rooted teeth extend from the crest of the alveolar bone to the cementum between the roots of the teeth (Fig. 11.10). These fibres also resist occlusal forces and prevent the luxation of the tooth.

11.3.6 Oxytalan Fibres of the PDL

The PDL also incorporates a subordinate fibre system comprising oxytalan fibres. The ultra-structural features of these fibres indicate that these fibres are immature elastic fibres. They are predominantly seen to run longitudinally in the PDL proper and cross the oblique fibres. These fibres are believed to stabilise the blood vessels as they are found to be associated with them.

11.4 Gingival Group of Fibres

Another distinct group of fibres associated with the gingiva's lamina propria is the gingival group of fibres. These fibres are discussed here as they play a role in maintaining the integrity of the periodontium. However, they are not strictly a part of the periodontal ligament

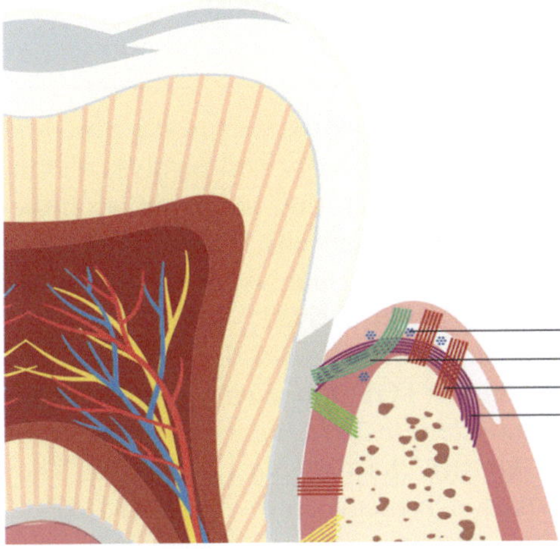

■ **Fig. 11.11** Schematic diagram of gingival fibres

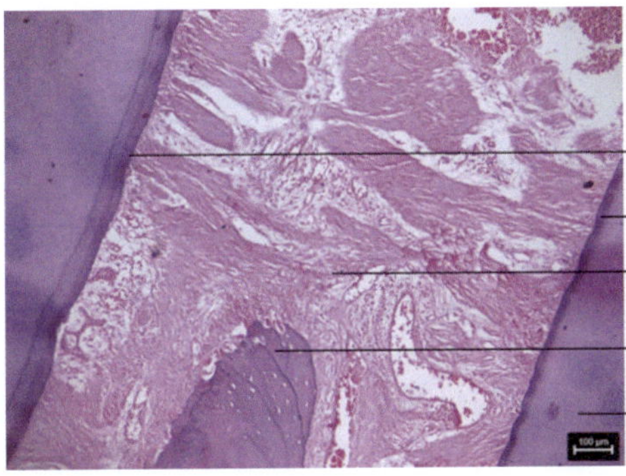

■ **Fig. 11.12** Histological section of tooth showing a transseptal group of fibres. (Reproduced with permission of Dr. Pooja Kamath, Dr. Treville Pereira, DY Patil University School of Dentistry, Navi-Mumbai, India)

(■ Fig. 11.11). The five groups of gingival fibres are described below:

11.4.1 Dentogingival Fibres

Dentogingival fibres are the most numerous gingival fibres that extend into the lamina propria of free and attached gingiva from the cervical cementum. These fibres help hold the gums around the tooth's cervical portion (■ Figs. 11.11 and 11.12).

11.4.2 Alveologingival Fibres

Alveologingival fibres radiate from the alveolar crest into the lamina propria of the free and attached gingiva. These fibres also serve to hold the free gingiva around the tooth (■ Figs. 11.11 and 11.12).

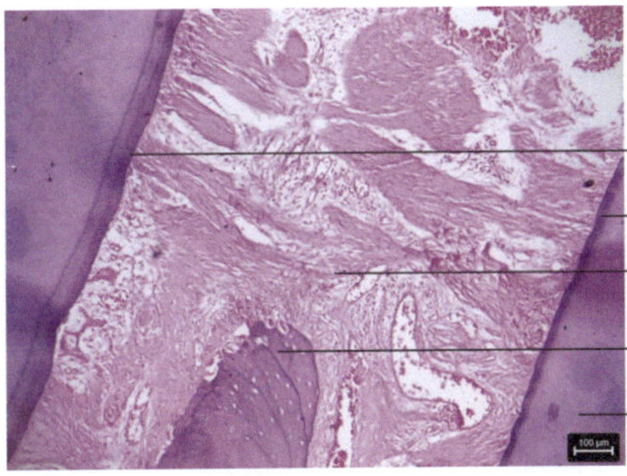

■ **Fig. 11.13** Histological section of tooth showing dentogingival and circular group of fibres. (Reproduced with permission of Dr. Harshvardhan S. Jois)

11.4.3 Dentoperiosteal Fibres

Dentoperiosteal fibres extend across the alveolar crest from the cementum and insert into the periodontium of the outer cortical plates of the alveolar process (■ Fig. 11.11).

Circular fibres form a band around the cervical portion of the tooth. They intermingle with the other fibres in this region and help bind the gingiva against the tooth (■ Figs. 11.11 and 11.12).

11.4.4 Transseptal Fibres

Transseptal fibres extend from one tooth's cementum to the adjacent tooth's cementum, crossing the alveolar bone's crest. These fibres act as transseptal ligaments, stabilising the interdental region (■ Fig. 11.13).

11.5 Cellular Composition of PDL and Ground Substance

Like most connective tissues, the PDL comprises fibroblasts, cementoblasts, osteoblasts, and inflammatory cells admixed within the fibrous tissue. Fibroblasts are the most prominent cells seen in the PDL. They are required to continuously renew the fibrous support system to maintain the adaptive response system to the occlusal load. Fibroblasts are arranged parallel to the fibres and contain abundant cell organelles associated with protein synthesis, responsible for the active secretion of collagen and the required matrix. The fibroblast can be seen uniformly distributed throughout the PDL and possesses well-developed cytoskeleton and gap junctions, which actively communicate with collagen fibres. Periodontal fibroblasts are also accountable and equipped for collagen degradation. The fibroblasts are known to possess cilia, which are believed to control the cell cycle.

11.6 Cells and Ground Substance

▪ Epithelial Cells

Remnants of Hertwig's epithelial root sheath (HERS) cells, referred to as cell rests of Malassez, can be seen in the PDL tissue. The rest cells are seen as closely packed clusters of cells separated from the rest of the tissue by the basal lamina. The cell rests of Malassez can be the source of pathological lesions and give rise to odontogenic cysts and tumours in the jawbones.

▪ Bone and Cementum Cells

PDL tissue also consists of osteoblasts, osteocytes, cementoblasts, and cementocytes. A cellular layer of osteoblasts is seen on the periodontal surface of the alveolar bone, and then, cementoblasts are noted on the periodontal surface of the cementum. These cells will be discussed in their respective topics.

▪ Defence Cells

Defence cells are mainly composed of macrophages, mast cells, and eosinophils. They are similar to defence cells in other connective tissues.

▪ Progenitor Cells

PDL tissue, analogous to other connective tissues, has progenitor cells that can divide and differentiate into required cells. These cells are believed to be responsible for the periodontal regeneration and repair process associated with periodontium.

▪ Ground Substance

The ground substance or the extracellular matrix (ECM) mainly comprises water, glycoproteins, and proteoglycans, which surround the collagen fibres and cells. These act as a medium and aid in exchanging nutrients from the blood capillaries like any other connective tissue. The PDL ground substance is estimated to be 70% water, and its composition is subject to the functional status of the PDL. An increase in the fluid and matrix is associated with an increase in the function of the PDL.

11.7 Mechanism of Periodontal Homeostasis

The turnover of periodontal tissue (production and destruction) happens continuously and involves a complex interaction of molecules that are mainly synthesised by fibroblasts and other cells. The cells produce growth factors and cytokines such as fibroblast growth factors (FGFs), platelet-derived growth factors (PDGFs), insulin-like growth factor 1 (IGF-1), transforming growth factors (TGFs), bone morphogenic protein (BMP), and interleukin-1 (IL-1), which are believed to monitor and control the fibroblast cell cycle. They actively secrete the matrix metalloproteinase-1(MMP-1), TGF-β, and tissue inhibitors of matrix metalloproteinases (TIMPs), which control collagen production by the fibroblasts. Cellular homeostasis within tissues is achieved through a delicate equilibrium involving intricate interactions between opposing and cooperative molecules, in which cytokines, metalloproteinases (MMPs), and natural MMP inhibitors play pivotal roles.

These molecules have specific functions that play a role in the maintenance of periodontal homeostasis in many ways, as mentioned below:

- The FGFs stimulate cell division, collagen synthesis, angiogenesis, osteogenesis, and cell migration.
- PGDF stimulates cell migration and cell division.
- TGF-β stimulates the synthesis of connective tissue matrix components, such as collagen, fibronectin, proteoglycan, and glycosaminoglycans.
- IL-1 mediates tissue remodelling, repair, and inflammation.

11.8 Functions of Periodontal Ligament

The functions of the periodontal ligament can be explained under the following aspects:

▪ Supportive

The primary supportive function of the PDL is through the following means mentioned below:

- Transmission of occlusal forces to the bone
- Attachment of the teeth to the bone
- Maintenance of the gingival tissues in their proper relationship to the teeth

- Resisting the impact of occlusal forces (shock absorption)
- Providing a soft-tissue 'casing' to protect the vessels and nerves from injury by mechanical forces

- **Sensory**

The PDL is abundantly supplied with a sound sensory nerve supply capable of transmitting tactile and pressure impulses with appropriate protective responses. The PDL provides a most efficient proprioceptive mechanism, allowing the identification of the amount of force applied, and helps maintain the PDL's health.

- **Homeostasis**

The cells of the periodontal ligament play an essential role in maintaining a balance between constant formation and renewal/remodelling of the PDL collagen fibres, alveolar bone, and cementum to maintain the functional ability of PDL. This is achieved by finely regulated activity of the area's cells to maintain the periodontium's physiological and functional homeostasis. The remarkable ability of the PDL to maintain a constant width of PDL is evidence of this process.

- **Eruptive**

PDL tissue is responsible for and facilitates the eruptive movements of the teeth and post-eruptive movements of the teeth.

11.9 Clinical Application of Periodontal Ligament, Including Age Changes

11.9.1 Age Changes in the Periodontal Ligament

Compared to all other tissues of the body, the PDL also shows common age-related changes. The number of cells and their associated function reduces with advancing age. Loss of gingival health and chronic effects on the periodontium promote destructive changes in the PDL (13).

Calcified masses in the PDL can be noted (◘ Fig. 11.14). Acellular cementum deposits in the PDL, formed due to disrupted appositional growth of cementum, are called cementicles. They are believed to be age-associated and, usually, appear like psammoma bodies, like calcifications in the cementum (◘ Fig. 11.14).

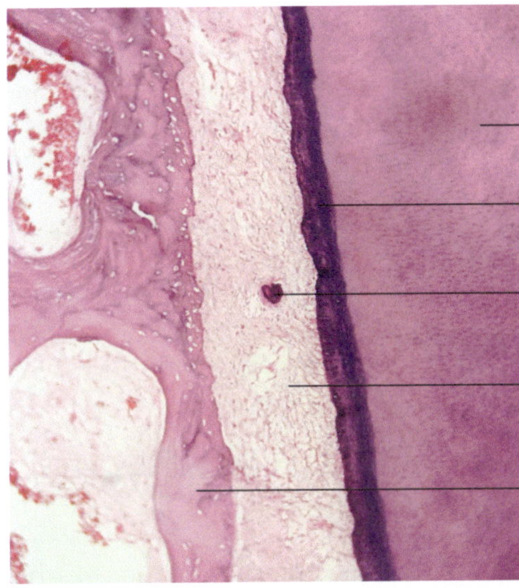

◘ **Fig. 11.14** Histological section of tooth showing calcified masses in the PDL space. (Reproduced with permission of Dr. Harshvardhan S. Jois)

11.9.2 PDL Tissue Adaptation to Functional Demand

PDL can adapt when subjected to an increase in functional demand. Generally, the amount of PDL tissue and the width of the PDL increase and decrease in accordance with the increase and decrease of demand. Such functional stimulation will also result in adaptive changes in adjacent cementum and alveolar bone. The clinical application of this is noted in restorative dentistry when a long-standing, out-of-function tooth and its supporting functions are restored. The associated periodontal tissues need time to adapt to the new functional demand obtained due to the new prosthesis. Orthodontic teeth movement also brings about changes in the functionality of the periodontal tissues, which bring about changes in the functionality of the periodontium and adapt the tooth to its new position.

11.10 Molecular Insights: Mineralisation in PDL

PDL is a specialised connective tissue as it does not undergo calcification under normal circumstances despite being closely associated with alveolar bone and cementum. The PDL also maintains a constant width throughout life despite changes in bone and cementum. This is because of the advanced molecular signalling, which exists in the PDL. Evidence indicates that the prostaglandin, bradykinin, and thrombin, secreted by fibroblasts, may play a role in the inhibition of the mineralisation of the connective tissue. However, ankylosis can happen when this system fails, and PDL gets calcified.

The studies have shown that the mean thickness of the periodontal ligament ranges from 0.15 to 0.38 mm. The PDL is thinnest at the middle portion of the tooth. The thickness varies with the age and function of the tooth.

11.10.1 Molecular Changes of the Ground Substance in the PDL

During periodontal diseases like periodontitis, the molecular composition of the ground substance in the PDL undergoes significant changes. Inflammatory mediators, such as pro-inflammatory cytokines and matrix metalloproteinases, lead to an imbalanced matrix turnover, causing the degradation of critical components like proteoglycans and collagen. These alterations impact the PDL's gel-like consistency and its ability to provide resistance to compressive and tensile forces.

Furthermore, advanced glycation end products and oxidative stress contribute to abnormal collagen cross-linking and tissue damage. Dysregulated fibroblast activity, cell signalling changes, and matrix maintenance enzyme imbalances further disrupt the PDL's structural and functional integrity.

The cumulative effect of these molecular changes in the PDL's ground substance results in the breakdown of periodontal tissues, leading to tooth mobility and, in severe cases, tooth loss. Understanding the molecular components of the ground substance and how they interact is essential for periodontics researchers and clinicians to develop effective treatments and therapies for maintaining healthy periodontal tissues and preventing tooth loss.

11.11 Periodontal Pathology

Inflammation from the pulp spreads to the apical periodontal ligament and brings about inflammatory changes at that location. Some examples are apical periodontitis, periapical granuloma, abscess, and cyst formation.

Finally, the most common clinical implication of PDL tissue is inflammation-induced periodontal disease. The polymorphic nature of the etiological factors and the host immune response is associated with diverse variations related to susceptibility to periodontal disease and response to the disease progression.

11.12 Summary

The periodontal ligament is an indispensable component of the dentition and the periodontium. It plays an essential role in providing stability to the teeth and attachment of the teeth to the bone. Its unique structural and functional characteristics make it an essential tissue in maintaining oral health and tooth function. Understanding the basic structure and functions of the PDL is vital for dental students and professionals.

Acknowledgements

The authors would like to thank the contributors, mentioned below, for the histological pictures of the chapter.

1. Dr. Pooja Kamath, Dr. Treville Pereira. DY Patil University School of Dentistry, Navi-Mumbai. India.
2. Schematic Pictures have been designed using assets from ▶ Freepik.com.
3. Dr. Harshvardhan S. Jois, Professor And Head, Dept of Oral Pathology & Microbiology, Army College of Dental Sciences, Hyderabad, Telangana, India.

Further Reading

Beertsen W, Mcculloch CAG, Sodek J. The periodontal ligament: a unique, multifunctional connective tissue. Periodontol 2000. 1997;13(1):20–40. https://doi.org/10.1111/j.1600-0757.1997.tb00094.x.

Berkovitz BKB, Moxham BJ, Newman HN. The periodontal ligament in health and disease 1982:470.

Berkovitz BKB, Holland GR, Moxham BJ. Oral anatomy, histology, and embryology. p. 462.

Birk DE, Zycband E. Assembly of the tendon extracellular matrix during development. J Anat. 1994;184(Pt 3):457.

Bosshardt DD, Schroeder HE. Cementogenesis reviewed: a comparison between human premolars and rodent molars. Anat Rec. 1996;245:267–92. https://doi.org/10.1002/(SICI)1097-0185(199606)245:2<267::AID-AR12>3.0.CO;2-N.

Coolidge ED. The thickness of the human periodontal membrane. J Am Dent Assoc Dent Cosm. 1937;24(8):1260–70.

de Jong T, Bakker AD, Everts V, Smit TH. The intricate anatomy of the periodontal ligament and its development: lessons for periodontal regeneration. J Periodontal Res. 2017;52(6):965–74. https://doi.org/10.1111/jre.12477.

Grant D, Bernick S. Formation of the periodontal ligament. J Periodontol. 1972;43(1):17–25. https://doi.org/10.1902/jop.1972.43.1.17.

Hand AR, Frank ME. Fundamentals of oral histology and physiology. https://www.wiley.com/en-sg/Fundamentals+of+Oral+Histology+and+Physiology-p-9781118342916.

Johnson R, Martinez RH. Synthesis of Sharpey's fiber proteins within rodent alveolar bone. Scanning Microsc. 1998;12(2):317–27. https://www.ecmjournal.org/smi/pdf/smi98-2-06.pdf.

Kumar GS. Orban's oral histology & embryology. 2011. https://www.elsevier.com/books/orbans-oral-histology-and-embryology/kumar/978-81-312-2819-7.

Mikola OJ, Bauer WH. Cementicles and fragments of cementum in the periodontal membrane. Oral Surg Oral Med Oral Pathol. 1949;2(8):1063–74. https://doi.org/10.1016/0030-4220(49)90220-0.

Nanci A. Ten Cate's oral histology: development, structure, and function. Mosby; 2012. p. 344.

Periodontal ligament: definition of periodontal ligament by Medical dictionary. https://medical-dictionary.thefreedictionary.com/periodontal+ligament.

Reed DA, Diekwisch TGH. Morphogenesis and wound healing in the periodontium. Stem Cell Biol Tissue Eng Dent Sci. 2015:445–58.

Histology of Bone and the Jawbones

Shankargouda Patil, Vidya Gurram Shankar, and David F Wilson

Contents

S R Prabhu et al. (eds.), *Oral Histology and Oral Histopathology*, https://doi.org/10.1007/978-3-031-77481-2_12

12.1 Introduction

Bone is a porous, mineralised, and specialised connective tissue, which makes up the skeleton of the body. It is one of the hardest body structures and is endowed with elasticity and the power of regeneration and repair. In this chapter, the various forms of bone and their associated terminology at macroscopic and microscopic levels are described.

12.2 Functions of Bone

- Structural function: Bone provides shape, support, and a framework to the body, is the site of attachment for muscles and tendons and protects vital organs such as the lungs, heart, and brain.
- Metabolic function: Bone is involved in the maintenance of mineral homeostasis in the body.
- Locomotion function: Individual bones of the skeleton provide levers for muscles and ligaments and, thus contribute to body movement.
- Reservoir function: The skeleton is a repository for cytokines and growth factors such as insulin-like growth factors (IGFs), transforming growth factor-beta (TGF-β) and bone morphogenetic proteins (BMPs). Bones are also reserve sites for minerals such as calcium and phosphate and house the red and yellow bone marrows.

12

12.3 General Structure of Bone

As a tissue, bone is made up of a calcified organic matrix and supporting soft, fibrous connective tissue (bone stroma) constituents. The latter provides the required neurovascular and lymphatic tissues and also acts as a reservoir for the precursors of bone cells. The calcified component of bone is made up of calcium hydroxyapatite crystals (Ca5(PO4)3OH) (67%) embedded in an organic matrix (33%). The organic component consists of 28% collagen, chiefly type 1 collagen and the remaining 5% of non-collagenous proteins. The non-collagenous proteins are either of an endogenous source (produced by bone cells) and include osteocalcin, osteopontin, bone sialoprotein and osteonectin or derived from a non-endogenous source.

12.4 Histological Methods Used to Study Bone

Understanding and being able to visualise the physiological and pathological microstructure of bone are of immense importance for better understanding normal bone biology, diagnosis of bone diseases and evaluation of biomaterial or drug effects. In addition, knowledge of bone structure is important in anthropology, medico-legal cases and in forensics.

Bone sections for light microscopic examination are of two types:

- Ground sections, which are thin sections of undecalcified bone that are produced using various techniques
- Decalcified sections, which are produced by the process of removing the mineralised matrix from the organic matrix of bone, making it comparatively soft and flexible, enabling easy sectioning of the specimen using routine histological techniques. The common decalcifying agents used are strong mineral acids, weaker organic acids and cheating agents. Decalcified sections can be stained with conventional dyes and immunohistochemically.

Histological stains that can be used to stain bone sections include:

- Haematoxylin and eosin: Bone stains a pink colour.
- Toluidine blue O: If mineralised, bone stains dark blue, and if non-mineralised, bone stains pale blue.
- Methylene blue/acid fuchsin: Bone stains bright pink and surrounding soft tissues stain blue–purple.
- Masson trichrome stain.
- Von Kossa/Van Gieson stain: It distinguishes mineralised bone matrix (stained black) from non-mineralised matrix (stained red).
- Alizarin red: It is specific for bone (stained red).
- Immunohistochemical stains.
- Histochemical stains: Examples are tartrate-resistant acid phosphatase (TRAP) and alkaline phosphatase.

12.5 Classification of Bone Types and Terminologies Applied to Bone

Bones may be broadly described using various criteria, such as (a) on their gross morphology (e.g. long, flat, short and irregular bones); (b) development origin (e.g. endochondral or intramembranous) and (c) microscopic appearance.

The nomenclature (terminology) applied to bone depends upon whether a bone is being examined macroscopically (i.e. with the naked eye) or microscopically. When describing "a bone", a particular terminology is applied. The outer zone of a bone is referred to as the cortex (◘ Fig. 12.1a) and is a variably thick layer of dense, compact bone called cortical bone. The dense cortical bone encloses less dense bone (medullary bone) made up of a network of relatively fine, interconnected trabeculae of bone (◘ Fig. 12.1b), fibrous connective tissue and, depending upon patient age, haematopoietic

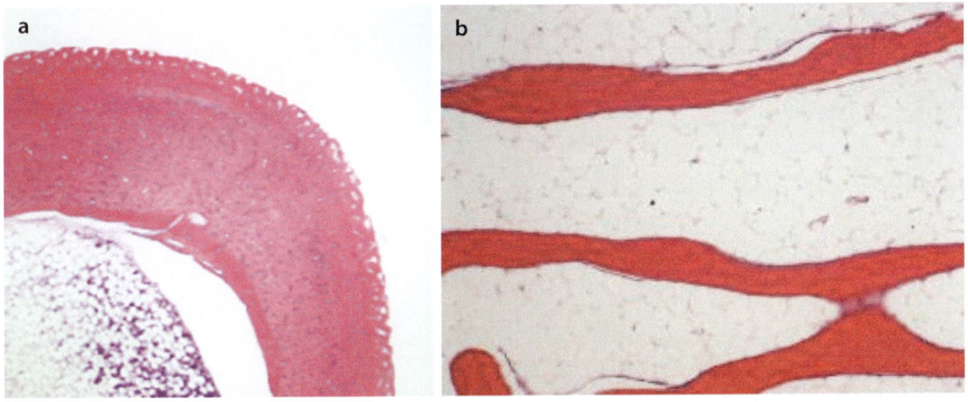

Fig. 12.1 Decalcified bone sections. **a** Low-power image of the cortex of a bone showing that it is composed of dense (compact) bone. **b** Photomicrograph of medullary bone showing that it is composed of thin trabeculae of bone. In this case, the stromal tissue consists of fatty marrow

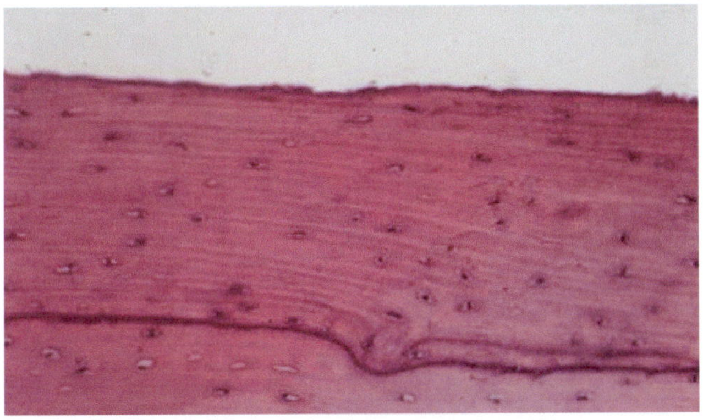

Fig. 12.2 Decalcified bone showing parallel arrays of thin bone lamellae on an outer cortical surface. Note that the osteocytes are aligned along the lamellae

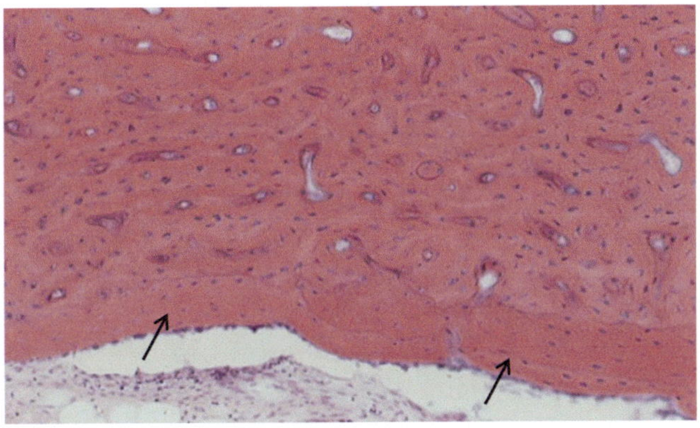

Fig. 12.3 Decalcified bone showing lamellar bone (arrow) lining the endosteal surface of a bone. The remainder of the bone in the photomicrograph consists of lamellar bone in the Haversian pattern

or fatty marrow. Macroscopically, the medullary bone can also be referred to as "cancellous bone", "trabecular bone" or "spongy bone".

When being described microscopically, a different terminology is employed. At this level, the following terms are used to describe the bone type observed:

- Lamellar bone
- Woven bone
- Bundle bone

In the normal adult skeleton, the greatest majority of bones is lamellar bone. This form of bone makes up both the cortex and trabeculae of individual bones. Lamellar bone is so called because its basic structure is that of multiple, tightly packed and repeating layers with aligned osteocytes. Two basic patterns of lamellar bone can be microscopically observed. The first pattern can be seen on the outer (periosteal) surface of bones (Fig. 12.2) and, sometimes, lining the inner (endosteal) cortical surface (Fig. 12.3).

The second pattern of lamellar bone is called Haversian bone. Histologically, this type of bone is characterised by tightly packed and concentrically arranged lamellae, formed around individual central canals called Haversian canals (Fig. 12.4), which provide the bone with a neurovascular supply and, hence, its vitality. Each Haversian unit is called an osteon. Osteons are characterised by their concentric lamellae and osteocytes aligned at the junctions between each lamella. Osteocytes reside in "spaces" called lacunae and interconnect with one another by means of very fine channels called canaliculi. Because of constant bone remodelling, osteons can have an irregular shape and vary in size. Areas between osteons are filled with parallel lamellae called interstitial lamellae (Fig. 12.5). The details of Haversian bone are best seen in undecalcified sections.

Woven bone can occur in various situations:

- During embryogenesis

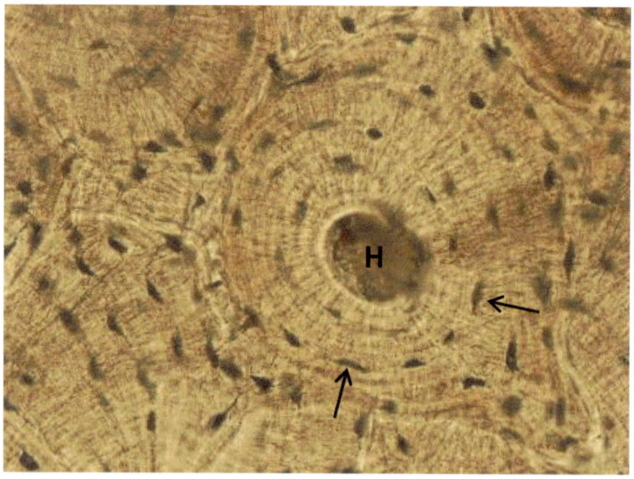

Fig. 12.4 Undecalcified bone section. An approximately circular-shaped osteon can be seen characterised by a central Haversian canal (H) surrounded by circular, concentric lamellae containing aligned osteocytes (arrows)

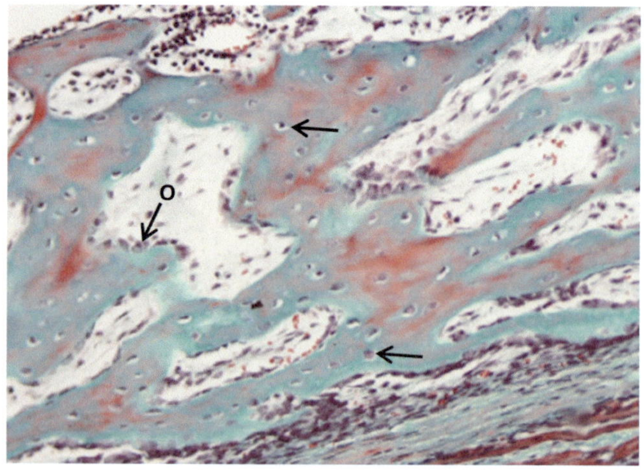

Fig. 12.6 Woven bone. Decalcified section showing interconnected trabeculae of woven bone with dispersed osteocytes (arrows). Osteoblasts (O arrow) are seen lining some regions of the trabeculae

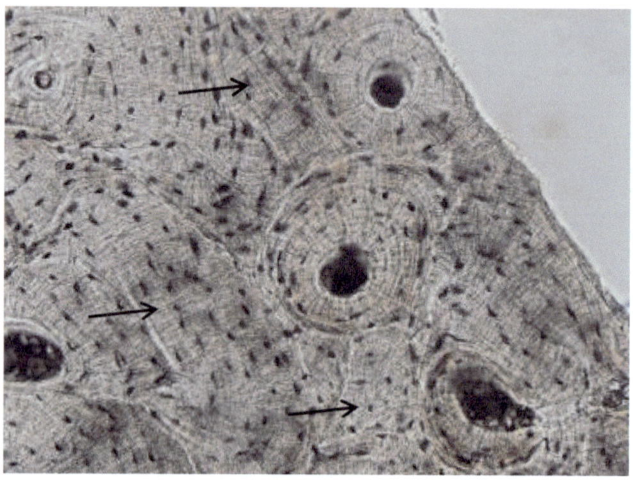

Fig. 12.5 Undecalcified bone section. Interstitial lamellae (arrows) are seen between variously sized osteons

- During bone healing
- In a range of non-neoplastic bone diseases
- In bone tumours

Woven bone (Fig. 12.6) is a rapidly formed bone and is the predominant type of bone seen in the forming skeleton during embryogenesis where skeletal bone formation is occurring by the process of endochondral ossification, for instance, in long bones, (Fig. 12.7) or in parts of the skeleton where bone formation begins with a framework of woven bone. Woven bone is also found in healing-fracture and tooth-socket sites and in a variety of pathological lesions of bone. Histologically, woven bone consists of irregularly shaped and sized trabeculae of condensed collagen matrix that lacks the osteon/lamella structure of adult lamellar bone.

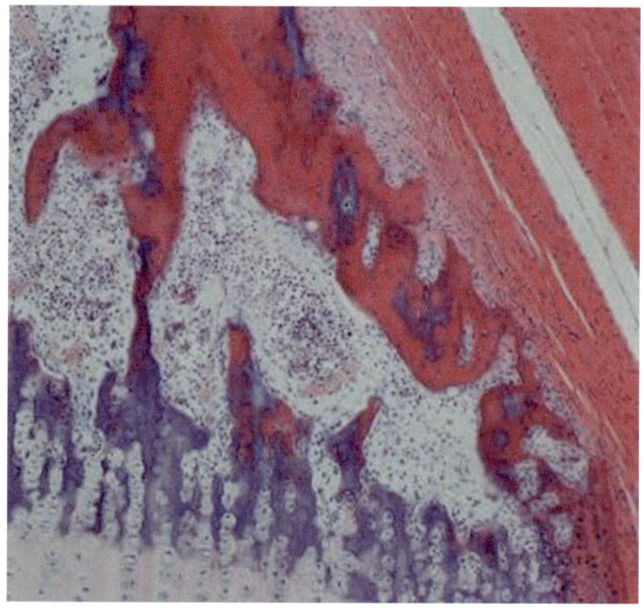

Fig. 12.7 Photomicrograph showing woven bone (red) replacing cartilage (blue) during the process of endochondral ossification in a long bone. The woven bone is later replaced by mature lamellar–Haversian bone as the skeleton develops. The description "bundle bone" is applied to a thin layer of bone lining the tooth sockets of the alveolus of both the mandible and maxilla. The histological features of this type of bone are described in section 12.8

Depending upon the rate at which woven bone is being laid down, it may appear as a relatively coarse collagenous matrix or a relatively homogeneous matrix in decalcified, haematoxylin- and eosin-stained sections. Also, depending upon whether or not the woven bone is being actively formed (e.g. as in a healing bone fracture/tooth socket, a bone tumour and during embryogenesis) or is in a relatively quiescent phase, the periphery of the matrix will be seen to be lined by either plump osteoblasts or flattened osteoblasts or appear to be devoid of matrix-lining cells.

12.6 Cellular Components of Bone

12.6.1 Osteoblasts

Osteoblasts (◘ Fig. 12.8) are the bone-forming cells in both woven bone and lamellar–Haversian bone. The primary function of these cells is to synthesise osteoid, the precursor to mineralised bone, composed predominantly of type 1 collagen. They are derived from osteoprogenitor cells (OPC) of mesenchymal origin, either from the bone marrow, endosteum or periosteum (determined OPC) or from other connective tissues when stimulated (inducible OPC). Osteoblasts are aligned linearly on the bone-forming surfaces or on remodelling bones.

Osteoblasts are mononucleated, differentiated cells that can undergo mitosis. They have well-developed protein production-associated organelles such as Golgi complexes and rough endoplasmic reticulum. Actin, myosin and cytoskeletal proteins are present within the cells, which assist in attachment and cell shape maintenance. Gap junctions occur between osteoblasts, but junctional complexes are lacking. The nucleus is located eccentrically farther away from the bone surface.

Osteoblasts secrete a variety of components—both collagen and non-collagenous proteins—that form osteoids such as type 1 collagen, type 5 collagen, non-collagenous proteins (participate in mineralisation) and cytokines (BMP) and growth factors (IGF) that regulate cellular function and bone formation. Osteoblasts are also proposed to act as a barrier to control ion influx over the bone-forming surface. Osteoblasts are also known to regulate osteoclasts and are also involved in bone remodelling and mineral metabolism.

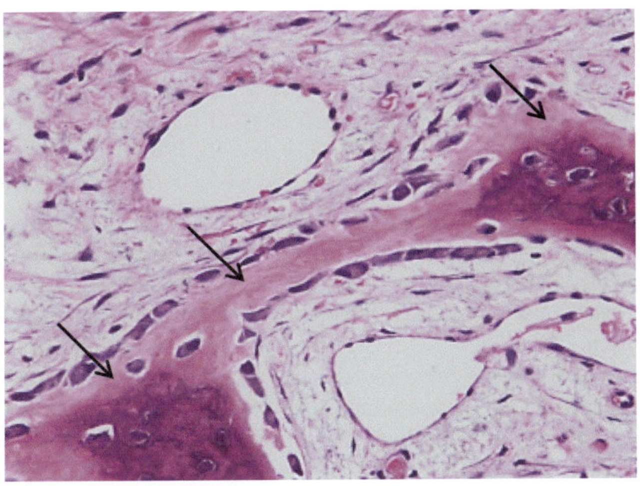

◘ **Fig. 12.8** Photomicrograph showing plump osteoblasts forming and lining an osteoid seam (arrows) joining two partially calcified trabeculae and also lining the partially calcified trabeculae. Note the osteoblasts that have been incorporated in the osteoid and calcified bone as osteocytes. The darker, basophilic colour in the trabeculae is indicative of the calcification of the matrix

Osteoblast differentiation from stem cell and their function are regulated by RUNX2 (also known as Cbfa1) and osterix. BMPs possess the ability to initiate osteoblastogenesis from the progenitor cells. insulin-like growth factor (IGF 1&2), fibroblast growth factor (FGF 1&2), platelet-derived growth factor (PDGF) and vascular endothelial growth factor (VEGF) promote osteogenesis.

Osteoblasts may end up being either of the following:

(a) Bone-lining cells when bone formation ceases. The osteoblasts flatten in shape, contain few organelles, align themselves along the bone surface and are termed bone-lining cells, which cover most of the bones in the adult skeleton. It is hypothesised that as these cells retain gap junctions with osteocytes, they create a network to control homeostasis and ensure bone vitality.
(b) Embedded within the bone matrix as osteocytes.

12.6.2 Osteocytes

Osteocytes are derived from entrapped osteoblasts within the mineralised or unmineralised matrix of bone. Woven bones and bones at the sites of repair tend to present an increased number of these cells owing to the rate of formation of these types of bone. Osteocytes form greater than 90% of the total number of bone cells in the skeleton; this fact alone implies that osteocytes have a major role in skeletal and mineral homeostasis.

Osteocyte cells are reduced in size when compared to osteoblasts and are individually located in lacunae which is a space occupied by the cell in the matrix. Each lacuna is characterised by the presence of large numbers of very fine, contiguous canaliculi that house dendrite-like osteocyte processes, which extend from each cell body (◘ Fig. 12.9). Each dendrite-like osteocyte extension within a canaliculus is in contact with its neighbours via gap junctions such that osteocytes in an osteon in lamellar–Haversian bones are in contact with one another. Via these dendritic-cellular extensions, osteocytes are also in contact with osteoblasts in both woven and lamellar–Haversian bones.

The proposed transformation mechanism of osteoblasts to osteocytes may either be the self-burial of stationary osteoblasts into osteocytes or the dynamic selection of certain osteoblasts to transform into osteo-

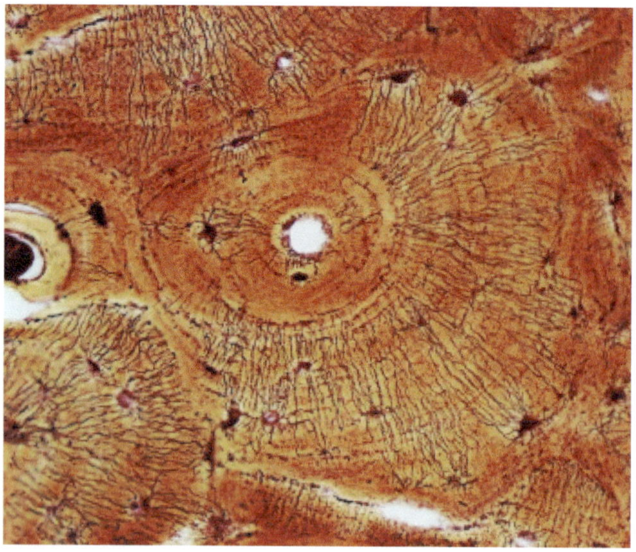

Fig. 12.9 Undecalcified bone section illustrating the network of very fine canaliculi arising from osteocyte lacunae in osteons within Haversian bone

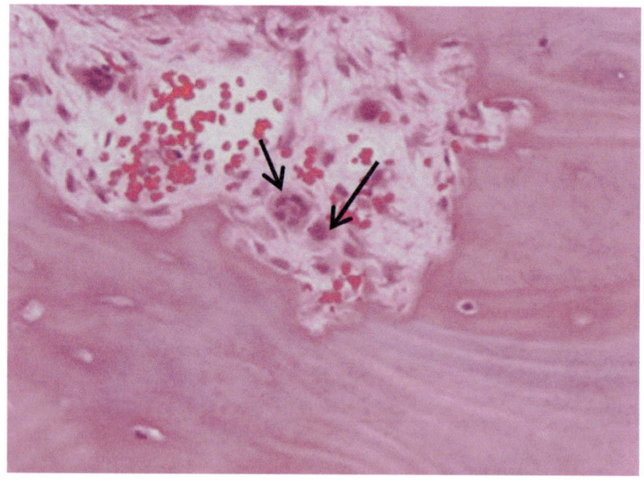

Fig. 12.10 Decalcified bone section. The bone surface exhibits a "chewed-out" appearance due to osteoclast cell activity. Osteoclasts (arrows) are indicated

cytes by the secretory activity of the former. RUNX2, osterix, leptin and TGF-β-related signalling mechanisms are a few of the factors that play a role in the transformation of osteoblasts into osteocytes.

The average half-life of osteocytes is around 25 years.

Details of the functions of osteocytes are still being elucidated. However, there is an extensive body of research showing that osteocyte networks in bones perform a variety of important functions related to bone homeostasis, bone remodelling and repair and mineral (e.g. calcium and phosphorus) metabolism in the body. These functions are affected by means of an extensive array of signalling molecules, which have been identified by in vivo and in vitro research studies. A detailed description of osteocyte functions is beyond the scope of this chapter. However, as an example, osteocytes act as mechanosensors, wherein the cells, along with their protoplasmic extensions in the canaliculi, are able to sense the surrounding biochemical and mechanical environments and respond accordingly. Resultant molecular signalling can either instruct osteoclasts to resorb bone or osteoblasts to form bone, thus, regulating bone dynamics. In the context of the latter, osteocytes produce sclerostin which inhibits osteoblasts. If osteocytes detect, for example, increased mechanical stresses, they can increase sclerostin production and, thus, activate osteoblasts to produce additional bone.

12.6.3 Osteoclasts

Osteoclasts are bone-resorbing cells that exert their bone removal functions when activated.

Osteoclasts are derived from haematopoietic precursors of the monocyte/macrophage lineage. Osteoblasts and marrow cavity stromal cells modulate osteoclast differentiation through molecular secretions and even direct cell-to-cell interaction. Receptor-activated nuclear factor κB, its ligand RANK and macrophage colony-stimulating factor (M-CSF) play a crucial role in monitoring osteoclastogenesis. Osteoprotegerin, secreted by osteoblasts, interferes with the formation of osteoclasts.

Osteoclasts are large multi-nucleated cells (15–20 nuclei) (Fig. 12.10) containing numerous cytoplasmic vacuoles and vesicles, which possess tartrate-resistant acid phosphatase (TRAP). Mitochondria are numerous in number but absent near the bone surface to be resorbed (ruffled border). When active, the cell surface facing towards the bone surface is deeply folded, forming a ruffled border. The periphery of the ruffled border opposed to the bone surface is devoid of cell organelles and creates a seal zone or clear zone with the aid of integrin-mediated cell adhesion proteins such as actin. The sealing zone is responsible for (a) attachment of the cell to the mineralised bone surface and (b) creation of a micro-environment between the cell and the bone surface.

Osteoclasts are rich in acid phosphatase and other lysosomal enzymes, which are synthesised in the rough endoplasmic reticulum and transported to the ruffled border through Golgi complexes. Proton pumps in the ruffled borders facilitate the introduction of hydrogen ions into the sealed zone and, hence, the dissolution of the apatite mineral in bone. Collagenases, including cathepsin and other enzymes, remove the organic component of bone during active resorption. As they resorb bone, the osteoclasts create shallow concavities along

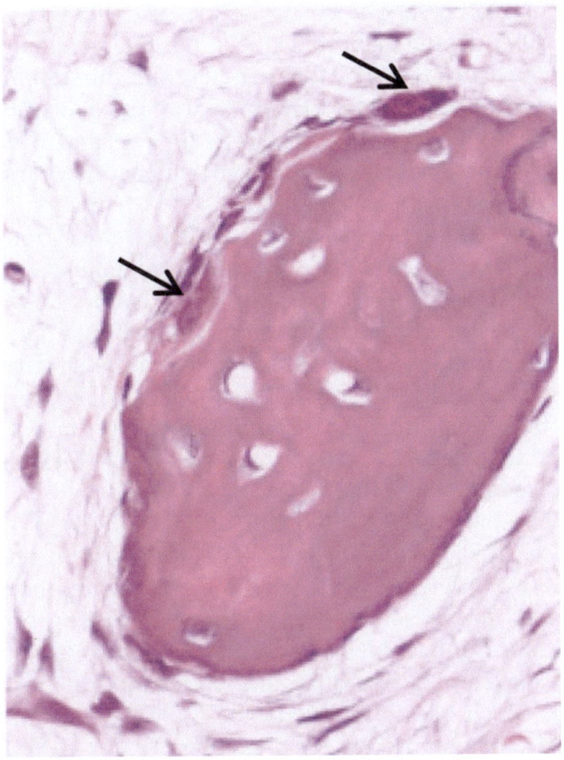

◘ **Fig. 12.11** Decalcified bone section. Osteoblasts (arrows) are seen occupying shallow depressions on the bone surface. These depressions are Howship's lacunae and represent areas where bone has been removed by the osteoclasts

the resorbing bone surface. These concavities are called Howship's lacunae (◘ Fig. 12.11).

Systemic factors can influence osteoclast activity. For example, oestrogen prevents bone loss by reducing osteoclastic activity. Vitamin D3 and parathyroid hormone promote bone resorption in high concentrations. Calcitonin prevents bone resorption as it is an inhibitor of osteoclast activity. Bisphosphonates do not suppress osteoclastogenesis but cause the apoptosis of osteoclasts.

12.7 Bone Remodelling and Repair

Physiological bone remodelling is constantly occurring in response to normal functional demands in order to maintain skeletal and bone homeostasis. Bone remodelling also occurs in the jaws in response to the forces applied during orthodontic therapy.

The processes associated with bone repair occur in relation to bone fractures and the repair of tooth sockets following tooth extraction. Here the granulation tissue that forms to replace the initial blood clot is replaced by woven bone, with the latter eventually being replaced by mature lamellar–Haversian bone.

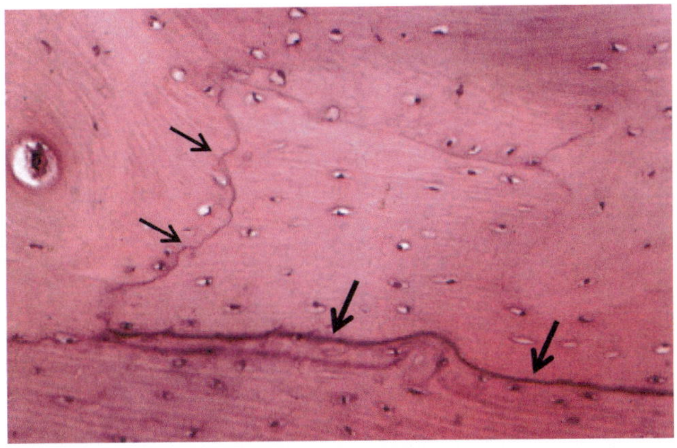

◘ **Fig. 12.12** Decalcified bone section. Photomicrograph showing reversal (small arrows) and resting lines (large arrows) in remodelled bone

Histological evidence of physiological bone remodelling is seen in decalcified bone sections in the form of resting lines and reversal lines (◘ Fig. 12.12). These are basophilic lines in areas of bone where the process of bone formation (apposition) has paused or where there has been osteoclastic resorption of a bone face followed by new bone formation. Resting lines are smooth, flat lines within the bone, whereas reversal lines are scalloped due to the presence of Howship's lacunae.

12.8 Jawbones

The macroscopic and microscopic characteristics of the adult jaws, including the alveolar processes, are essentially the same as other bones of the skeleton. At the macroscopic, clinical level, the maxilla and mandible exhibit an outer cortex and an inner medullary area of trabecular (cancellous or spongy) bone. Microscopically, the bone of the maxilla and mandible consists of lamellar–Haversian bone, with the added presence of a special bone type called bundle bone that lines the tooth sockets of the alveolar bone of both jaws.

The alveolar bone is the part of the jaw bones that forms and supports the tooth sockets. It not only houses and anchors the tooth roots but also aids in the absorption and distribution of occlusal forces. Further, it encloses and protects the developing permanent tooth buds and organises an eruptive pathway for both dentitions.

During the late bell stage of tooth development, individual tooth germs are separated by developing bony septae and bridges, thereby encasing them in the respective bony compartments. Dental follicle cells differentiate into cementum and periodontal ligament; some cells also differentiate into osteoblasts and form alveolar bone proper. Later, root development and tooth eruptions are responsible for the increase in alveolar bone height. While tooth development and eruption are responsible for alveolar process formation, loss of teeth leads to gradual loss of alveolar height.

The alveolar bone proper is the part of the alveolar bone that lines individual tooth sockets. It is a combination of perforated, lamellar and bundle bones that surround tooth roots and provide attachment to periodontal ligament principal fibres. This component of the alveolar bone is termed the cribriform plate. The perforations in the cribriform plates provide a pathway for the neurovascular tissue of the periodontal ligament. Zuckerkandl and Hirschfeld's nutrient canals are present within the interdental and interradicular septae.

Bundle bone (◻ Fig. 12.13) forms a thin and, sometimes, interrupted lining of the cribriform plates. Microscopically, bundle bone appears as an amorphous form of bone that is structurally composed of calcified Sharpey's fibre bundle ends that are embedded in an amorphous calcified bone matrix. Sharpey's fibres are the ends of the principal fibres of the periodontal ligament that insert into the cementum and into the bundle bone, thus, tethering tooth roots to the alveolar bone.

The supporting alveolar bone is composed of cortical plates, which form the outer and inner plates of the alveolar process. The cortical plates are thinner in the maxilla than the mandible, thickest in the premolar and molar buccal region of the mandible and thinnest in the anterior tooth region of both jaws. Trabecular bone occupies the region between cortical plates and alveolar bone proper and includes marrow rich in adipocytes and pluripotent mesenchymal cells.

12

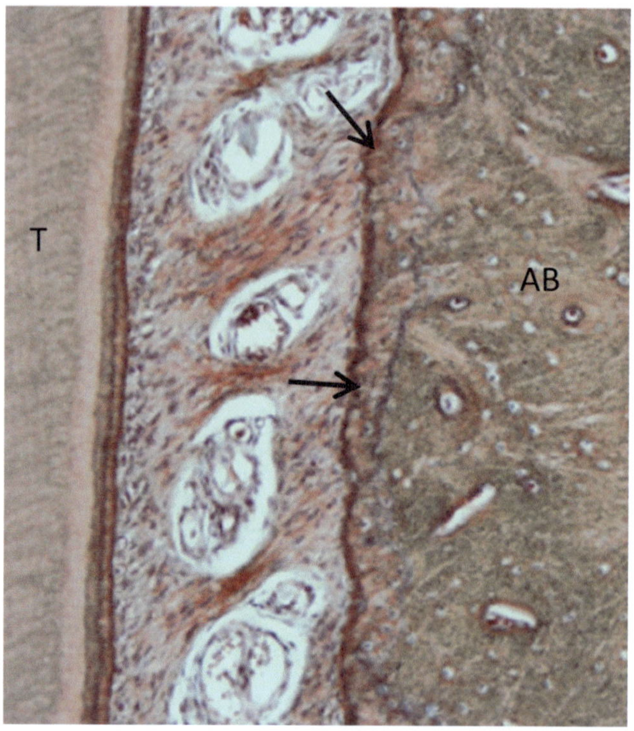

◻ **Fig. 12.13** Decalcified bone section showing a thin layer of bundle bone (arrows) forming the innermost layer of alveolar bone proper (AB). T is the tooth root and PL is the periodontal ligament

The mandible, or lower jaw, is the largest, strongest and movable bone of the face and is antagonistic to the maxilla. Anatomically, the mandible is connected to the temporal bone through the temporomandibular joint. It is innervated by the mandibular branch of the trigeminal nerve and predominantly supplied by the inferior alveolar blood vessels. It serves many important functions, such as mastication, deglutition and speech and is involved in facial expressions.

The mandible is the second bone in the body to ossify and begins forming around 6 weeks in utero. It undergoes two different ossification processes during embryogenesis. The intramembranous bone formation occurs in relationship to Meckel's cartilage and forms the bulk of a developing mandible and endochondral ossification, which occurs mainly in the upper portion of the ramus and mandibular condyle.

The maxilla is the second-largest bone of the face and forms the upper jaw. It also contributes to the formation of the nose, mouth, orbit and infratemporal and pterygopalatine fossae. Each side of the maxilla is composed of a body (pyramidal in shape, which encloses the maxillary sinus) and four processes, namely frontal, alveolar, palatine and zygomatic. It articulates with the nasal, lacrimal, frontal, palatine, ethmoid and zygomatic bones and those at the opposite side of the maxilla.

Embryologically, the maxilla forms in relation to an ossification centre in the mesenchyme of the maxillary process of the first arch. Although no arch cartilage exists in the maxillary process, its ossification centre is associated with the nasal capsule cartilage. A secondary cartilage (zygomatic/malar cartilage) also contributes to its development. The maxilla predominantly forms as intramembranous bone with ossification centres in the maxilla proper (above canine fossa) and premaxillary regions (one above incisive fossa). The premaxilla may persist as a separate bone due to the persistence of the suture until middle age.

12.9 Summary

Bone is a vital, calcified connective tissue that forms the skeleton of the human body. It is one of the hardest body structures and is endowed with a specific degree of elasticity and the power of regeneration and repair.

The terminology of bone varies depending upon whether mature, adult bone is being described or whether the bone being considered is embryonic or repair bone. In addition to providing postural support to the body and the means for movement of body parts mediated by muscles and tendons, bone also plays an important role in relation to mineral homeostasis in the body.

Further Reading

Avery JK, Chiego DJ. Essentials of oral histology and embryology: a clinical approach. Reed Elsevier; 2007.

Chow DH, Zheng L, Tian L, Ho KS, Qin L, Guo X. Application of ultrasound accelerates the decalcification process of bone matrix without affecting histological and immunohistochemical analysis. J Orthop Transl. 2019;17:112–20.

Clarke B. Normal bone anatomy and physiology. Clin J Am Soc Nephrol. 2008;3(Suppl 3):S131.

Corrieri B, Márquez-Grant N. What do bones tell us? The study of human skeletons from the perspective of forensic anthropology. Sci Prog. 2015;98(4):391–402.

Crockett JC, Rogers MJ, Coxon FP, Hocking LJ, Helfrich MH. Bone remodelling at a glance. J Cell Sci. 2011;124(7):991–8.

Garg K, Chaurasia BD. BD Chaurasia's Human anatomy for dental students/edited by Krishna Garg.

Goh YC, Tan CC, Lim D. Coronoid hyperplasia: a review. J Stomatol Oral Maxillofac Surg. 2020;121(4):397–403.

Hadjidakis DJ, Androulakis II. Bone remodeling. Ann N Y Acad Sci. 2006;1092(1):385–96.

Hosoya A, Hoshi K, Sahara N, Ninomiya T, Akahane S, Kawamoto T, Ozawa H. Effects of fixation and decalcification on the immunohistochemical localization of bone matrix proteins in fresh-frozen bone sections. Histochem Cell Biol. 2005;123:639–46.

Jenita G, Gheena S, Ganapathy D. Histological comparison of ground section, decalcified section and resin embedded section of bone-a review. Ann Romanian Soc Cell Biol. 2021:2608–13.

Kenkre JS, Bassett JH. The bone remodelling cycle. Ann Clin Biochem. 2018;55(3):308–27.

Khan IA, Bordoni B. Histology, Osteoclasts. In: StatPearls. StatPearls Publishing; 2022.

Kini U, Nandeesh BN. Physiology of bone formation, remodeling, and metabolism. Radionuclide and hybrid bone imaging.

Koenig LJ, Tamimi D, Perschbacher SE. Diagnostic imaging: oral and maxillofacial E-book. Elsevier Health Sciences; 2017.

Kular J, Tickner J, Chim SM, Xu J. An overview of the regulation of bone remodelling at the cellular level. Clin Biochem. 2012;45(12):863–73.

Kumar GS. Orban's oral histology & embryology-E-BOOK. Elsevier Health Sciences; 2015.

Lee SK, Kim YS, Oh HS, Yang KH, Kim EC, Chi JG. Prenatal development of the human mandible. Anat Rec. 2001;263(3):314–25.

Malhan D, Muelke M, Rosch S, Schaefer AB, Merboth F, Weisweiler D, Heiss C, Arganda-Carreras I, El Khassawna T. An optimized approach to perform bone histomorphometry. Front Endocrinol. 2018;9:404664.

Nanci A, editor. Ten Cate's oral histology-e-book: development, structure, and function. Elsevier Health Sciences; 2017.

Olszta MJ, Cheng X, Jee SS, Kumar R, Kim YY, Kaufman MJ, Douglas EP, Gower LB. Bone structure and formation: a new perspective. Mater Sci Eng R Rep. 2007;58(3–5):77–116.

Parada C, Chai Y. Mandible and tongue development. Curr Top Dev Biol. 2015;115:31–58.

Parvizi J. Osteoblasts. In: High yield orthopaedics E-book. Elsevier Health Sciences; 2010.

Qin Q, Li Y, Zhou Y. An improved method for preparing stained ground teeth sections. PeerJ. 2023;11:e15240.

Rentsch C, Schneiders W, Manthey S, Rentsch B, Rammelt S. Comprehensive histological evaluation of bone implants. Biomatter. 2014;4(1):e27993.

Rider KA, Flick LM. Differentiation of bone and soft tissues in formalin-fixed, paraffin-embedded tissue by using methylene blue/acid fuchsin stain. Anal Quant Cytol Histol. 2004;26(5):246–8.

Rigueur D, Lyons KM. Whole-mount skeletal staining. Humana Press; 2014.

Sangeetha R, Uma K, Chandavarkar V. Comparison of routine decalcification methods with microwave decalcification of bone and teeth. J Oral Maxillofac Pathol. 2013;17(3):386.

Shim MJ. Bone changes in femoral bone of mice using calcein labeling. Korean J Clin Lab Sci. 2016;48(2):114–7.

Singh I. Human embryology. JP Medical Ltd; 2014.

Sivapathasundharam B, Rajendran A. Shafer's textbook of oral pathology. Elsevier Health Sciences; 2012.

Veselá B, Švandová E, Bobek J, Lesot H, Matalová E. Osteogenic and angiogenic profiles of mandibular bone-forming cells. Front Physiol. 2019;10:124.

White TD, Black MT, Folkens PA. Human osteology. Academic press; 2011.

Histology of the Temporomandibular Joint

Tabita Joy

Contents

S R Prabhu et al. (eds.), *Oral Histology and Oral Histopathology*, https://doi.org/10.1007/978-3-031-77481-2_13

13.1 Introduction

The temporomandibular joint (TMJ) is the most complex synovial joint in the body. The right and left TMJs work synchronously. They are anatomically located in the maxillofacial area, providing articulation between the mandible and the cranium on each side (◘ Fig. 13.1).

The TMJ is a composite anatomical joint that performs a simple gliding motion (ginglymus, which is a 'hinge' movement during opening and closing of the mandible), and the other element has a sliding motion (arthrodial–axial during lateral excursions of the mandible) and is, therefore, called a 'ginglymoarthrodial' joint.

The TMJ differs from all other movable joints in that the articulating bone surfaces (◘ Fig. 13.1) of the mandibular condyle and the glenoid fossa and eminence are, as described later, fibrous connective tissue rather than hyaline cartilage. The body of one of the articulating bones (mandible) houses teeth that require specific modes of articulation during rest and mastication. Functionally, the TMJ depends upon the complex interactions of the bony components of the joint along with muscles, ligaments, an articular disc, synovial tissues and fluid, and a fibrous capsule, which encompasses the joint.

13.2 Development of the Temporomandibular Joint

The histodifferentiation and organisation of the TMJ occur between the 10th and the 12th week. During the 10th week, the two joint cavities form, thereby, defining the intervening articular disc.

The inferior compartment forms first (at 10 weeks), separating the future disk from the developing condyle, and the upper compartment starts to appear at about 11½ weeks. By the 16th week, the TMJ unit acquires a definite form. The connective tissue between the developing condyle and temporal bone becomes organised into primitive synovial membranes, synovial cavities, the articular disk, and the bilaminar area.

In early infancy, the articular fossa is shallow, and the eminence is ill-defined (◘ Fig. 13.2). In early childhood, the fossa deepens, and the eminence elongates. Only after the eruption of the permanent dentition at 7 years does the articular tubercle begin to become prominent. Most rapid growth occurs between the ages of 10 and 11, and thereafter, the TMJ completes its development.

The joint structures grow laterally, concomitant with the widening of the neurocranium. The temporal element, rather than the condyles, is critical in establishing this lateral growth.

13

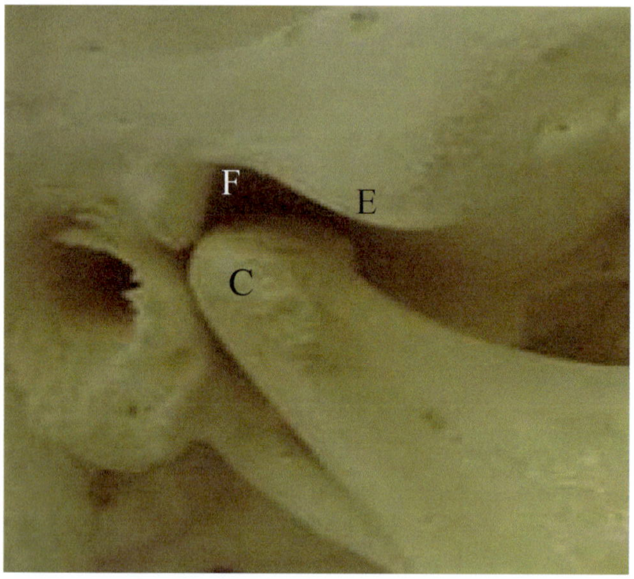

◘ **Fig. 13.1** The bony components of the TMJ are the mandibular condyle (C), the concave glenoid fossa (F), and the articular eminence (E). (Image courtesy of Professor David F Wilson, Adelaide, Australia)

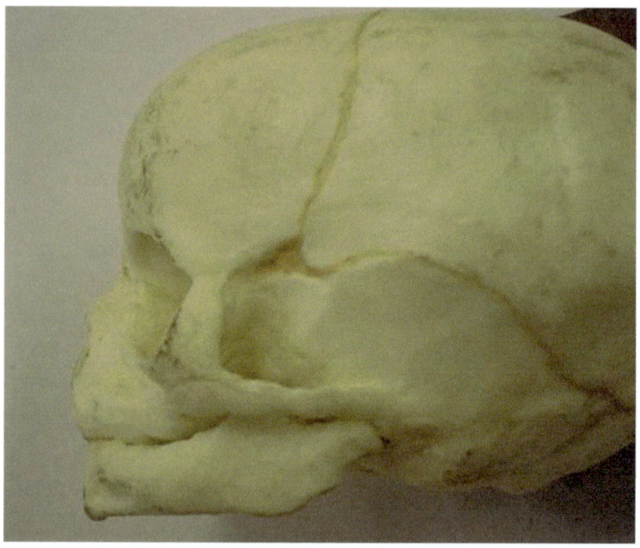

◘ **Fig. 13.2** The foetal skull and mandible show the relative absence of the mandibular ramus, the absence of an articular eminence, and a very shallow glenoid fossa. (Image courtesy of Professor David F Wilson, Adelaide, Australia)

Defective development of the TMJ results in ankylosis, producing immobilisation and impaired mandibular formation.

13.3 Anatomy of Temporomandibular Joint

The bones of the temporomandibular articulation are the glenoid fossa (on the under-surface of the squamous part of the temporal bone) and the condyle (supported by the condylar process of the mandible).

The articulating area of the TMJ on the temporal bone is located on its inferior aspect, seen prominently from the base of the skull. This area includes the articular eminence and the articular (glenoid) fossa. The articular eminence is positioned anterior to the articular fossa and consists of a smooth, rounded protuberance on the inferior aspect of the zygomatic process (◘ Fig. 13.3).

As stated earlier, there are several components to the TMJ articular unit (◘ Fig. 13.4). These are as follows:

1. The TMJ capsule
2. Bone components:
   (a) Temporal bone components: Glenoid fossa and the articular eminence
   (b) Mandibular component: the condyle
3. Articulating disc
4. Synovial cavities, membrane, and fluid
5. Muscles and ligaments

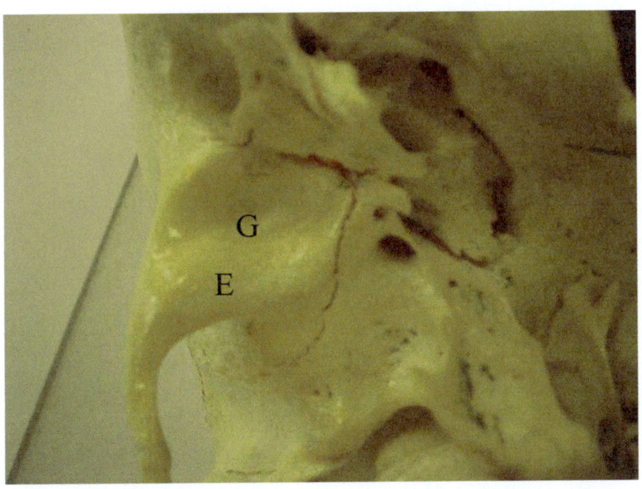

◘ **Fig. 13.3** Photograph of one side of the base of the skull showing the concave glenoid fossa (G) and the more anteriorly placed articular eminence (E). (Image courtesy of Professor David F Wilson, Adelaide, Australia)

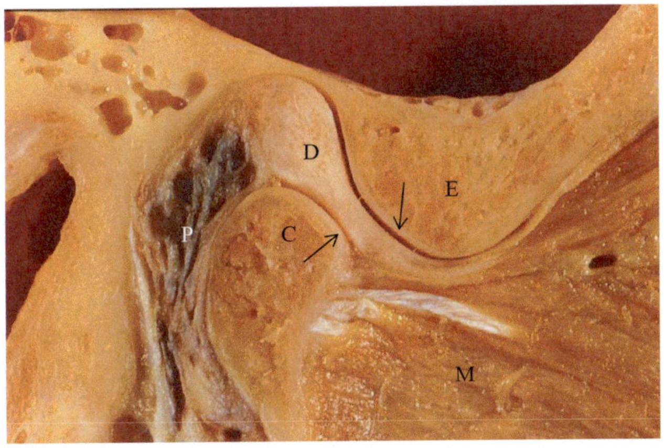

◘ **Fig. 13.4** Gross anatomic specimen showing some of the components of the TMJ articular complex. C is mandibular condyle. D is articular disc, the bulk of which is sitting in the glenoid fossa in this specimen. The narrow superior and inferior joint spaces are seen on the superior and inferior aspects of the disc. E is articular eminence. M is pterygoid muscle tissue. P denotes the highly vascular posterior attachment tissues, which are evident. Thin zones of pale articular tissue (arrows) are seen lining the head of the condyle and the articular eminence. (Image courtesy of Dr. Caroline Crowley, Adelaide, Australia)

13.4 Histology of Temporomandibular Joint (◘ Fig. 13.5)

13.4.1 Articular Capsule

The macroscopic structure reveals a girdling structure covering the components of the TMJ called the articular capsule or capsular ligament. The capsule encloses the margin of the temporal bones, articular eminence, and articular fossa superiorly. Inferiorly, the capsule wraps around the circumference of the neck of the condyle. Posteriorly, the capsule is attached to the temporal bone and anteriorly to the external auditory canal above and the posterior aspect of the condyle below. Above the disk, the capsule is lax, whereas below, it is attached tightly to the condyle. As the condylar head slides along the articular plane during function, the capsule is described as loose, and it is supported by a medial ligament (sphenomandibular), a lateral ligament (temporomandibular), and a posterior ligament (stylomandibular). It is a very thin, relatively avascular, and fibrous non-elastic membrane. It consists of a dense collagenous membrane that seals the joint space and provides passive stability, enhanced by increased local thickenings in its walls to form anatomically recognisable ligaments, as well as active stability from pro-

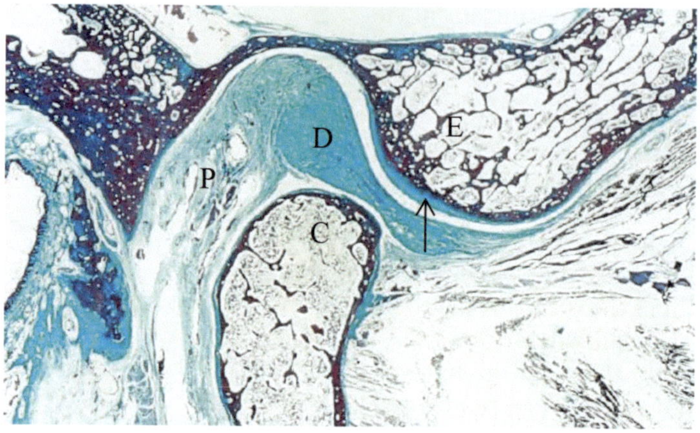

Fig. 13.5 Lower-power microscopic view of the TMJ. C is condylar head, D is disc, E is articular eminence, and P is posterior attachment connective tissue. Articular soft tissue (arrow) is evident, lining the articular eminence, as are the superior and inferior joint spaces. (Image courtesy of Dr. Caroline Crowley, Adelaide, Australia)

prioceptive nerve endings in the capsule. The posterior capsule is highly vascular, where a number of blood vessels appear, known as the vascular triangle and often called pis vasculosa.

13.4.2 Temporal Bone

The temporal bone consists of a thin zone of compact bone overlying cancellous bone (see Fig. 13.5). The surface facing the superior joint space of compact bone is covered by the periosteum. The innermost part of the bone consists of the endosteum and the medullary cavity with its bone marrow. The articulating bony surfaces are covered by fibrocartilage immediately overlying the periosteum. The section through the temporal bone shows a very thin lining of the articular surface of the glenoid fossa, while the section through the articular eminence shows a thick articular covering (Fig. 13.5).

13.4.3 Articular Eminence and Glenoid Fossa

The articulating surface of the temporal bone is convex at the tubercle (eminence) and concave posteriorly at the glenoid fossa. The articulating surface of the condyle and the opposing surfaces of the temporomandibular fossa, including the articular tubercle, are covered by fibrocartilage. Chondrocytes in the posterior aspect of the mandibular condylar region are exposed to greater tensional forces than compression. These express collagen types I and II. Experimental studies indicate that mechanical forces acting on the mandibular condyle play a significant role in the proliferation, differentiation, and rate of maturation of chondrocytes in the articular soft tissue.

13.4.4 Mandibular Condyle

In a mature adult, each condyle consists of compact bone overlying cancellous bone.

Fibrocartilage overlies the articulating aspect of the condyle. The bony trabeculae at the head of the condyle are grouped in such a way that they radiate from the neck of the mandible and reach the cortex at right angles, thus, enhancing the strength of the condyles. In contrast to the temporal bone, a growth centre is present in the head of the mandibular condyle before an individual reaches maturity. This growth centre consists of hyaline cartilage deep into the articulating surface of the condyle. This is the last growth centre of bone in the body and is multidirectional in its growth capacity. Over time, the cartilage is replaced by bone using endochondral ossification.

Four distinct layers have been described covering the bony head of the adult condyle (Fig. 13.6):

1. The most superficial layer facing the inferior joint space forms the articular surface and is composed of fibrous tissue (mainly collagen, but with some elastin fibres). Fibroblasts/fibrocytes within the surface layer are sparsely distributed.
2. Beneath the articular surface layer is a more cellular zone (cell-rich zone).
3. Beneath the cell-rich zone is a zone where the cells are rounded and have the appearance of cartilage-like cells; this layer is generally referred to as the fibrocartilaginous layer.
4. Immediately covering the bone is a thin zone of calcified cartilage, distinguished from the underlying bone of the mandibular condyle by its different staining properties. This calcified cartilage is a remnant of the secondary condylar cartilage.

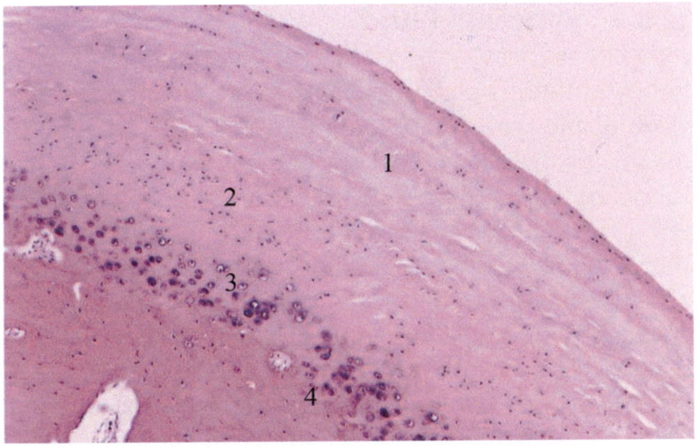

Fig. 13.6 Photomicrograph of an adult condylar head showing the identifiable articular zones. (1) Articular surface zone, (2) cell-rich zone, (3) fibrocartilage zone, and (4) calcified cartilage zone. (Image courtesy of Professor David F Wilson, Adelaide, Australia)

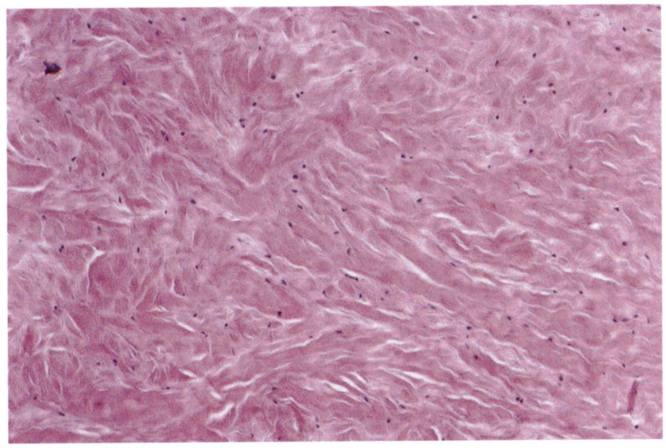

Fig. 13.7 Photomicrograph of a TMJ disc illustrating the arrangement of the collagen into coarse fibrous bundles. (Image courtesy of Professor David F Wilson, Adelaide, Australia)

13.5 Articulating Disc (Meniscus)

The TMJ disc is a fibrocartilage tissue, biconcave and elliptical with two faces, superior and inferior; two margins, medial and lateral; and two extremities, anterior and posterior. The disc is anchored around its lateral borders to the articular capsule and anteriorly to the external pterygoid muscle by a fibroblastic connective tissue. The masseter and temporalis muscles also have fibrous connections to the anterior and lateral edges of the articular disc. In the early developmental stage of the TMJ, the disc is composed of fibrocartilage. As maturation progresses, the fibrocartilage is replaced by dense fibrous connective tissue.

The articular disc has two layers: the fibrous connective tissue layer and the synovial membrane layer. The fibrous connective tissue layer is firm and non-elastic and is surrounded by ligaments.

The principal fibres are coarse collagen bundles (Fig. 13.7), while elastic fibres occur only in small amounts. The collagen fibre bundles in the intermediate region of the disc are aligned parallel in an antero-posterior plane. The fibre bundles of the anterior and posterior segments of the disc, however, do not exhibit a preferred orientation. In some regions, the collagen fibres appear wavy, which is believed to be related to their ability to accommodate tensional force.

The articular disc contains spindle-shaped cells that combine the properties of chondrocytes and fibroblasts. The cells possess numerous fine processes, many extending for considerable distances. These processes are rich in the gap-junction protein connexin 43. This may allow for the passage of nutrients and fluid from the peripheral blood vessels to the central avascular regions of the disc. These cells synthesise collagen types I, II, and IX and cartilage-specific proteoglycans. They also express the matrix metalloproteinases (MMPs) and tissue inhibitors of matrix metalloproteinases needed for turnover and repair of the fibrocartilaginous extracellular matrix (ECM). The surface of the articular disk is covered by a cell-free, proteoglycan-rich lamina.

Collagen fibres in the thinner, central region of the intra-articular disc (also known as the intermediate zone) run mainly in an antero-posterior direction. In the thicker anterior and posterior portions (also known as the anterior and posterior bands, respectively), prominent fibre bundles also run transversely (medio-lateral orientation) and supero-inferiorly, giving the fibres a much more convoluted appearance. Around the periphery of the disc, the collagen fibre bundles are arranged circumferentially. When viewed in polarised light, the collagen fibres show alternating dark and light bands, indicating that they are wavy or crimped.

The ground substance of the disc comprises about 5% of its dry weight. The principal glycosaminoglycans are chondroitin sulphate and dermatan sulphate, which, due to their anionic charge, can absorb water and help resist compressive loading.

13.6 Synovial Cavities, Membrane, and Fluids

13.6.1 Synovial Cavities

The superior synovial cavity is located between the upper surface of the articular disk and the articulating surface of the squamous temporal bone. The cavity extends from the articular eminence back to the posterior margin of the fossa.

The inferior synovial cavity is positioned between the condyle and the inferior surface of the disk and is semicircular in profile.

13.6.2 Synovial Membrane

The synovial cavities are lined by a thin tissue sheet of the synovial membrane (synovium and stratum synoviale). The synovial membrane is stretched and flattened during joint movements, while at rest, it shows folding. It has considerable ability to regenerate. There are two synovial membranes in the joint: one lines the capsule above the disc, and the other lines the capsule below the disc. The synovial membrane folds to form synovial villi, which project into the joint spaces. It is neither an epithelial lining nor an actual membrane; rather, it is composed entirely of connective tissue rich in collagen V. It is well vascularised with numerous fenestrated capillaries. The synovium consists of a bilaminar discontinuous intimal layer of synoviocytes that overlie a loose subintimal layer of connective tissue rich in blood capillaries. The lining layer of the synovial membrane in the temporomandibular joint contains two types of lining cells: macrophage-like type A and fibroblast-like type B cells. Type A cells exhibit significant phagocytic properties derived from blood monocytes and remove wear and tear debris from the synovial fluid. Type A cells have surface filopodia, many plasma membrane invaginations, and associated pinocytotic vesicles. Their cytoplasm contains numerous mitochondria and lysosomal elements and a prominent Golgi complex and little or no rough endoplasmic reticulum (RER). Type B cells produce synovial fluid and are sometimes called secretory S cells. They are rich in RER. Type B cells synthesise the hyaluronate found in synovial fluid.

The subintima is a loose connective tissue containing vascular elements together with scattered fibroblasts, macrophages, mast cells, fat cells, and some elastic fibres, which prevent the folding of the membrane. The intima varies in structure, having one to four layers of synovial cells embedded in an electron-dense, amorphous-material, fibre-free intercellular matrix.

The synovial membrane is richly supplied with blood vessels. Three types of synovial capillaries are found in the synovial membrane: continuous, fenestrated, and discontinuous. The fenestrated types are found in the matrix of the synovial membrane. Lymphatic vessels drain into the capsular, collecting lymphatic vessels.

13.6.3 Synovial Fluid

Synovial fluid is elaborated from the rich capillary network of the synovial membrane, which is augmented by mucin, probably secreted by the synovial cells. It is a lubricant and nutrient fluid for the avascular tissues covering the condyle, the articular eminence, and the disc, filling the joint cavity. The fluid is a dialysate of lymph and plasma consisting of a protein–mucopolysaccharide complex. It is not completely acellular but contains mostly lymphocytes and monocytes.

The synovial fluid is characterised by physical properties of viscosity, elasticity, and plasticity. It is a transparent, clear, straw-coloured viscous fluid. The viscosity of the fluid is believed to be a result of mucin produced by certain cells of the synovial membrane. The hyaluronic acid is also secreted by the macrophage-like cells (Type A cells) of the synovial membrane, has a high viscosity, and provides lubricating properties to the synovial fluid.

13.7 Ligaments

The TMJ has one major and two minor ligaments. The temporomandibular ligament is the major ligament, while the sphenomandibular and stylomandibular ligaments are minor ligaments. The lateral aspect of the capsule is thickened to form a fan-shaped ligament known as the temporomandibular ligament, which runs obliquely backwards and downwards from the lateral aspect of the articular eminence to the posterior aspect of the condylar neck.

13.8 Innervation and Blood Supply to the Joint

Blood is supplied to the TMJ through branches of the superficial temporal, deep auricular, anterior tympanic, and ascending pharyngeal arteries. These branches converge into the capsule joint.

Small arteries, arterioles, and capillaries pass into the peripheral third of the articular disc. The central portion of the joint reveals that the thin portion of the disc is avascular.

The nerve supply to the TMJ is through the mandibular division of the trigeminal nerve. The neural branches are the auriculotemporal, masseteric, and deep temporal nerves. Nerves containing myelinated and non-myelinated fibres enter the capsule and disc to supply the anterior, posterior, medial, and lateral regions of the joint. The thin central portion of the disc is free of nerves. Both myelinated and non-myelinated nerves are found in the connective tissue core of the synovial folds.

13.9 Temporomandibular Joints of Aged Individuals

With age, the articular surface of the fossa and tubercle becomes more fibrous and less vascular. In postnatal life, as the articular tubercle grows, the disk changes shape and becomes more compact, less cellular, and more collagenous. The mature disk is avascular and aneural in its central portion but is filled with vessels, nerves, and elastic fibres posteriorly, attaching it to the squamotympanic suture.

With advancing age, the quality of synovial fluid decreases, and the synovial villous projection increases, more prominent in joints affected by a pathological process.

13.10 Changes in the Articular Eminence Morphology with Dental Functions

The TMJ does not operate independently of the surrounding muscles. Changes in occlusion from various causes may produce displacement of the condyle-disc-to-disc-fossa relation and irritate the peripheral disc areas and associated nerve receptors.

13.11 Pathologies Associated with the Temporomandibular Joint

Abnormalities of the TMJ may develop as part of a generalised systemic disease, or they may arise because of local causes. The most common pathologic condition is degenerative arthritis, characterised by degenerative changes in the articular surfaces. Histopathological changes in the articular disk include neovascularisation, cell clustering, and fibrillation. Haemorrhage and fibrosis of the condyle and papillomatous hyperplasia of the synovial membrane are also evident following anterior displacement. Systemic diseases that affect TMJ are osteoarthritis and rheumatoid arthritis. The TMJ may also be affected by congenital and developmental anomalies, traumatic injuries, internal derangements, and various forms of benign and malignant neoplasms.

13.12 Summary

The temporomandibular joint is a unique joint located bilaterally in the maxillofacial region. It is formed by the articulating surfaces of the mandibular condyles and glenoid fossa and articular eminence of the temporal bone. The histology of the temporal joint consists of the TMJ capsule; the bony components, the temporal bone components (the glenoid fossa and the articular eminence) and; the mandibular component (the condyle); the articulating disc; and the synovial cavities, membrane, and fluid, along with the muscles and ligaments. Each component has its own importance and functionality in maintaining the smooth movements of the joint from infancy to adulthood. A few physiological changes occur in the architectural and histological structure of TMJ. The synovial fluid secreted by the cells of the synovial membrane nourishes and lubricates the joint.

13.12.1 Clinical Consideration

Congenital and developmental anomalies, trauma, infection, degenerative disorders, and neoplasms, both benign and malignant, can involve the TMJ.

Further Reading

Avery JK, Bernick S. Structure and function of the temporomandibular joint. In: Oral development and histology. 3rd ed. New York: Thieme Stuttgart; 2001. p. 353–63.

Chiego DJ Jr. Essentials of oral histology and embryology. 6th ed. Elsevier Health Sciences; 2023.

Fehrenbach M, Popowics T. Illustrated dental embryology, histology, and anatomy. Elsevier Health Sciences; 2019.

Garant P. Cartilage and temporomandibular joint. In: Oral cells and tissues. Quintessence Books; 2003. p. 321–33.

Hardiman R, Kujan O, Kochaji N. Normal variation in the anatomy, biology, and histology of the maxillofacial region. In: Farah C, Balasubramaniam R, McCullough M, editors. Contemporary Oral medicine: a comprehensive approach to clinical practice. Springer International Publishing AG; 2019. p. 1–66.

Laskin DM. Temporomandibular joint. In: Provenza DV, editor. Fundamentals of oral histology and microbiology. 2nd ed. Lea and Febiger; 2022. p. 283–96.

Nanci A. Ten cate's oral histology: development, structure, and function. Elsevier Health Sciences; 2007.

Sperber H. Craniofacial development and growth. Hamilton; 2001.

Histology of the Oral Mucosa

Monica Charlotte Solomon

Contents

S R Prabhu et al. (eds.), *Oral Histology and Oral Histopathology*, https://doi.org/10.1007/978-3-031-77481-2_14

14.1 Introduction

The oral mucosa is a unique organ—a moist, mucous membrane that lines the surface of the oral cavity. The oral mucosa extends from the skin of the lips to the moist lining of the intestinal mucosa. Hence, its structure has features of skin and the intestinal mucosa. Moreover, its structure varies in different parts of the oral cavity to adapt to the functional needs of that area.

14.2 Development

The oral mucosa begins to form around the sixth week of intrauterine life and the entire oral mucosa is formed by the 20th week of intrauterine life. The oral mucosa membrane develops from both the ectoderm and endoderm—the part that lines the anterior part of the oral cavity is derived from the ectoderm and the portion of the oral mucosa that arises from the branchial arches is derived from the endoderm.

14.3 Classification

- Based on the function
- Based on the structure

Based on the Function

- Masticatory mucosa
- Gingiva and hard palate
- Lining or reflecting mucosa
  Lips and cheek
  Alveolar mucosa
  Floor of the mouth
  Soft palate
- Specialized mucosa
  Dorsum of the tongue—taste buds

Based on the Structure

- Keratinized mucosa
  Masticatory mucosa
  Vermilion border of the lip
- Nonkeratinized
  Lining mucosa
  Specialized mucosa

14.4 Keratinized Mucosa

The gingiva and the hard palate, which are masticatory mucosa, are lined by an epithelium that is keratinized. This keratinized epithelium comprises keratinocytes, the cells that produce keratin. The keratinocytes are arranged in four layers: stratum basale, stratum spinosum, stratum granulosum, and stratum corneum. A keratinocyte migrates from stratum basale through all the layers up to the stratum corneum. As it passes through the layers, it undergoes morphological and biochemical modifications and becomes a differentiated cell. At the surface of the epithelium, the keratinocyte sheds off or is cast off—it desquamates. This time that a keratinocyte takes to divide and migrate through the entire thickness of the epithelium is called the turnover time or rate. The turnover time varies for different regions of the oral cavity.

14.5 Stratum Basale

The basal layer comprises a single layer of cuboidal cells; however, there are two populations of cells. One population of cells is serrated, packed with tonofilaments, and prepared for adaption and anchorage. These cells have protoplasmic processes that project from their basal surface toward the connective tissue.

The second population of cells consists of nonserrated cells that synthesize DNA and undergo mitosis, providing slowly cycling stem cells. These stem cells give rise to slowly dividing cells that protect the genetic information and many amplifying cells that undergo maturation. Sometimes, mitotic figures can be seen in the cells beyond the basal layer. Thus, the basal and the parabasal layers are referred to as stratum Grgminativum, albeit only the cells of the basal layer can undergo cell division.

Ultrastructurally, the basal cells show ribosomes, rough endoplasmic reticulum, and tonofilaments. The basal cells are attached to the basal lamina through hemidesmosomes. The hemidesmosomes comprise a single attachment plaque and the adjacent plasma membrane of the cell. The basal cells are connected to each other by desmosomes. Desmosomes are made up of transmembranous proteins and proteins within the cells. The transmembranous proteins are desmoglein and desmocollins that are of the cadherin family. These proteins are attached to the cytoskeleton of the keratinocytes via cytoplasmic attachment plaque proteins, desmoplakin, and plakoglobin.

14.6 Stratum Spinosum

The spinous cells make up the second layer of the epithelium. This layer comprises cells that are polyhedral in shape and larger than the basal cells. These polyhedral cells resemble a cocklebur or a sticker that has a spine ending at a desmosome. These cells are very active in protein synthesis. They also synthesize additional proteins that are different from those that are made by the basal cells. This alteration indicates the biochemical modifications that are taking place during the process of keratinization.

The spinous appearance of the cells is due to the shrinkage of the cells during tissue preparation, causing them to separate from each other except at the points where desmosomes anchor them together. The intercellular spaces are large and distended, making the desmosomes more prominent. This gives the cells a prickly appearance.

The tonofilament cytoskeleton of the keratinocytes and the desmosomes form the tensile strength of the epithelium. Under a light microscope, it appears as if the tonofilaments course from cell to cell across the intercellular bridges (the desmosomes). Yet, electron microscopic examination shows that the tonofilaments turn or loop around the attachment plaque. The filaments do not cross over to the adjacent cell. A type of agglutinating material attaches the tonofilaments to the desmosomes. The desmosome's attachment plaque contains the polypeptides desmoplakin and plakoglobin. The intercellular spaces contain glycoproteins, glycosaminoglycans, and fibronectin.

14.7 Stratum Granulosum

14

The cells of stratum granulosum are larger than the cells of the spinous layer. They are also flatter and wider. The cells contain many basophilic granules known as keratohyalin granules. The tonofilaments are dense and are associated with these keratohyalin granules.

Although the nuclei of these cells show degenerative and pyknotic changes, the cells still produce keratin, but the rate of their synthesis varies from that of the cells of the spinous layer.

The superficial cells of the stratum spinous and the cells of the stratum granulosum contain a membrane coated by lamellar granules called keratinosomes or Odland bodies. These lamellar granules contain glycolipids and discharge their content in the intracellular spaces, and this contributes to the permeability barrier of the epithelium.

As differentiation continues, the inner unit of the cell membrane thickens and forms a 10 nm-thick cornified cell envelope layer. This cornified cell envelope is made up of involucrin, loricrin, periplakin, and envoplakin. An enzyme, transglutaminase, cross-links involucrin, periplakin, and envoplakin. On this scaffold, loricrin and small proline-rich proteins and sulfur-rich proteins are added that stabilize the cell envelope.

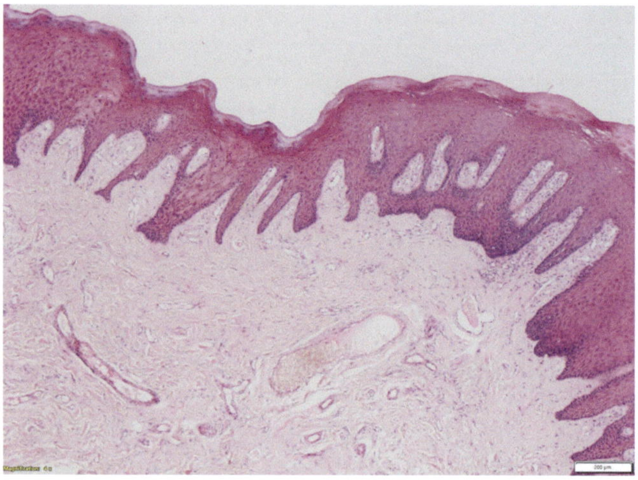

Fig. 14.1 Histology of the gingiva showing a para-keratinized stratified squamous epithelium, elongated rete ridges, and a dense connective tissue stroma (H&E 4×). (Courtesy: Department of oral and maxillofacial pathology and oral microbiology, Manipal College of Dental Sciences, Manipal)

14.8 Stratum Corneum

This layer is made up of cells that are flatter and larger than the granular cells. The cells do not produce proteins and, hence, the nucleus, ribosomes, and mitochondria disappear.

Ortho-keratinized epithelium: The cells are acidophilic and amorphous. The cells have a protein called filaggrin that forms a matrix in the cell. In this matrix, tonofilaments are densely packed through cross-linking with disulfide bonds. The keratinized cells become dehydrated and compact and cover a greater area than the basal cells. These cells do not synthesize proteins.

Ultrastructurally, the cells of the stratum corneum are densely packed with tonofilaments that are coated with filaggrin. The cell surface and the desmosomes are altered. The plasma membrane is thicker.

Para-keratinized: The nucleus is pyknotic and condensed. The cytoplasmic organelles are partially lysed.

14.9 Non-keratinocytes

Epithelium also contains a small group of cells that do not contain cytokeratin filaments. These cells do not produce keratin, form desmosomal junctions, or undergo maturative changes or desquamate. These cells migrate from the neural crest cells or from the bone marrow. The non-keratinocytes that are seen in the oral epithelium are melanocytes, Merkel cells, and Langerhans cells.

14.10 Melanocytes

Melanocytes are derived from the neural crest and migrate into the epithelium at around 11 weeks of gestation. Melanocytes, through their dendritic process, establish contact with 30–40 keratinocytes. Melanocytes produce melanin and transfer them to the adjacent keratinocytes. Melanocytes are identified by the dopa reaction or the silver staining methods. The dopa reaction recognizes the tyrosinase dopa oxidase enzyme present in the melanocytes. The melanocytes have a spider-like dendritic appearance stained with silver stains. In H&E stain, the melanocytes appear as clear cells. Thus, melanocytes are referred to as clear cells or dendritic cells. The most specific stain for melanocytes is the "Mason- Fontana" stain. The number of melanocytes vary in number in different regions. The degree of pigmentation varies in different parts of the oral cavity. This variation in the degree of pigmentation depends on the dispersal of the melanosomes, quantity of melanin within the melanosomes, and the rate of degradation of the pigment.

14.11 Merkel Cells

Merkel cells migrate from the neural crest to the oral epithelium, are also seen among the basal cells, and are specialized neural pressure-sensitive receptor cells. They respond to touch sensation. They are usually seen in the masticatory mucosa. These cells do not possess dendritic processes. Electron-microscopically, the nucleus shows a deep invagination and a characteristic rodlet. The cells contain many electron-dense granules. The function of these granules is in still not known. The Merkel cells are well recognized by the periodic acid Schiff stain.

14.12 Langerhans Cells

The Langerhans cells are both clear cells and dendritic cells that are located in the superficial layers of the epithelium. These cells have a convoluted nucleus and rod-like granules called Birbeck granules in their cytoplasm. They contain vimentin-type intermediate filaments. Langerhans cells are recognized via gold chloride stain, ATPase stain, and immunofluorescent markers. This cell is hematopoietic in origin. They migrate from the lamina propria to the epithelium. Langerhans cells play a pivotal role in the immune response. These cells migrate to the epithelium in response to the chemotactic factors released by the keratinocytes or an antigenic challenge from bacterial plaque. These cells function by recognizing the antigen and presenting it to the lymphocytes either locally or at the lymph nodes. Langerhans' cells present the "specific antigen" to helper T lymphocytes, and the interleukin-1 produced by the keratinocytes stimulates the T cells to produce interleukin-2.

14.13 Basement Membrane and Basal Lamina

The basal lamina is a cell-free zone that is 1–4 μm wide, which forms the interface between the epithelium and the connective tissue. This zone contains neutral mucopolysaccharides, especially glycosaminoglycans, and, hence, stains positive for periodic acid Schiff stain.

The basal lamina is composed of lamina and fibers. The lamina lucida is a clear zone, which is just below the epithelial cells, while lamina dense is a dark zone, adjacent to the connective tissue.

Lamina lucida: The lamina lucida is a 20–40 nm wide glycoprotein layer that contains laminin and bullous pemphigoid antigen and type IV collagen.

Lamina densa: The lamina dense contains type IV collagen coated with heparan sulfate in a chicken-wire pattern. Type IV collagen fibers, as anchoring fibrils, form loops and are inserted in the lamina densa. Type I and type III collagen fibers run through the loops of the anchoring fibrils.

14.14 Lamina Propria

The lamina propria is a connective tissue that supports the epithelium; it is divided into a papillary portion and a reticular portion.

The papillary portion is between the epithelial ridges and is of variable depth. The papillary portion may not be present in a few areas such as the alveolar mucosa. The interlocking arrangement of the epithelial ridges and the connective tissue increases the area of contact between lamina propria and epithelium and facilitates the exchange of nutrients from the blood vessels to the epithelial cells.

The reticular layer is below the papillary portion of the lamina propria. This layer contains fine immature argyrophilic reticular fibers. The reticular layer contains collagen fibers arranged in a net-like manner.

The ground substance of the lamina propria contains glycoproteins and proteoglycans. The prominent proteoglycans are hyaluronan, heparan sulfate, versican, decorin, biglycan, and syndecan, to name a few. The fibers that are seen in the lamina propria are type I and type III collagen and elastic fibers. The elastic fibers are more often seen in the lining epithelium and help in restoring the form of the tissues after they stretch. The lamina propria may be attached to the periosteum of the underlying bone or lies just above the submucosa.

14.15 Nonkeratinized Epithelium

The nonkeratinized epithelium does not produce keratin and, hence, does not have the cornified layer. The cellular layers of the nonkeratinized epithelium are stratum basale, stratum intermedium, and stratum granulosum.

Stratum basale: The cells of the stratum basale comprise a single layer of cuboidal cells.

Stratum intermedium: The cells are polyhedral in shape and larger than those that are in the stratum spinosum of the keratinized epithelium. The cells do not have a prickly appearance because the intercellular space is not distended. The cells do contain a sparse amount of cytokeratin filaments. These filaments are biochemically different from those of the keratinized epithelium. The cells of the stratum intermedium are attached by desmosome junctions.

Stratum superficial comprises flat or squamous cells. They contain a lesser number of tonofilaments and lack keratohyaline granules. They are also nucleated cells. The cells ultimately desquamate just like the cornified squames of the keratinized epithelium. The epithelium does not contain a stratum granulosum or a stratum corneum.

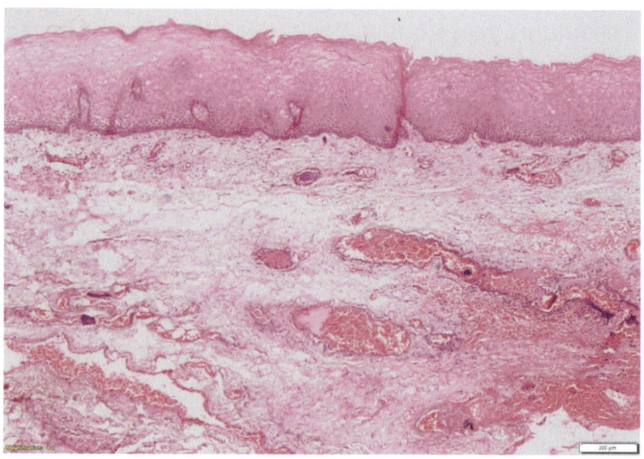

Histology of the buccal mucosa showing a nonkeratinized epithelium and a delicate submucosa (H&E 4×). (Courtesy: Department of oral and maxillofacial pathology and oral microbiology, Manipal College of Dental Sciences, Manipal)

14.16 Specialized Mucosa

14.16.1 Dorsal Surface of the Tongue

The dorsal surface of the tongue is rough and irregular. There is a V-shaped groove that divides the tongue into an anterior part, which is the body of the tongue, and a posterior part, which is the base of the tongue. The body of the tongue makes up two-thirds of the entire length and is papillary, while the base of the tongue makes up one-third of the tongue and is predominantly lymphoid in structure.

14.16.2 Circumvallate Papillae

Circumvallate papillae are seen just in front of the V-shaped terminal sulcus between the body and the base of the tongue. They are usually 8–10 in number. They do not rise above the surface, but they have a deep circular furrow around them. They are connected to the surface of the tongue only at their base. There are numerous taste buds in the epithelium on the lateral surface of the papilla. There are several small serous glands called von Ebner's glands within the papilla. These ducts open into the trough and drain their secretions. The serous secretions from the von Ebner gland are rich in salivary lipase.

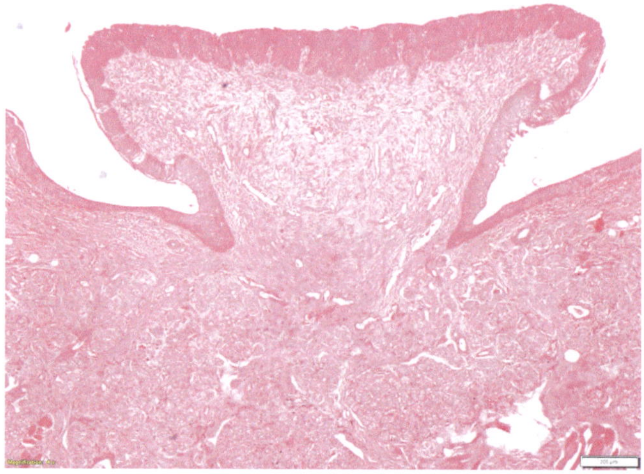

Histology of the circumvallate papillae with taste buds (H&E 4×). (Courtesy: Department of oral and maxillofacial pathology and oral microbiology, Manipal College of Dental Sciences, Manipal)

14.16.3 Fungiform Papilla

Fungiform papillae are mushroom-shaped papillae that are interspersed between the filiform papillae. They are round and pinkish protuberances on the surface of the tongue. They appear pink because of their rich capillary network that is visible through the thin epithelium. They also contain a few taste buds on their dorsal surface.

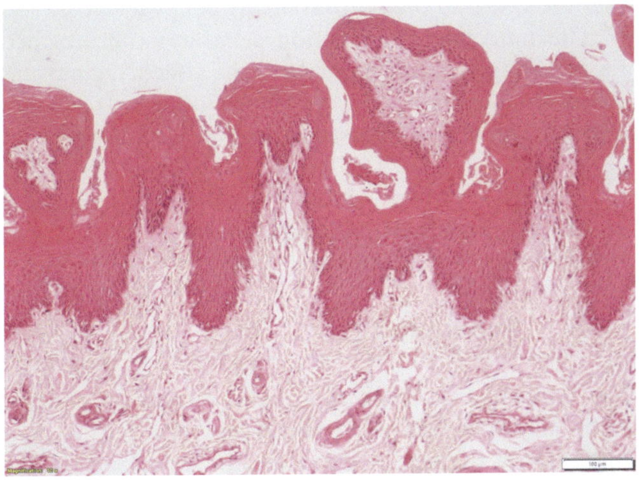

Histology of the fungiform papilla (H&E 4×). (Courtesy: Department of oral and maxillofacial pathology and oral microbiology, Manipal College of Dental Sciences, Manipal)

14.16.4 Filiform Papillae

Filiform papillae are found on the anterior part of the tongue. These papillae are fine, pointed, and cone-shaped and have a velvet-like appearance. These papillae are thread-like epithelial projections with a core of connective tissue at the center. The overlying epithelium is keratinized and forms tufts at the apex of the papilla.

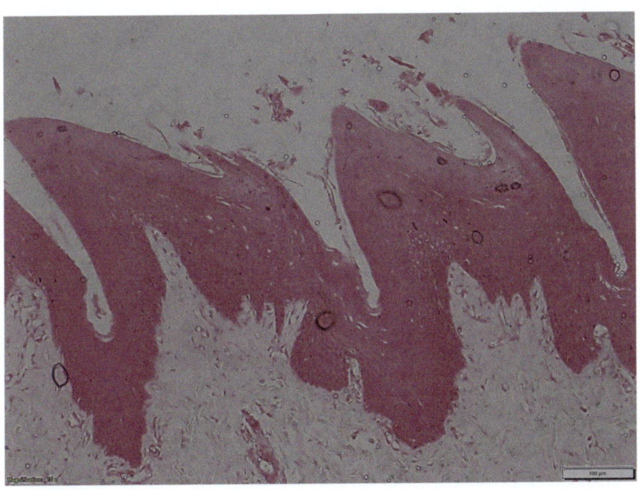

Histology of the filiform papilla (H&E 4×). (Courtesy: Department of oral and maxillofacial pathology and oral microbiology, Manipal College of Dental Sciences, Manipal)

14.16.5 Taste Buds

Taste buds are unique structures that are seen within the epithelium of the papillae of the tongue. They are present on the inner wall of the trough surrounding the circumvallate papillae, within the folds of the foliate papillae, and in a few of the fungiform papillae. They are small, ovoid or barrel-shaped, and about 80 μm high and 40 μm thick. They extend from the basement membrane to the surface of the epithelium. The taste bud comprises a taste pore, which is a small opening. This taste pore is surrounded by a few flat epithelial cells. The taste pore leads into a narrow space that is also lined by the supporting cells of the taste bud.

The taste bud comprises 30–80 spindle-shaped cells. There are three different types of cells in the taste buds. The light cells or type I cells are supporting cells that are at the periphery and arranged like the staves of a barrel. These cells comprise half the number of cells of the taste buds. These cells comprise granular endoplasmic reticulum, vesicles, vacuoles, and mitochondria. These cells contain a less dense spherical nucleus.

The dark cells or type II cells are neuroepithelial cells. The dark cells are elongated cells with numerous fine cytoplasmic filaments that are arranged as bundles, Golgi apparatus, mitochondria, endoplasmic reticulum, and membrane-bound vesicles in the cytoplasm. These cells have dense nuclei. These cells carry finger-like projections at their superficial end, which reach into the space beneath the taste pore.

A rich plexus of nerves is found below the taste buds; a few nerve fibers enter the epithelium and are in contact with the sensory cells.

14.17 Keratinized Epithelium

14.17.1 Hard Palate

Macroscopic appearance: The hard palate is pink in color just like the gingiva.

Microscopic appearance: The palate is made up of a uniform well-keratinized epithelium. There is an increase in the number and length of the desmosomes, the density of the tonofilaments, and the complementary grooves and ridges. These features are an adaptation of the keratinizing epithelium to resist masticatory forces and to attach the epithelium firmly to the underlying lamina propria.

The lamina propria has numerous long papillary projections and is thicker in the anterior than in the posterior part of the hard palate. The submucosa of the palate varies at different parts of the hard palate and has been designated as different zones:

- Gingival region
- Palatine raphe that extends from the incisive papilla to the palatine uvula
- Anterolateral area, a fatty zone that lies between the palatine raphe and the gingiva
- Posterolateral area, a glandular zone that lies between the palatine raphe and the gingiva

The submucosa is a wide region which is firmly attached to the periosteum of the maxillary and palatine bones. This submucosa comprises dense bands and trabeculae of fibrous connective tissue. The submucosa is divided into irregular intercommunicating compartments. In the anterior part, the submucosa is filled with adipose tissue and the posterior part with glandular tissue. The lamina propria is fixed to the periosteum by dense bands of fibrous connective tissue. These bands are at right angles to the surface.

The anterior palatine vessels and nerves within a loose connective tissue are present at the junction of the alveolar process and the horizontal part of the hard palate. This wedge-shaped area is larger in the posterior part and smaller in the anterior part.

14.17.2 Incisive Papilla

The incisive papilla is formed of dense connective tissue. It contains vestigial nasopalatine ducts. These ducts vary in length and are lined by simple or pseudostratified columnar epithelium. The epithelium also contains several goblet cells. Small mucous glands open into the lumen of the ducts. Most often, the ducts are surrounded by irregular islands of hyaline cartilage.

14.17.3 Palatine Rugae

The palatine rugae are irregular, asymmetric ridges of oral mucosa extending from the incisive papillae. The core of the palatine rugae is made up of dense connective tissue layer with fine interwoven fibers.

14.17.4 Gingiva

Gingiva is a masticatory mucosa that extends from the dento-gingival junction to the alveolar mucosa. The gingiva is normally pink, but at times it may have a grayish tint. The color of the gingiva depends on the degree of keratinization and the thickness of the epithelium.

The gingiva is divided into:

- Gingival sulcus
- Free gingiva
- Free gingival groove
- Attached gingiva
- Mucogingival junction
- Alveolar mucosa
- Interdental papilla

A free gingival groove separates the free gingiva from the attached gingiva. The free gingival groove is parallel to the margin of the gingiva at a distance of 0.5–1.5 mm, and it is apical to the bottom of the gingival sulcus.

The mucogingival junction separates the attached gingiva and the alveolar mucosa. The attached gingiva is about 4–6 mm and the mucogingival junction is 3–5 mm below the level of the crest of the alveolar mucosa.

14.18 Microscopic Appearance

14.18.1 Epithelium

The epithelium is para-keratinized in 75% of the ginigva, ortho-keratinized in 15%, and nonkeratinized in 10%. The color of the gingiva depends on the thickness of the keratinization. When the layer of keratin is thick, the epithelium appears whiter and is less translucent. The presence of melanin that is produced by the melanocytes gives a brownish–black pigmentation to the gingiva.

Portions of the epithelium of the gingiva are elevated and between the elevations are shallow depressions. This results in the clinical appearance of stippling of the gingiva. There may be protuberances of the epithelium along with the stippling of the epithelium. These are functional adaptations to withstand mechanical forces.

The interdental papilla is that part of the gingiva that is present between two adjacent teeth. The interdental papilla between the posterior teeth is tent-shaped, while the interdental papilla between the anterior teeth is pyramidal in shape. Among the posterior teeth, the buccal and lingual part is high, while the central area is like a valley. This valley-like central area is called col. A thin nonkeratinized epithelium covers the col.

14.18.2 Lamina Propria

The lamina propria of the gingiva comprises reticular and a papillary component. The connective tissue is dense with a few lymphocytes, plasma cells, and macrophages. In the papillary portion the connective tissues are long, slender, and numerous. The connective tissue comprises dense collagenous fibers, mainly type I and type III collagen fibers. They support the free gingiva and are divided into four groups:

- Dento-gingival: These are the most numerous of collagen fibers. They extend from the cementum into the laminal propria of the gingiva
- Alveolo-gingival: These collagen fibers arise from the alveolar crest and extend into the lamina propria
- Circular: These collagen fibers encircle the tooth and interlace with each other
- Dento-periosteal: These collagen fibers run from the cementum into the periosteum of the alveolar crest
- Circular:
- Semicircular: These fibers connect the cementum on one side of the tooth to the opposite side after passing through the free gingiva
- Interdental: These fibers connect the buccal and lingual papillae
- Longitudinal
- Vertical: These fibers run vertically from the alveolar mucosa or attached mucosa to the marginal mucosa
- Transgingival

In addition, there are other accessory collagen fibers such as the transseptal fibers, which are seen in the interdental region. These fibers pass from the cementum of one tooth to the marginal gingiva of the adjacent tooth and run above the crest of the alveolar bone.

Elastic fibers are few in the lamina propria and are usually in the walls of the blood vessels. Oxytalan fibers are also present in the lamina propria of the gingiva.

The fibroblasts that are present in the lamina propria have minimal contractile protein and lack alkaline phosphatase. The ground substance has more of hyaluron and a lower turnover rate. The ground substance releases prostaglandin in response to histamine.

14.18.3 Dento-gingival Junction

This is the junction between the tooth and the gingiva. The epithelium of the gingiva that is attached to the tooth is called attachment epithelium.

The junctional epithelium looks just like the reduced enamel epithelium with a basal layer of cells and a few layers of flattened cells. This epithelium is nonkeratinized. The junctional epithelium extends up to 2 mm on the surface of the tooth. This epithelium has the highest turnover rate of 5 or 6 days. This epithelium has large intercellular spaces and, hence, is highly permeable and permits neutrophils to pass in and out of the epithelium. It also permits the flow of crevicular fluid.

The mechanical strength of the dento-gingival junction is due to both the connective tissue and the epithelium that is attached to enamel.

The junctional epithelium plays a significant role in maintaining the health of the gingiva. This junction is unique as it is one of both a hard tissue and a soft tissue. The dense lamina propria takes up the masticatory forces. When the epithelium is injured, the injury is repaired by the turnover of the cells and their ability to migrate. When the connective tissue is injured, the ribosomes within the fibroblasts produce procollagen molecules and ground substance to heal the injury.

There are lymphocytes and plasma cells in the connective tissue beneath the gingival sulcus and the attachment epithelium. When there is an infection or inflammation, Langerhans cells migrate to the gingival sulcus. The lysosomes that are present in the lymphocytes have a phagocytic potential and can defend the gingival sulcus from microbial infection.

14.19 Development of the Dento-gingival Junction

When odontogenesis is complete, the basal lamina of the enamel organ remains as a thin membrane on the surface of the tooth called a primary enamel cuticle. The enamel organ is reduced to a few layers of flattened cuboidal cells and is called the reduced enamel epithelium. This reduced enamel epithelium covers the entire crown of the tooth. When the tooth erupts, the tip of the tooth comes close to the oral epithelium and the reduced enamel epithelium and the oral epithelium fuse with each other. The epithelium that covers the tip of the tooth degenerates in the center, and the crown of the tooth emerges into the oral cavity. Once the tooth emerges into the oral cavity, the reduced enamel epithelium is called primary attachment epithelium. As the tooth erupts, the reduced enamel epithelium becomes shorter, and finally, a shallow groove called the gingival sulcus is formed between the gingiva and the surface of the tooth. This sulcus is bound by the attachment epithelium at its base and the gingival margin laterally. As the tooth erupts, the reduced enamel epithelium detaches from the tooth.

14.20 Shift of the Dento-gingival Junction

There is a gradual shift in the location of the dento-gingival junction that takes place with time. When the crown emerges into the oral cavity, the attachment epithelium separates from the surface of the enamel. During the process of eruption, when the tooth reaches the plane of occlusion, one-third to one-fourth of the crown is covered with the attachment epithelium. Then a gradual exposure of the crown takes place.

When the reduced enamel epithelium is still present, the cells of the oral epithelium join them by forming desmosomes. Later, the reduced enamel epithelium is lost, and the cells of the oral epithelium form hemidesmosomes and a lamina lucida and attach themselves to the tooth. This new attachment is called the secondary attachment epithelium.

- In the first stage, the gingival sulcus is present on the enamel-covered crown, and the apical end of the attachment epithelium is at the cemento-enamel junction.
- In the second stage, the gingival sulcus is still on the enamel, and the apical end of the attachment epithelium is on the surface of the cementum.
- In the third stage, the bottom of the gingival sulcus is at the cemento-enamel junction, and the epithelial attachment is completely on the cementum. The entire enamel-covered crown is fully exposed.
- In the fourth stage, there is recession of the gingiva. The entire attachment is on the cementum.

The rate of exposure of the crown and the recession of gingiva vary for different people.

14.21 Lip

A non keratinized, stratified squamous epithelium forms the epithelium of the lip and cheek. The lamina propria comprises dense connective tissue with irregular papillae. The underlying muscle is attached to the lamina propria through the submucosa. The submucosa comprises of strands of dense collagen fibers, along with fat cells and small mixed salivary gland tissues. The strands of connective tissues limit the mobility of the mucous membrane. The mixed salivary glands are in the submucosa of the lips. In the cheeks, the glands are larger and found between the muscles of the buccinator muscle. The buccal mucosa at the corner of the mouth may contain isolated sebaceous glands called Fordyce spots.

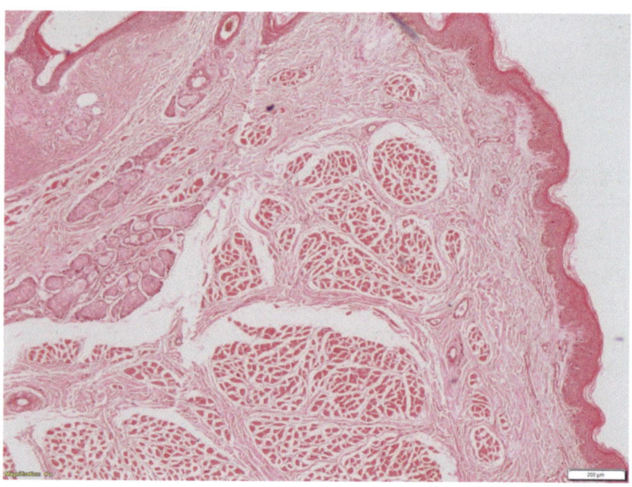

Histology of the vermilion border of the lip (H&E 4×). (Courtesy: Department of oral and maxillofacial pathology and oral microbiology, Manipal College of Dental Sciences, Manipal)

14.22 Vestibular Fornix and Alveolar Mucosa

The gingiva is separated from the alveolar mucosa by the mucogingival junction. The epithelium of the alveolar mucosa is thin and nonkeratinized. The lamina propria contains papillae that are low. The submucosa is thin and a well-defined loose connective tissue with mixed salivary gland tissue.

14.23 Ventral Surface and Floor of the Mouth

The ventral surface of the tongue contains a dep lingual vein on both sides of the midline. The tongue is attached to the floor of the mouth through the lingual frenum. The mucosa of the inferior surface of the tongue is smooth and thin. The epithelium is nonkeratinized, and the papillae are numerous but short.

The mucosa of the floor of the mouth is thin and loosely attached to the underlying structures. This makes the floor of the mouth free and mobile. The epithelium is nonkeratinized and the papillae of the lamina propria is short. The submucosa contains adipose tissue and sublingual mixed salivary glands.

14.24 Soft Salate

The epithelium is nonkeratinized, stratified squamous epithelium. The lamina propria are few and short and contain elastic fibers. The submucosa is relatively loose and contains mucous glands. Taste buds are also present in the submucosa. The submucosa is highly vascularized and imparts a reddish color to the soft palate.

14.25 Vascularity

The vascularity of the oral mucosa is derived from the arteries that are present in the submucosa and from the periosteum. The blood vessels in the reticular layer the arteries give off smaller branches of arteries that anastomose with adjacent vessels. The vessels reach the papillary layer and come to lie subjacent to the basal epithelial cells. In the buccal mucosa, the capillaries follow a tortuous path with numerous branches that pass through each of the papillae of the lamina propria. In the filliform papilla, there are numerous capillaries, while in the fungiform and circumvallate papillae there are larger arterioles.

The flow rate of the blood in the oral mucosa is greater than that in the skin and is the greatest in the gingiva. The postcapillary venules in the gingival sulcus express ELAM and ICAM, which play a vital role in leukocyte mobility. As there are no arterio–venous shunts in the gingiva, it does not have a role in the regulation of the temperature. Yet, due to the extensive vascularity and the anastomoses of the arteries and capillaries, healing of tissue of the oral mucosa takes place rapidly.

14.26 Neural Innervation

The nerve supply to the oral mucosa is predominantly sensory in nature. The neural innervation mediates voluntary and reflexive activities of the oral mucosa such as swallowing, speaking, and gagging. The nerve supply to the oral mucosa is derived from the maxillary and mandibular nerve branches of the trigeminal nerve. In addition, the facial nerve, glossopharyngeal nerve, and the vagus nerve also contribute to the neural innervation of the oral cavity.

Free nerve endings of the sensory nerves are seen in the lamina propria and in the epithelium. In the epithelium, the nerve endings are associated with the Merkel cells. In the lamina propria, organized nerve endings are seen in the papillary region. The sensations that are perceived in the oral cavity are warmth, cold, touch, pain, and taste. The nerve endings that are in the oral mucosa are specialized and have varied morphology. They are Meissner's or Ruffini's corpuscles that are responsible for touch sensation and the Krause's bulbs that are sensitive to cold stimuli. The touch sensation is more pronounced in the anterior part of the tongue and the hard palate. The touch receptors in the soft palate are responsible for swallowing, gagging, and retching sensations. The Krause's bulbs are present in the vermilion border of the lip and the tip of the tongue. The pain sensation is derived due to activation of the polypeptides in the interstitial fluid, which, in turn, stimulate the free nerve endings of the slow-conducting unmyelinated nerves and the thin myelinated nerves.

14.27 Molecular Aspects

The cytoskeleton of the keratinocyte is the presence of keratin tonofilaments. The cytokeratins that are present in the keratinized stratified squamous epithelium are cytokeratins 1, 6, 10, and 16. In the nonkeratinized epithelium are cytokeratins 4, 13, and 19. The cytokeratins in the stratified epithelium has a molecular weight of 67 KDa. The keratinocytes also possess several cell-surface receptors.

14.28 Age Changes of the Oral Mucosa

The epithelium becomes dry and smooth as the salivary secretion also decreases. The epithelium gradually losses its sensitivity to thermal, chemical, and mechanical stimuli and taste perception. The epithelium becomes thin as the thickness of the epithelial ridges is reduced. The number of filiform papillae is also less. Varicose veins may be seen on the ventral aspect of the tongue and are called lingual varices. The cellularity of the epithelium also decreases, as well as the amount of collagen in the submucosa and the lamina propria.

14.29 Functions of the Oral Mucosa

- Defense: The oral mucosa forms a protective barrier for the underlying tissues against bacterial invasion. Even though the oral cavity is a normal harbor for microbes, the bacteria or their toxins are prevented from penetrating the epithelium and causing infection. In addition, the cells of the epithelium produce antibodies and, hence, facilitates cellular and humoral immunity.
- Lubrication: The secretions of the minor salivary glands in the oral cavity keep the oral mucosa moist to help in speech, mastication, swallowing, and perception of taste.
- Sensory: The oral mucosa is a sensory organ with receptors for touch, pressure, pain, temperature, and taste. Reflexes such as swallowing, gagging, and salivation are initiated by these receptors.
- Protective: The underlying vital structures are protected from the masticatory forces by the oral mucosa.

14.30 Clinical Considerations

The structure of the submucosa in different parts of the oral cavity has a great influence in the clinical scenario.

In areas where the submucosa is loose like in the cheek and lips:

- Infection can spread rapidly and widely.
- When there is edema and hemorrhage, it can cause swelling of the tissues.
- Since the submucosa is lightly attached to the underlying structures, an incision will cause a gaping wound that requires suturing.
- Infiltration of a medicament is easy and less painful, and the fluid can easily disperse into the tissues.

In the masticatory mucosa where the submucosa is firmly attached to the underlying tissues:

- An Incision in this mucosa does not result in the formation of a gaping wound.
- Infiltration of a local anesthetic is tough and painful.

Drug Delivery: The floor of the mouth is an ideal site for placement of medicaments. This the region in the oral cavity with a high tissue permeability.

The turnover rate of the epithelium of the oral mucosa is higher than that of the skin. This helps in healing of the oral mucosa, and in addition, there is scar formation in the oral cavity.

The oral mucosa is a common site for the first manifestation of various systemic disorders, autoimmune conditions, and nutritional deficiencies. The oral cavity is the most common site for the occurrence of squamous cell carcinomas.

Further Reading

Kumar GS. Orban's oral histology and embryology. 12th ed. Elsevier.
Kumar GS. Orban's oral histology and embryology. 15th ed. Elsevier.
Ten Cate R. Oral histology, development structure and function. 5th ed. Mosby.

Histology of Salivary Glands

Jumma Alkhabuli and Sadeq Ali Al-Maweri

Contents

S R Prabhu et al. (eds.), *Oral Histology and Oral Histopathology*, https://doi.org/10.1007/978-3-031-77481-2_15

15.1 Introduction

Salivary gland (SG) development involves epithelial-mesenchymal interactions through multiple coordinated progressive mechanisms leading to a branching morphogenesis process that ends up with secretory endpieces and duct formation.

Salivary glands play a major role in the maintenance of the oral cavity structures and homeostasis. They secrete saliva that lubricates oral mucosa and provide essential salivary electrolytes, enzymes such as salivary amylase, and antimicrobial complexes to protect the soft and hard oral tissues.

Human SGs are broadly categorized into minor and major glands. The latter glands are comprised of pairs of parotids, submandibular, and sublingual glands, while the minor glands consist of 600–1000 tiny submucosal glands. About 1.5 L of saliva is released per day, of which 90% of the total saliva comes from the major glands while the remaining 10% is secreted by the minor SGs.

Histologically, the parenchyma of each gland is comprised of two main elements, namely the secretory endpieces (acini) and ducts. Acinus is the basic functional unit of the gland comprised of acinar cells, which are either of serous or mucous secretion. Mucous acini with a few attached serous acinar cells "serous demilune" are also found, particularly in submandibular and sublingual glands.

This chapter aims to describe the basic microscopic histology of the major salivary glands in light of the recent available information.

15

15.2 Histology

The major SGs have fundamentally similar structures; the secretory endpieces (acini) and branched multiple ducts. Each major gland is surrounded by a capsule of fibrous connective tissue extending into the body of the gland dividing it into lobes and lobules (◘ Fig. 15.1). The parotid and submandibular glands have single excretory ducts opening into the oral cavity called Stenson's and Wharton's ducts, respectively, whereas the sublingual gland invariably possesses multiple tiny ducts (ducts of Rivinus) that open directly into the sublingual fold. In some individuals, abnormal development of ducts of Rivinus leads to a single duct (Bartholin duct) opening anteriorly.

A salivary gland comprises a course of branched ducts that end in a tubular or spherical secretory unit or acinus (◘ Fig. 15.2). A bunch of grapes is probably the best analogy that simulates salivary gland histology with the stem representing ducts and grapes resembling secretory endpieces. The opening of the excretory duct in the oral cavity branches off into smaller interlobar and interlobular excretory ducts.

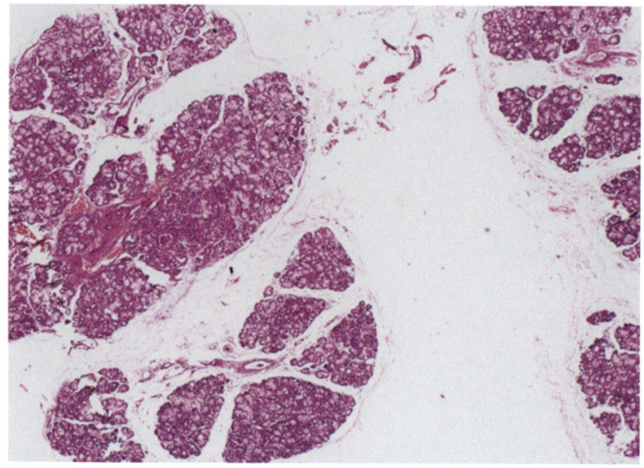

◘ **Fig. 15.1** Light micrograph section (×4) showing the lobular organization of the submandibular gland

15.2.1 Fibrous Connective Tissues (Capsule)

Major SGs are wrapped by a thick fibrous capsule that extends into the gland dividing it into large segments "lobes" and smaller parts (lobules). The thick fibrous tissue partition (septa) divides the gland into multiple lobes and is continuous with the capsule, which encompasses the blood vessels and nerves supplying the gland (◘ Fig. 15.3). The fine connective tissue partitions surround the ducts and endpieces within the lobules. The extracellular matrix is made of collagen and elastic fibers along with glycoproteins and proteoglycan. Fibroblasts and other inflammatory cells constitute the main cellular components. The parotid gland is the first gland to develop a capsule and remains the last to complete encapsulation. The sublingual gland has a poorly developed capsule.

15.2.2 Secretory Cells

The secretory cell is the smallest functioning unit present in a gland. Essentially, two main types of secretory cells exist in salivary glands; serous and mucous cells. These cells vary in basic microscopic structure and types of molecular secretions. Serous cells primarily contain glycoproteins, which have many enzymatic activities, whereas mucous cells contain mucin glycoproteins, which are different in structure from serous cell glyco-

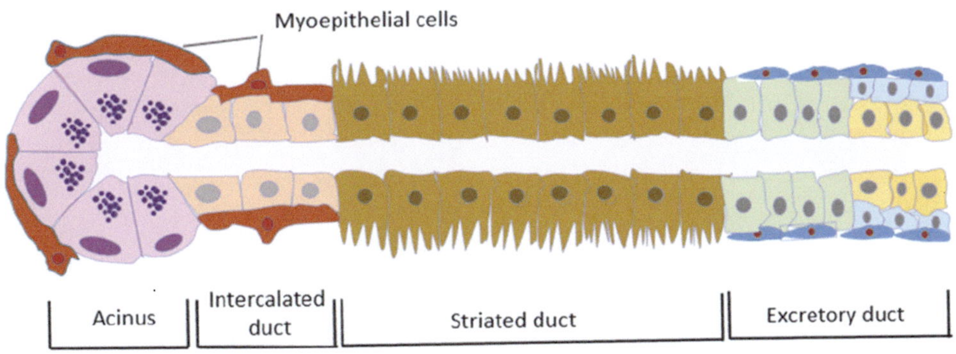

Fig. 15.2 Schematic diagram showing details of the parenchymal myoepithelial cells surrounding mucous acinus and associated intercalated, striated, and excretory ducts

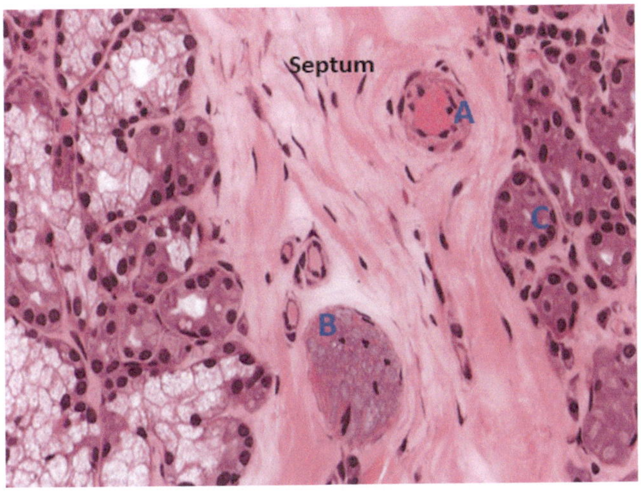

Fig. 15.3 Light micrograph, sublingual (SG) H&E section (×20) showing blood vessel **a**, nerve **b**, and acinus **c** within the interlobular septum

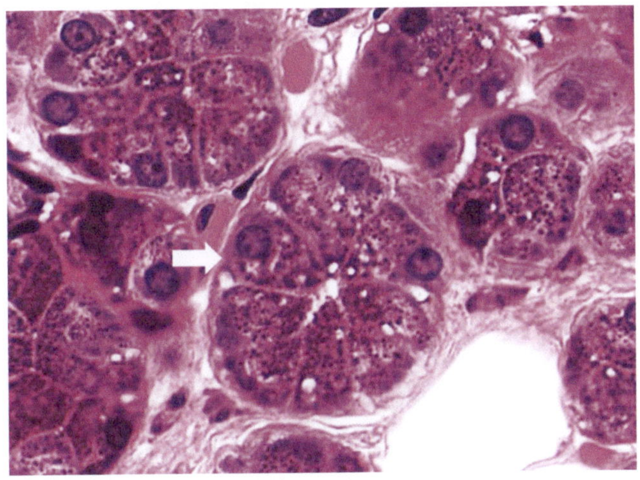

Fig. 15.4 Light micrograph of the parotid gland, H&E section (×40). Arrow showing serous acinus

proteins. Mucins mainly lubricate the oral soft tissues and act as a barrier against microbial aggregation on mucosal surfaces.

15.2.2.1 Serous Cells

A serous secretory endpiece (acinus) is comprised of 8–12 serous cells, exhibiting a spherical shape arranged circumferentially around a central lumen (Fig. 15.4). Each cell has a pyramidal shape with the narrow apex forming part of the central lumen. The acinar lumen extends between adjacent secretory cells as "intercellular canaliculi". The nuclei have a round shape, located in the basal half of the cell. It is not uncommon to see binucleated cells. The cytoplasm possesses various secretory granules (zymogen granules) storing several saliva proteins. The granules are mostly present in the apical portion of the cells. The other intracellular organelles including rough endoplasmic reticulum, mitochondria, cytoskeletal components, and lysosomes are abundantly present. The lateral and basal cell membranes exhibit regular folds extending laterally to interdigitate with similar processes of the adjacent cells. The folds increase the cell surface area thus increasing the ionic exchange processes (Fig. 15.5).

The acinar cells in both mucous and serous acini are joined together through several intercellular adhesion molecules, including tight junctions, adhering junctions, and desmosomes. The tight junction in particular functions as a selective regulator for the passage of water and ions. The secretory cells are intimately attached to the underlying basal lamina and adjacent connective tissue by hemidesmosomes. The various adhesion molecules act to hold adjacent cells together. The adhesion molecules play a major role in transmitting cellular signals. The tight junction possesses several proteins involved in the regulation of cytoskeletal organization and signaling to and from the nucleus. The gap junctions on the cellular lateral surfaces permit the passage of the small molecules between cells. Microscopically, in standard hematoxylin and eosin-stained sections, the serous cells are stained purple with the basic dye hema-

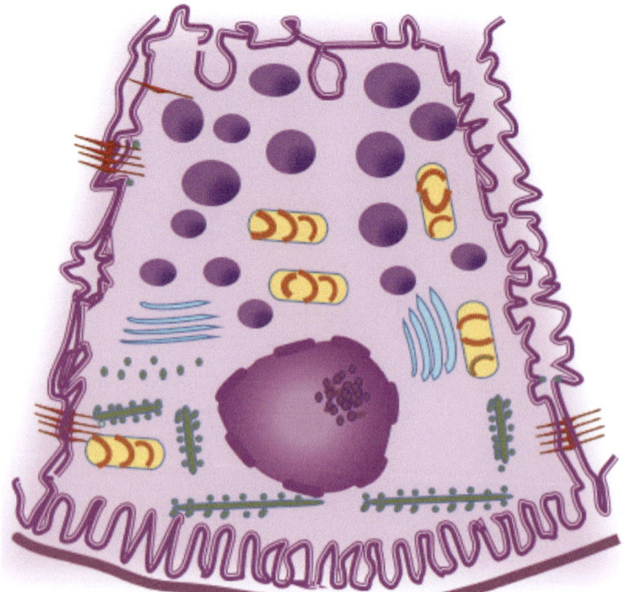

Fig. 15.5 A schematic view showing a longitudinal section of a serous cell, intercellular canaliculi, basal cell membrane infolds, and intracellular organelles

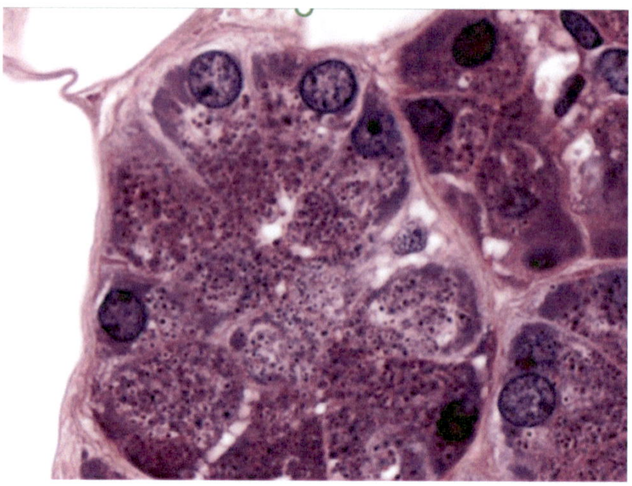

Fig. 15.6 Light micrograph of a parotid gland, H&E section (×40) demonstrating stained zymogen granules at the cells apex

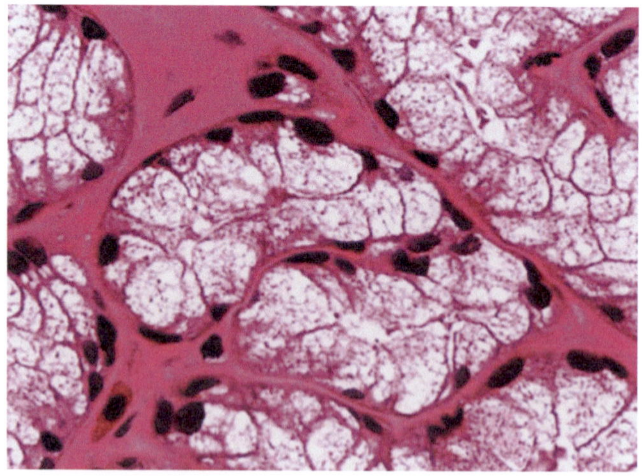

Fig. 15.7 Light micrograph of a sublingual gland, H&E section (×40) demonstrating tubular mucous acini and mucous cells

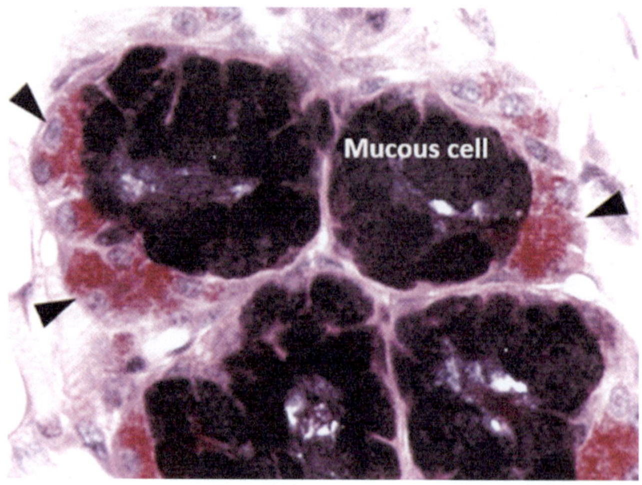

Fig. 15.8 Light micrograph section (×40) of mucous acini with serous demilune (arrowheads) stained with periodic acid Schiff (PAS), Alcian blue, and haematoxylin. PAS and Alcian blue stain mucous cells in dark purple. The serous demilunes stain only with PAS (magenta). (*From Hand AR. Salivary glands. In Provenza DV, Seibel W, editors: Oral histology: inheritance and development, ed 2, Philadelphia, 1986, Lea and Febiger*)

toxylin (H&E) due to their high content of cytoplasmic RNA and the zymogen granules stand out conspicuously at their apex (Fig. 15.6).

15.2.2.2 Mucous Cells

The mucous secretory endpieces have a tubular configuration in cross-section. The central lumen size is relatively larger than the serous acini lumen (Fig. 15.7). Mucous secretory acini may have a few serous secretory cells attached in the form of crescent-shaped caps (demilunes). These serous demilunes are commonly seen in the submandibular, sublingual, and less commonly in minor salivary glands. The serous demilunes are identical to the main secretory endpieces. The contents of the demilunes reach the central lumen via the intercellular canaliculi of the mucous cells. The cytoplasm of mucous cells possesses an abundant amount of carbohydrate-rich mucous granules in the apical two-thirds of the cells compressing the nuclei and the other organelles towards the basal cell membrane. In routine H&E-stained sections, the mucous cells appear clear or with bubbly cytoplasm and nuclei. However, when a special stain such as the Periodic Acid-Schiff (PAC) or Alcian blue is used the cell contents are intensely stained (Fig. 15.8). Electron microscope examination of mucous cells reveals that the secretory granules are fused to one another, and their contents appear lucent, although filamentous material may be seen. In fact, the typical mucous granules appearance is believed to be an artifact induced during the fixation process. These mucous acinar cells mainly produce mucin and a few other macromolecules and their secretion rate is inferior to serous acinar cells.

15.2.2.3 Serous Demilunes

In submandibular, sublingual glands, and to a lesser extent minor glands, some of the mucous acini are capped with a few crescent-shaped serous cells called serous demilunes. They are more predominant in the submandibular gland compared to sublingual glands (◘ Figs. 15.9a, b).

15.2.3 Ducts

In addition to carrying saliva from acinar cells to the oral cavity, ducts play a major role in modifying saliva from the secretory status (isotonic) to hypotonic. Essentially, there are three main types of ducts, namely intercalated, striated, and excretory ducts. The intercellular canaliculi between cells of the secretory endpieces are considered part of the salivary gland ductal system.

15.2.3.1 Intercalated Ducts

These ducts are in intimate contact with the secretory endpiece, and are comprised of a single layer of low cuboidal cells possessing scanty cytoplasm. The duct cells have a simple structure displaying a few RER, small Golgi complexes, and a few secretory granules (◘ Fig. 15.10a, b). The apical portion of the cells exhibits short microvilli projecting towards the lumen. They are the smallest ducts and relatively long in parotid and submandibular glands compared to sublingual glands. Ionic exchanges occur in this duct where bicarbonate ions are secreted while chloride ions are absorbed from saliva. It is thought that the intercalated duct cells contribute to saliva formation, release lactoferrin, and lysozymes as well as differentiation into other gland cells through the in-house stem cells. The intercalated ducts are covered by myoepithelial cells towards the basal side

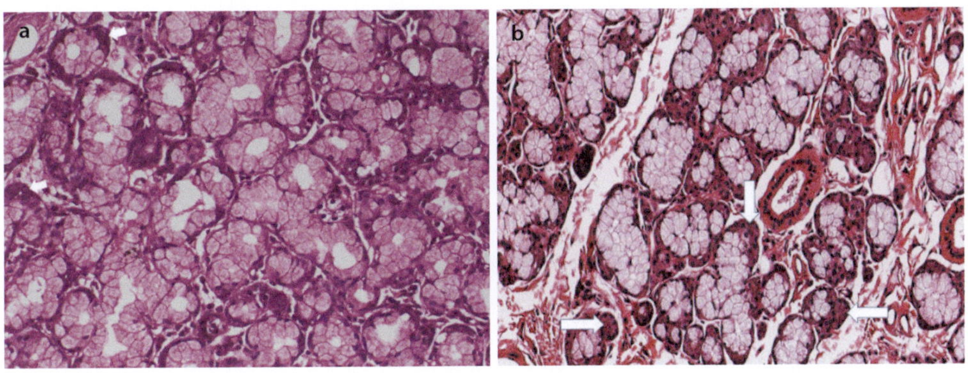

◘ **Fig. 15.9** **a** Light micrograph section (×40), H&E, and submandibular gland section demonstrating the serous demilunes attached to mucous acini (arrows). **b** Light micrograph sublingual gland section (×40), H&E, demonstrating serous demilunes attached to mucous acini (arrows)

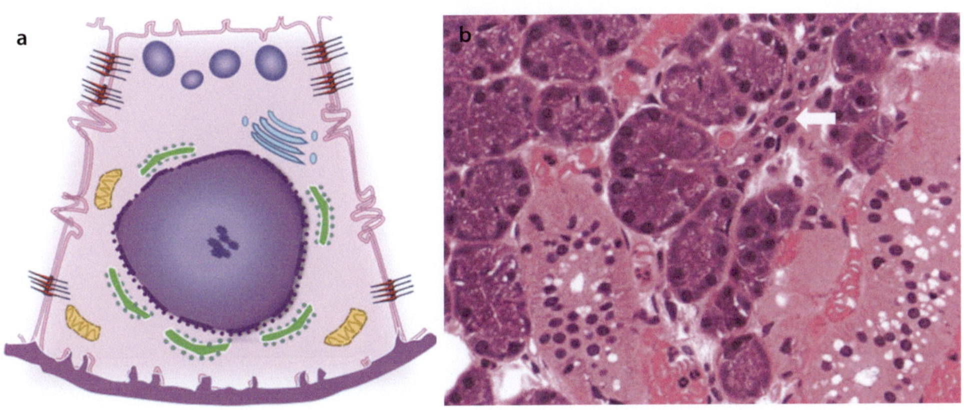

◘ **Fig. 15.10** **a** A schematic diagram showing a longitudinal section of a low cuboidal intercalated duct cell. Note the few intracellular organelles. **b** Light micrograph of parotid gland section (×20), H&E, showing the intercalated duct and the associated serous acini (arrow)

providing support to the duct cells and enhancing saliva transportation (◘ Fig. 15.11). Microscopically, the intercalated ducts are very small and compact, thus difficult to recognize easily.

15.2.3.2 Striated Ducts

Striated ducts receive the primary saliva from the intercalated ducts. They are comprised of columnar cells featuring basolateral membrane invaginations providing the characteristic feature of duct striations. The stacking of elongated mitochondria between the infolds of the basolateral cell membranes is responsible for the striation appearance (◘ Fig. 15.12a, b). The duct cell has a centrally located nucleus and the cytoplasm shows the presence of abundant mitochondria, lysosomes, and a few vesicles or secretory granules apically. Some smooth endoplasmic reticulum may be present at the apical cytoplasm but the rough endoplasmic reticulum is scarce. Striated ducts comprise the major part of the intralobular duct system, and the apical portion of the cells shows microvilli facing the lumen, which is larger than that of the intercalated ducts. In addition to saliva transportation, the striated ducts play an important role in the modification of saliva from isotonic to hypotonic through the basolateral membrane ion channels, where the Na^+ is reabsorbed and K^+ is secreted in the saliva. The apical granules in the duct cells are able to store and release kallikrein, and capable of proteins endocytosis process.

15.2.3.3 Excretory Ducts

Excretory ducts are located in the interlobular connective tissue septum and are the largest among all salivary gland ducts. The lumen wall is lined by pseudo-stratified columnar epithelial cells and several small basal cells (◘ Fig. 15.13). The basal cells sit on the basal lamina but do not reach the lumen. Presumably, these cells have

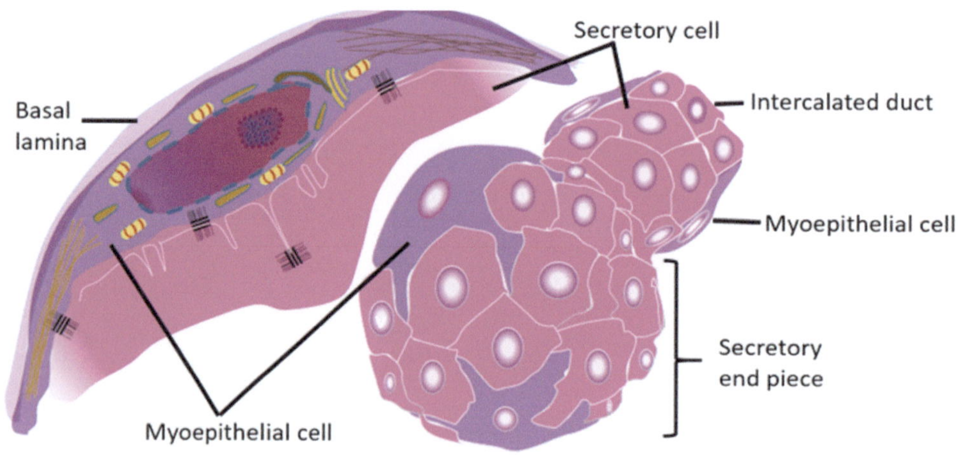

15

◘ **Fig. 15.11** A model representing the association of myoepithelial cells with the secretory endpiece

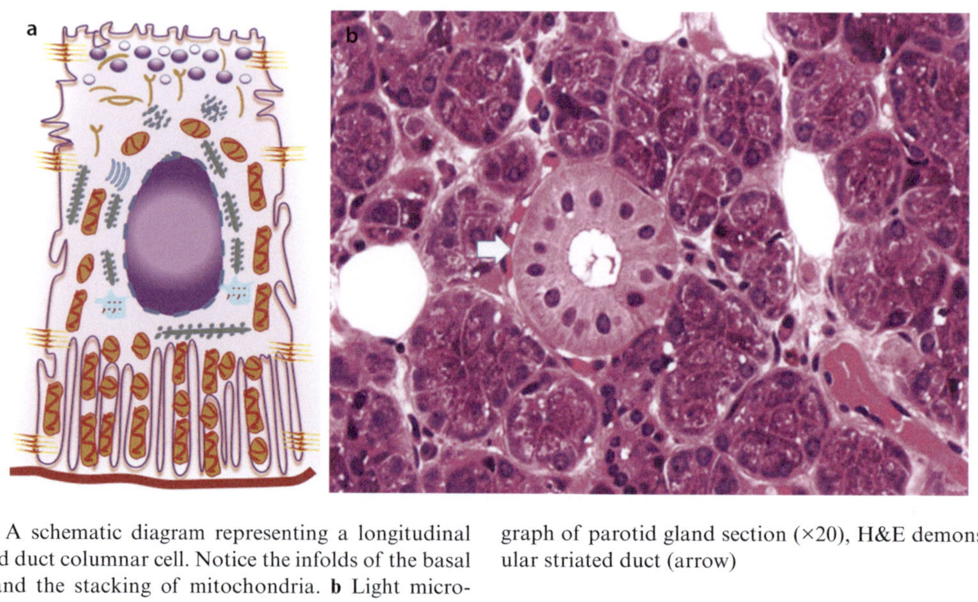

◘ **Fig. 15.12** **a** A schematic diagram representing a longitudinal section of striated duct columnar cell. Notice the infolds of the basal cell membrane and the stacking of mitochondria. **b** Light micrograph of parotid gland section (×20), H&E demonstrating intralobular striated duct (arrow)

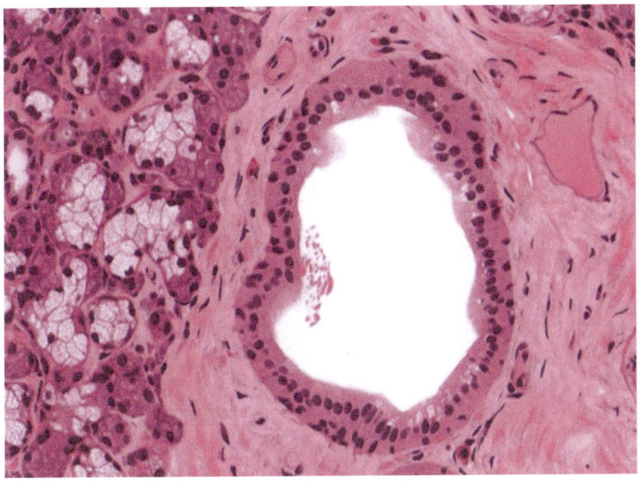

■ **Fig. 15.13** Light micrograph of lingual gland section (×20), H&E demonstrating interlobular excretory duct. Mucous acini with serous demilunes are also seen close to the duct

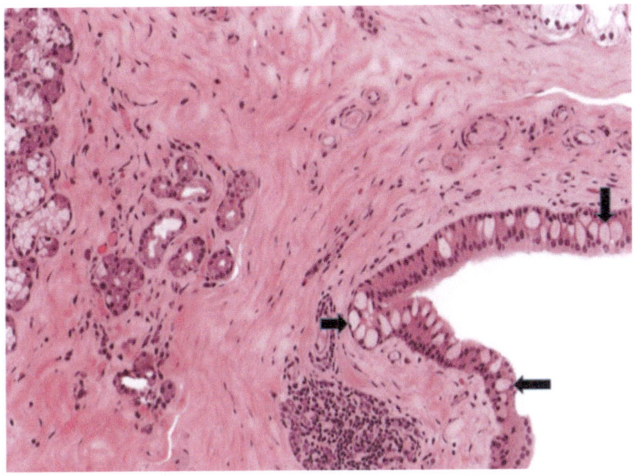

■ **Fig. 15.14** Light micrograph of lingual gland section (×10), H&E demonstrating Goblet cells in the main excretory duct wall (arrows)

the ability to differentiate and replace the columnar cells. The lumen wall of the main excretory duct shows the presence of scattered mucous goblet cells (■ Fig. 15.14). Tuft (brush) cells and dendritic (antigen-presenting) cells are also present. Stratified cuboidal or stratified columnar epithelium may be present in large excretory duct sizes. As the duct approaches the oral cavity, the lining epithelium may show modification and becomes a stratified epithelium. The interlobular connective tissue around the ducts is rich in blood vessels and nerves.

15.2.4 Myoepithelial Cells

These are contractile epithelial cells embracing the secretory endpieces and intercalated ducts. The cells assume a stellate shape exhibiting processes containing myosin, actin, and cytokeratin proteins. Myoepithelial cells are derived from epithelial cells residing on the basal lamina and have similar functional and structural characteristics to smooth muscle cells. The main function of the myoepithelial cells is to provide support to the endpiece secretory cells and their contraction expels saliva from the acinar cells to the ductal system. Other functions include providing signals to the secretory cells required for maintaining cell polarity and structural organization of the secretory endpiece. It is thought that myoepithelial cells synthesize several proteins including proteinase inhibitors and anti-angiogenesis factors, which have tumor suppressor activity.

Microscopically, the myoepithelial cell processes extend from the body of the cell and surround the secretory endpiece. The processes are filled with actin filaments and soluble myosin. A few mitochondria and short cisternae of rough endoplasmic reticuli are present in the perinuclear cytoplasm (■ Fig. 15.11). Of note, it is not easy to identify myoepithelial cells in an H&E-stained section, and myoepithelial immunohistochemical markers are required.

Myoepithelial cells seem to dominate the submandibular glands more than the parotid glands, and this may be attributed to the nature of saliva secretion of the submandibular glands.

15.3 Histology of the Major Salivary Glands

15.3.1 Parotid Gland

The secretory endpieces in the parotid glands are purely serous (■ Figs. 15.5 and 15.15). The acinar cells have a pyramidal shape with a round, basally oriented nucleus encircling a central lumen. In H&E-stained sections, the basal cytoplasm takes basophilic dyes, while the apical secretory granules stain with acidophilic dyes. Fat cell spaces are frequently seen in parotid gland sections.

The parotid gland has several long-intercalated ducts, lined by cuboidal epithelial cells. The striated ducts are acidophilic of large diameter lined by simple columnar epithelium, with round, centrally placed nuclei. The duct exhibits fine striations, demonstrating the infolded basal cell membranes and mitochondria. Excretory ducts are present in the interlobular connective tissue septum. The duct is lined by pseudostratified columnar epithelium with basal and goblet cells.

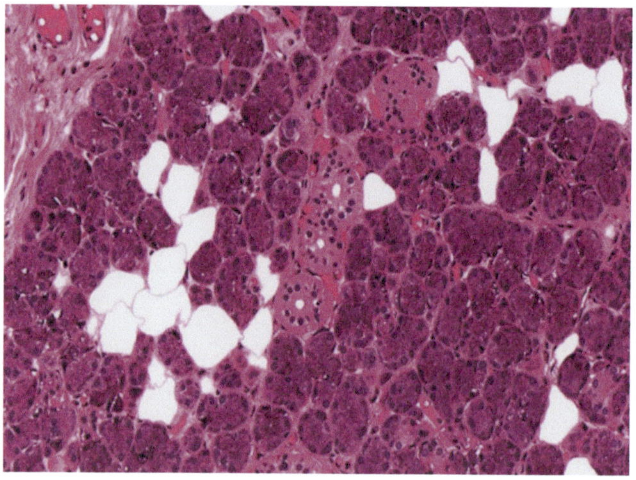

■ **Fig. 15.15** Light micrograph of parotid gland section (×10), H&E demonstrating pure serous acini. The white empty spaces represent fat cells

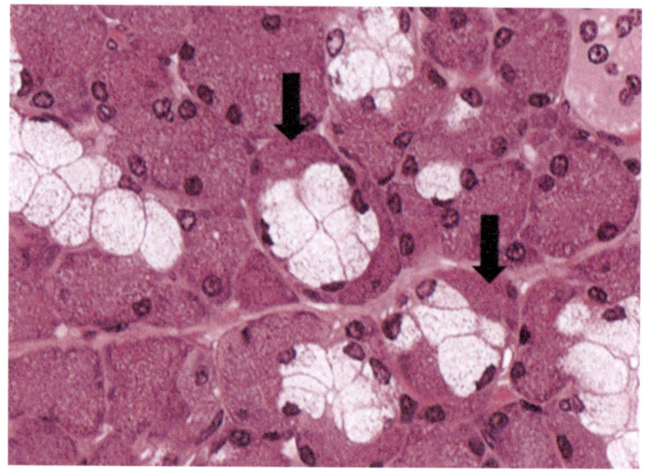

■ **Fig. 15.16** Light micrograph of submandibular gland section (×40), H&E demonstrating serous demilune capping mucous acini

15.3.2 Submandibular Gland

The submandibular gland secretory endpieces are mostly serous (95%) with only 5% being mucous. The gland is encapsulated by fibrous connective tissue that extends into the gland dividing it into multiple lobes and further into lobules. The parenchyma comprises the functional component of the gland that consists of secretory cells and ducts. The serous secretory cells are arranged in a tube or acinus. In these polarized cells, the base has a spherical nucleus and rough endoplasmic reticulum (basophilic), while the apex part contains abundant secretory granules (eosinophilic).

15

The mucous secretory cells are polarized cells with flattened nuclei compressed against the basal cell membrane. They stain faintly with a "foamy" appearance owing to the extracted mucous during the tissue processing. The cells contain densely stained chromatin. The lumen of mucous acini is larger than that of the serous acini. Some of the mucous acini are capped by crescent-shaped serous cells; the serous demilune (■ Fig. 15.16). The serous demilunes have a comparable structure to the serous endpiece cells but their secretions pass through small intercellular canaliculi present between the mucous acinar cells to reach the tubule lumen.

Intercalated and striated ducts are present within the lobules (intralobular ducts), and although less numerous compared to parotid glands they are structurally similar. The intercalated ducts are the smallest ducts that insert into and drain individual acini. The duct cells are low cuboidal and stain lighter with H&E compared to the acinar cells. The striated ducts arise from intercalated ducts and their cells are columnar with basal striations (■ Fig. 15.12a, b). The interlobular or excretory ducts are located out of the lobules and lined by simple cuboidal or columnar epithelial cells that undergo a gradual transition into pseudostratified, stratified cuboidal, or columnar epithelia. The opening of the duct in the oral cavity is lined with stratified squamous epithelium.

15.3.3 Sublingual Gland

Sublingual glands are the smallest pair of major salivary glands and the last to develop. They are located inferolateral to the tongue, right beneath the mucous membrane of the floor of the mouth, and above the mylohyoid muscles. They present predominantly mucous acinar cells and the serous acini are extremely rare (■ Fig. 15.17). It is thought that the appearing serous acini are likely sections through the serous demilunes. About 65% of sublingual gland secretion is mucous and 35% is serous. The sublingual gland exhibits several excretory ducts found near the lingual frenum (ducts of Rivinus). The intralobular ducts are fewer in number compared to other salivary glands. Unlike parotid and submandibular glands, sublingual glands lack proper encapsulation, and the intercalated and striated ducts are infrequent. Saliva drains directly into the oral cavity through the ducts of Rivinus or occasionally via a single excretory duct (Bartholin's duct).

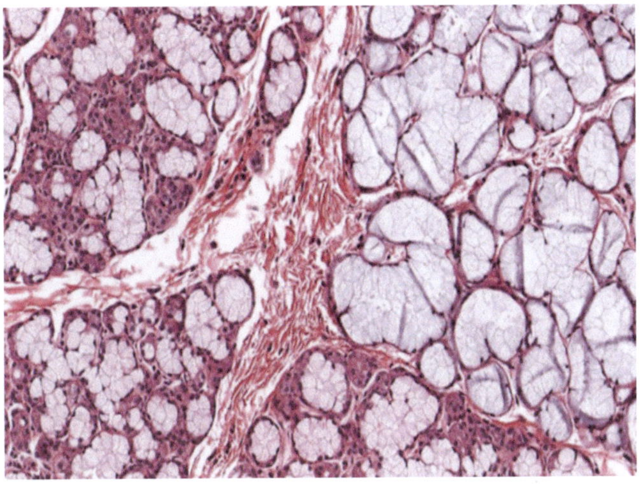

Fig. 15.17 Light micrograph section of the sublingual gland (×10), H&E demonstrating serous demilune capping mucous acini and pure mucous acini

15.4 Histology of the Minor Salivary Glands

Minor salivary glands are comprised of around 600–1000 small submucosal glands scattered throughout the oral cavity and oropharynx. They consist of secretory endpieces and duct aggregates arranged into lobule-like structures, intermingling muscle fibers of the tongue and connective tissue of the submucosa. The majority of minor salivary glands are of pure mucous acini and a few with serous demilunes. The only pure serous aggregates are von Ebner's lingual serous glands which are associated with the circumvallate papillae on the dorsum of the tongue and the foliate papillae on the posterolateral surface of the tongue. Secretions of Ebner's gland are released in the troughs surrounding the circumvallate papillae where many taste buds are present. The serous secretion is thought to be essential to clean the taste bud receptors for the next stimulant. The individual minor glandular aggregates have excretory ducts that drain saliva directly onto the oral mucosa surface. Both, the intercalated and striated ducts are often poorly developed and lack the typical structure found in the major glands.

Acknowledgments We would to thank and appreciate the help and support of T. Clark Brelje and Robert L. Sorenson" ▸ www.HistologyGuide.org', Department of Genetics, Cell Biology and Development, University of Minnesota, Minneapolis, MN, for providing permission to use some micrographic images of the salivary glands.

Further Reading

Amano O, Mizobe K, Bando Y, Sakiyama K. Anatomy and histology of rodent and human major salivary glands. Acta Histochem Cytochem. 2012;45(5):241–50. https://doi.org/10.1267/ahc.12013.

Carpenter GH. The secretion, components, and properties of saliva. Annu Rev. Food Sci Technol. 2013;4(1):267–76. https://doi.org/10.1146/annurev-food-030212-182700.

Chibly AM, Aure MH, Patel VN, Hoffman MP. Salivary gland function, development, and regeneration. Physiol Rev. 2022;102(3):1495–552. https://doi.org/10.1152/physrev.00015.2021.

de Paula F, Teshima THN, Hsieh R, Souza MM, Nico MMS, Lourenco SV. Overview of human salivary glands: highlights of morphology and developing processes. Anat Rec. 2017;300(7):1180–8. https://doi.org/10.1002/ar.23569.

Ghannam MG, Singh P. Anatomy, head and neck, salivary glands. In: StatPearls. Treasure Island, FL: StatPearls Publishing; 2023.

Grewal JS, Bordoni B, Shah J, Ryan J. Anatomy, head and neck. Sublingual Gland; 2020. https://www.ncbi.nlm.nih.gov/books/NBK535426/.

Guillemot L, Paschoud S, Pulimeno P, Foglia A, Citi S. The cytoplasmic plaque of tight junctions: a scaffolding and signalling center. Biochim Biophys Acta Biomembranes. 2008;1778(3):601–13. https://doi.org/10.1016/j.bbamem.2007.09.032.

Hand AR. Salivary glands, anatomy and histology. In: Encyclopedia of gastroenterology. 2004. pp. 313–7. https://doi.org/10.1016/b0-12-386860-2/00628-6.

Histologyguide.com. Endocrine glands | histology guide. https://histologyguide.com/slidebox/12-exocrine-glands.html#salivary-glands. Accessed 16 Oct 2023.

Holmberg KV, Hoffman MP. Anatomy, biogenesis and regeneration of salivary glands. Monogr Oral Sci. 2014;24:1–13. https://doi.org/10.1159/000358776.

Maruyama C, Monroe M, Hunt J, Buchmann L, Baker O. Comparing human and mouse salivary glands: a practice guide for salivary researchers. Oral Dis. 2019;25(2):403–15. https://doi.org/10.1111/odi.12840.

Nanci A. Ten Cate's oral histology development, structure, and function. 9th ed. Elsevier; 2016. pp. 236–59. https://shop.elsevier.com/books/ten-cates-oral-histology/nanci/978-0-323-48518-0. Accessed 16 Oct 2023.

Tucker AS. Salivary gland development. Semin Cell Dev Biol. 2007;18(2):237–44. https://doi.org/10.1016/j.semcdb.2007.01.006.

Oral Histopathology

Contents

Developmental Defects of Teeth

Devaki Sundararajan

Contents

S R Prabhu et al. (eds.), *Oral Histology and Oral Histopathology*, https://doi.org/10.1007/978-3-031-77481-2_16

16.1 Introduction

Dental development is a highly regulated biological process. Several specific and highly regulated sequences of steps are involved in the developmental process of teeth. If any developmental processes are disturbed or exaggerated, numerical and structural changes in the teeth can occur. Dental anomalies are caused by complex interactions between genetic, epigenetic, and environmental factors during dental development. The developmental anomalies to be discussed in this chapter include those related to the number, shape, and size of the teeth, as well as those with defective structures. History, and clinical and radiographic examinations provide diagnostic information of developmental disorders of teeth. Histological diagnosis is usually not required. Rarely, however, diagnosis of structural defects such as amelogenesis imperfecta, dentinogenesis impaerfecta and dentinal dysplasia may be confirmed histologically.

16.2 Classification of Developmental Disorders of Teeth

16.2.1 Developmental Anomalies Related to the Number, Size, and Shape of Teeth

1. Anodontia, Hypodontia, and Oligodontia
2. Hyperdontia (Supernumerary Teeth)
3. Microdontia and Macrodontia
4. Gemination, Fusion, and Concrescence
5. Taurodontism and Dilaceration
6. Enamel Pearl
7. Talon Cusp
8. Hutchinson's Incisors and Mulberry Molars
9. Supernumerary Roots

Definitions and key features with an emphasis on histopathological structures are discussed in this chapter.

16.2.1.1 Anodontia, Hypodontia, and Oligodontia

- **Definition**

- Tooth agenesis is defined as the absence of teeth due to the failure of teeth to develop.
- Anodontia represents the complete absence of all teeth.
- Hypodontia refers to the absence of up to five teeth.
- Oligodontia refers to the absence of six or more teeth.

- **Key Features**

- Tooth agenesis can occur due to genetic mutations in specific genes.
- Can be multifactorial with genetic mutations and environmental factors such as trauma, infections, and toxins.
- Oligodontia can occur as an isolated trait or be part of a syndrome.
- Oligodontia is associated with over 60 syndromes, including hypohydrotic ectodermal dysplasia (HED).
- Syndromic oligodontia may occur due to mutations in WNT10A and PAX9, which are the most reported genetic aetiologies for isolated oligodontia.
- The syndromes associated with oligodontia include Rieger syndrome, Down syndrome, Van der Woude syndrome (BCDS), Axenfeld–Rieger syndrome (ARS), Witkop syndrome, Ellis–van Creveld syndrome (EVCS), Branchio-oculo-facial syndrome, and oculofaciocardiodental syndrome.
- No treatment is required for a single missing tooth. When multiple teeth are missing, removable or fixed prosthodontics or implants may be necessary.

16.2.1.2 Hyperdontia (Supernumerary Teeth)

- **Definition**

Supernumerary teeth represent a dental anomaly in which additional teeth besides the normal dentition are present in the oral cavity.

- **Key Features**

- Both genetic and environmental factors influence this dental anomaly.
- Approximately 75% of the cases represent single tooth hyperdontia, 15% show two supernumerary teeth, and three or more supernumerary teeth are noted in <10% of the cases.
- Supernumerary teeth are more common in the maxillary incisor region and often fail to erupt.
- The maxillary and mandibular fourth molars are the next common supernumerary teeth.
- Multiple non-syndromic supernumerary teeth most frequently occur in the mandible.
- Supernumerary teeth can be unilateral or bilateral.
- Supernumerary teeth can be supplemental (normal size and shape) or rudimentary (abnormal size and shape).
- A supernumerary tooth in the maxillary anterior incisor region is called mesiodens.
- A supernumerary fourth molar is called distomolar or distodens.
- A supernumerary tooth located buccally or lingually to a molar tooth is called a paramolar.

- Extragnathic supernumerary teeth have been reported in other sites such as the gingiva, soft palate, nasal cavity, maxillary sinus, orbit, and brain.
- Impacted supernumerary teeth are often discovered in radiographs when wide spaces are noted between erupted teeth or when misalignment of erupted teeth is seen.
- A radiographic evaluation or advanced imaging such as cone-beam computed tomography (CBCT) may be necessary for a definitive diagnosis.
- The treatment depends on the location and number of supernumerary teeth. Surgical removal may be indicated if the extra tooth interferes with the eruption of a normal tooth, during orthodontic treatment to correct malocclusion, or if it is associated with pathology such as a cyst or tumour.

16.2.1.3 Microdontia and Macrodontia

- **Definition**
- Microdontia refers to teeth that are smaller in size than normal size.
- Macrodontia represents teeth that are larger than normal tooth size.

- **Key Features**
- Microdontia is more common than macrodontia.
- Compound odontoma may be considered as a collection of microdonts.
- Genetic and hereditary factors may affect the size of teeth.
- Microdontia is often associated with agenesis and is more common in women.
- Micodontia affecting one tooth is common. The most affected tooth is the maxillary lateral incisor with a peg-shaped crown and normal root. The next common tooth to be affected is the third molar.
- Microdontia affecting multiple teeth is uncommon but may be seen in conditions such as Down syndrome and pituitary dwarfism.
- Macrodontia is often associated with hyperdontia and is more common in men.
- Macrodontia can be unilateral or bilateral.
- Macrodontia affecting one single tooth is more common in incisors, canines, second premolars, and third molars.
- Macrodontia affecting all the teeth or multiple teeth is rare and can be noted in conditions such as pituitary gigantism and otodental syndrome.
- Macrodontia (unilateral involvement) can be noted in hemifacial hyperplasia.
- Abnormal elongation of the roots is called radiculomegaly and is often noted in oculo-facio-cardio-dental syndrome.
- No treatment is necessary for microdontia or macrodontia unless restoration of the tooth to normal size is necessary due to esthetic concerns.

16.2.1.4 Gemination, Fusion, and Concrescence

- **Definition**
- Gemination refers to an enlarged tooth in which the tooth count is normal when the affected tooth is counted as one tooth.
- Fusion refers to an enlarged tooth when the count reveals one missing tooth.
- Concrescence represents the union of two adjacent roots of teeth by cementum.

- **Key Features**
- Gemination and fusion represent developmental alterations involving the shape of the tooth.
- Gemination and fusion can occur in both the deciduous and permanent dentition.
- Gemination and fusion are more common in the permanent anterior teeth.
- Gemination and fusion may lead to caries, malalignment, and asymmetry. These abnormalities can cause functional and esthetic problems.
- Gemination is more common in the maxilla, and fusion is more common in the mandible.
- Most cases of gemination and fusion are unilateral but bilateral involvement can occur rarely.
- Thc diagnosis of gemination and fusion is mainly based on the tooth count as the affected teeth can present as bifid crowns with one or two roots or as one enlarged crown with one or two roots. The roots can be separated or fused.
- Concrescence represents fusion of roots of two adjacent teeth by cementum.
- Concrescence mostly involves the maxillary molar teeth. Most reported cases of concrescence are between a maxillary second molar and an impacted maxillary third molar tooth.
- Concrescence may occur as a developmental alteration or due to periapical inflammatory process.
- The management options for gemination, fusion, and concrescence include no treatment, orthodontics, prosthodontics, or extraction based on individual cases.
- Concrescence may cause difficulties during orthodontic treatment with movement of teeth and complications during extractions.

16.2.1.5 Taurodontism and Dilaceration

- **Definition**

- Taurodontism represents an abnormality of tooth structure where the body of the tooth and the pulp chamber are enlarged with apically displaced pulpal floor and furcation.
- Dilaceration refers to an abnormal curve in the root and rarely the crown of the tooth.

- **Key Features**

- In taurodontism, the elongation of the pulp chamber of teeth causes displacement of furcation in multi-rooted teeth apically resulting in alteration to the shape of the affected tooth.
- The affected tooth exhibits a rectangular shape with short roots.
- Although deciduous teeth can be affected, this condition most commonly affects the permanent molar teeth.
- The crown looks normal clinically, and the abnormality is discovered on radiographic examination.
- Can be unilateral or bilateral and multiple teeth may be affected.
- Can occur as an isolated trait or can be part of a syndrome. Taurodontism is often noted in patients with hypodontia or cleft lip and palate.
- During root development the Hertwig's epithelial root sheath may fail to invaginate to produce bifurcation or trifurcation area resulting in taurodontism.
- Based on the degree of apical displacement of the pulpal floor, taurodontism can be classified as mild, moderate, or severe.
- No treatment is required. Complications may arise during endodontic therapy due to the shortened pulp canal.
- Dilaceration frequently involves the tooth root but rarely can involve the crown of the tooth.
- Although the cause may be unknown, trauma to the tooth germ during tooth development may result in bend in the tooth root.
- Pathology such as a cyst or tumour can also cause dilaceration of a developing tooth.
- Dilaceration is typically discovered on radiographic examination.
- No specific treatment is necessary for dilaceration. Complications may arise during endodontic treatment or extraction of a tooth exhibiting dilaceration.

16.2.1.6 Enamel Pearl

- **Definition**

Enamel pearl represents ectopic circumscribed protrusion of enamel on the root surface.

- **Key Features**

- Most cases of enamel pearl are noted at the root furcation.
- Enamel pearls can be composed entirely of enamel, enamel and dentine or may contain enamel, dentine, and pulp.
- Mostly involves the permanent maxillary and mandibular molars. Frequently detected in maxillary second and third molars.
- Other permanent teeth or deciduous teeth are rarely affected.
- Enamel pearl often appears as a well-defined radiopaque change on the radiograph. Three-dimensional imaging, such as cone-beam computed tomography (CBCT), can help distinguish an enamel pearl from an odontoma, pulp stone, or calculus.
- Periodontal attachment to the tooth is impaired due to the presence of enamel pearl, which results in plaque accumulation. This can result in periapical or periodontal lesions with angular bone loss along the surface of the root.
- No specific treatment is recommended. Optimal oral hygiene should be encouraged to prevent loss of periodontal attachment.
- Removal of enamel pearl should be done carefully as vital pulp tissue may be present in some cases.

16.2.1.7 Talon Cusp

- **Definition**

Talon cusp is an additional cusp projecting on the lingual or labial surface of an anterior deciduous or permanent tooth.

- **Key Features**

- Talon cups are composed of enamel, dentin and in some cases may also contain pulp.
- It is more common in the maxillary anterior permanent teeth. The maxillary lateral incisor is the most affected tooth.
- The accessory cusp is most seen on the palatal surface of a maxillary anterior tooth. Rarely can involve the facial surface of an anterior tooth.
- Can affect deciduous dentition, but it is uncommon.
- Increased prevalence of talon cusp is noted in syndromes including Rubinstein-Taybi, Ellis-van Creveld, and Sturge-Weber syndrome.
- A developmental groove may be present where the cusp fuses with the surface of the tooth.
- Complications from talon cusps include caries, periodontal problems, and interference with occlusion in case of talon cusps involving the palatal surfaces of the maxillary anterior teeth.
- Removal of talon cusp can be achieved with periodic reduction and covering the exposed dentin with calcium hydroxide.

16.2.1.8 Hutchinson Incisors and Mulberry Molars

- **Definition**

Hutchinson teeth are dental malformations affecting the permanent incisors and permanent molars in congenital syphilis.

- **Key Features**

- Syphilis is a chronic infection caused by Treponema pallidum.
- Congenital syphilis represents manifestations of the infection in the foetus from maternal transmission.
- Congenital syphilis is characterised by the Hutchinson's triad—Hutchinson's teeth, ocular interstitial keratitis, and eighth nerve deafness. Hutchinson triad is a late manifestation of congenital syphilis noted 2 years after birth.
- Premature loss of primary teeth and palatal perforation have also been reported as manifestations of congenital syphilis.
- An inflammatory reaction in response to the Treponema pallidum infection causes the dental defect. The exact mechanism by which the infection causes disruption to the tooth crown formation for only a short duration is unclear.
- The permanent incisors and molars are affected as Treponema pallidum crosses the placenta only after the 16th week of intrauterine life.
- Hutchinson's incisors show altered incisor edges with either a deep vertical notch or a screwdriver-shaped appearance when the notch is lost through wear. The affected teeth are short and narrow towards the incisal edge.
- Hutchinson incisors are more commonly seen involving the upper central incisors.
- The permanent first molar teeth can appear small and dome-shaped with closely placed cusps. The occlusal surface is narrow and smooth, with the absence of grooves between the cusps. These molar teeth are termed moon or bud molars.
- Mulberry molar represents a molar tooth defect in congenital syphilis where deep groves are noted around the base of each cusp caused by enamel hypoplasia producing the appearance of a mulberry fruit.
- The affected incisors and molar teeth often show non-specific severe enamel hypoplasia.

16.2.1.9 Supernumerary Roots

- **Definition**

Supernumerary roots represent the development of an increased number of roots compared to normal tooth anatomy.

- **Key Features**

- Supernumerary roots can be seen in both deciduous and permanent dentitions.
- Any tooth can be affected.
- Most frequently affects the permanent molars, especially the third molars, followed by the canines and premolars.
- The supernumerary root may be long and divergent or short and narrow.
- Depending on the size and location of the supernumerary root, it may be visible in the radiographs or obscured by other tooth roots.
- No specific treatment is required for supernumerary roots.
- Detection of the supernumerary roots using radiographs or other imaging techniques is necessary during endodontic treatment or extraction.

16.2.2 Developmental Anomalies Related to the Structure of Teeth

1. Amelogenesis Imperfecta
2. Dentinogenesis Imperfecta
3. Dentine Dysplasia (Dentinal dysplasia)
4. Regional Odontodysplasia (Ghost Teeth)
5. Dens Invaginatus and Dens Evaginatus
6. Fluorosis (Mottled Enamel)
7. Tetracycline-induced discoloration of teeth

16.2.2.1 Amelogenesis Imperfecta

- **Definition**

Amelogenesis imperfecta (AI) represents developmental alterations in the structure of enamel without any association with systemic conditions or syndromes.

- **Key Features**

- Amelogenesis imperfecta can be associated with other dental anomalies, such as pulpal calcification and taurodontism.
- Hypoplastic AI is caused by inadequate deposition of enamel matrix. The affected teeth may show surface pits, thinning of the enamel or complete absence of enamel. The affected teeth may also show a generalised or localised pattern.
- Hypomineralized AI can exhibit enamel showing normal thickness, but the enamel is weak and chips off easily.
- Hypomineralized AI can be subdivided into hypomaturation AI and hypocalcified AI. Hypomaturation AI occurs because of incomplete protein removal, and the enamel appears brittle. Hypocalcified AI occurs due to inadequate calcium deposition, resulting in soft enamel that can be lost easily.

- AI can be transmitted by an autosomal dominant (AD) and diffuse autosomal recessive (AR) or X-linked mode of inheritance. Multiple gene alterations have been identified.
- A universally acceptable classification system for AI does not exist because of different phenotypes (clinical appearance) and molecular patterns.
- Several genetic mutations (about 15 genes) associated with various phenotypes of amelogenesis imperfecta have been recognised and include *AMELX, ENAM, AMBN, KLK4, MMP20, FAM83H, Dlx3, WDR72, C4orf26, SLC24A4, ITGB6, LAMB3,* and *FAM20A*.
- <UNK> Genetic heterogeneity and overlapping phenotypes make classifying and diagnosing AI based on its clinical appearance impossible without genetic testing.
- Most cases show diffuse involvement of deciduous and permanent dentition.
- Radiographically, the enamel shows a thin peripheral outline over the dentine and may exhibit resorptive changes.
- Treatment options are based on the clinical presentation and severity. Apart from esthetics, the complications associated with AI include caries, impaction, delayed eruption, sensitivity, loss of vertical dimension, and open bite. Full crowns and facial veneers can help protect the tooth and improve esthetics.

16.2.2.2 Dentinogenesis Imperfecta

▪ **Definition**

Dentinogenesis imperfecta (DI) represents a developmental disturbance of dentine without any associated systemic disorders.

▪ **Key Features**

- DI is associated with several different mutations in the *DSPP* gene.
- An updated classification system proposed by de La Dure-Molla in 2015 favours a designation of mild, moderate, and severe DI based on the phenotype.
- This disorder is inherited as an autosomal dominant trait. It can occur in any race.
- DI can affect both deciduous and permanent dentition.
- The affected dentition shows yellow-brown or grey-blue discolouration with translucence.
- The enamel separates easily from the underlying defective dentine. The exposed dentine undergoes rapid attrition.
- Ultrastructural studies show changes to the surface topography, quantity, organisation, and orientation of the collagen fibres in DI.
- Radiographically, the affected teeth show bulbous crowns, cervical constriction, and thin roots. The pulp chambers show rapid obliteration following the eruption.
- In the mild form of DI, the deciduous teeth show blue or brown discolouration and translucence. The radiographs show the classic features of DI-bulbous crowns, cervical constriction, thin roots, and early pulp obliteration. The permanent teeth in mild form of DI show normal colour crown. Radiographically, the affected teeth show apically extended enlarged pulp chambers. These pulp chambers are described as thistle tube-shaped or flame-shaped pulp chambers. Pulp stones are often seen.
- The severe form of DI, which is also called shell teeth, shows normal thickness enamel, thin dentine involving both the crown and root, or only the root and significantly enlarged pulp.
- Premature loss of teeth due to defective dentine in DI can result in hearing loss.
- A mild form of DI can be managed with full crowns. In severe attrition cases, rebuilding the vertical dimension using composite restorations may be considered. Premature tooth loss is common, and the affected patients may be treated with full dentures or implants.

16.2.2.3 Dentine Dysplasia (Dentinal Dysplasia)

▪ **Definition**

Dentine dysplasia (DD) is a rare genetic developmental disorder affecting dentine production in teeth. It commonly exhibits an autosomal dominant inheritance. There are two types: DD Type 1(radicular type) and DD Type II (Coronal type).

▪ **Key Features**

- Defective dentine sialoprotein gene is the cause for both types.
- Dentine dysplasia affects both primary and permanent teeth.
- The crowns of teeth in DD-I appear morphologically normal with standard shape and colour, but the roots appear short and conical or may be absent (rootless tooth).
- Patients with DD-I often present with pain and periapical radiolucencies, extreme mobility, short or absent roots, and premature loss of teeth.

- Occasionally, DD-I exhibits near-normal root length with a visible pulp chamber and large pulp stones located in the coronal portion of the canal and a few periapical radiolucencies.
- Dentine dysplasia-II shows translucent grey-brown discolouration of the tooth crown, thin roots, and pulp obliteration.
- Radiographically, DD-II crowns appear bulbous, and pulp chambers may be obliterated.
- The treatment for DD-1 depends on the length of the root and the presence of periapical inflammatory disease. Complete dentures and implant-supported prostheses are fabricated for patients with premature loss of teeth.
- The treatment of DD-II is directed towards the specific symptoms that are apparent in each patient.

Histopathological Features

The histopathological description is limited to the standard type of DD, the radicular type. The coronal enamel and dentin appear normal. The central portion of the root that is apical to the area of disorganised dentine shows whorls of tubular dentine and atypical osteodentine surrounded by a peripheral layer of normal dentine, giving the root an appearance of a "stream flowing around boulders" (◘ Fig. 16.1).

16.2.2.4 Regional Odontodysplasia (Ghost Teeth)

Definition

Regional odontodysplasia (ROD) is a rare developmental abnormality that affects the development of enamel, dentine, and pulp.

Key Features

- Regional odontodysplasia is a rare developmental disorder characterised by hypoplasia and hypocalcification of enamel and dentine.
- The term odontodysplasia was first used by Zegarelli et al. in 1963. Pindborg added "regional" to the term "odontodysplasia" as this condition typically affects only one quadrant.
- ROD usually affects several adjacent teeth in one quadrant but rarely may cross the midline involving more than one quadrant.
- ROD can affect both deciduous and permanent dentition.
- Patients are usually diagnosed between the ages of 2 and 11 when the deciduous and permanent teeth erupt.
- There may be a slight female predominance but no racial predilection.
- The maxilla is affected more commonly than the mandible.
- Etiopathogenesis has not been established. The suggested etiologic factors include local trauma, circulatory disorders, ischemia, radiation therapy, metabolic disturbances, nutritional deficiencies, activation of latent virus during tooth development, childhood illness with hyperpyrexia, and local somatic mutations.
- The aetiology may be multifactorial with local and systemic factors. Several cases of ROD have been reported in patients with vascular nevi of the head and neck.
- ROD can show a variety of clinical manifestations and is associated with distinctive clinical, radiological, and histopathological findings.
- Some patients may have mild facial asymmetry or hyperplasia of the soft tissues overlying the affected teeth. Several contiguous teeth are affected **in** one quadrant, and many of the affected teeth may be impacted.
- The erupted teeth affected by ROD are hypoplastic and hypocalcified and clinically appear as yellow or brown malformed teeth. These teeth are prone to significant tooth structure loss and caries associated with periapical infection.
- Radiographically, the affected teeth show "ghost-like" appearance due to the thin hypoplastic and hypomineralized enamel and dentine forming a wispy outline of the tooth crown. There is no distinction between the enamel and dentin as both exhibit similar radiodensities. The pulp chamber is large and often contains calcifications. The roots appear short with open apices.
- The treatment depends on the severity of the odontodysplasia and may include extraction of the affected teeth.
- In the absence of infection and symptoms, the affected teeth may be preserved to promote normal development of the affected jaw.
- A removable partial prosthesis is often fabricated to preserve the alveolar ridge height to enable skeletal growth in younger patients. Unerupted teeth are left in place while erupted teeth may be covered with stainless steel crowns or restorations.
- Severely malformed fragile or infected teeth that cannot be saved are often extracted. In adult patients, the affected teeth can be extracted and replaced with implants.

Histopathological Features

The ground sections of the affected tooth show enamel of varying thickness exhibiting an irregular surface

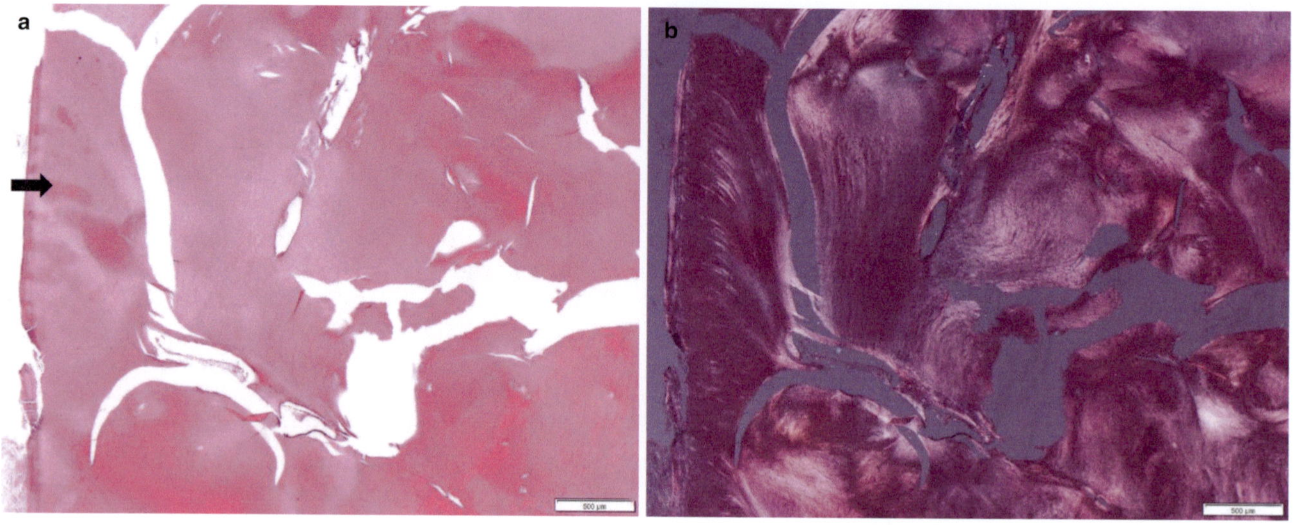

Fig. 16.1 (**a**, **b**) Photomicrograph of a tooth with dentine dysplasia type 1 showing a disorganised mixture of tubular dentine and osteodentine surrounded by normal dentine (black arrow) (**a**) and the same section under the polarised light (**b**)

architecture. The dentine shows a combination of poorly organised globular dentin and amorphous material. The pulp tissue often contains calcifications that may exhibit lamellations. Histopathological examination of the hyperplastic dental follicle surrounding the crown of the affected tooth shows foci of collections of basophilic, circular and ovoid, enamel-like calcifications called enameloid conglomerates. Islands and cords of odontogenic epithelium can be seen scattered throughout the lesional tissue (Fig. 16.2).

16.2.2.5 Dens Invaginatus and Dens Evaginatus

- **Definition**

- Dens invaginatus represents a developmental tooth abnormality characterised by an infolding of the enamel organ into the dental papilla prior to mineralisation.
- Dens evaginatus is a tooth anomaly presenting as an accessory cusp on the occlusal surface of a posterior tooth.

16

- **Key Features**

- These dental anomalies occur because of genetic or environmental factors.
- The aetiology of these conditions has not been well understood.
- Dens invaginatus can occur because of the invagination of the inner enamel epithelium into the interior aspect of the developing tooth bud before mineralisation.
- The invagination originates in the tooth crown and may extend into the root giving the appearance of a "tooth within a tooth" radiographically.
- Dens invaginatus can involve any tooth, but the permanent maxillary lateral and central incisors are most affected.
- Dens invaginatus has various clinical presentations. The invagination may be limited to the coronal aspect of the tooth or may extend beyond the CEJ, or the invagination of dental tissue may extend into the root canal, sometimes resulting in multiple apical foramina.
- Accumulation of bacterial microorganisms in the invagination predisposes the affected tooth to development of caries and subsequent pulpal necrosis.
- Sealing of the opening to the invagination with calcium hydroxide is recommended to preserve the vitality of the tooth.
- Endodontic treatment may be attempted if pulpal inflammation or necrosis occurs. However, due to the complex anatomy, preservation of the tooth with endodontic therapy may not be possible. In such cases, extraction of the affected tooth may be necessary.
- Dens evaginatus presents a cusp-like protrusion or tubercle from the occlusal surface of a posterior tooth.
- Dens evaginatus can occur due to abnormal proliferation of the dental papilla into the stellate reticulum of the enamel organ during tooth development.
- Often seen bilaterally involving the premolars.
- Higher incidence of dens evaginatus is noted in people of Asian descent, Alaskan Natives, and American Indians.

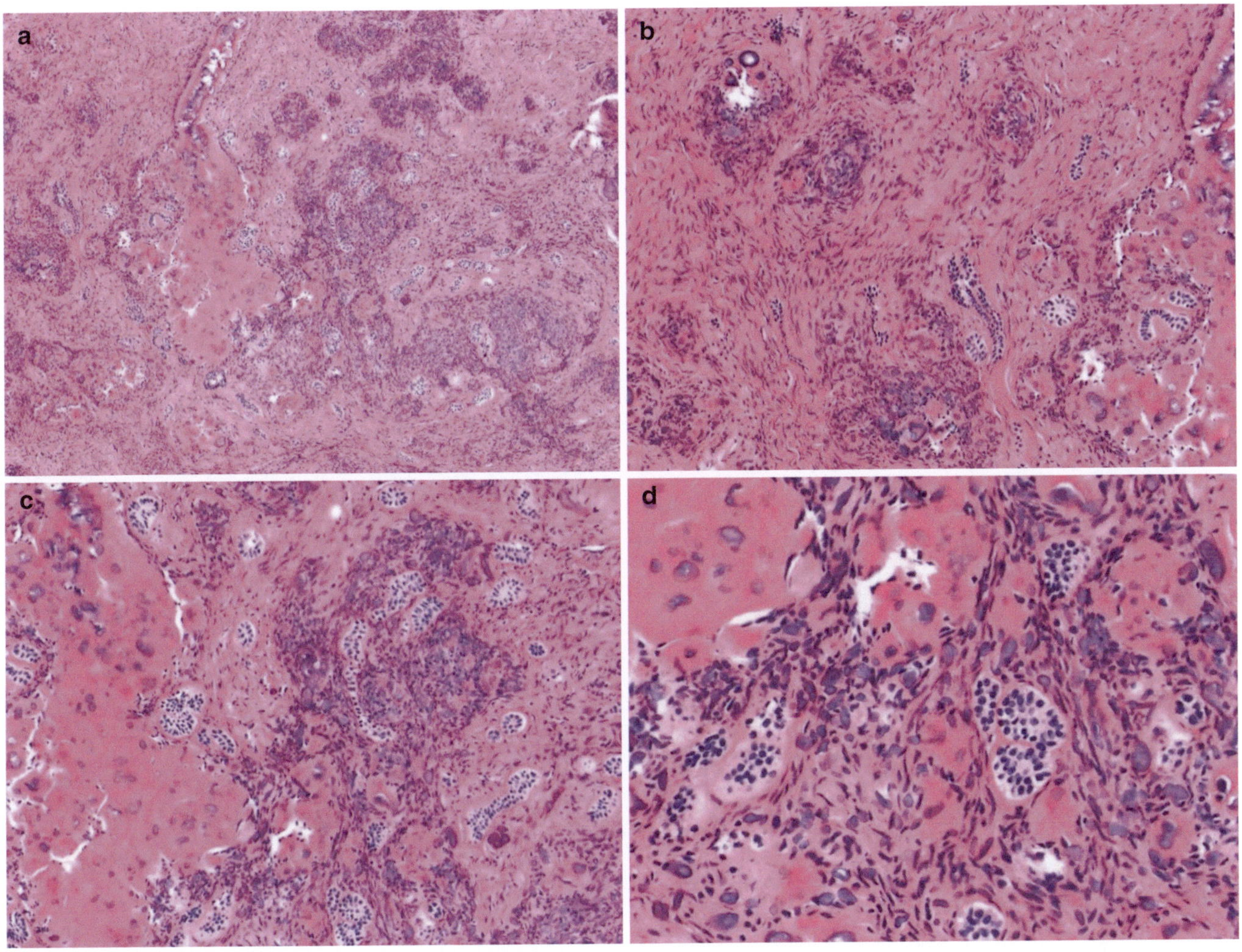

Fig. 16.2 (a–d) Low, medium, and high power view images showing follicular tissue in regional odontodysplasia exhibiting collections of enameloid conglomerates and islands of odontogenic epithelium scattered throughout the lesional tissue

- The tubercle is typically composed of enamel and dentine and often contains pulp tissue.
- The accessory cups can cause occlusal interference and show rapid wear resulting in pulp exposure and periapical pathology.
- Removal of the accessory cusp with direct or indirect capping may be indicated to prevent pulp necrosis.

16.2.2.6 Fluorosis (Mottled Enamel)

Definition

Dental fluorosis represents enamel defects due to ingesting greater than optimal amounts of fluoride during tooth development.

Key Features

- Patients exposed to fluoride concentrations >2–4 ppm develop noticeable enamel defects.
- Fluoride ingestion occurs through fluoridated water, fluoride in toothpaste, fluoride supplements, and fluoride in infant formula.
- Retention of amelogenin protein in the enamel structure causes enamel defects in fluorosis.
- The enamel alterations can show a chronologic pattern as ingesting excess fluoride affects only the teeth forming at the time of exposure.
- The white, chalky areas noted in fluorosis represent hypomineralized enamel.
- The severity of fluorosis depends on the amount of fluoride exposure during tooth development.
- Mild cases of fluorosis only show colour abnormalities. The enamel may show yellow-brown discolouration, with white or opaque areas.
- Moderate to severe cases of fluorosis show clinically noticeable enamel defects with pits, fissures and missing enamel. Mottled enamel is an older term to describe teeth affected by moderate to severe fluorosis.

- Enamel hypoplasia may be present as brown discolouration with deep or rough pits.
- Although caries is rare in teeth affected by fluorosis, the enamel is weak and can easily flake off.
- The diagnosis is based on the history of ingesting excess fluoride and bilateral symmetric distribution of the enamel changes.
- Patients' major concern is esthetics, especially when it involves the anterior teeth. Affected teeth can be treated with dental veneers, crowns, or light-cured resin restorations.

16.2.2.7 Tetracycline-Induced Discolouration of Teeth

▪ **Definition**

Tetracycline-induced discolouration of the teeth represents intrinsic staining of the developing teeth due to exposure to tetracycline.

▪ **Key Features**

- Clinically visible discolouration of the teeth can occur due to the incorporation of tetracycline into the developing tooth.
- The severity of the discolouration is dependent on the dose and duration of the medication use.
- The colour of the affected teeth ranges from bright yellow to dark brown. The affected teeth may show bright yellow fluorescence under ultraviolet light.
- The development of deciduous tooth crowns occurs from the fourth month of gestation to approximately the 12th month of life. The development of crowns of the permanent teeth begins from birth until approximately 8 years of age. Ingestion of tetracycline during the development of tooth crowns can cause clinically visible discolouration of teeth.
- To prevent tetracycline-related teeth discolouration, the medication should not be administered during pregnancy or in children younger than 8 years of age.
- No treatment is necessary. The affected teeth may be covered with crowns and veneers for esthetic purposes.

Further Reading

Abdel-Kader MA, Abdelazeem AF, Ahmed NE-MB, Khalil YM, Mostafa MI. Oral rehabilitation of a case with regional odontodysplasia using a regenerative approach-a case report and a review of literature. Spec Care Dentist. 2019;39(3):330–9. https://doi.org/10.1111/scd.12378.

Alani A, Bishop K. Dens invaginatus. Part 1: classification, prevalence and aetiology. Int Endod J. 2008;41:1123–36.

Andrade-Maia G, Pereira TS, Clementino LC, et al. Developmental defects of enamel: a bibliometric analysis of the top 100 most-cited papers. Caries Res. 2024;58(2):104–10. https://doi.org/10.1159/000535856.

Buchanan GD, Tredoux S, Schouwstra C-M, Nel C, Gamieldien MY. Double gemination or fusion of a permanent mandibular second molar: a case report. Chin J Dent Res. 2021;24(3):199–202. https://doi.org/10.3290/j.cjdr.b1964973.

Castilho NL, Resende KKM, Santos JAD, et al. Oligodontia in the clinical spectrum of syndromes: a systematic review. Dent J (Basel). 2023;11(12):279. https://doi.org/10.3390/dj11120279.

Chen D, Li X, Lu F, Wang Y, Xiong F, Li Q. Dentin dysplasia type I-A dental disease with genetic heterogeneity. Oral Dis. 2019;25(2):439–46. https://doi.org/10.1111/odi.12861.

Chen J-W, Huang GT-J, Bakland LK. Dens evaginatus: current treatment options. J Am Dent Assoc. 2020;151(5):358–67. https://doi.org/10.1016/j.adaj.2020.01.015.

de La Dure-Molla M, Fournier BP, Berdal A. Isolated dentinogenesis imperfecta and dentin dysplasia: revision of the classification. Eur J Hum Genet. 2015;23(4):445–51. https://doi.org/10.1038/ejhg.2014.159.

Decaup P-H, Garot E, Rouas P. Prevalence of talon cusp: systematic literature review, meta-analysis and new scoring system. Arch Oral Biol. 2021;125:105112. https://doi.org/10.1016/j.archoralbio.2021.105112.

Gadi LSA, Chau DYS, Parekh S. Morphological and ultrastructural collagen defects: impact and implications in dentinogenesis imperfecta. Dent J (Basel). 2023;11(4):95. https://doi.org/10.3390/dj11040095.

Gallacher A, Ali R, Bhakta S. Dens invaginatus: diagnosis and management strategies. Br Dent J. 2016;221:383–7.

Garvey MT, Barry HJ, Blake M. Supernumerary teeth—an overview of classification, diagnosis and management. J Can Dent Assoc. 1999;65(11):612–6.

Herrera-Rojas NA, de Priego GAP-M. Amelogenesis imperfecta. Case report. Rev Cient Odontol (Lima). 2023;11(2):e156. https://doi.org/10.21142/2523-2754-1102-2023-156.

Jafarzadeh H, Abbott PV. Dilaceration: review of an endodontic challenge. J Endod. 2007;33(9):1025–30. https://doi.org/10.1016/j.joen.2007.04.013.

Jain A, Sisodia S, Rana KS, Gupta C, Ansari I, Dholakia PP. The study of prevalence and distribution of shape anomalies of teeth in Indian population on the basis of age and gender. Cureus. 2022;14(8):e28532. https://doi.org/10.7759/cureus.28532.

Ji Y, Wang Y, Huang S, Zhang F. Regional odontodysplasia on the left side of the mandible: report of an unusual case. J Clin Pediatr Dent. 2023;47(5):176–80. https://doi.org/10.22514/jocpd.2023.068.

Keuning MW, Kamp GA, Schonenberg-Meinema D, Dorigo-Zetsma JW, van Zuiden JM, Pajkrt D. Congenital syphilis, the great imitator-case report and review. Lancet Infect Dis. 2020;20(7):e173–9. https://doi.org/10.1016/S1473--3099(20)30268-1.

Levitan ME, Himel VT. Dens evaginatus: literature review, pathophysiology, and comprehensive treatment regimen. J Endod. 2006;32(1):1–9. https://doi.org/10.1016/j.joen.2005.10.009.

MacDonald D. Taurodontism. Oral Radiol. 2020;36(2):129–32. https://doi.org/10.1007/s11282-019-00386-1.

Marya A, Sharan J, Mandava P, El-Hassanein E-HH. Complications associated with the surgical removal of non-syndromic supernumerary premolar tooth buds in the mandible. J Surg Case Rep. 2023;2023(5):rjad304. https://doi.org/10.1093/jscr/rjad304.

Mladenovic R, Arsic Z, Velickovic S, Paunovic M. Assessing the efficacy of AI segmentation in diagnostics of nine supernumerary teeth in a pediatric patient. Diagnostics (Basel). 2023;13(23):3563. https://doi.org/10.3390/diagnostics13233563.

Nijakowski K, Woś P, Surdacka A. Regional odontodysplasia: a systematic review of case reports. Int J Environ Res Public Health. 2022;19(3):1683. https://doi.org/10.3390/ijerph19031683.

Nissanka-Jayasuriya EH, Odell EW, Phillips C. Dental stigmata of congenital syphilis: a historic review with present day relevance. Head Neck Pathol. 2016;10(3):327–31. https://doi.org/10.1007/s12105-016-0703-z.

Pessoa L, Galvão V. Clinical aspects of congenital syphilis with Hutchinson's triad. BMJ Case Rep. 2011;2011:bcr1120115130. https://doi.org/10.1136/bcr.11.2011.5130.

Putrino A, Caputo M, Galeotti A, Marinelli E, Zaami S. Type I dentin dysplasia: the literature review and case report of a family affected by misrecognition and late diagnosis. Medicina (Kaunas). 2023;59(8):1477. https://doi.org/10.3390/medicina59081477.

Revelo-Mejía IA, Hardisson A, Rubio C, Gutiérrez ÁJ, Paz S. Dental fluorosis: the risk of misdiagnosis-a review. Biol Trace Elem Res. 2021;199(5):1762–70. https://doi.org/10.1007/s12011-020-02296-4.

Sánchez AR, Rogers RS 3rd, Sheridan PJ. Tetracycline and other tetracycline-derivative staining of the teeth and oral cavity. Int J Dermatol. 2004;43(10):709–15. https://doi.org/10.1111/j.1365-4632.2004.02108.x.

Schultz KM, Penner CR. A review of selected dental anomalies with histologic features in the pediatric patient. Pediatr Dev Pathol. 2023;26(6):572–82. https://doi.org/10.1177/10935266231207045.

Sullivan M, Noonan V, Sundararajan D, Gallagher G. Dens invaginatus (dens in dente). J Mass Dent Soc. spring 2017;66(1):50.

Wang S-K, Lee Z-H, Aref P, Chu K-Y. A novel ODAPH mutation causing amelogenesis imperfecta and its expression in human dental tissues. J Dent Sci. 2024;19(1):524–31. https://doi.org/10.1016/j.jds.2023.09.020.

Zengin AZ, Sumer AP, Ozturk G, Noujeim M. Imaging characteristics of enamel pearls on CBCT and their co-relation with supernumerary tooth. Oral Radiol. 2022;38(3):370–7. https://doi.org/10.1007/s11282-021-00567-x.

Zhang Y, Jin X, Zhang Z, et al. A novel approach to full-mouth rehabilitation of dentinogenesis imperfecta type II: case series with review of literature. Medicine (Baltimore). 2024;103(4):e36882. https://doi.org/10.1097/MD.0000000000036882.

Zhang Z, Zou X, Feng L, et al. Splicing mutations in AMELX and ENAM cause amelogenesis imperfect. BMC Oral Health. 2023;23(1):893. https://doi.org/10.1186/s12903-023-03508-8.

Zilberman U, Abramov J, Smith P. Supernumerary roots in maxillary deciduous canines: a rare anomaly with a long history. Arch Oral Biol. 2021;132:105292. https://doi.org/10.1016/j.archoralbio.2021.105292.

Histopathology of Dental Caries

Norman A Firth and Muhammed Yakin

Contents

S R Prabhu et al. (eds.), *Oral Histology and Oral Histopathology*, https://doi.org/10.1007/978-3-031-77481-2_17

17.1 Introduction

Dental caries is one of the most prevalent diseases worldwide. Despite being a preventable disease, it remains responsible for major tooth loss. The bacterial metabolism of sugars results in subsurface demineralisation of teeth by acids. This leads to the breakdown of enamel and dentine, resulting in an open route for bacteria to reach the dental pulp. This leads to inflammation of the pulp (pulpitis) and inflammation of the periodontal tissues. Cariogenic bacteria are in an adherent biofilm called dental plaque. Tooth brushing removes dental plaque from accessible sites but not from inaccessible surfaces inter-proximally or occlusal pits. Cariogenic bacteria are able to produce a pH low enough to decalcify tooth substance. Strains of *Streptococcus mutans* are the organisms most commonly associated with dental caries and have multiple cariogenic properties. These include the ability to produce lactic acid from sucrose, live at a pH lower than 5.0, adhere to pellicle and contribute to plaque formation.

17.2 Enamel Caries

Enamel caries is caused by an alteration in the composition of the bacterial biofilm, which leads to an imbalance between the demineralisation and remineralisation processes in the tooth enamel.

Key Features

- Enamel is the most highly mineralised tissue and is, therefore, a barrier to bacterial attack.
- Once the enamel has been breached, dental caries spread more readily through dentine, initially along the dentinoenamel junction (DEJ) and then down dentinal tubules.
- The carious process in enamel involves both demineralisation and remineralisation of enamel, and as a result, the early solubilisation of enamel occurs in the subsurface.
- Early enamel caries can be seen on smooth surfaces as a white opaque lesion immediately beneath the contact point. When probed, this area is still hard and smooth.
- Caries that forms on the occlusal surfaces of the posterior teeth is called pit and fissure caries.
- In both smooth-surface and pit and fissure caries, the process appears to go through phases of demineralisation and remineralisation.
- Bacteria cannot physically penetrate the enamel until cavitation occurs, i.e. the intact surface layer is lost. Once this occurs, the process favours demineralisation, and the carious process progresses towards the dentine, reaching the dentino-enamel junction.
- Diagnostic and management protocols for enamel caries are beyond the scope of this chapter, and the reader should refer to other sources in the literature.

Histopathology

The study of enamel caries microscopically is limited as the conventional decalcification process results in the loss of all enamel. Thin ground sections through teeth can be prepared, and with the use of polarised light, enamel caries can be observed. Four zones can be visualised: the surface zone, the body of the lesion, dark zones and the translucent zone where the deepest demineralisation has occurred. Of these, the surface zone (Fig. 17.1) is most important as it remains more highly mineralised than the body and dark zones and is subject to remineralisation from calcium and phosphate from either the surface plaque or the deeper demineralised zones.

The same processes occur in pit and fissure caries (Fig. 17.2), resulting in the same zones visible on either side of the fissure.

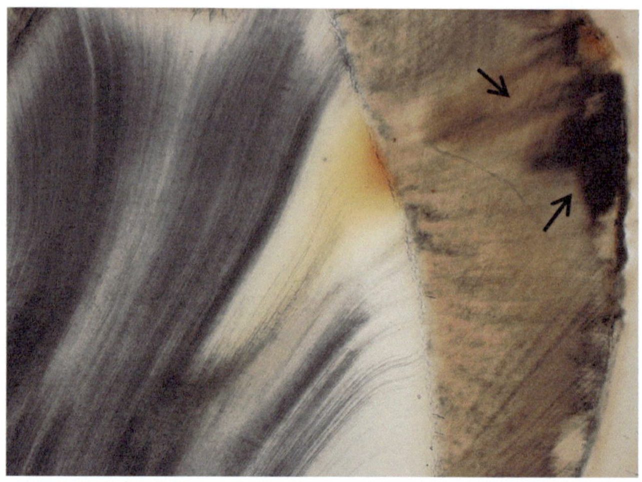

Fig. 17.1 Undecalcified section showing a smooth-surface carious lesion with an intact surface. The dark area (arrows) in the enamel points to the dark zone of the lesion. The zones of an early carious lesion seen in polarised, decalcified sections are not identifiable in plain transmitted light sections such as this. Discolouration in the dentine indicates caries. (Courtesy of Professor David F Wilson, Adelaide, Australia)

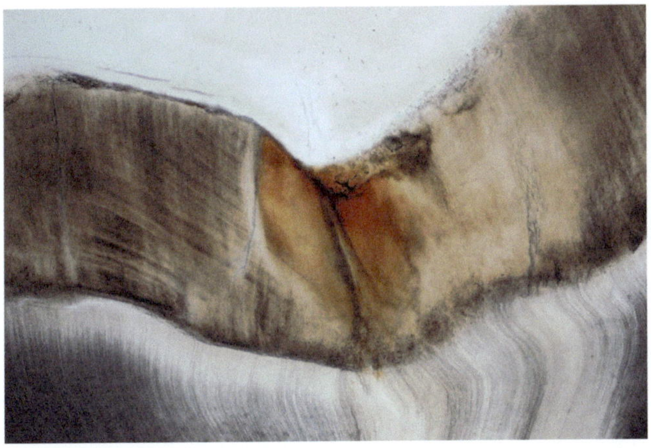

Fig. 17.2 Undecalcified tooth crown section showing discolouration of the intact enamel indicative of fissure caries. (Courtesy of Professor David F Wilson, Adelaide, Australia)

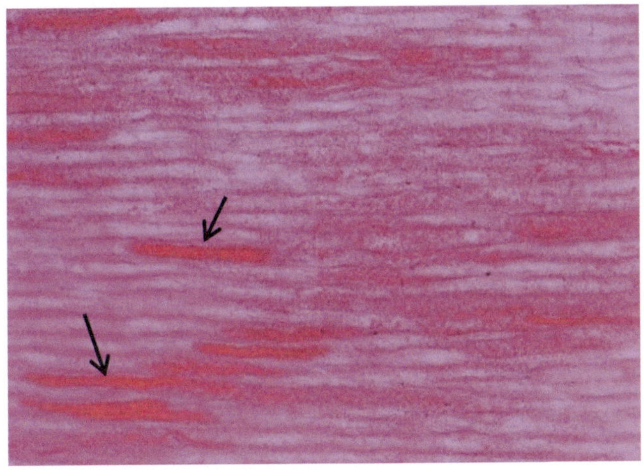

Fig. 17.3 Decalcified haematoxylin and eosin–stained section of carious dentine. The initial signs of dentine caries include the presence of linear arrays of bacteria (arrows) invading the dentine tubules. (Courtesy of Professor David F Wilson, Adelaide, Australia)

17.3 Dentinal Caries

Key Features

- As soon as the carious process reaches the dentinoenamel junction (DEJ), it spreads laterally and more rapidly due to the lower percentage of inorganic content and easier progression.
- Because the environment in dentine is different to that of enamel in terms of the structural organisation and the ratio of the organic and inorganic content, there is a change in the profile of the bacterial species in dentine caries, which turns into facultative and strict anaerobes, which are more dependent on degradation of organic content for their metabolism as opposed to ingested carbohydrates.

Histopathology

Caries at the DEJ initially spread only as wide as the width of enamel caries. Once the bacteria breach the DEJ, they enter the dentine through the tubules (Fig. 17.3), particularly in the absence of reactionary changes in dentine to rapidly progressing lesions.
The small bacterial colonies appear as clusters of basophilic granules in haematoxylin and eosin (H&E) sections that track along the dentinal tubules. With time, acid production by the bacterial colonies leads to further demineralisation of the dentine, degradation of the organic content and widening of the tubules, resulting in the formation of liquefactive foci (Fig. 17.4a) along the axis of the dentinal tubules, which become progressively larger.

In advanced dentine caries, the bacterial colonies also migrate into and widen the lateral branches of the dentinal tubules, called canaliculi, and lead to large liquefactive foci called transverse clefts perpendicular to the long axis of the dentinal tubules (Fig. 17.4b).

Microscopically, the later stages of dentine caries are characterised by more obvious destruction of the dentine matrix and its replacement by bacterial colonies (Fig. 17.5a, b).

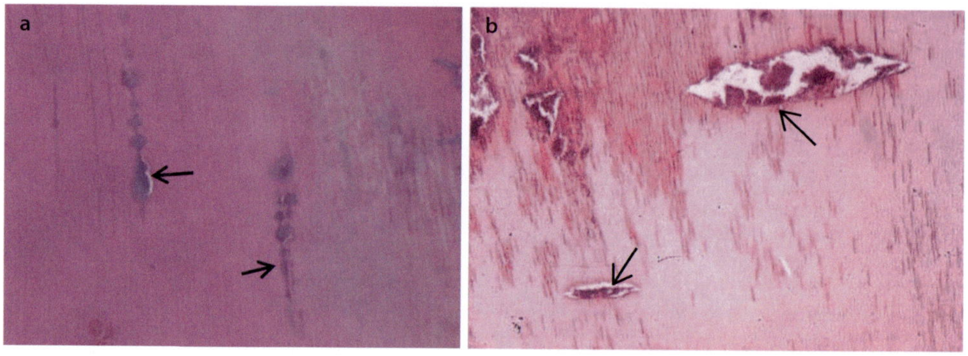

Fig. 17.4 Decalcified haematoxylin and eosin-stained sections of dentine caries. **a** Small, rounded protuberances (arrows) aligned with dentinal tubules are evident. These are liquefaction foci. **b** Large, bacteria-filled defects (arrows) orientated at right angles to the tubule direction in the dentine are called transverse clefts. These clefts extend across many tubules. (Courtesy of Professor David F Wilson, Adelaide, Australia)

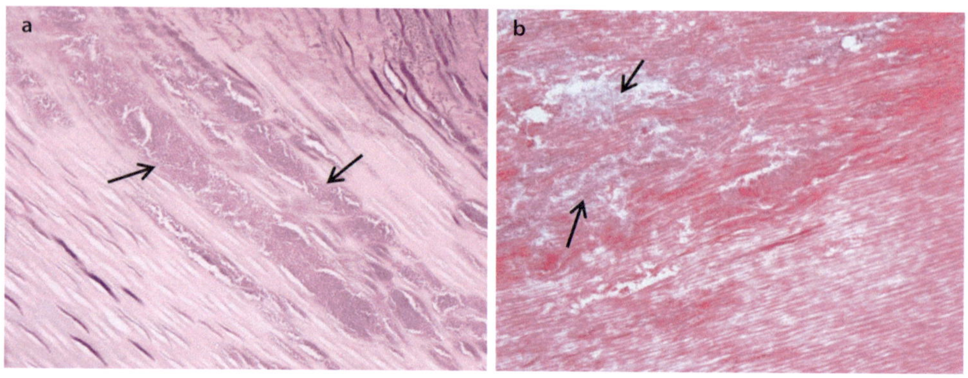

Fig. 17.5 Decalcified haematoxylin and eosin–stained section of dentine caries. **a** Prominent, linear arrays of bacterial colonies (arrows) aligned along the tubule direction are seen replacing the destroyed dentine matrix. **b** More advanced dentine caries show generalised loss of dentine matrix and replacement by bacterial colonies (arrows) along with fragmentation of residual dentine matrix. (Courtesy of Professor David F Wilson, Adelaide, Australia)

17.4 Root Surface Caries

17

- **Key Features**

- Unlike typical carious lesions involving the crown of the tooth, root surface caries develop on the tooth's root due to factors like gingival recession, which exposes the roots to plaque and bacteria. These areas are more vulnerable because they lack the protective enamel covering found on the crown.
- Age, hyposalivation and inadequate oral hygiene increase the risk of root surface caries. Prevention involves diligent oral care, regular dental check-ups and addressing underlying factors contributing to gingival recession to safeguard the roots from decay.
- Detection is straightforward when extensive gingival recession allows easy visualisation of root surfaces but can be difficult when root exposure is minimal.
- Cementum is readily decalcified and prevents little protection from invading microorganisms.
- The initial invading microorganisms include *S. mutans*, Actinomyces species and anaerobic bacteria considered periodontal pathogens. Invasion is along Sharpey's fibres or between fibre bundles and then spread laterally.
- Early detection and treatment are crucial to prevent further damage and maintain oral health.

- **Histopathology**

Following decalcification, the process is similar to that in dentine, with softening and destruction of tissue (Fig. 17.6). The flora invading dentine are likely to be identical to those seen in coronal caries, with progression in dentine and reactionary changes in the pulp. Due to the curvature of dentinal tubules, reactionary dentine apical to the lesion will result. While bacteria penetrate dentine early in root caries lesions, preventive measures rather than operative procedures often arrest the carious process.

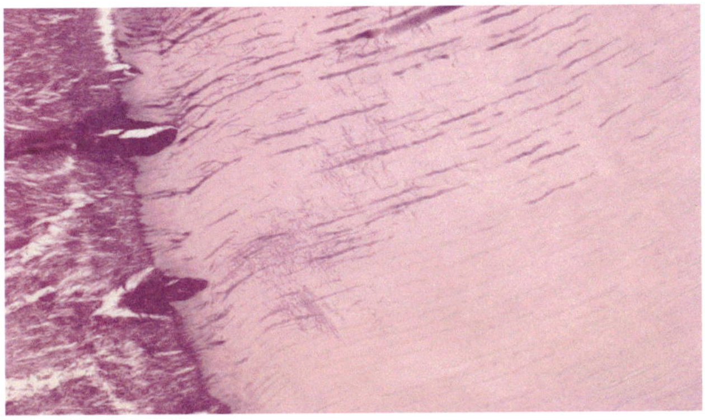

Fig. 17.6 Micrograph of early root caries. (Courtesy of Professor David F Wilson, Adelaide, Australia)

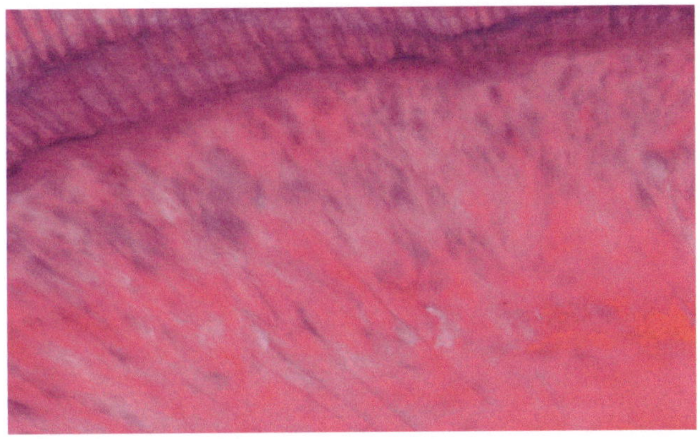

Fig. 17.7 A decalcified haematoxylin and eosin-stained section of dentine shows irregular reparative dentine abutting normal dentine. The reparative dentine shows few tubules. (Courtesy of Professor David F Wilson, Adelaide, Australia)

17.5 Dentinal Reactionary Changes

Stimulation of dentine evokes reactionary changes in dentine and pulp. Irritants include caries, erosion, attrition, abrasion and restorative procedures. Reactionary dentine is initially laid down by viable odontoblasts as peritubular dentine or within the pulp before cavitation in enamel occurs. This is a slow process, which is more likely to be significant in slowly progressing lesions. With the death of odontoblasts, odontoblast-like cells can differentiate in vital pulp and form reactive dentine more quickly. This can continue until pulp vitality is lost. The term tertiary dentine encompasses these changes.

The four reactionary changes in dentine are as follows:

- Translucent dentine, in which reactionary dentine within tubules reduces their diameter and, therefore, reduces bacteria's penetration. This reaction occurs near the dentino-enamel junction and extends laterally from the sides of thc caries lesion. It is often visible radiographically and clinically during the excavation of the carious lesion.
- Regular reactionary dentine forms at the interface between the pulp and dentine. Odontoblasts are responsible for their formation, and they reduce the stimulation of odontoblasts and cells in the pulp by increasing the thickness of dentine between the caries and the pulp, e.g. by obliterating pulp horns.
- Irregular reparative dentine is produced and consists of dentine composed of irregular tubules and disorganised mineralised tissue resembling bone.
- Dead tract formation occurs when odontoblasts die and dentinal tubules are sealed off. This may be protective against advancing caries if peritubular dentine was formed in a significant amount prior to odontoblast death, in which case the dentinal tubules become sclerotic. Conversely, if not, caries can advance more rapidly.

Histopathology

Irregular reparative dentine (Fig. 17.7) is laid down by differentiated cells from the pulp. It is variable, with appearances ranging from dentine with irregular tubules to a disorganised bone-like mineralised tissue. This response is usually moderate or severe carious stimulation i.e. more rapidly evolving lesions than those evoking regular, reactionary dentine formation. This irregular dentine does not provide much protection from an invasive carious front.

17.6 Summary

Dental caries is one of the most common diseases worldwide. Caries is a microbial disease of the calcified tissues of the teeth, characterised by demineralisation of the inorganic portion and destruction of the organic substance of the tooth. Over 150 years of research have been done, yet many aspects of the aetiology of this disease are obscure and efforts at prevention are only partly successful. It is convenient to think of caries as a multifactorial disease, but essential to the process are dietary sugar intake and other factors that are dependent on it. The pathological features of dental caries have been described, and thorough knowledge is required to correlate these features with clinical progression and current treatment practices.

Further Reading

Odell EW. Chapter 4. Cawson's essentials of oral pathology and oral medicine. Elsevier; 2017. p. 53–72.

Ritter AV. Sturdevant's art & science of operative dentistry. Elsevier Health Sciences; 2017.

Warreth A. Dental caries and its management. Int J Dent. 2023;2023:9365845. https://doi.org/10.1155/2023/9365845.

17

Histopathology of the Diseases of the Dental Pulp

Nagamani Narayana

Contents

S R Prabhu et al. (eds.), *Oral Histology and Oral Histopathology*, https://doi.org/10.1007/978-3-031-77481-2_18

18.1 Introduction

Pulpal diseases are usually the sequelae of caries and trauma. Trauma leading to inflammatory pulp pathology can be due to insufficient cooling during the preparation of or deep metal restorations with no restorative lining. Very rarely, acute physical trauma to teeth, usually anterior teeth, can lead to the severance of the apical blood supply, leading to sterile necrosis of the pulp. Low-grade, chronic injuries of indeterminate origin can lead to pulp fibrosis and, on occasion, internal tooth resorption. Pulpal diseases are mainly classified based on their clinical symptoms. Usually, the pulp is not biopsied for diagnosis.

18.2 Inflammatory Pulp Disease

Inflammatory pulpal disease is called pulpitis. This is classified based on the correlation of clinical symptoms with histopathology. The American Association of Endodontists has classified inflammatory pulpal diseases as pulpitis, reversible and irreversible pulpitis, and pulpal necrosis. Both reversible and irreversible pulpitis may be sub-classified as acute or chronic. Different authorities have developed classifications that include other descriptors, such as acute or chronic pulpitis or open or closed pulpitis (see Fig. 18.1).

18.3 Variables That Can Affect the Quality of Pulp Histopathology

The dental pulp is enclosed by dense, calcified tissues and the small diameter root apex opening to the periodontal ligament connective tissues. The process of preparing histological sections of pulp involves fixation of an extracted tooth followed by decalcification of the tooth in acid prior to the specimen being embedded in paraffin, sectioned, and then stained. Inadequate pulp fixation can easily occur since the fixative solution has to diffuse through the small diameter root apex, unlike the situation in a normal soft tissue specimen where the fixative agent has easy access to all surfaces of the specimen. Sufficient fixation leads to well-recognised changes in the odontoblast layer, referred to as "wheat sheafing" (Fig. 18.2), and to poor preservation of cellular detail. Over-decalcification of a tooth specimen can also lead to disruptive changes to pulp constituents, including the poor staining of pulp cells. Difficulties encountered during the sectioning of teeth can also lead to disruptions in pulp architecture, such as tearing of the soft tissue pulp components and separation of the pulp from the dentine. The existence of these variables can affect the appearance of the pulp when it is being assessed for signs of pathology, such as inflammatory pathology.

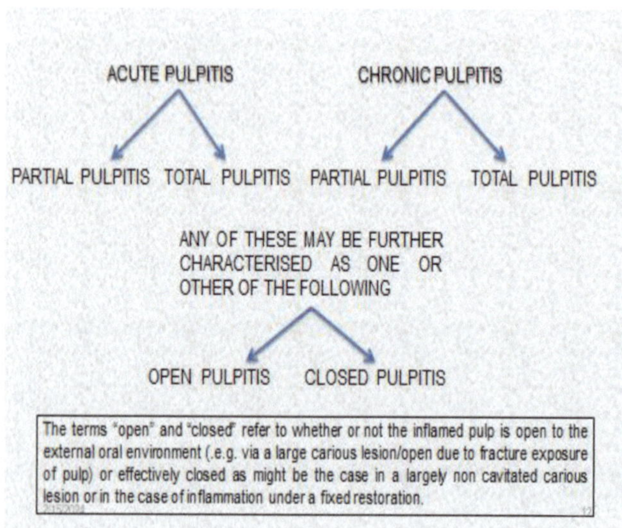

Fig. 18.1 Showing variations in the classification of pulpitis

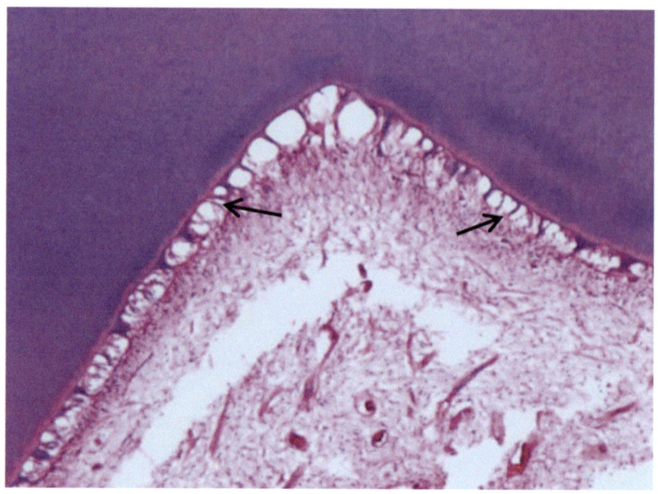

Fig. 18.2 Inadequate pulp fixation. This decalcified tooth section shows coronal pulp and dentine. Note the oedematous and clumped nature of the odontoblast layer (arrows), which is referred to as wheat sheafing. Also, note the tears in the pulp tissue resulting from poor fixation and sectioning difficulties

18.4 Reversible Pulpitis

Reversible pulpitis is characterised by mild sensitivity to heat/cold and sweet foods due to reversible inflammatory changes in the tooth.

Key Features

- Pain is of short duration and not spontaneous.
- There are no radiographic changes at the apex of the tooth, while the tooth may have deep restoration or caries.
- Pulp responds to vitality tests, and there is no tenderness associated with percussion.
- Pulp returns to normal in 3 months. If symptoms persist, then a diagnosis of irreversible pulpitis should be considered.

Histopathology

The histopathological features of reversible pulpitis vary and can be subtle. In some cases, the pulp may appear generally normal but exhibits dilated blood vessels and scattered inflammatory cells. These changes may be generalised or focal and can be subtle (Fig. 18.3).

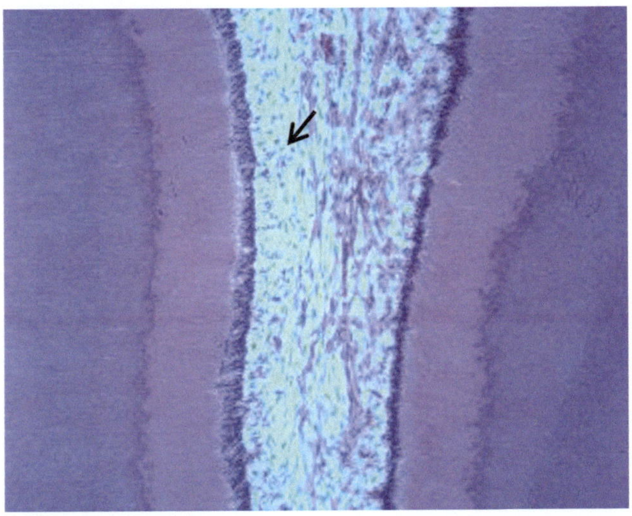

Fig. 18.3 Reversible pulpitis. In this micrograph, there are signs of oedema on the left-hand side of the section and a scattering of inflammatory cells (arrow). (Courtesy of Professor David F Wilson, Adelaide, Australia)

18.5 Irreversible Pulpitis

Irreversible pulpitis is characterised by a constant severe pain that arises without provocation.

Key Features

- The classic clinical feature is lingering pain even after the stimulus is removed (stimuli are thermal stimuli (heat/cold).
- Spontaneous pain wakes the patient up at night, or pain is exacerbated on lying down.
- Pain may be referred to, making it difficult to locate the involved tooth.
- Pulp may respond early or does not respond to vitality tests.
- Tooth may be tender to percussion if periapical tissues are involved.
- Tooth may present with deep caries with or without pulpal exposure.

Histopathology

Microscopically, irreversible pulpitis (Figs. 18.4a, b and 18.5) will exhibit distinct evidence of an acute or chronic inflammatory cell infiltrate of variable severity. Some lesions show evidence of loss of odontoblasts, along with varying degrees of fibrosis, with fibrosis a feature of longer-standing lesions. Acute irreversible pulpitis is characterised by an intense acute-chronic inflammatory cell infiltration with possible areas of necrosis.

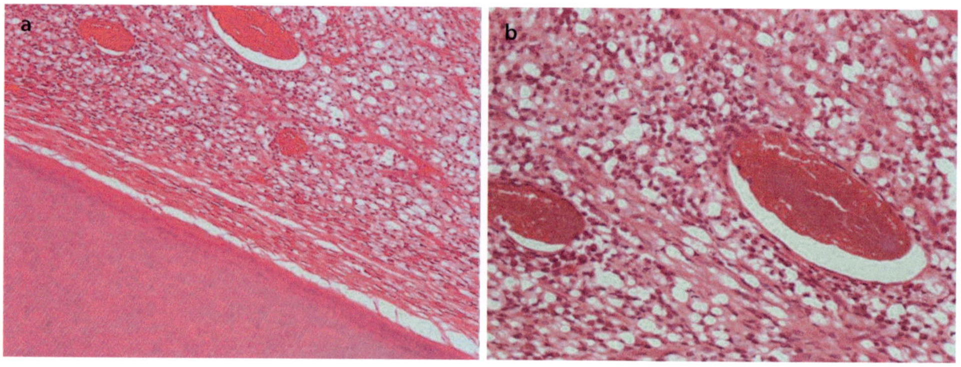

■ **Fig. 18.4** a and b Irreversible pulpitis. The pulp exhibits diffuse oedema, congested and dilated blood vessels and an absence of odontoblasts **a**. More clearly illustrated diffuse inflammatory cell infiltrate and obvious oedema are seen **b**. The grossly dilated and congested blood vessels, along with the evidence of severe inflammation, would probably indicate that the pulp is undergoing necrosis

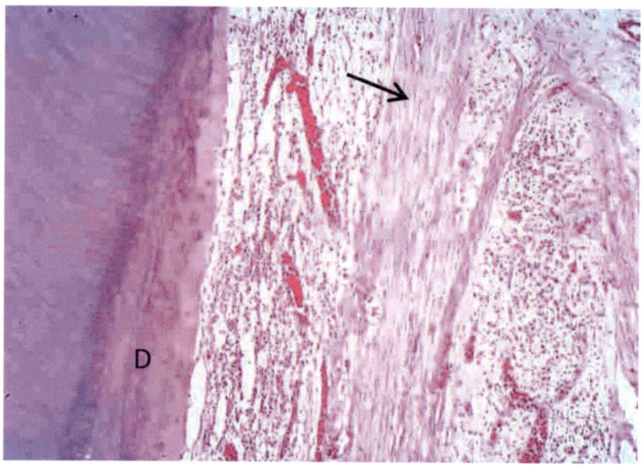

■ **Fig. 18.5** Irreversible pulpitis. In contrast to ■ Fig. 18.4a, b, the pulp in this instance exhibits less intense but still very prominent evidence of inflammation along with fibrosis (arrow). Note the absence of odontoblasts and the presence of reparative–tertiary dentine (D), indicating that the pulp had previously responded to some form of injury before the odontoblasts were lost. (Courtesy of Professor David F Wilson, Adelaide, Australia)

18.6 Pulpal Necrosis

Pulpal necrosis (cell and tissue death) can occur by two mechanisms. The most common cause of pulpal necrosis is necrosis consequent to severe pulpal inflammation, usually due to caries. The second mechanism of pulp necrosis occurs when the apical blood supply to the pulp is severed, thus resulting in an absence of blood flow to the pulp. This phenomenon is a consequence of severe physical trauma to a tooth. It is usually encountered in anterior teeth, which have suffered significant physical trauma and sometimes intrusion because of accidental trauma. This form of pulp necrosis is referred to as sterile necrosis.

Key Clinical Features

- The tooth does not respond to vitality tests.
- There may be a history of trauma to the tooth resulting in discolouration of the tooth crown or the presence of deep decay.

Histopathology

In cases of inflammatory necrosis, all or some of the normal pulp is replaced by a dense mass of inflammatory cells and an absence of normal pulp features (■ Fig. 18.6).

18

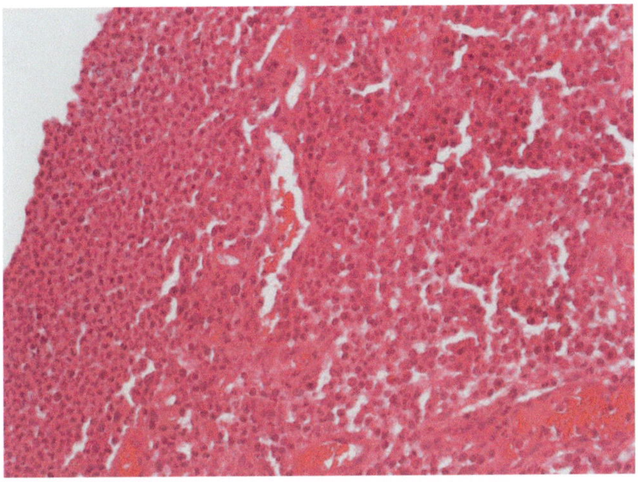

Fig. 18.6 Inflammatory pulp necrosis shows the replacement of normal pulp by an intense accumulation of dead and dying inflammatory cells

18.7 Chronic Hyperplastic Pulpitis (Pulp Polyp)

Chronic hyperplastic pulpitis, also known as pulp polyp or proliferative pulpitis, is an uncommon and specific type of inflammatory hyperplasia associated with nonvital teeth.

Key Clinical Features

- Clinically presents with a red/pinkish nodule protruding from the tooth.
- Tooth does not respond to vitality tests.
- Seen in younger patients with a grossly carious tooth.
- Hyperplastic tissue is painless and may bleed on probing.
- It needs to be differentiated from a gingival polyp, where the soft tissue is attached to the marginal gingiva.

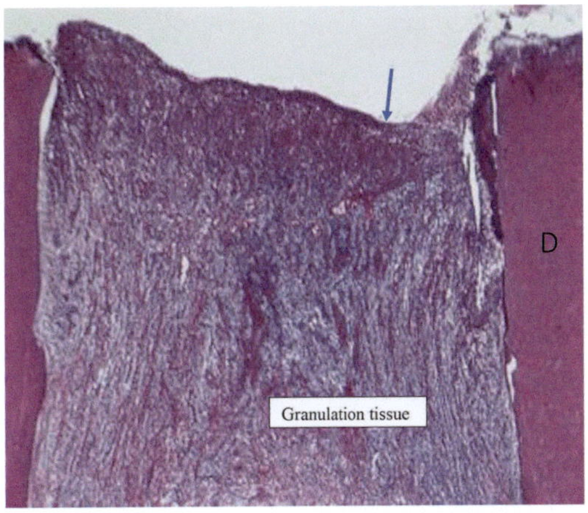

Fig. 18.7 Granulation tissue covered by epithelium (arrow) replacing normal pulp surrounded by dentine (D)

Histopathology

Normal pulp is replaced by granulation tissue; the surface of the polyp may be covered by stratified squamous epithelium (Fig. 18.7).

18.8 Pulp Stones (Pulp Calcifications)

Pulp stones are discrete calcifications within the pulp of healthy or diseased teeth, which may exist freely within the pulp tissue or attached to the dentine.

Key Features

- Pulp stones may be true or false.
- True pulp stones show dentinal tubules and may be free or attached to the dentine wall.
- Amorphous dystrophic calcifications (Fig. 18.8) devoid of dentinal tubules can occur.
- Pulp stones and calcifications may obstruct endodontic treatment.

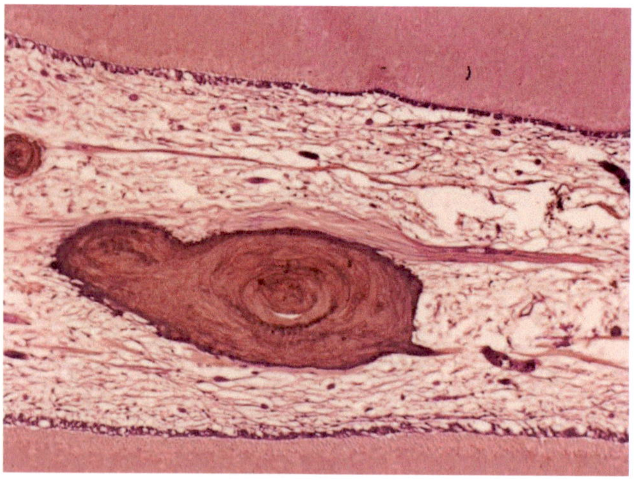

▣ Fig. 18.8 Pulp stone in normal pulp

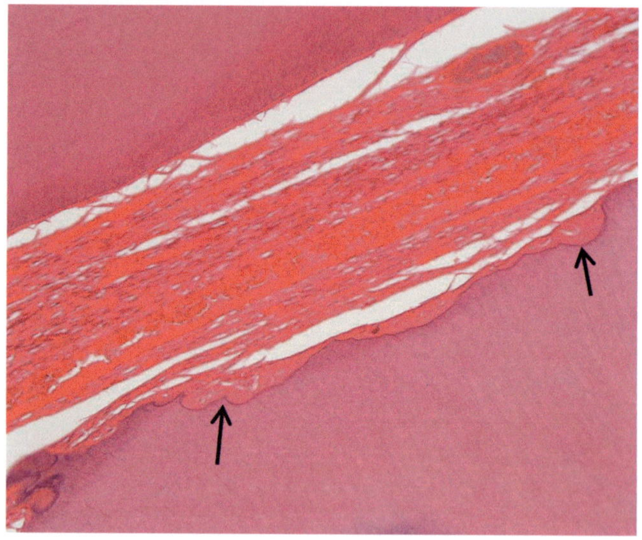

▣ Fig. 18.9 Photomicrograph showing evidence of resorption of the dentine indicated by "resorptive bays" (arrows) and replacement by an eosinophilic matrix. The normal pulp in this specimen has been replaced by dense fibrous tissue. Pulp fibrosis can be a consequence of ageing and/or the effects of low-grade chronic injury to the pulp. (Courtesy of Professor David F Wilson, Adelaide, Australia)

18.9 Internal Resorption

Although rare, resorption of the internal aspect of the dentine is well recognised.

Key Features

- Internal resorption usually occurs because of a continuous chronic inflammatory process.
- Usually asymptomatic.
- Usually occurs either in the mid or apical area of the root.
- They are discovered by chance on routine radiographs or by the clinical sign of a "pink spot" on the crown. The pink spot is the result of the resorptive process that has extended to the cervical area of the crown.
- The most common type is the presence of a focal area of dentine resorption with or without replacement by amorphous, bone matrix-like material.
- Instances where there has not been replacement of dentine can present on a radiograph as a focal radiolucency in the dentine.
- Less prominent signs of dentine resorption (▣ Fig. 18.9) can occasionally be seen in decalcified tooth specimens during routine histological examination.

18

Histopathology

An internal resorption lesion mainly consists of granulation tissue. The pulpal connective tissue is highly vascularised with varying degrees of chronic inflammatory cell infiltration with lymphocytes, macrophages, neutrophilic leukocytes, and plasma cells. "Resorptive bays" with numerous odontoclasts are also seen (▣ Fig. 18.9).

18.10 Summary

Inflammatory diseases of the pulp as a response to caries and trauma to the tooth are discussed.

The accuracy of pulpal diagnoses is limited due to subjective data obtained at history taking. Visual inspection, radiographic examination, and pulp tests should corroborate subjective data for an accurate diagnosis. Studies have shown no clear association between clinical examination and histopathology of the pulp.

Further Reading

Abbott PV, Yu C. A clinical classification of the status of the pulp and the root canal system. Aust Dent J. 2007;52(1 Suppl):S17–31. https://doi.org/10.1111/j.1834-7819.2007.tb00522.x.

Cawson RA, Odell EW. Cawson's essentials of oral pathology and oral medicine. 8ht ed. Elsevier; 2002. p. 60–6.

Goldberg M. The dental pulp. Biology, pathology and regenerative therapies. Springer; 2014. p. 125–54.

Goldberg M. Understanding dental caries from pathogenesis to prevention and therapy. Springer; 2016. p. 127–52. https://doi.org/10.1007/978-3-319-30552-3_1.

Naseri M, Khayat A, Zamaheni S, Shojaeian S. Correlation between histological status of the pulp and its response to sensibility tests. Iran Endod J. 2017;12(1):20–4. https://doi.org/10.22037/iej.2017.04.

Ricucci D, Loghin S, Siqueira JF Jr. Correlation between clinical and histologic pulp diagnoses. J Endod. 2014;40(12):1932–9. https://doi.org/10.1016/j.joen.2014.08.010. Epub 2014 Oct 12.

Zuza EP, Carrareto AL, Lia RC, Pires JR, de Toledo BE. Histopathological features of dental pulp in teeth with different levels of chronic periodontitis severity. ISRN Dent. 2012;2012:271350. https://doi.org/10.5402/2012/271350. Epub 2012 Apr 10.

Histopathology of Gingival and Periodontal Diseases

Emily Ming-Chieh Lu

Contents

S R Prabhu et al. (eds.), *Oral Histology and Oral Histopathology*, https://doi.org/10.1007/978-3-031-77481-2_19

We now understand that the presence of pathogenic biofilm, while a crucial requirement for the development of periodontitis, is alone insufficient to cause disease. The host immune response against the microbial challenge, in cooperation with the junctional epithelium (JE), is central to the pathoaetiology of periodontitis. Within the periodontium, the most significant immune protective mechanism is the recruitment of the neutrophils which along with the sustained release of pro-inflammatory cytokines, drives alveolar bone loss, leading to further tissue destruction.

Thus, the disease develops from intricate interactions between the biofilm and the host immune response. The outcome of the microbial challenge from the dental plaque depends, therefore, on the balance between the protective and destructive aspects of the host response. Fluctuations in the host–parasite relationship upset the balance between the protective and destructive aspects of the host response. Therefore, while gingivitis can remain stable for an extended period in a number of individuals, it can progress to periodontitis in susceptible individuals where there is an imbalance between the host and microbial factors.

In this chapter, the histopathological features of periodontal disease will be described through a series of stages: initial lesion gingivitis, early lesion gingivitis, established lesion gingivitis, and advanced lesion. It is important to note that these histopathological changes occur constitute a continuum. Additionally, histopathological features of acute periodontal abscesses and necrotising periodontal diseases are discussed. It is important that the reader relates these histopathological features to the clinical presentation of the disease.

19.1 Introduction: The Periodontium in Health

In health, a balance exists between the microbial challenge from the plaque biofilm and the host defence mechanisms. The junctional epithelium (JE) serves to provide attachment to the tooth, creating a seal which is essential in maintaining periodontal health. The JE is a permeable tissue, allowing both the ingress of bacteria and their by-products, as well as the emigration of immune cells, as part of the outflow of gingival crevicular fluid (GCF). Thus, in healthy gingivae, there is a continuous low-level emigration of polymorphonuclear neutrophils (PMNS) into the gingival sulcus. For more detailed information on the histology of the normal periodontal tissues, the reader is encouraged to refer to oral histology texts.

19.2 Aetiology of Gingival and Periodontal Diseases: The Dental Plaque Biofilm

Dental plaque biofilm is a complex microbial community that develops on the tooth surface (and other hard non-shedding materials), embedded in a matrix of polymers of bacterial and salivary origin. The formation of dental biofilm confers protective mechanisms for the microorganisms against the host's innate immunity and thus this results in ineffective attempts at phagocytosis.

The microbial composition of the plaque biofilm changes from health to disease. In gingival health, there is an abundance of Gram-positive facultative anaerobic cocci (streptococci). In disease, the composition of the plaque changes such that there are increases in proportions of Gram-negative facultative anaerobic rods and eventually Gram-negative obligate anaerobes which predominate the chronic gingivitis or periodontitis lesion.

Over the years, different plaque theories have been proposed to explain how the accumulation of plaque biofilm can result in the development of periodontal diseases. These include the non-specific plaque theory, the specific plaque theory, ecological plaque theory (for detailed descriptions, the reader should refer to oral microbiology or pathology texts).

The Keystone Plaque Hypothesis is now the widely accepted theory and proposes that keystone pathogens such as *Porphyromonas gingivalis* disrupt the symbiotic relationship between microorganisms and host immune response, thus enabling pathobionts (opportunistic bacteria) to thrive. Therefore, these keystone pathogens while present in relatively low numbers can have a disproportional effect on their environment.

More recently, the "inflammation-mediated polymicrobial emergence and dysbiotic-exacerbation" (IMPEDE) model was recently proposed (Van Dyke et al. 2020). This theory emphasises the inflammatory state as the driver of plaque-induced gingivitis and periodontitis. Thus, if the host immune and inflammatory response is controlled and regulated, gingivitis will not progress to periodontitis. However, if the inflammatory response becomes dysregulated, tissue damage occurs.

Nevertheless, failure to regularly and mechanically disrupt the accumulation of dental biofilm through effective oral hygiene practices can result in the onset of gingivitis.

19.3 Gingivitis

Gingivitis is defined by an inflammatory lesion resulting from interactions between the dental plaque biofilm and the host's immune-inflammatory response. It is charac-

Table 19.1 Classification of periodontal diseases and conditions (based on the 2017 World Workshop)

Periodontal diseases and conditions	Periodontal health, gingival diseases and conditions	Periodontal health and gingival health
		Gingivitis: biofilm-induced
		Gingival diseases: Non-dental biofilm-induced
	Periodontitis	Necrotising periodontal diseases
		Periodontitis
		Periodontitis as a manifestation of systemic diseases
	Other conditions affecting the periodontium	Systemic diseases or conditions affecting the periodontal supporting tissues
		Periodontal abscesses and endodontic-periodontitis lesions
		Periodontal abscesses and endodontic-periodontic lesions
		Mucogingival deformities and conditions
		Traumatic occlusal forces
		Tooth and prosthesis-related factors

Adapted from Caton 2018, J Clin Periodontol. 2018. ► https://doi.org/10.1111/jcpe.12935

terised by red, swollen gingivae, that may bleed on gentle probing, all of which are hallmarks of acute inflammation (► Box 19.1). These clinical features appear 1–2 weeks after the initial accumulation of plaque at the gingival margin. The diagnosis, based on the 2017 World Workshop classification is dental plaque biofilm-induced gingivitis (Table 19.1).

Importantly, the inflammatory conditions remain contained within the gingiva and do not extend apical to the mucogingival junction and the remaining supporting tissues (cementum, periodontal ligament, and alveolar bone) are unaffected. There is no clinical attachment loss (CAL) and radiographs also confirm no alveolar bone loss.

Gingivitis is a reversible condition. The experimental gingivitis studies (Loe 1965) showed that there is a one-to-one relationship between dental plaque and the development of gingivitis. Once plaque biofilm is removed, the inflammatory stimuli is removed, resulting in the resolution of inflammation and tissue healing. Thus, gingivitis is managed through mechanical removal of the plaque biofilm and effective oral hygiene measures by the patient. The reversal of gingivitis following removal of the plaque biofilm also confirms the gingivitis diagnosis.

While all individuals with periodontitis will have had suffered from gingivitis at one point, not all patients with gingivitis will necessarily progress to periodontitis. However, it may be difficult to identify individuals with gingivitis who may progress.

Box 19.1. Key Features of Dental Plaque Biofilm-Induced Gingivitis

- Red, swollen gingivae
- Bleeding on probing
- Reversible condition-gingivitis is reversed following removal of plaque biofilm
- There is no clinical attachment loss and radiographs also confirm no alveolar bone loss.

19.3.1 Histopathology

The histopathology of the development of gingivitis based on Page and Schroeder (1976) as initial, early, and established will be described first. The final stage is the advanced stage under the subsection on periodontitis. A summary of the key histopathological features at each stage of the lesion is outlined in Table 19.2.

Table 19.2 Summary of the histopathological features of gingivitis and periodontitis

Gingivitis	Initial lesion (2–4 days)	– Increased vascular dilation and increased vascular permeability. – Increase recruitment and emigration of PMNs into the gingival sulcus. – The inflammatory infiltrate largely consists of neutrophils with few lymphocytes. – Increased GCF flow
	Early (4–7 days)	– Marked increase in vascular dilation and permeability. – The inflammatory infiltrate predominately consists of lymphocytes and macrophages. – Increase recruitment and emigration of PMNs into the gingival sulcus. – Increased GCF flow – Loss of collagen – No attachment loss. No bone loss and no pocket formation
	Established gingivitis	– Proliferation of JE and SE – Loss of collagen – Importantly, there is no loss of attachment and no pocket formation. – The majority of lymphocytes are B cells, although up to 30% may be T cells. – Significant PMN recruitment and migration – The volume of the inflammatory infiltrate increases with apical and lateral extension. – Plasma cells predominate in the inflammatory infiltrate. – However, there is no loss of alveolar bone – No connective tissue attachment loss – This stage is characterised by continued cellular emigration and increased tissue turnover.
Periodontitis	Advanced – Pocket formation – Pocket contains subgingival calculus, plaque and inflammatory exudate, consisting of fluid and cells, mainly PMN. – Pocket epithelium shows areas of irregular hyperplasia and rete ridge formation, alternating with areas of thinning and ulceration. – Significant increases in vascular dilation and vascular permeability – Significant recruitment and emigration of PMNs – Loss of connective tissue attachment – Loss of collagen	– Marked apical migration and proliferation of the JE with areas of ulceration. – Loss of connective tissue attachment – Extensive chronic inflammatory infiltrate in connective tissue adjacent to the JE – Destruction of PDL fibres which inert in the alveolar bone and cementum – Loss of ground substance and damage to the fibroblasts. – Alveolar bone loss – Pocket formation

19.4 Initial Lesion Gingivitis (2–4 days After Plaque Accumulation)

The initial lesion of gingivitis is characterised by an acute inflammatory response. The vascular events which accompany this include increase in vasodilation and increase in vascular permeability. Additionally, there is also apparent PMN emigration to the gingival sulcus, an increase in the flow of GCF and loss of collagen. The inflammatory infiltrate is characterised by mainly neutrophils in the gingival crevice and adjacent CT. This contrasts to the relatively small numbers of lymphocytes in the first week which becomes more marked in the infiltrate as the lesion progresses to established gingivitis.

In the first 2–4 days after plaque accumulation, the predominant microorganisms are mostly Gram-positive aerobic and saccharolytic. Microorganisms increase the permeability of the JE enabling both the ingress of bacterial products and emigration of GCF, which at this stage is still mainly interstitial fluid.

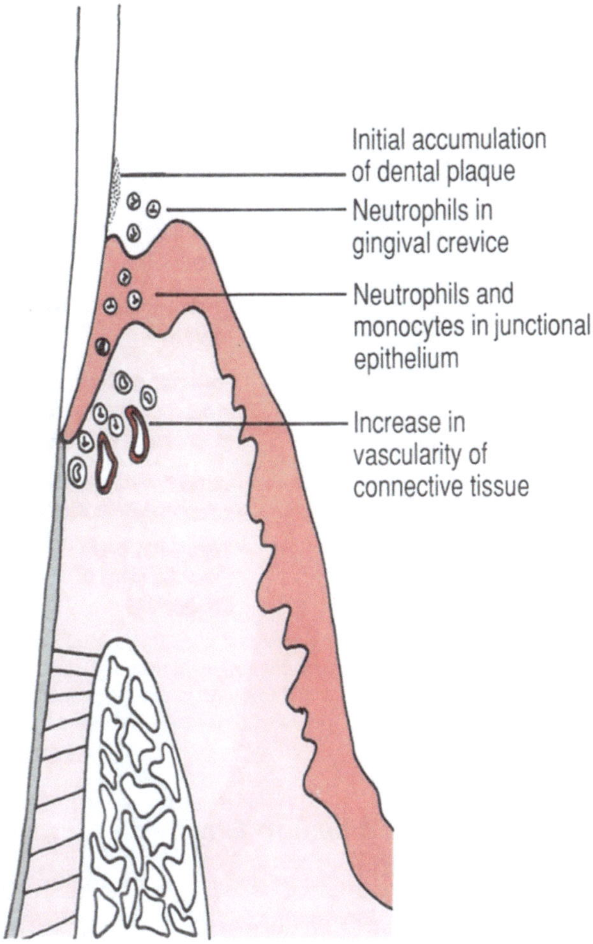

Fig. 19.1 Initial lesion showing presence of neutrophils in response to initial plaque accumulation. There is also increased vascularity of the connective tissues

In response to chemoattractants from plaque bacteria and inflammatory mediators, neutrophil recruitment and emigration are increased. Once in the gingival sulcus, there is a "failed" attempt by the PMNs at phagocytosis, resulting in the release of lysosomal enzymes and thus local disintegration of collagen. However, this is a failed attempt at phagocytosis as the formation of the plaque biofilm acts as a protective mechanism against neutrophils.

Additionally, PMNS form neutrophil extracellular traps (NETs) that trap and kill microbial pathogens and can lead to severe tissue damage.

Pro-inflammatory stimuli found in the gingival sulcus, such as lipopolysaccharide (LPS), IL-8, TNF-α, and streptococcal M protein, can all induce NET. IL-8 is a strong chemoattractant, promoting the chemotaxis of PMNs into the gingival sulcus, is a strong stimulus for NET formation, thus positive feedback loop, as the body attempts to contain the bacterial infection. The inflammatory state is sustained by the release of pro-inflammatory cytokines during NETosis which increase cell adhesion molecules such as endothelial cell leukocyte adhesion molecules (ELAM-1) and intercellular adhesion molecule-1 (ICAM-1). These chemoattracts, along with an increase in IL-8 production by epithelial cells favour an escalation of neutrophil recruitment and emigration through the junctional epithelium into the gingival sulcus. The key events of the initial lesion are summarised in Fig. 19.1 and ▶ Box 19.2.

Box 19.2. Histopathological Features of the Initial Lesion (2–4 days)

- Increased vascular dilation and increased vascular permeability.
- Increase recruitment and emigration of PMNs into the gingival sulcus.
- The inflammatory infiltrate largely consists of neutrophils with few lymphocytes.
- Increased GCF flow

19.5 Early Lesion Gingivitis (4–7 days)

The early lesion is characterised by an increase in the influx of inflammatory cells recruited to the area, which largely consists of T and B lymphocytes and macrophages. Cytokines produced from T helper cells stimulate the B lymphocytes to transform into antibody-specific plasma cells. The lymphocytic infiltrate expands apically and laterally apical to the JE and is accompanied by a significant loss of collagen. However, there is no loss of attachment (Figs. 19.2 and 19.3, and ▶ Box 19.3).

There is a marked increase in vascular dilation and vascular permeability, resulting in an increase in GCF flow. The GCF is essentially an inflammatory exudate and consists of plasma proteins, immunoglobulins, and complement components. However, it is modified during its passage through the crevice by the addition of bacterial products and components derived from connective tissue breakdown.

These immunologic responses are accompanied by localised proliferation and the increase in permeability of the JE and sulcular epithelium (SE). The widening of the intercellular spaces between epithelial cells further promotes the ingress of bacterial products into gingival tissues, escalating the inflammatory response and deepening of the gingival crevice. The latter encourages the

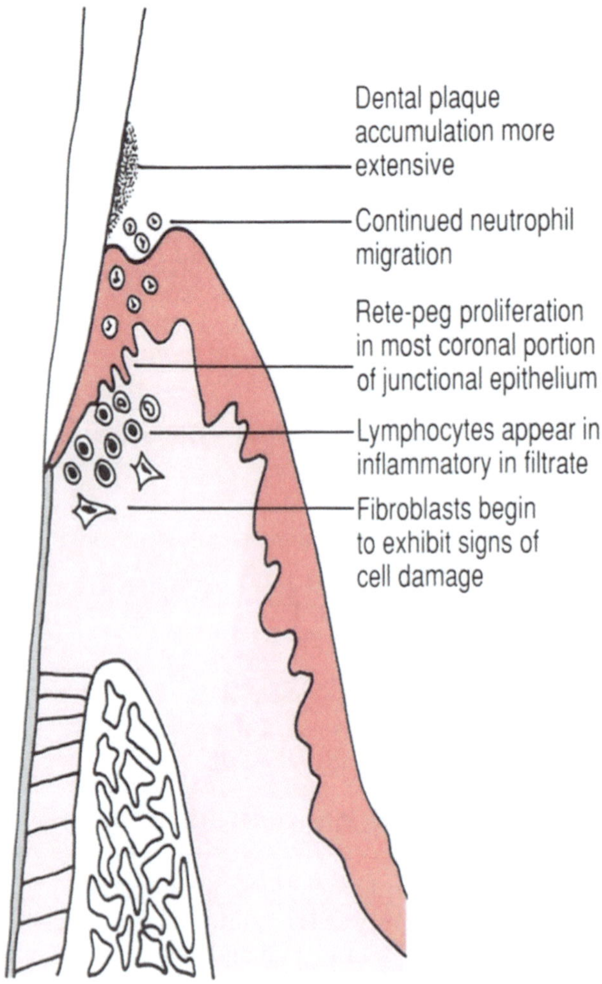

Fig. 19.2 Early lesion showing increased neutrophil migration and proliferation of junctional epithelium (JE). Lymphocytes also appear in the inflammatory infiltrate and there are no early signs of damage to the collagenous tissue

proliferation of anaerobic Gram-negative organisms in the plaque. These organisms produce endotoxins and proteolytic enzymes, which will stimulate the inflammatory response further.

> **Box 19.3. Histopathological Features of the Early Lesion (4–7 days)**
> - Marked increase in vascular dilation and vascular permeability.
> - The inflammatory infiltrate predominately consists of lymphocytes and macrophages.
> - Increase recruitment and emigration of PMNs into the gingival sulcus.
> - Increased GCF flow
> - Local proliferation of JE and SE

19

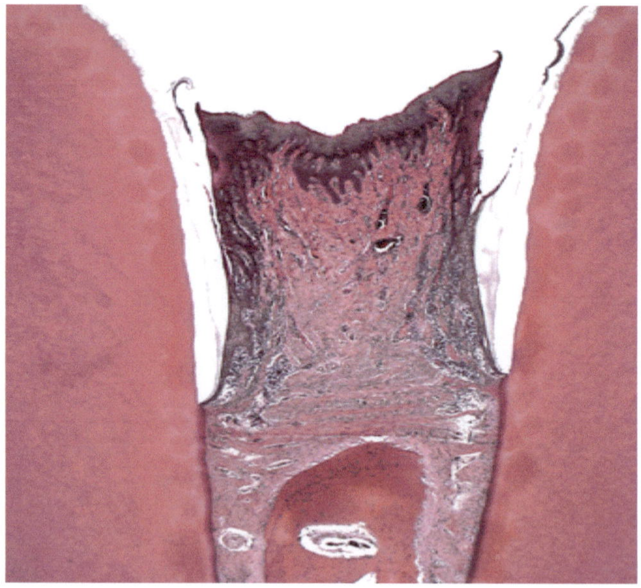

Fig. 19.3 Initial or early lesion gingivitis. There is a deepened gingival crevice, but no pocket formation, as the epithelial attachment still remains on the enamel. There is evidence of JE rete hyperplasia. The presence of the inflammatory cells is concentrated around the region of the JE and extends apically into the CT. There is no alveolar bone loss

19.6 Established Lesion Gingivitis (2–3 weeks)

If the plaque biofilm is allowed to persist, thus sustaining the immunologic response, the early gingivitis may progress to become established gingivitis, which is the advanced stage of gingivitis.

The established lesion is characterised by an inflammatory infiltrate consisting predominately of plasma cells, thus highlighting a change in the quality of the infiltrate from a predominantly lymphocyte one, as observed in early gingivitis (Figs. 19.4 and 19.5).

The increase in the extent of the inflammatory infiltrate is accompanied by marked collagen loss in the involved connective tissue. There is also further proliferation of the JE, which is heavily infiltrated by inflammatory cells migrating into the gingival crevice (▶ Box 19.4).

Cytokines released by immune cells and epithelial cells enhance the recruitment and emigration of PMNs, lymphocytes, and macrophages into the area. Activation of these immune cells further drives the production of pro and anti-inflammatory cytokines, thus leading to both protective and damaging effects on the host. The latter is also reflected in the evidence of healing (angiogenesis and fibrosis) as well as inflammation, and this is typical of the chronicity of the lesion.

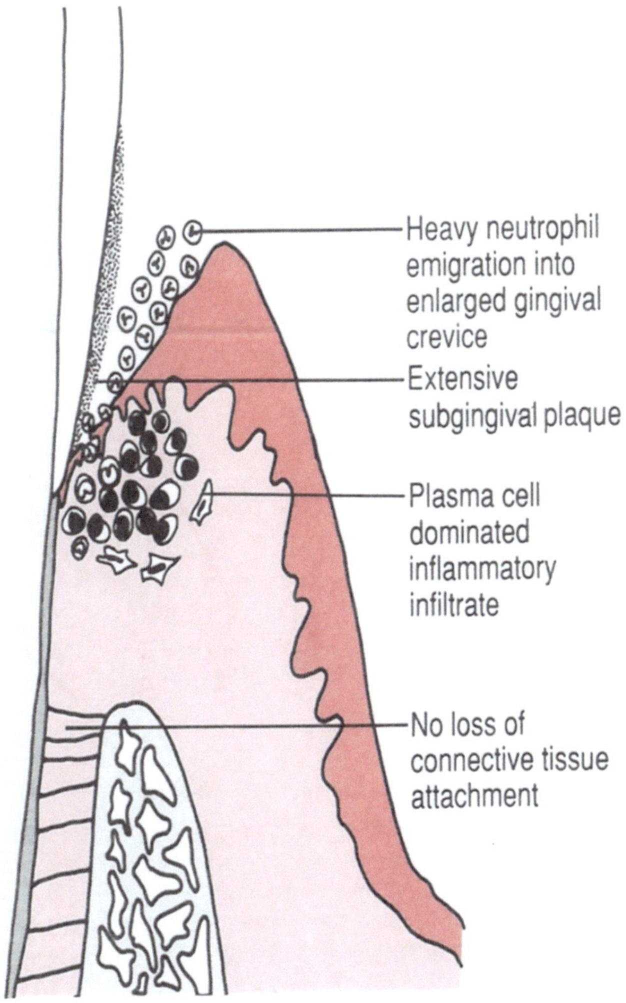

Fig. 19.4 Established gingivitis. The inflammatory infiltrate consists predominately of plasma cells There are also increased concentrations of neutrophil recruitment and emigration to the gingival sulcus. However, there is no loss of connective tissue attachment

It is important to remember, that there is a complex interplay between microbial factors and host responses in the pathogenesis of periodontal disease. Where the microbial challenge is contained by host the immune response, the periodontal disease remains at the established but stable gingivitis stage for a substantial period.

However, thorough mechanical removal of plaque biofilm will predictably result in tissue healing and resolution of inflammation in most individuals with no inherited immunodeficiency diseases. Therefore, while the established lesion is the most advanced stage of gingivitis, this stage of the continuum is still reversible, meaning there will be no irreversible damage to the tissue architecture once the removal causative agent has been removed.

Progression to the advanced lesion occurs where the microbial challenge has overwhelmed the host defence mechanisms, thus resulting in tissue destruction and periodontitis.

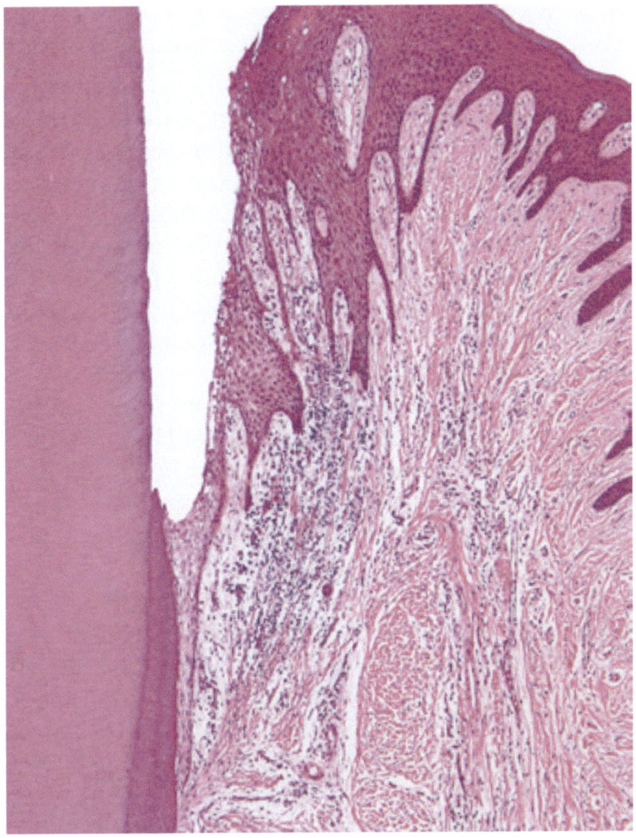

Fig. 19.5 Established gingivitis. The lining of the junctional epithelium shows evidence of epithelial hyperplasia and rete ridges, which are normally absent. Inflammatory cells are localised to the gingival crevice. There is no formation pocket yet

Box 19.4. Histopathological Features of Established Gingivitis

- Proliferation of JE and SE
- Loss of collagen
- Importantly, there is no loss of attachment and no pocket formation
- The majority of lymphocytes are B cells, although up to 30% may be T cells.
- Significant PMN recruitment and migration
- The volume of the inflammatory infiltrate increases with apical and lateral extension
- Plasma cells predominate in the inflammatory infiltrate.
- However, there is no loss of alveolar bone
- No connective tissue attachment loss
- This stage is characterised by continued cellular emigration and increased tissue turnover.

19.7 Periodontitis

Periodontitis is a chronic inflammatory disease with a high prevalence of 50% overall and is the sixth most common human disease. It is caused by the presence of dysbiotic plaque biofilm, which triggers an inadequate immune-inflammatory response, and results in the progressive destruction of the supporting tissues of the teeth, ultimately leading to tooth loss. Therefore, the periodontitis phenotype is characterised by an excessive, yet ineffective and non-resolving inflammation, resulting in tissue damage.

Periodontitis is typically preceded by gingivitis which progresses to periodontitis in susceptible individuals where there is an imbalance between the host and microbial factors. In a small minority of patients, it can advance rapidly leading to significant bone loss at a young age.

While dental plaque biofilm results in gingivitis, periodontitis is characterised by three clinical features:

- The loss of periodontal tissue support, manifested through clinical attachment loss (CAL) and radiographic signs of alveolar bone loss
- The presence of periodontal pockets
- Gingival bleeding

The case definition of periodontitis based on the 2017 World Workshop classification, as well as the clinical features of periodontitis is outlined in ▶ Boxes 19.5 and 19.6, respectively.

Management of periodontitis essentially involves (1) implementation of effective oral hygiene measures and behavioural change for OH improvement, (2) professional mechanical plaque removal (PMPR), (3) management of risk factors such as smoking cessation and diabetes control, and (4) ongoing monitoring and consider referral to periodontist.

Periodontitis is also associated with multiple systemic conditions such as cardiovascular disease, diabetes mellitus, adverse pregnancy outcomes, rheumatoid arthritis, inflammatory bowel disease, metabolic syndrome, chronic kidney disease, respiratory diseases, cognitive decline, Alzheimer's disease, and cancers. Therefore, successful treatment of periodontal disease is important for both oral and systemic health.

19

Based on pathophysiology, three different forms of periodontitis have been identified:

1. Periodontitis
2. Necrotising periodontitis
3. Periodontitis as a direct manifestation of systemic diseases

The histopathology of periodontitis and periodontitis as a manifestation of systemic diseases will be described under "Advanced lesion" below. The histopathology of necrotising periodontitis will be outlined separately in the latter part of this chapter.

Box 19.5. Case Definition of Periodontitis, Based on the 2017 World Workshop Classification

A patient is a periodontitis case where:

- Interdental CAL is detectable at ≥2 non-adjacent teeth, or
- Buccal or oral CAL ≥3 mm with pocketing >3 mm is detectable at ≥2 teeth.

Additionally, the observed CAL cannot be ascribed to non-periodontal causes such as: (1) gingival recession of traumatic origin, (2) dental caries extending in the cervical area of the tooth, (3) the presence of CAL on the distal aspect of a second molar and associated with malposition or extraction of a third molar, (4) an endodontic lesion draining through the marginal periodontium, and (5) the occurrence of a vertical root fracture.

Box 19.6. Key Features of Periodontitis

- Pocket formation
- Clinical attachment loss
- Radiographic signs of alveolar bone loss
- Gingival bleeding
- Gingival recession
- Mobility
- Risk of tooth loss

19.8 Advanced Lesion

The advanced lesion is characterised by irreversible destruction of connective tissue attachment, collagen loss, and alveolar bone loss. A key feature is the proliferation and apical migration of the JE, thus resulting in the formation of pockets (◘ Figs. 19.6, 19.7, and 19.8).

This inflammatory infiltrate extends below the base of the JE into the CT above the crest of the alveolar bone and consists of a high concentration of plasma cells and numerous T lymphocytes and macrophages. The inflammatory infiltrate while similar in composition compared to established gingivitis, is more extensive. As the size and intensity of the infiltrate increase, the disease progresses into the supporting tissues, leading to the disintegration of collagen in the supracrestal CT and the destruction of PDL fibres (◘ Fig. 19.9). The foci of inflammatory cells may be separated by bands of fibrous tissue, suggesting the body's attempts at repair. However,

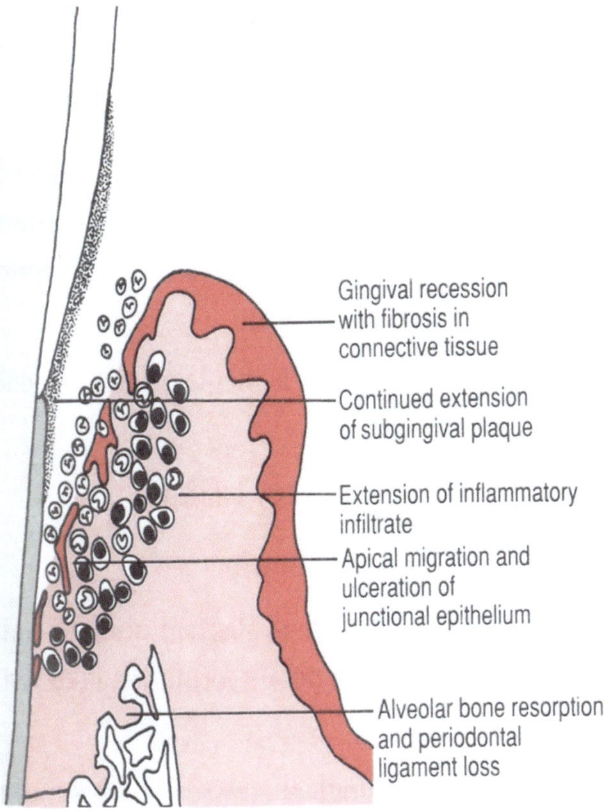

Fig. 19.6 The advanced lesion is characterised by apical migration of the junctional epithelium, alveolar bone loss, connective tissue, and periodontal ligament breakdown, as well as expansive inflammatory infiltrate

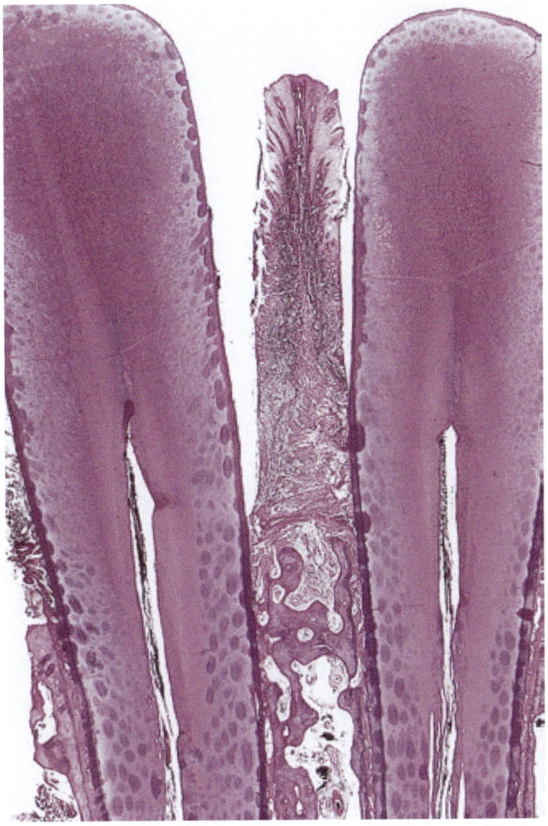

Fig. 19.7 Periodontitis. The periodontal pocket has extended onto the cementum, accompanied by a dense inflammatory infiltrate in the interdental gingiva

the newly formed collagen bundles do not simulate the architecture of the original fibres.

Periodontal destruction is characterised by periods of activity interspersed by periods of quiescence. During the quiescent phase, osteoblasts are not present in significant numbers on the surface of the alveolar bone adjacent to the inflammatory infiltrate. However, during active bone resorption, there is a marked increase in osteoclastic activity. A summary of the key histopathological features of the advanced lesion is outlined in ► Box 19.7.

Box 19.7. Histopathological Features of Advanced Lesion

The main difference between advanced and established lesions is the obvious loss obvious connective tissue attachment and alveolar bone.

- Pocket formation
- Pocket contains subgingival calculus, plaque and inflammatory exudate, consisting of fluid and cells, mainly PMN.
- Pocket epithelium shows areas of irregular hyperplasia and rete ridge formation, alternating with areas of thinning and ulceration.
- Significant increases in vascular dilation and vascular permeability
- Significant recruitment and emigration of PMNs
- Loss of connective tissue attachment
- Loss of collagen
- Alveolar bone loss
- Dense inflammatory infiltrate in the CT, the composition of which is similar to that in established gingivitis.

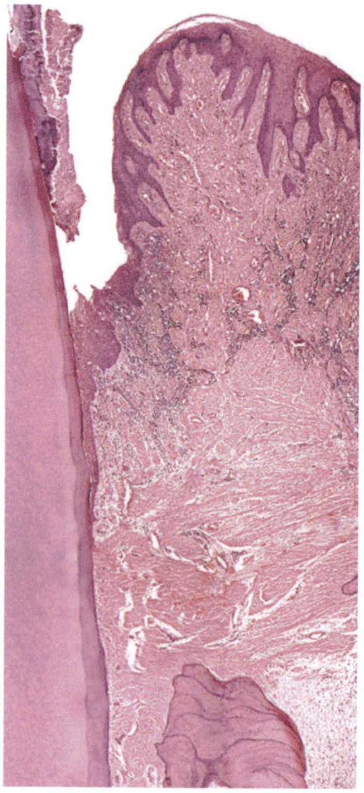

■ **Fig. 19.8** Periodontitis. Pocket formation within which there is evidence of subgingival calculus and plaque. The epithelium of the pocket wall is hyperplastic showing rete processes at the base of the pocket. There is evidence of alveolar bone loss. Supracrestally, there is a band of fibrous tissue which separates the alveolar bone from the inflammatory infiltrate

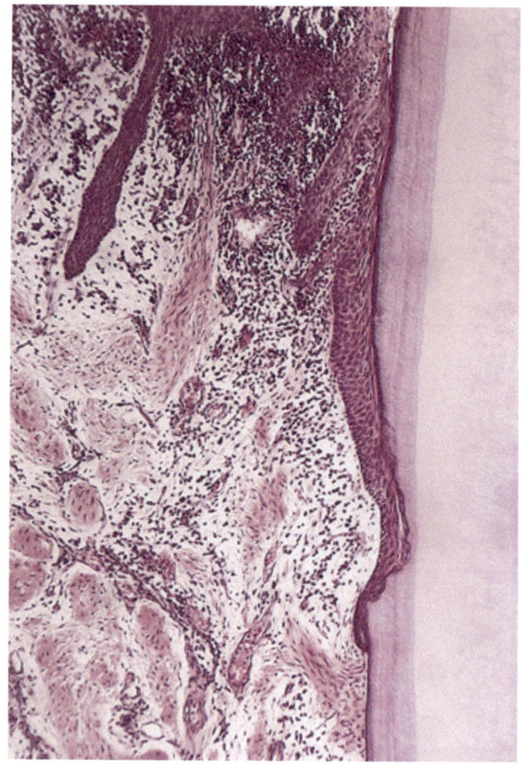

■ **Fig. 19.9** Periodontitis. Higher power view showing loss of collagen in areas with the dense inflammatory infiltrate

19.9 Apical Migration of the JE

The molecular mechanisms responsible for the apical migration are unclear. Recent findings suggest the presence of an inhibitory signal within the connective tissues that is responsible for the integrity and anatomical position of the JE. Thus, it was proposed that during periodontitis, damage to the connective tissues removes its inhibitory effect on epithelial growth, resulting in the proliferation and the apical migration of the JE.

19.10 Mechanisms of Tissue Destruction

It is now widely accepted that the main mechanisms of tissue destruction are related to host immune responses which are responsible for nearly 80% of the risk associated with tissue damage. By contrast, the direct action of the bacteria accounts for only 20% of the tissue damage. Thus, most of the tissue destruction in periodontal disease is thought to be due to inappropriate activation of the host response to microbial plaque, resulting in an upregulation of tissue degradation systems.

19.10.1 Collagen and Connective Tissue Destruction in Periodontal Disease

Connective tissue destruction involves a family of proteolytic enzymes, known as matrix metalloproteinases (MMPs), which are produced by fibroblasts and some immune cells. Of the MMPs, MMP-8 is the most well studied.

In health the normal remodelling of the CT is tightly controlled, resulting in a balance between rates of synthesis and degradation which reflects the balance between the activity of the MMPs and their inhibitors. The main group of inhibitors present in the tissues are known as tissue inhibitors of metalloproteinases (TIMPs) and they are also mainly produced by fibroblasts and macrophages. The destruction of CT in periodontitis reflects an imbalance between the levels of MMPs and TIMPs in the tissues, thus resulting in a relative increase in MMP activity.

The production of MMPs and TIMPs is influenced by a variety of factors, particularly cytokines. Thus IL-1β and TNF-α are mediators of connective tissue destruction.

19.10.2 Bone Resorption in Periodontal Disease

Both bacterial and host-derived factors act locally to trigger osteoclastic activity resulting in bone resorption. When bone resorption is not balanced by bone deposition, net bone loss occurs.

Key host-derived factors which mediate bone resorption include:

- Cytokines: IL-1β, TNF-α, IL-6, Prostaglandin E2 (PGE_2)
- Prostaglandin E2 (PGE_2)

Bacterial-derived factors (such as cell wall components) may also play a role in this process, by stimulating the release of host-derived factors.

19.11 Acute Periodontal Abscesses

Periodontal abscesses most frequently occur in preexisting periodontal pockets. This is likely caused by factors that disturb the balance between the host and bacterial microorganism. An acute periodontal abscess is characterised by a localised accumulation of pus within the periodontal pocket. Without intervention to drain the abscess, rapid tissue destruction and severe bone loss can ensue compromising tooth prognosis.

19.11.1 Management

Drain abscess, PMPR, followed by reinforcement of oral hygiene. Systemic antibiotics may also be appropriate if there are signs of systemic involvement.

19.11.2 Histopathology

During this acute phase, the bony wall outlining the pocket undergoes alveolar bone resorption by osteoclasts, with loss of connective tissue attachment and consequently rapid deepening of the pocket, which can extend towards the apex. Concomitantly, the pocket and its surrounding area show a dense infiltration of neutrophils and the formation of pus (Fig. 19.10).

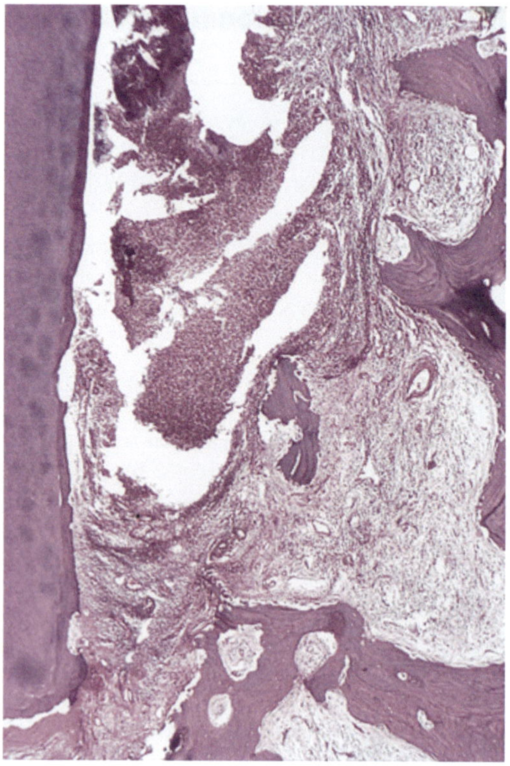

■ Fig. 19.10 Acute periodontal abscess showing pocket formation, within which contains plaque and calculus. Dense concentrations of neutrophils are present forming pus and inflammation, thus resulting in bone resorption of the bony walls associated with the periodontal pocket

19.12 Necrotising Periodontal Diseases

Necrotising periodontal diseases, based on the 2017 World Workshop classification (■ Table 19.1) are a group of conditions that can lead to significant damage to the periodontal tissues and are primarily caused by anaerobic infections. Typically, it is observed in young individuals who are otherwise healthy but may be associated with factors such as smoking, poor plaque control, and stress. However, it can also develop in children undergoing immunosuppressive treatment and in patients with HIV. Historically, this condition was referred to as "trench mouth" due to its prevalence among soldiers during World War I. However, it is now rarely seen in developed nations.

19

Necrotising periodontitis is characterised by a history of pain, ulcerated gingival margins, and "punched-out" gingival papillae, and is diagnosed via a combination of history and clinical presentation (▶ Box 19.8).

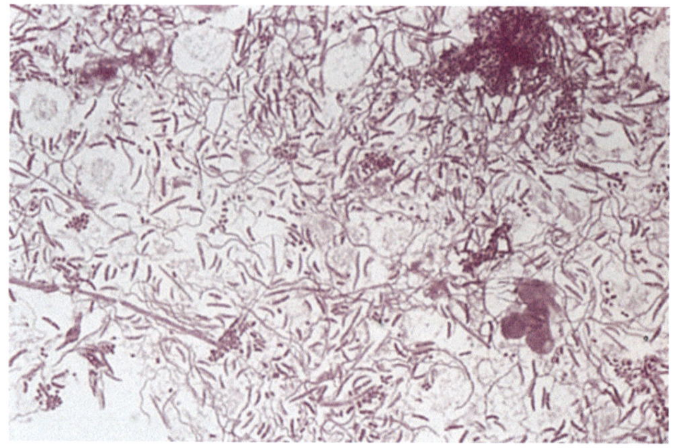

■ Fig. 19.11 Necrotising periodontal disease, showing dense concentrations of Treponema spp. and Fusobacterium nucleatum

19.12.1 Aetiology

Characterised by the presence of spirochetes and fusiforms, treatment with metronidazole antibiotic is effective.

19.12.2 Management

Removal of plaque biofilm, effective oral hygiene measures, in combination with systemic application of metronidazole. As the initial implementation of OH may be quite painful for the patient, anti-septic mouthwash may be appropriate in the initial stages.

19.12.3 Histopathology

The histopathology is characterised by invasion of tissues by spirochetes and fusiforms (■ Fig. 19.11). The epithelium and connective tissue exhibit a high concentration of neutrophils. Ulcers are coated with a layer of slough that harbours abundant bacteria. The remaining tissue displays shallow necrosis, with bacteria penetrating the upper layers. However, the deeper tissues are still viable and are infiltrated by plasma cells and macrophages. The key histopathological features of necrotising periodontal diseases are outlined in ▶ Box 19.9.

> **Box 19.8. Key Clinical Features of Necrotising Periodontal Diseases**
> - Papilla necrosis
> - Bleeding
> - Pain
> - Observed in an individual with a compromised host response.

> **Box 19.9. Histopathology of Necrotising Periodontal Diseases**
> - Invasion of spirochetes and fusiforms
> - Ulcerated gingival epithelium and pocket lining.
> - High concentration of neutrophils
> - Presence of necrotic tissue

19.13 Summary

- A symbiotic relationship between plaque biofilm and host immune system promotes gingival health.
- If the biofilm is allowed to accumulate this will increase the development of gingival inflammation, leading to incipient dysbiosis.
- However, a balance between the microbial challenge and host defence mechanisms in non-susceptible individuals reduces the risk of progression from gingivitis to periodontitis.
- In susceptible individuals, incipient dysbiosis can trigger an inappropriate and often exaggerated immune response. This imbalance between microbial and host response leads to tissue destruction and periodontitis.
- Mechanical removal of the biofilm is necessary to reduce inflammation and thus promotes the symbiotic relationship between the microbial species and host defence mechanism, which favours health.
- The most significant immune protective mechanism is the recruitment of the neutrophils; which along with the sustained release of pro-inflammatory cytokines, drives alveolar bone loss, leading to further tissue destruction.
- Therefore, most of the tissue damage is caused by the indirect actions of the host response and only a minority by the direct action of the bacteria or bacterial products.

Further Reading

Chapple ILC, Mealey BL, Van Dyke TE, Bartold PM, Dommisch H, Eickholz P, et al. Periodontal health and gingival diseases and conditions on an intact and a reduced periodontium: consensus report of workgroup 1 of the 2017 world workshop on the classification of periodontal and peri-implant diseases and conditions. J Periodontol. 2018;89(Suppl 1):S74–84.

Gao Z, Mackenzie IC. Patterns of phenotypic expression of human junctional, gingival and reduced enamel epithelia in vivo and in vitro. Epithelial Cell Biol. 1992;1:156–67.

Graves DT, Cochran D. The contribution of interleukin-1 and tumor necrosis factor to periodontal tissue destruction. J Periodontol. 2003;74:391–401.

Hajishengallis E, Hajishengallis G. Neutrophil homeostasis and periodontal health in children and adults. J Dent Res. 2014;93(3):231–7.

Hajishengallis G, Darveau RP, Curtis MA. The keystone-pathogen hypothesis. Nat Rev. Microbiol. 2012;10(10):717–25.

Jin LJ, Lamster IB, Greenspan JS, Pitts NB, Scully C, Warnakulasuriya S. Global burden of oral diseases: emerging concepts, management and interplay with systemic health. Oral Dis. 2016;22(7):609–19.

Loe H, Theilade E, Jensen SB. Experimental gingivitis in man. J Periodontol (1930). 1965;36:177–87. https://doi.org/10.1902/jop.1965.36.3.177. PMID: 14296927.

Lu E, Hobbs C, Dyer C, Ghuman M, Hughes FJ. Differential regulation of epithelial growth by gingival and periodontal fibroblasts in vitro. J Periodontal Res. 2020;55:859.

Meyle J, Chapple I. Molecular aspects of the pathogenesis of periodontitis. Periodontol 2000. 2015;69(1):7–17.

Papapanou PN, Sanz M, Buduneli N, Dietrich T, Feres M, Fine DH, et al. Periodontitis: consensus report of workgroup 2 of the 2017 world workshop on the classification of periodontal and peri-implant diseases and conditions. J Periodontol. 2018;89(Suppl 1):S173–82.

Van Dyke TE, Bartold PM, Reynolds EC. The nexus between periodontal inflammation and dysbiosis. Front Immunol. 2020;11:511.

Histopathology of the Cysts of the Jawbones

Hardeep Chehal

Contents

S R Prabhu et al. (eds.), *Oral Histology and Oral Histopathology*, https://doi.org/10.1007/978-3-031-77481-2_20

20.1 Introduction

Jawbones are unique as they contain the teeth. The mandible is formed by the fusion of the right and left mandibular prominences. The maxilla is formed by the fusion of the right and left maxillary bones with the anterior premaxilla. A true cyst is an epithelial-lined pathologic cavity. True cysts of the bones are commonly encountered in the jawbones. The lining may originate from the epithelium trapped in areas of jawbone fusion or from the cystic degeneration of odontogenic epithelium.

20.1.1 Classification

Based on aetiology, jawbone cysts are classified as inflammatory or developmental. Based on the origin of the cyst lining epithelium, they are also classified as odontogenic and non-odontogenic. Inflammatory cysts include radicular cysts, residual cysts, and buccal bifurcation cysts. Developmental cysts include dentigerous cysts, lateral periodontal cysts, ortho-keratinised odontogenic cysts, odontogenic keratocysts (OKC), glandular odontogenic cysts, calcifying odontogenic cysts, and eruption cysts. Non-odontogenic cyst includes nasopalatine duct cyst.

20.2 Radicular (Periapical) and Residual Cysts

- **Key Features**
- An inflammatory odontogenic cyst developing at the apex of a non-vital tooth. It arises due to the proliferation and cystic degeneration of the epithelial cell remnants within the periodontal ligament (rests of Malassez). Other sources of the lining epithelium include crevicular epithelium, sinus lining or epithelium lining the sinus tract. This stimulation of the epithelial rests is a reactionary process in response to the noxious products exuded from the apex of the necrotic non-vital tooth.
- Variations include lateral radicular cyst and residual periapical cyst. As the name suggests, a lateral radicular cyst is evident on the lateral aspect of a non-vital tooth with a lateral foramen. A residual cyst results from the incomplete curettage of the periapical lesional tissues after the tooth is removed.
- The mean age of development of a radicular cyst is 40.5 years, with most cases seen in relation to anterior maxillary teeth, the maxillary lateral incisor being most involved. Both deciduous and primary teeth may be involved.
- Most patients are asymptomatic and do not present with a bony expansion. This is a slow-growing lesion. Cyst enlargement is due to the increasing hydrostatic pressure of its contents.
- Radiographically, it presents as a well-defined radiolucent lesion at the apex of a tooth (1) (periapical cyst), along the lateral surfaces of roots (2) (lateral radicular cyst) or in edentulous areas (3) (residual cyst). All three variants have sclerotic borders and may vary in size. Loss of lamina dura and root resorption is common.

- **Histologic Features**
- All three variants have identical histopathologic features.
- *Cyst lining*: It is usually composed of non-keratinised stratified squamous epithelium showing areas of hyperplasia, spongiosis, or neutrophilic exudation. Occasionally, the lining shows respiratory or mucous cells. In maxillary cysts, the respiratory epithelial lining can originate from nasal or sinus mucosa adjacent to the tooth. In mandibular cysts, the presence of respiratory or mucous cells is attributed to the pluripotent nature of the odontogenic epithelium. Occasionally, Rushton bodies with granular or homogenous eosinophilic calcifications of various shapes and sizes are present within the epithelial lining. They are of little significance or prognostic value and are a common feature of inflammatory cysts. Rarely, the epithelial lining (◘ Figs. 20.1 and 20.2) may become dysplastic.
- *Cyst wall*: An inflammatory cyst has lymphocytes, neutrophils, plasma cells, histiocytes, and occasionally mast cells and eosinophils within the cyst wall. Cholesterol clefts with adjacent multinucleated giant

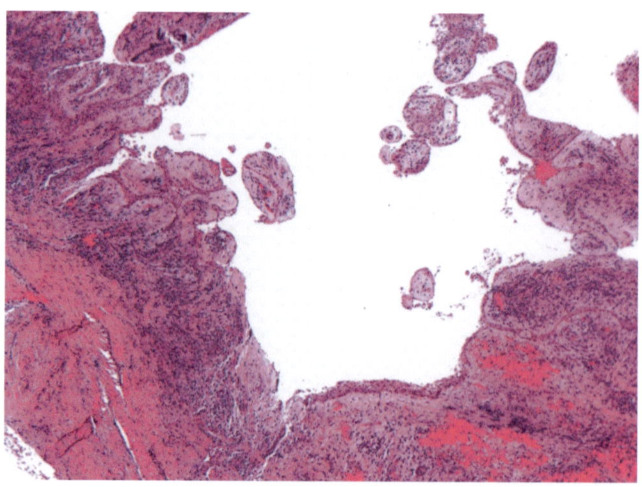

◘ **Fig. 20.1** Periapical cyst. Cyst lined by stratified squamous epithelium. Connective tissue cyst wall contains a chronic inflammatory infiltrate

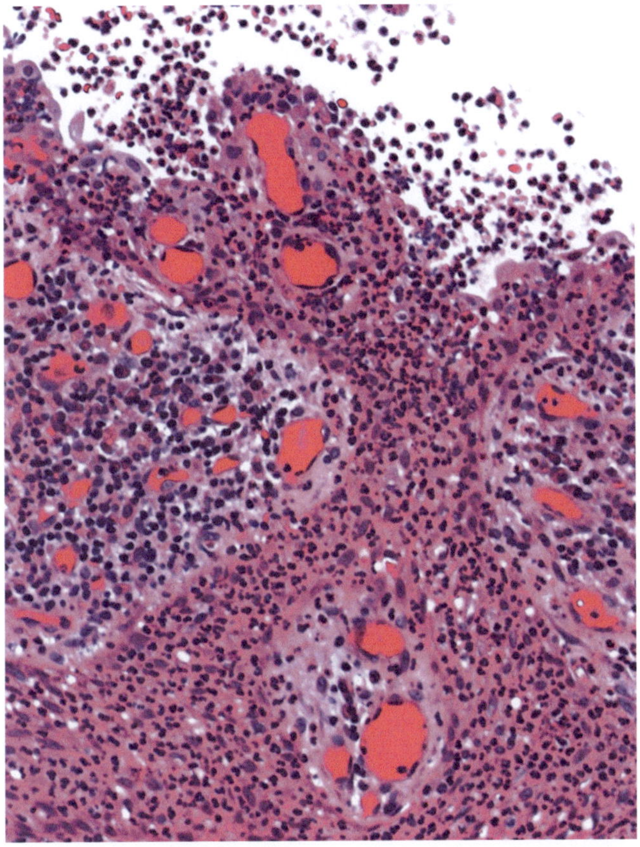

Fig. 20.2 Periapical cyst. Cyst wall with an inflammatory cell infiltrate containing lymphocytes intermixed with neutrophils, plasma cells, histocytes, and eosinophils

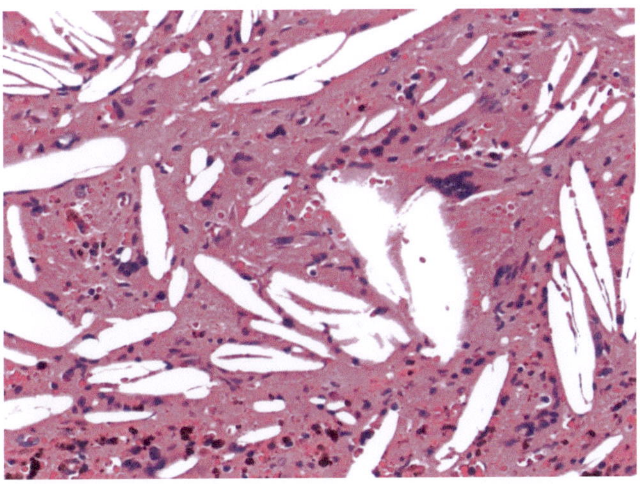

Fig. 20.3 Periapical cyst. Connective tissue wall containing cholesterol clefts

cells may also be present, leading to delayed healing of the cyst despite appropriate treatment because cholesterol cannot be removed by the giant cells and macrophages. Other substances seen in the wall

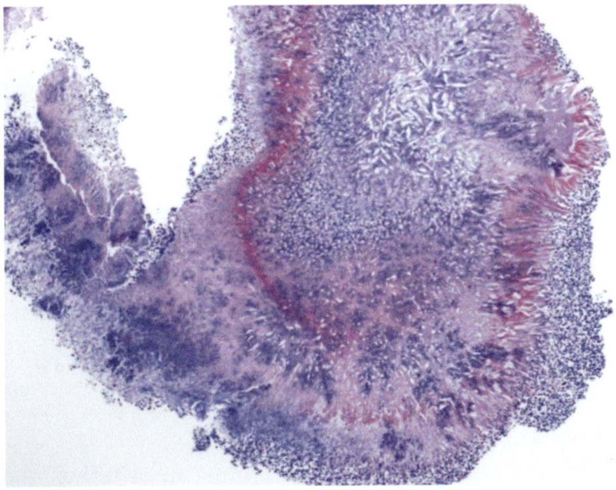

Fig. 20.4 Periapical cyst. Bacterial colony (Actinomyces) seen within the cyst wall

include hemosiderin, bacterial colonies, foreign material, and dystrophic calcifications (Figs. 20.3 and 20.4).

- *Cyst lumen*: It may contain fluid, and/or cellular debris. Hemosiderin, bacterial colonies (actinomyces), foreign material, and dystrophic calcifications have also been seen.

20.3 Dentigerous Cyst

- **Key Features**
- A developmental odontogenic cyst arising at the crown of an impacted tooth; it is attached to the tooth at the cementoenamel junction. The lesion arises due to the separation of the reduced enamel epithelium from the crown of the involved tooth. The average radiographic follicular space is 3–4 mm. A dentigerous cyst is suspected when the space exceeds 5 mm. Occasionally, periapical inflammation from the overlying deciduous tooth results in a dentigerous cyst in the underlying permanent tooth.
- This cyst, almost exclusively, occurs in permanent teeth, with the mandibular third molar being the most involved tooth, followed by the maxillary third molar, maxillary canine, and mandibular second premolar. Rarely, an impacted deciduous tooth or a supernumerary tooth may be involved.
- Most patients have a slight male predilection in the second or third decades of life.
- Most cases are asymptomatic and detected as incidental radiographic findings. Secondary infection may cause swelling and/or pain, and a large cyst can cause facial asymmetry.

- Eruption cyst is the soft tissue counterpart of the dentigerous cyst, appears clinically as a soft gingival nodule and is not routinely examined histologically.
- Radiographically, it presents as a well-defined unilocular radiolucent lesion associated with the crown of an unerupted tooth and attaching to the tooth at the cementoenamel junction. The border is usually corticated. In cases where the cyst arises due to an inflammatory process, the borders tend to be ill-defined. A large cyst may displace or resorb the roots of adjacent teeth.

Histologic Features

- Histopathology varies depending on whether the cyst is inflamed or not.
- *Cyst lining of a dentigerous cyst*: the epithelial lining is composed of three to five layers of non-keratinised squamous cells. This epithelium is pluripotent and can differentiate into mucous cells, ciliated cells, and/or glandular cells (Figs. 20.5 and 20.6).
- *Cyst lining of an inflamed dentigerous cyst*: the epithelial lining composed of non-keratinised squamous cells shows variable amounts of hyperplasia, spongiosis, and rete ridges. The epithelial lining may be disrupted.
- *Cyst wall of a developmental dentigerous cyst*: the wall is composed of loose fibrous connective tissue with a myxoid background containing glycosaminoglycans. Inactive islands of odontogenic epithelium may be present in the wall. Inflammatory cells are scanty and the interface between the epithelium and connective tissue is flat.
- *Cyst wall of an inflamed dentigerous cyst*: the wall is composed of fibrous connective tissue showing variable amounts of acute and chronic inflammatory cells. Cholesterol granulomas, foreign body giant cells, haemorrhage and fragments of bone may be seen in the cyst wall (Fig. 20.7).
- *Cystic lumen of a developmental dentigerous cyst*: may contain serosanguineous fluid and/or cellular debris.
- *Cystic lumen of an inflamed dentigerous cyst*: may contain fluid and/or cellular debris. Hemosiderin, bacterial colonies (actinomyces), foreign material, and dystrophic calcifications may also be seen.

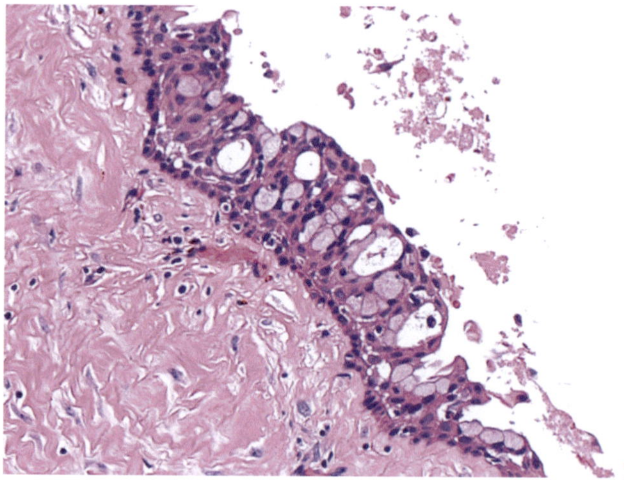

Fig. 20.6 Dentigerous cyst. Scattered mucous cells can be seen in the epithelial lining. Epithelium and connective tissue interface are flat

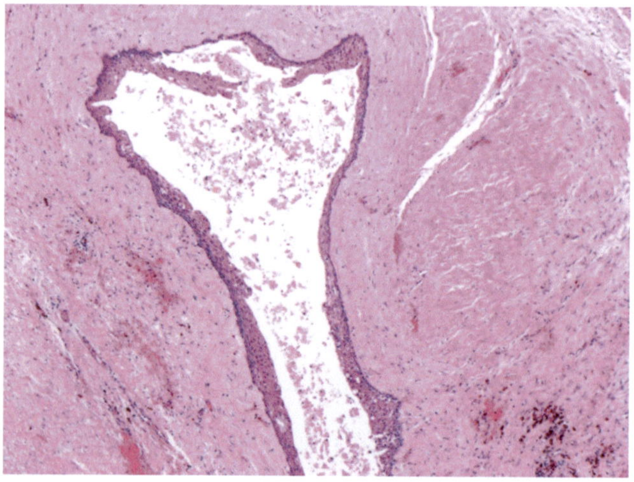

Fig. 20.5 Dentigerous cyst. Non-inflamed dentigerous cyst showing a thin, non-keratinising epithelial lining

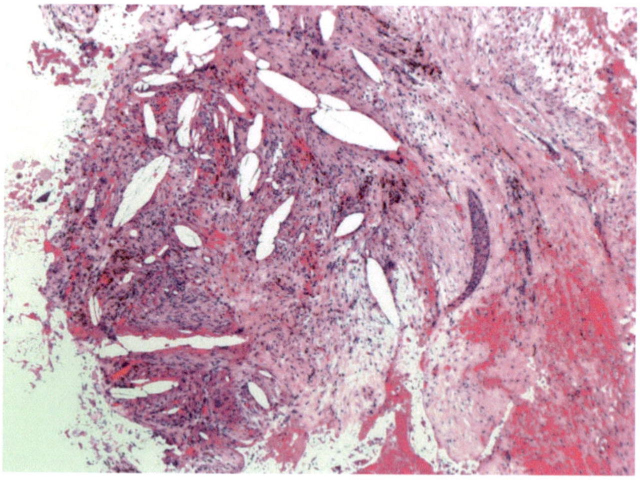

Fig. 20.7 Dentigerous cyst. Inflamed dentigerous cyst showing cholesterol clefts and inflammatory cells within the cyst wall

20

20.4 Odontogenic Keratocyst

Key Features

- A potentially aggressive developmental odontogenic cyst arises due to the proliferation and cystic degeneration of the cell rests of the dental lamina. This cyst shows a greater growth potential, a higher recurrence rate, and a possible association with nevoid basal cell carcinoma syndrome compared with other odontogenic cysts.
- Inactivating mutation of the PTCH1 gene has been reported in most sporadic and syndromic cases. The suprabasilar cell layer also shows a greater expression of proliferating cell nuclear antigen (PCNA) and Ki-67, both proliferation markers.
- The mean age of development of sporadic odontogenic keratocyst is 37 years, and most patients range between 10 and 40 years of age. The posterior mandible and ramus are the favourable sites. A syndromic cyst arises at a younger age. Male predilection is evident in both sporadic and syndromic cases.
- Most lesions are discovered as incidental findings. As this cyst grows in an anterior-posterior direction, some large cysts may not be detected clinically. Lesions are asymptomatic; pain, drainage, and swelling may be present in some instances. In sporadic cases, the presence of a unifocal cyst is the norm. Multifocal cysts are often syndromic.
- Radiographically, the lesion presents as a well-defined unilocular or multilocular radiolucency with a corticated margin. In 25–40% of cases, an unerupted tooth is seen in association with the cyst. The resorption of adjacent teeth is an uncommon feature.

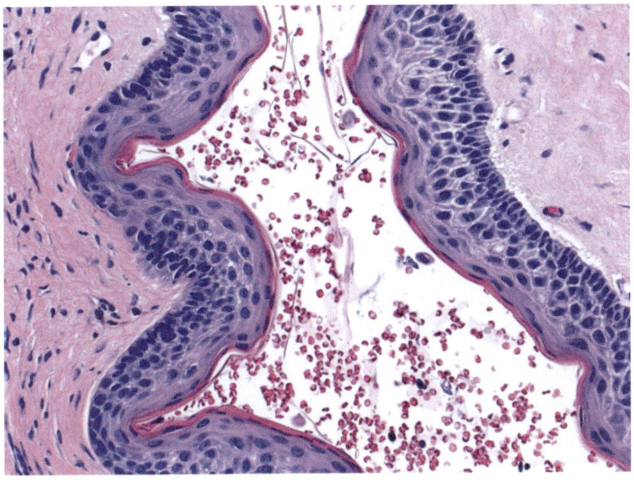

Fig. 20.8 Odontogenic keratocyst. The epithelial lining is composed of a uniform layer of stratified squamous epithelium. The epithelium and connective tissue interface is flat and devoid of inflammation

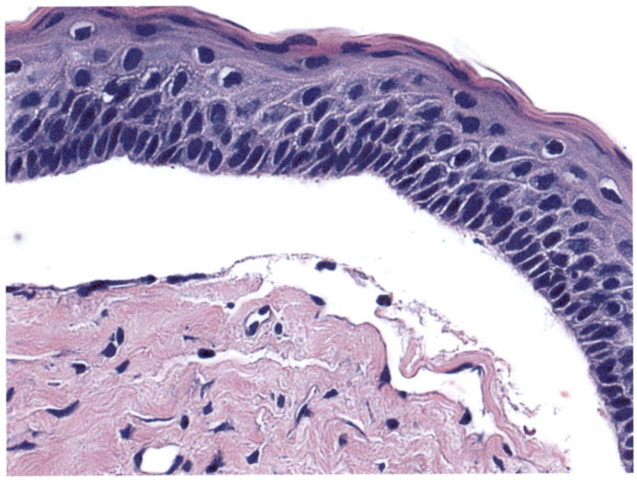

Fig. 20.9 Odontogenic keratocyst. The epithelial lining is six to eight cells thick with hyperchromatic and palisaded basal cell layer. The parakeratotic surface is corrugated

Histologic Features

- Both the syndromic and sporadic odontogenic keratocysts show the same distinctive and diagnostic histopathology pattern.
- *Cystic lining*: It is composed of five to ten cells thick parakeratotic and corrugated epithelial lining. The basal cell layer of the lining is columnar and has hyperchromatic and palisaded nuclei. This epithelial lining is fragile and leads to recurrence if not completely removed during surgery. Some odontogenic keratocysts show inflammatory changes very similar to other inflammatory odontogenic cysts—epithelial hyperplasia, spongiosis, or neutrophilic exostosis, formation of rete ridges, and lack of palisading of nuclei and parakeratin formation (Figs. 20.8 and 20.9).
- *Cystic wall*: This thin and friable fibrous connective tissue wall surrounds the lining and cystic lumen. The lining and wall interface is generally flat. Satellite cysts and odontogenic epithelium strands and islands are often visible. Rarely, cartilage may also be seen. Inflammatory changes are seen when inflammation is present.
- *Cystic lumen*: It may contain fluid, parakeratin, and/or cellular debris.

20.5 Lateral Periodontal Cyst

Key Features

- A rare developmental odontogenic cyst occurring on the lateral surface of the tooth. In most cases, it is an incidental finding on radiographs taken for other diagnostic purposes. The cystic epithelial lining orig-

inates from the proliferation and cystic degeneration of the cell rests of Malassez in the dental lamina.
- Variations of the lateral periodontal cyst are (1) gingival cyst of the adult; as the name suggests, it is histopathologically and pathologically similar but arises in the gingiva. (2) botryoid odontogenic cyst; an intrabody polycystic/multilocular lateral periodontal cyst.
- The median age is between the fifth and seventh decades of life. Very rarely is it seen in a person younger than 30 years. Most lesions arise in the mandibular premolar area, followed by the canine-lateral incisor area.
- Patients are asymptomatic and do not present with bony expansion.
- Radiographically, the lateral periodontal cyst presents as a well-defined round or oval radiolucent lesion measuring approximately 1.0–1.5 mm in greatest diameter on the lateral aspect of the tooth root. The lamina dura of the involved tooth is intact, and in most cases, the tooth is vital. Sometimes, an inflamed periapical cyst appearing lateral to a non-vital tooth may be radiographically confused with the lateral periodontal cyst.

- **Histologic Features**
- *Cyst lining*: The cyst has a three to eight cell layer thick epithelial lining of non-keratinised squamous or cuboidal cells. Focal areas of nodular epithelial thickenings composed of swirling glycogen-rich clear cells are noted in the lining (◘ Fig. 20.10).

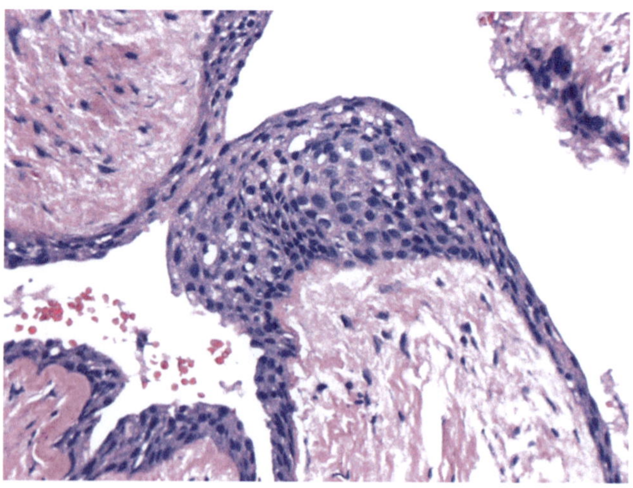

◘ **Fig. 20.10** Lateral periodontal cyst. Thin epithelial lining with focal nodular thickening. Foci of glycogen-rich clear cells and epithelial cells, arranged in a swirling pattern, are seen within the nodular thickening

20

- *Cyst wall*: It is composed of non-inflamed fibrous connective tissue containing foci of odontogenic epithelium. The interface between the wall and the cyst lining is flat.
- *Cyst lumen*: It may contain fluid and/or cellular debris.

20.6 Calcifying Odontogenic Cyst (Gorlin Cyst)

- **Key Features**
- Uncommon odontogenic cyst lined by ameloblastoma-like epithelium, ghost cells, and calcified ghost cells. They arise due to the proliferation and cystic degeneration of the epithelial cell remnants of the dental lamina or possibly the reduced enamel epithelium surrounding an unerupted tooth.
- In the 2022 World Health Organization classification, this cyst is categorised under ghost cell lesions. It may be associated with mutations of CTNNB1, which encodes for β-catenin. β-catenin plays a key role in the regulation of cell proliferation, differentiation, and apoptosis. This cyst is sometimes seen along with other odontogenic tumours such as an odontoma, adenomatoid odontogenic tumours, and ameloblastoma. Peripheral calcifying odontogenic cysts are seen on the gingiva and are less aggressive than their intraosseous counterpart.
- The mean age of occurrence is 30 years, and most cases are diagnosed in the second to fourth decades of life. For a cyst seen with an odontoma, the mean age is 17 years. Both the jaws have an equal predilection, and the anterior region of the jaws (incisor-canine region) is a preferred site of occurrence.
- A large cyst results in a painless bony expansion. Nasal stuffiness, epistaxis, and headaches may be the symptoms associated with a large maxillary calcifying odontogenic cyst.
- Radiographically, a well-defined unilocular or multilocular radiolucency with sclerotic margins is usually seen. Scattered radiopacities within the lesion are noted in 1/3rd of the cases. An impacted tooth, most often canine, may be seen in association with the lesion in a minority of cases. Root resorption or divergence has been reported.

- **Histologic Features**
- *Cyst lining*: It is composed of non-keratinised stratified squamous epithelial cells. This lining is four to ten cells thick, with the basal cells resembling amelo-

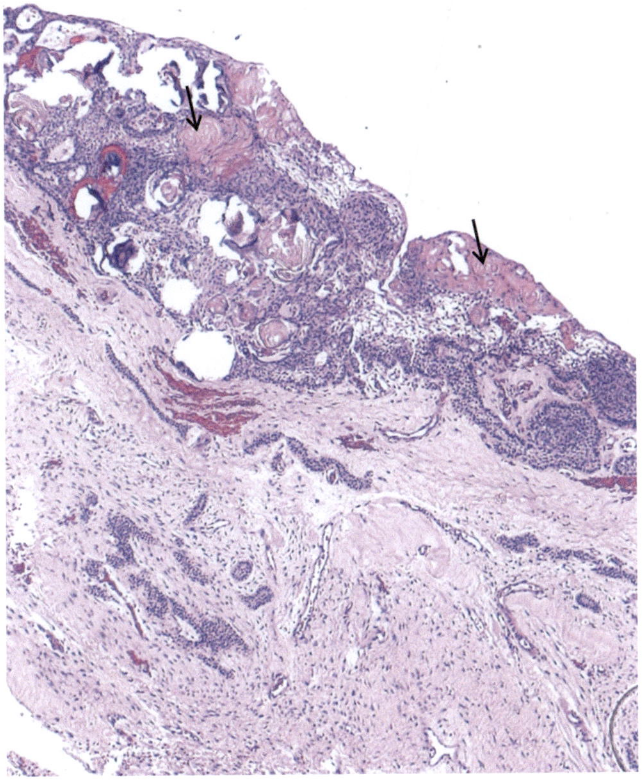

Fig. 20.11 Calcifying odontogenic cyst. The lining shows ameloblastoma-like epithelial cells, and eosinophilic ghost cells (arrows) are present within the epithelial lining. Connective tissue wall contains odontogenic epithelium cell islands and is mildly inflamed

blasts. The hyperchromatic cells of these basal cells are polarised away from the basement membrane. Epithelial cells overlying this basal layer resemble cells of the stellate reticulum of ameloblastoma. These cells are star-shaped and loosely arranged. The most striking feature is the presence of suprabasilar ghost cells—eosinophilic cells without a nucleus but with a preserved outline. Some of these ghost cells fuse and form an amorphous eosinophilic acellular mass. Calcifications within ghost cells are common (Figs. 20.11 and 20.12).

- *Cyst wall*: It consists of collagenised fibrous connective tissue containing scattered inflammatory cells. Multiple daughter cysts may be present in the cyst wall.
- *Cyst lumen*: It may be filled with masses of ghost cells and dystrophic calcifications.

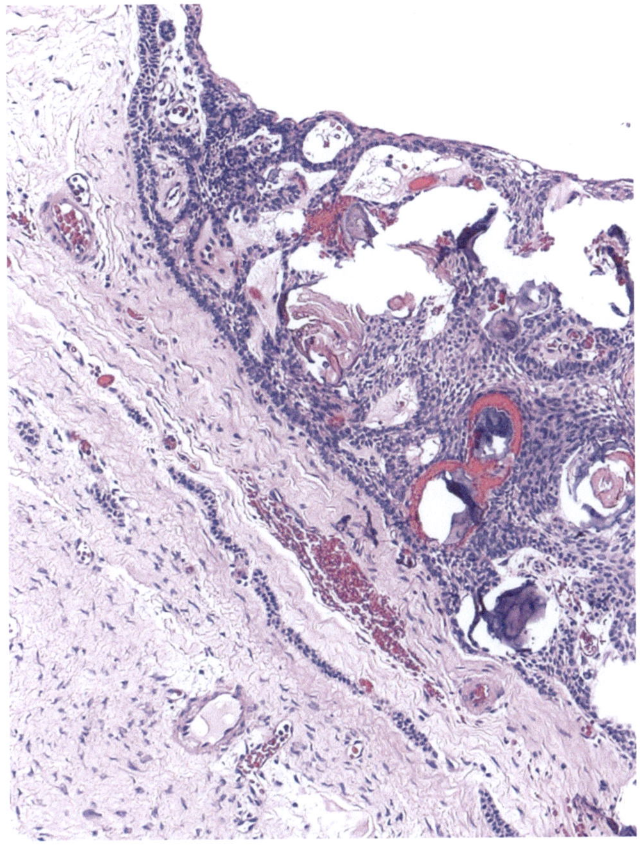

Fig. 20.12 Calcifying odontogenic cyst. The lining shows ameloblastoma-like epithelial cells with a columnar basal layer

20.7 Glandular Odontogenic Cyst

Key Features

- A rare and aggressive developmental odontogenic cyst showing odontogenic epithelium with glandular features. The presence of glandular characteristics in the cyst lining reflects the pluripotent nature of odontogenic epithelium. The cyst develops due to the proliferation and cystic degeneration of the epithelial cell remnants of the dental lamina.
- Manifests as an asymptomatic lesion which may show bony expansion and cortical perforation, if large. Tooth displacement and root resorption are seen in a few cases. It tends to recur.
- Mean age of development is 49.5 years. Most patients are between the fifth and seventh decades of life; it is rare to encounter this lesion before 20 years of age. This lesion shows a strong predilection for the anterior mandible and often crosses the midline, producing anterior mandibular expansion.

- Radiographically, it presents as a well-defined unilocular or multilocular radiolucent lesion with corticated borders. Cortical expansion and root resorption may be seen in some cases.

Histologic Features

- *Cyst lining*: It is composed of non-keratinised stratified squamous or basaloid epithelial cells with areas containing ciliated cells, mucous cells, duct-like structures, or microcystic spaces. Luminal epithelial cells are cuboidal and eosinophilic and often protrude into the cystic lumen in a hobnail or a papillary pattern, showing secretory activity. Clear and goblet cells containing mucous may also be seen within the lining epithelium. In some areas, the epithelial cells are hyperplastic and swirling, producing a plaque-like thickness. The microcystic spaces are lined by cuboidal epithelial cells and contain mucicarmine-positive fluid (Fig. 20.13a, b).

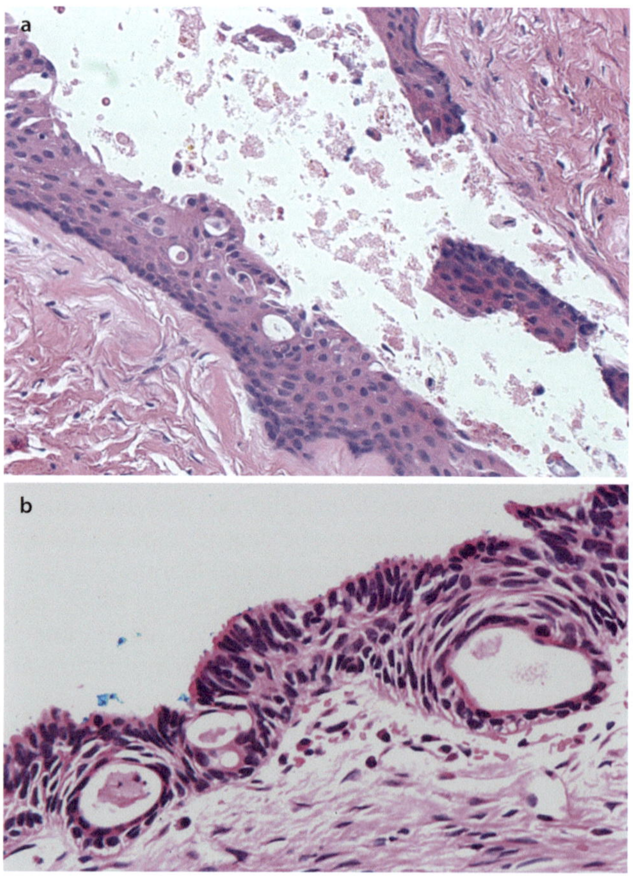

Fig. 20.13 **a** Glandular odontogenic cyst. Lined by stratified squamous epithelium that shows microcysts. Connective tissue wall is devoid of inflammation. **b** Glandular odontogenic cyst showing the duct-like spaces in the epithelial lining. (Courtesy: Professor David F Wilson, Adelaide, Australia)

- *Cyst wall*: *It* consists of collagenous fibrous connective tissue. It often contains epithelial islands showing cystic spaces and microcysts. No inflammatory cells are seen, and the interface between the wall and the epithelial lining is flat.
- *Cyst lumen*: It may contain mucicarmine + fluid and/or cellular debris.

20.8 Ortho-keratinised Odontogenic Cyst

Key Features

- A rare developmental odontogenic cyst characterised by the production of orthokeratin by its epithelial lining. They are due to the proliferation and cystic degeneration of the dental lamina rests.
- In 2017, the World Health Organization designated this cyst as a distinct entity from the odontogenic keratocysts (OKC).
- Most patients are in the third to fourth decades of life, and males are affected slightly more than females. The posterior mandible and ramus area are most commonly affected.
- This is a slow-growing, non-aggressive lesion. Clinical expansion may be seen; however, most patients are asymptomatic.
- Radiographically, it presents as a well-defined unilocular or multilocular radiolucent lesion. 75% of cases are associated with an impacted third molar tooth. The size variation ranges from 1 to 7 cm in greatest diameter.

Histologic Features

- *Cyst lining*: It is composed of 5–15 cells thick orthokeratinised stratified squamous epithelium, showing few areas of hyperplasia. Focal sebaceous differentiation of the epithelial cells has been reported. The upper epithelial cell layers show keratohyalin granules. The basal cell layer is cuboidal and lacks palisading of the nuclei (Fig. 20.14).
- *Cyst wall*: It is composed of collagenised fibrous connective tissue devoid of inflammatory cells. The epithelial lining and cyst wall interface is flat.
- *Cyst lumen*: *A* thick layer of orthokeratin is seen in the lumen.

20

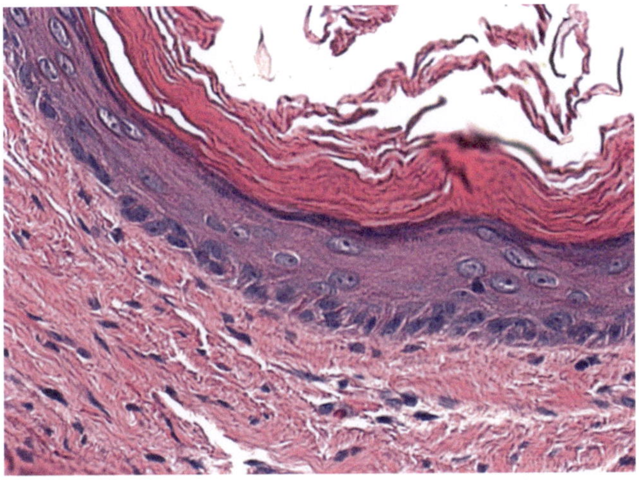

■ **Fig. 20.14** Ortho-keratinised odontogenic cyst. Thin epithelial lining without palisading of basal cell layer. A thick layer of ortho-keratin is seen on the luminal surface

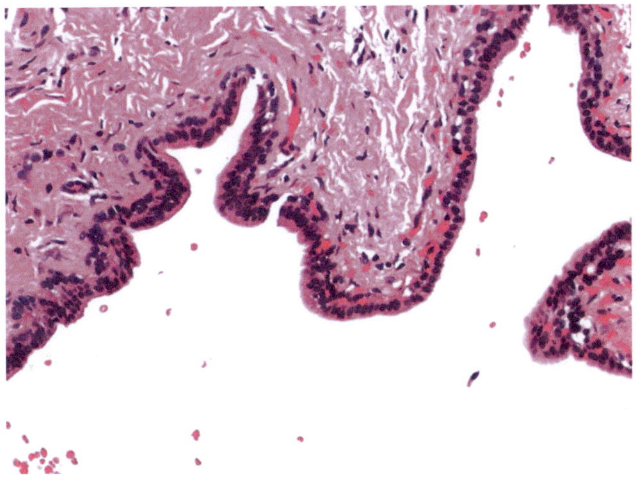

■ **Fig. 20.15** Nasopalatine duct cyst. Cystic lining showing pseudostratified columnar epithelial cells with cilia

20.9 Nasopalatine Duct Cyst (Incisive Canal Cyst)

Key Features

- It is the most common non-odontogenic cyst of the oral cavity, arising due to the proliferation and cystic degeneration of the epithelial cell remnants of the nasopalatine duct within the nasopalatine canal (incisive canal). The exact aetiology causing this proliferation and degeneration is not fully understood. However, the triggering factors include trauma or infection. The nasopalatine canal contains nasopalatine nerves and blood vessels.
- This cyst may develop at any age, but most patients are between the fourth and sixth decades; very rarely, it may be seen in the first decade of life. As the name suggests, it develops anywhere in the nasopalatine canal, which runs from the nasal floor on either side of the nasal septum to the anterior part of the hard palate in the incisive palate area. Studies have shown a male predilection.
- Manifests as an asymptomatic or symptomatic lesion, depending on its size and secondary inflammation. An asymptomatic cyst is found incidentally on radiographs taken for other purposes. A cyst with symptoms may produce an anterior palatal swelling, drainage, formation of a fistula, or paresthesia of the area due to compression of the nasopalatine nerve. When the cyst develops closer to the nasal floor, it may produce a swelling or discharge on the nasal floor.
- Radiographically, a well-defined round, oval, inverted pear-shaped, or heart-shaped radiolucent lesion with corticated margins is seen in the anterior maxilla, at or near the midline, between the apices of the central incisors. The lesion causes root diversion. Root resorption is uncommon. Any radiolucency in this area <6 mm is considered an incisive foramen, not a nasopalatine duct cyst.

Histologic Features

- *Cyst lining*: Depending on the vertical location of the cyst within the canal, the lining may be composed of a combination of the following cell types: pseudostratified epithelial cells, stratified epithelial cells, columnar epithelial cells, cuboidal epithelial cells, ciliated epithelial cells, goblet cells, or respiratory epithelial cells. The majority of the cysts are lined by stratified squamous epithelium. Cysts arising at the inferior aspect of the canal are lined by squamous epithelium, and those arising at the superior aspect are lined by respiratory epithelium (■ Fig. 20.15).
- *Cyst wall*: Lymphocytes, neutrophils, plasma cells, and histiocytes are present in various numbers within the fibrous tissue cyst wall. The contents of the cyst wall aid in the diagnosis of this cyst, as moderate-sized nerves and small muscular arteries and veins are seen in the nasopalatine duct cyst (■ Figs. 20.16 and 20.17).
- *Cyst lumen*: It may contain fluid, keratin, and/or cellular debris.

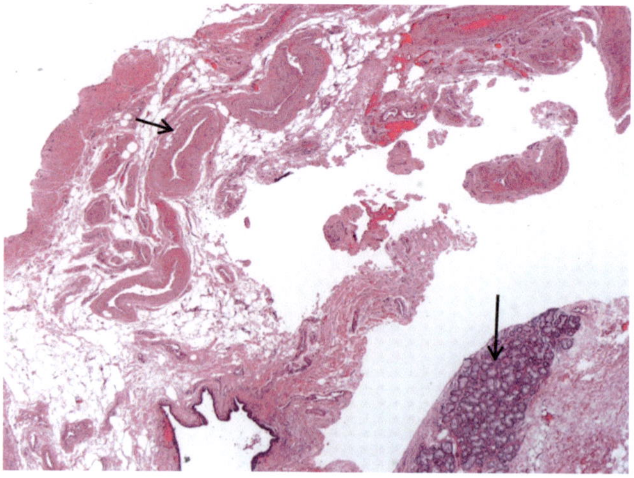

Fig. 20.16 Nasopalatine duct cyst. Flattened epithelial cell lining. Cyst wall showing blood vessels and minor salivary glands (arrows)

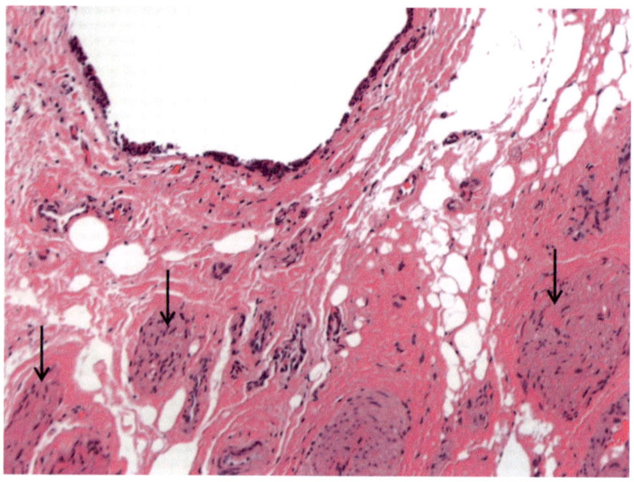

Fig. 20.17 Nasopalatine duct cyst. Cyst wall showing nerve bundles (arrows)

20.10 Summary

Odontogenic cysts are true cysts that originate from the odontogenic tissues in the jaw bones. The lesions are typically asymptomatic. Pain and bony swelling may be present in late stages of development. The radiographic presentation is that of a well-defined radiolucency or radiolucency with radiopacity. The gold standard for diagnosis is the histologic examination.

Further Reading

Chen J-H, Tseng C-H, Wang W-C, Chen C-Y, Chuang F-H, Chen Y-K. Clinicopathological analysis of 232 radicular cysts of the jawbone in a population of southern Taiwanese patients. Kaohsiung J Med Sci. 2018;34(4):249–54. https://doi.org/10.1016/j.kjms.2018.01.011.

Crane H, Da Forno P, Kyriakidou E, et al. Multiple orthokeratinized odontogenic cysts: a report of two cases and review of the literature. Head Neck Pathol. 2020;14:381–5. https://doi.org/10.1007/s12105-019-01042-0.

Nel C, Robinson L, Roza ALOC, Ker-Fox J, Gomes NR, Fonseca FP, Santos-Silva AR, Romañach MJ, Vargas PA, van Heerden WF. Clinical and radiologic spectrum of glandular odontogenic cysts: a multicenter study of 92 cases. Oral Surg Oral Med Oral Pathol Oral Radiol. 2022;133(5):593–603. https://doi.org/10.1016/j.oooo.2021.11.008. Epub 2021 Nov 27.

Perez A, Lenoir V, Lombardi T. Dentigerous cysts with diverse radiological presentation highlighting diagnostic challenges. Diagnostics. 2022;12(8):2006. https://doi.org/10.3390/diagnostics12082006.

Samir MC, Lamiae G, Bassima C. Calcifying odontogenic cyst of anterior maxillary: case report and review. Int J Surg Case Rep. 2021;85:106267. https://doi.org/10.1016/j.ijscr.2021.106267.

Subbappa A. Lateral periodontal cyst: a review of a rare presentations. J Med Dental Sci. 2015;4:9830–5. https://doi.org/10.14260/jemds/2015/1418.

Winters R, Garip M, Meeus J, Coropciuc R, Politis C. Safety and efficacy of adjunctive therapy in the treatment of OKC (odontogenic keratocyst): a systematic review. Br J Oral Maxillofac Surg. 2023;61:331. https://doi.org/10.1016/j.bjoms.2023.04.006.

Yeom HG, Kang JH, Yun SU, et al. Nasopalatine duct cyst with sebaceous differentiation: a rare case report with literature review. BMC Oral Health. 2021;21:419. https://doi.org/10.1186/s12903-021-01772-0.

Histopathology of Odontogenic Tumours of the Jawbones

Hardeep Chehal

Contents

S R Prabhu et al. (eds.), *Oral Histology and Oral Histopathology*, https://doi.org/10.1007/978-3-031-77481-2_21

21.1 Introduction

Tumours arising from the cells involved in tooth development are called odontogenic tumours. These tumours are found only within the jawbone or soft tissue overlying teeth. They are derived from epithelial, ectomesenchymal and/or mesenchymal tissues that constitute the tooth-forming apparatus. These tumours are generally benign, but several odontogenic tumours exhibit locally invasive behaviour with a high rate of recurrence. This chapter briefly discusses clinicopathologic aspects of odontogenic tumours, highlighting the histologic features.

21.2 Tumours of Odontogenic Epithelium

21.2.1 Classification

Classification of odontogenic tumours is based on the behaviour and origin (◘ Table 21.1).

◘ **Table 21.1** Classification of odontogenic tumours. (Source: ► WHO classification of head and neck tumours (4th edition), 2017. Gaillard F, Knipe H, Luong D, et al. WHO classification of odontogenic and maxillofacial bone tumours. Reference article, ► Radiopaedia.org (Accessed on 11 Feb 2024) ► https://doi.org/10.53347/rID-2278)

Classification of Odontogenic Tumours
Benign odontogenic tumours
Benign epithelial odontogenic tumours
– Ameloblastoma
– Ameloblastoma, unicystic type
– Ameloblastoma, extraosseous/peripheral type
– Metastasising ameloblastoma
– Squamous odontogenic tumour
– Calcifying epithelial odontogenic tumour
– Adenomatoid odontogenic tumour
Benign mixed epithelial and mesenchymal odontogenic tumours
– Ameloblastic fibroma
– Primordial odontogenic tumour
– Odontoma
– Dentinogenic ghost cell tumour
Benign mesenchymal odontogenic tumours
– Odontogenic fibroma
– Odontogenic myxoma
– Cementoblastoma
– Cemento-ossifying fibroma
Malignant odontogenic tumours
Odontogenic carcinomas
– Ameloblastic carcinoma
– Primary intraosseous carcinoma not otherwise specified
– Sclerosing odontogenic carcinoma
– Clear-cell odontogenic carcinoma
– Ghost cell odontogenic carcinoma
Odontogenic carcinosarcoma
Odontogenic sarcoma

21.3 Benign Epithelial Odontogenic Tumours

21.3.1 Ameloblastoma

- **Key Features**

- Ameloblastoma is the second most common odontogenic tumour after odontoma.
- Though classified as benign, ameloblastoma is locally aggressive, expansile, and recurrent, hence, considered the most common clinically significant odontogenic tumour.
- Ameloblastoma arises in the jawbone from four epithelial cell sources: the rest of the dental lamina, the developing enamel organ, the epithelial lining of an odontogenic cyst, or the basal cell layer of the oral epithelium.
- A vast majority of ameloblastomas (80%), show BRAF p.V600E mutation (valine substituted by glutamic acid at amino acid 600). BRAF is a protein that leads to a variety of cell mechanisms, such as metabolism and proliferation. The presence of BRAF V600E mutation is frequently present in a younger patient and is related to clinical behaviour, showing increased multilocularity, expansion, and recurrence.
- Based on different clinical presentations, prognosis, and treatment modalities, the three categories of ameloblastoma are (1) conventional solid or multicystic, (2) unicystic, and (3) peripheral.
- The conventional (multicystic) type is seen in most cases. The mean age of development of conventional ameloblastoma is 42 years, with most patients between the third and seventh decades of life. It is rare in the first decade and uncommon in teenagers.
- A unicystic ameloblastoma (see below) may arise de novo or from the neoplastic transformation of an intraosseous cyst lining. In such cases, a microscopic examination of the presumed cyst confirms the diagnosis. The mean age of unicystic ameloblastoma is 16 years, and most patients are in their second decade of life.
- Extraosseous (peripheral) ameloblastoma is uncommon. It arises from cells resting on the dental lamina outside of the jawbones and presents as a bump on the gum. Microscopically, it shows features of conventional (follicular) ameloblastoma. Peripheral ameloblastoma arises in later life, with a mean age of 52. Posterior mandibular bone/soft tissue is the preferred site for all three variants.
- Asymptomatic bony expansion is a characteristic feature of ameloblastoma. If not treated, the lesions continue to expand locally to a large size. Pain and alteration of sensation are not consistent features of conventional or unicystic ameloblastoma. Recent reports dispute that the unicystic ameloblastoma is less aggressive than the conventional one.
- Radiographically, conventional ameloblastomas are unilocular or multilocular radiolucencies showing well-defined corticated borders with buccal and lingual cortical expansion. The margins of the radiolucency often show irregular scalloping. An unerupted tooth may be associated with it. Root resorption of adjacent teeth is frequently seen. These radiographic changes are not detected in peripheral ameloblastoma.
- Desmoplastic ameloblastoma (see below) is a histopathologic variant of conventional ameloblastoma. It does not follow the typical clinical and radiographic features of ameloblastoma. It has a marked predilection for the anterior mandibular and maxillary region and shows a mixed radiolucent and radiopaque image due to osseous metaplasia within the dense fibrous septae.

- **Histologic Features**

1. There are six microscopic variations, with the follicular and plexiform patterns being the most common. The other four variants are acanthomatous, granular cell, desmoplastic, and basal cell type. Conventional ameloblastoma very often undergoes cystic degeneration.

   Neoplastic Odontogenic Epithelium. The neoplastic component of ameloblastoma is the odontogenic epithelium, showing various patterns:

   (a) **Follicular Ameloblastoma**: Epithelial cells form islands (◘ Fig. 21.1a–c). The outermost layer is composed of tall columnar cells. The nuclei of these cells are located opposite to the basement membrane (reverse polarity). This outermost layer of epithelium may also show areas where the cells resemble basal cells. The core of the island is composed of loosely arranged angular cells resembling the stellate reticulum of the developing enamel organ. Cystic degeneration of these neoplastic epithelial islands is often seen.

   (b) **Plexiform Ameloblastoma**: Epithelial cells form long anastomosing cords or large sheets (◘ Fig. 21.2a, b). The outermost layer is composed of columnar or cuboidal cells showing reverse polarity. The inner core is made of loosely arranged angular cells. Cystic degeneration is uncommon in this variant. Sometimes, the cuboidal cells form duct-like structures. If this duct-like structure shows dentinoid depositions, then the diagnosis is

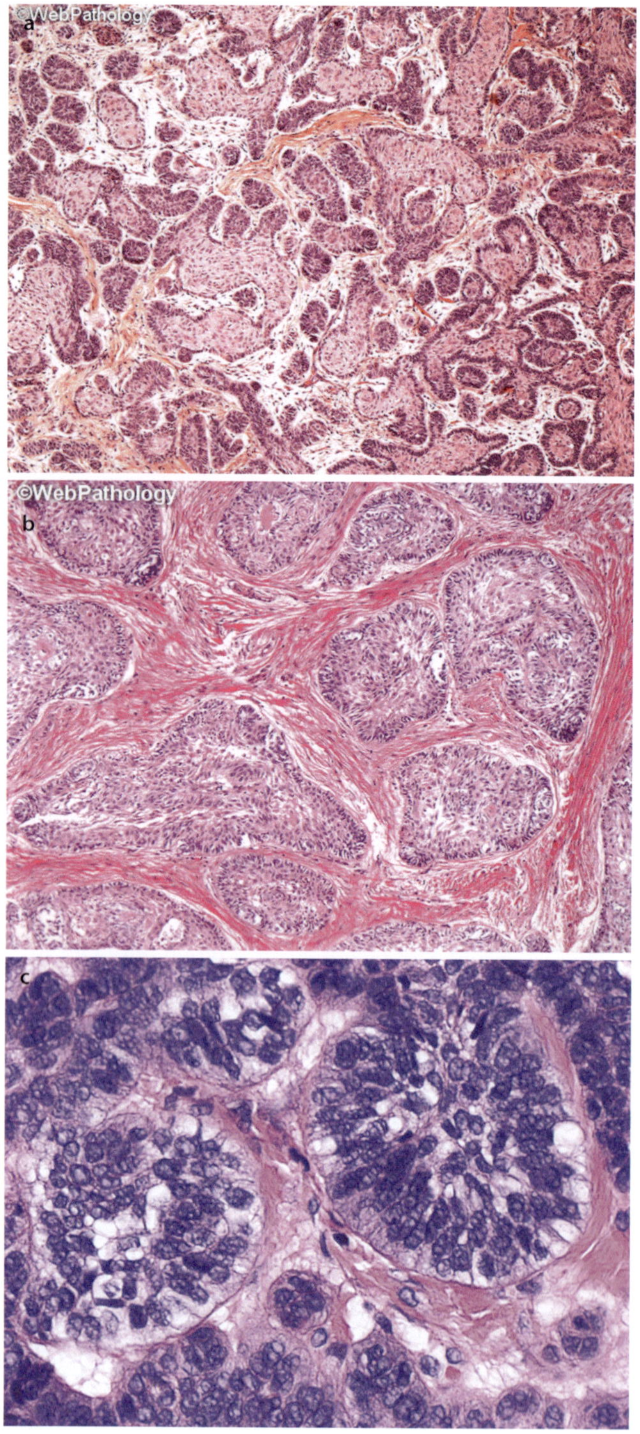

Fig. 21.1 Ameloblastoma **a**–**c**. Follicular pattern: This pattern consists of round, oval, or irregular islands of epithelium that mimic enamel organ epithelium. The nests and islands show peripheral palisading of columnar cells with reverse polarity i.e. their nuclei are polarised away from the basement membrane. The central portion of the islands consists of angulated cells resembling the stellate reticulum of the developing tooth germ. The nests are separated by mature fibrous connective tissue stroma. (Courtesy of Dr. Dharam Ramnani, USA ► Webpathology.com). **c** Ameloblastoma. Follicular type. The peripheral columnar cells of the neoplastic epithelial islands show reverse polarity. The central zone has loosely placed cells

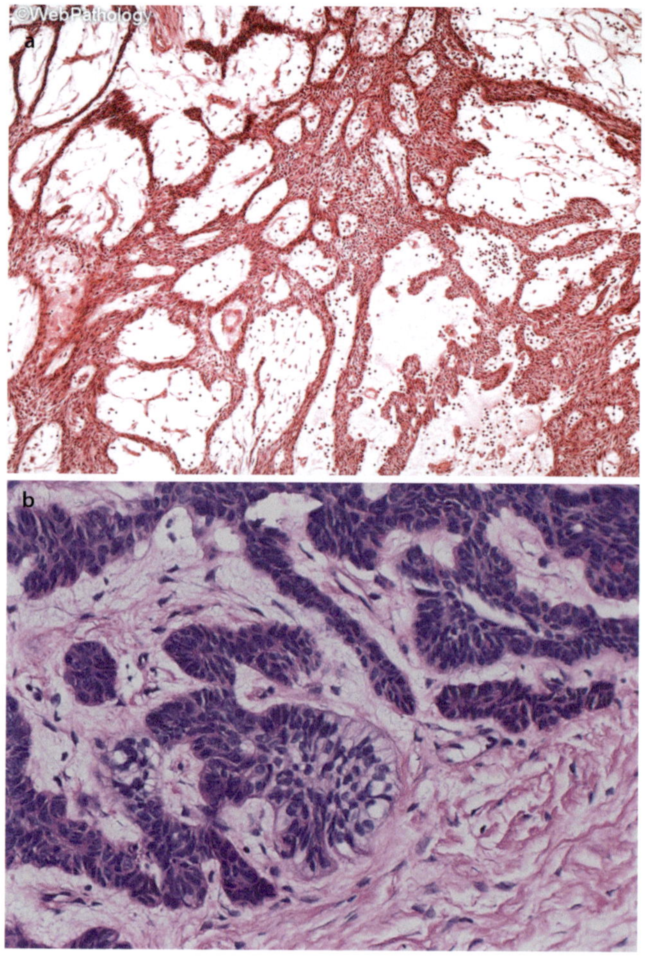

Fig. 21.2 **a** Ameloblastoma. Plexiform pattern. This consists of anastomosing interconnected thin strands or cords of basaloid cells, often without peripheral palisading and reverse nuclear polarity. Within these cords are more loosely arranged epithelial cells. The surrounding stroma is vascular and composed of loose connective tissue. Cyst formation is uncommon in the plexiform type. (Courtesy of Dr. Dharam Ramnani, USA ► Webpathology.com). **b** Ameloblastoma. Plexiform pattern. Anastomosing cords of odontogenic epithelium

adenoid ameloblastoma (an ameloblastoma-like) neoplasm. It has been reported that the BRAF p.V600E gene mutations are not present in adenoid ameloblastomas.

(c) **Acanthomatous Ameloblastoma**: The central core of epithelial island cells shows extensive squamous metaplasia with keratin formation (Fig. 21.3), sometimes resulting in a misdiagnosis of squamous cell carcinoma.

(d) **Granular Cell Ameloblastoma**: Epithelial cells show extensive granular changes. These granular cells have abundant eosinophilic granules in the cytoplasm (Fig. 21.4).

(e) **Basaloid Cell Ameloblastoma (Basal Cell Ameloblastoma)**: Epithelial cells form nests

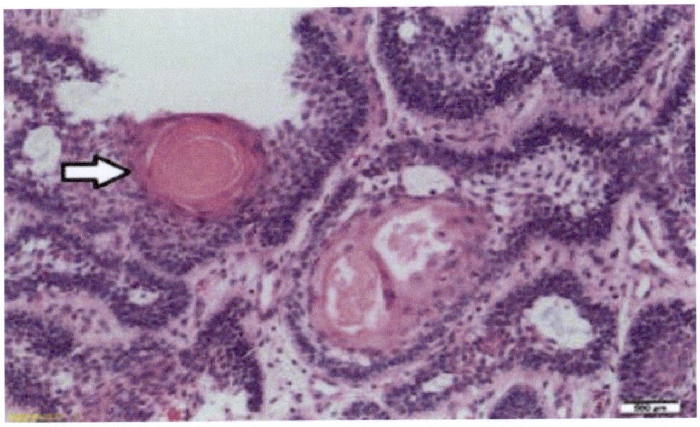

■ **Fig. 21.3** Ameloblastoma. Acanthomatous pattern. The epithelial island shows squamous metaplasia with keratin formation (arrow). (Courtesy of Dr. Fadi Titinchi. University of Western Cape, Cape Town, South Africa)

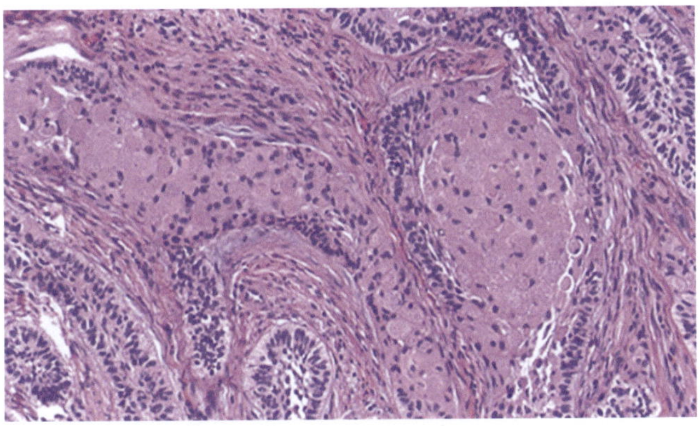

■ **Fig. 21.4** Ameloblastoma. Granular cell pattern. Central cells of tumour islands show prominent granular cytoplasm

of uniform basaloid cells. Central loose angular cells are absent, and the peripheral cells showing reverse polarity are cuboidal rather than columnar (■ Fig. 21.5).

(f) **Desmoplastic Ameloblastoma**: Epithelial cells form small islands and cords, while peripheral columnar ameloblast-like cells are inconspicuous (■ Fig. 21.6).

2. *Non-neoplastic Ectomesenchyme*: This is composed of mature vascular connective tissue stroma, loose and less collagenised in follicular pattern as compared to the densely collagenised desmoplastic ameloblastoma. This desmoplasia has been attributed to the production of transforming growth factor-β (TGF-β) by the tumour cells, which stimulates various cells, including fibroblasts, to produce extracellular matrices such as collagen, fibronectin, proteoglycans, and others. TGF-β is not expressed in other histologic variants of ameloblastomas.

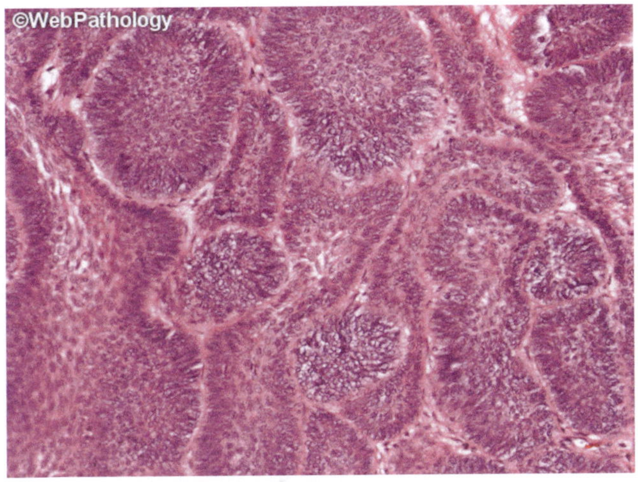

■ **Fig. 21.5** Ameloblastoma. Basaloid cell pattern. The basaloid type of ameloblastoma consists of islands of uniform basaloid cells. There is no central stellate reticulum in the islands. The hypercellularity, nuclear crowding, and nuclear hyperchromasia in such cases can be mistaken for basal cell carcinoma. (Courtesy of Dr. Dharam Ramnani, USA ► Webpathology.com)

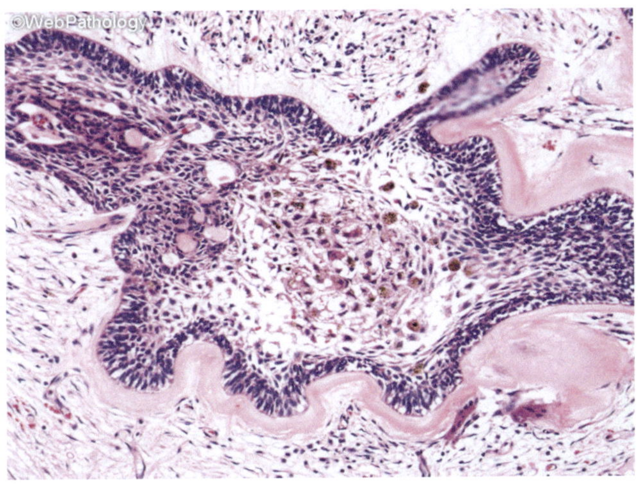

■ **Fig. 21.6** Ameloblastoma. Desmoplastic variant. This shows thin cords or strands of odontogenic epithelium in a densely collagenised stroma. Peripheral palisading may not be apparent. Secretion of transforming growth factor-beta is responsible for the dense sclerotic stroma. (Courtesy of Dr. Dharam Ramnani, USA ► Webpathology.com)

21.3.1.1 Unicystic Ameloblastoma

- Unicystic ameloblastoma is a slow-growing cystic lesion that shows clinical and radiologic characteristics of an odontogenic cyst.

■ **Histopathology**

- In histological examination, unicystic ameloblastoma shows a typical ameloblastomatous epithelium lining part of the cyst cavity (■ Fig. 21.7).
- Unicystic ameloblastoma is less aggressive than its solid or multicystic counterparts.

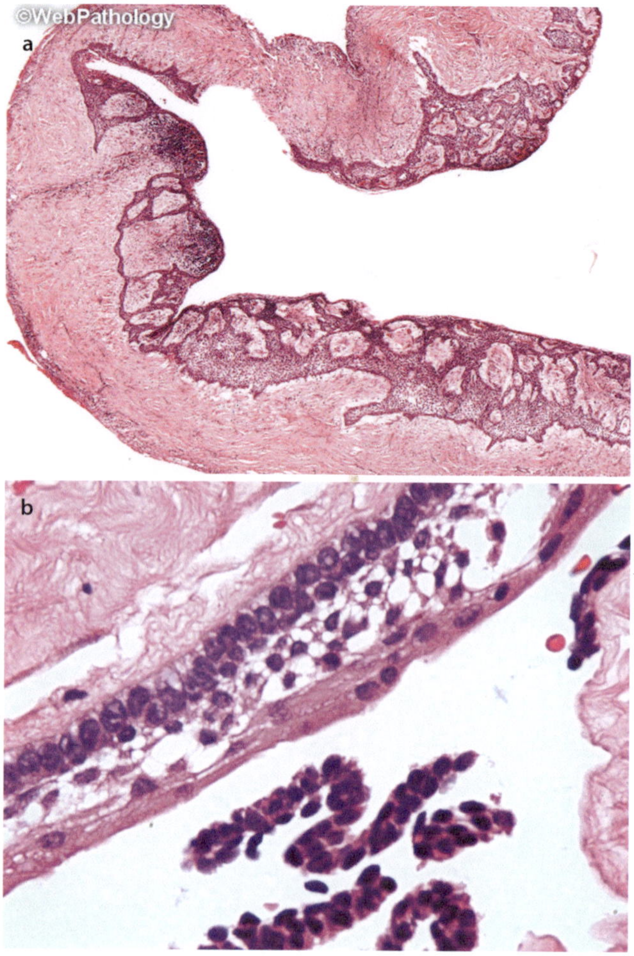

■ **Fig. 21.7** **a** Unicystic ameloblastoma. Luminal type: The neoplastic epithelium is confined to the luminal surface of the cyst, i.e. the lesion consists of a simple unilocular cyst with a fibrous wall lined partially or completely by multiple layers of ameloblastic epithelium. The basal portion of the lining epithelium is tall, columnar, or cuboidal with peripheral palisading and reverse polarity (nuclei oriented away from the basement membrane). The peripheral portion (towards the luminal aspect) is composed of loosely cohesive cells resembling stellate reticulum. (Courtesy of Dr. Dharam Ramnani, USA ▶ Webpathology.com). **b** Unicystic ameloblastoma. Luminal type. The cyst's lining has ameloblastic epithelium with a hyperchromatic and polarised basal cell layer. The underlying cells resemble the stellate reticulum. Luminal content shows epithelial lining stripped off from the adjacent cystic wall of the tumour

- According to the degree of ameloblastomatous epithelial extension, three histological types are recognised: luminal, intraluminal, and mural types.
  - In the luminal type, the ameloblastic growth is confined to the cystic lining, and no intraluminal or intramural extension of the tumour is present.
  - In the intraluminal type, the lining gives rise to a nodular ameloblastic proliferation projecting into the lumen.
  - The mural type exhibits tumour infiltration into the fibrous cyst wall.

21

21.3.1.2 Peripheral Ameloblastoma (Extraosseous Ameloblastoma)

Peripheral ameloblastoma (extraosseous ameloblastoma) is a rare benign odontogenic tumour that occurs commonly in the mandibular gingiva.

- The tumour arises from the cell rest of Serres, reduced enamel epithelium, and basal cells of the surface epithelium.
- Clinically, peripheral ameloblastoma mimics granuloma, peripheral ossifying fibroma, peripheral giant cell granuloma, and squamous papilloma.
- Peripheral ameloblastoma has similar histological patterns as the conventional type.

21.3.2 Squamous Odontogenic Tumour

- **Key Feature**
- Rare, benign, locally infiltrative epithelial odontogenic tumour. It may originate from enamel organs, dental lamina remnants, or the periodontal ligament.
- The average age of development is 34, with ages ranging from 9 to 67. A multifocal lesion may be seen in a single patient.
- Squamous odontogenic tumour manifests as a slow-growing, painless or painful bony expansion often associated with the mobility of teeth.
- Radiographically, this tumour is a well-defined, triangular radiolucent defect lateral to the root or roots of the teeth. Most of the defects are approximately 1.5 cm in diameter. A minority of cases have a corticated border or an ill-defined border.

- **Histology Features**
- *Neoplastic Component*: The squamous odontogenic tumour is composed of variable-sized islands of bland odontogenic squamous epithelial cells which are flat or cuboidal. Individual cell keratinisation, vacuolisation and microcystic spaces is frequently seen within the islands. Calcified structures and globular eosinophilic materials are also seen (■ Fig. 21.8).
- *Non-neoplastic Ectomesenchyme*: The vascular fibrous connective tissue is interspersed between the neoplastic odontogenic epithelial islands.

21.3.3 Calcifying Epithelial Odontogenic Tumour

- **Key Features**
- This uncommon epithelial odontogenic tumour, also known as the Pindborg tumour, has an uncertain origin. Some investigators suggest that it originates from the enamel organ, while others attribute its ori-

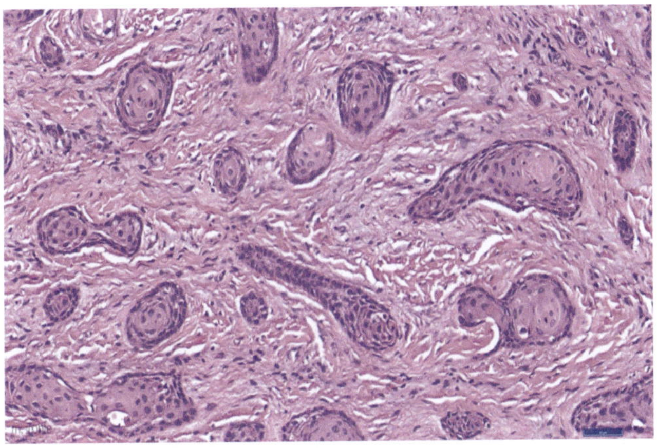

Fig. 21.8 Squamous odontogenic tumour. Bland epithelial islands in fibrous connective tissue stroma

gin to the dental lamina remnants. PTCH 1 gene (a tumour suppressor gene) mutation has been documented in a small series. Further research is required to explain the exact pathogenesis of calcifying epithelial odontogenic tumours.

- The mean age of development of this tumour is 40, with most patients between the second and fourth decades of life. However, it can be seen in a wide age range. Most cases develop in the posterior mandible.
- It manifests itself as a slow-growing, painless bony expansion. They may also arise peripherally as a sessile, asymptomatic mass on the gingiva, especially the anterior gingiva.
- Radiographically, a calcifying epithelial odontogenic tumour is a well-defined, unilocular or multilocular radiolucency or a radiolucent-radiopaque lesion. A minority of cases have a corticated border or an ill-defined border.

Histologic Features

- *Neoplastic Component*: Calcifying epithelial odontogenic tumour is composed of islands, sheets and strands of neoplastic odontogenic epithelial cells, which are large polygonal cells with eosinophilic cytoplasm and distinct outlines showing intercellular bridges. The nuclei of these cells show pleomorphism, but mitotic activity is scant.
- Extracellular amyloid-like material is always seen, and this material develops concentric calcifications (Liesegang ring calcification), which tend to fuse and form large masses.
- Variants of the basic histologic pattern include: (1) Cell-rich variant contains large sheets of epithelial cells with minimal production of amyloid-like material and calcifications. (2) Amyloid-rich variant with few epithelial cells. (3) A clear-cell variant, which has a prominent, clear-cell population (Figs. 21.9 and 21.10).

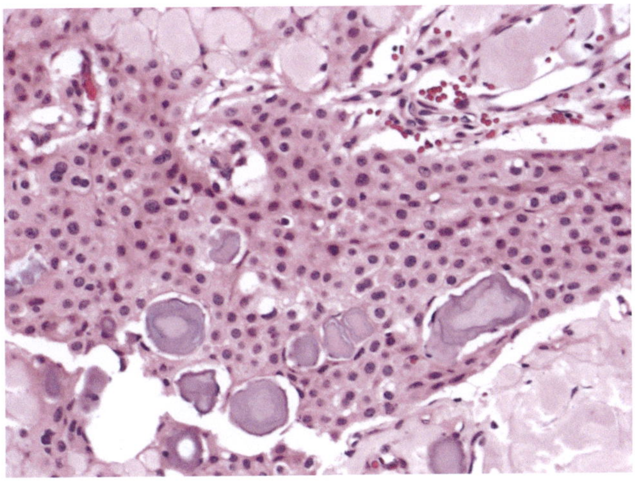

Fig. 21.9 Calcifying epithelial odontogenic tumour. Polyhedral cells showing eosinophilic cytoplasm and Liesegang ring calcifications

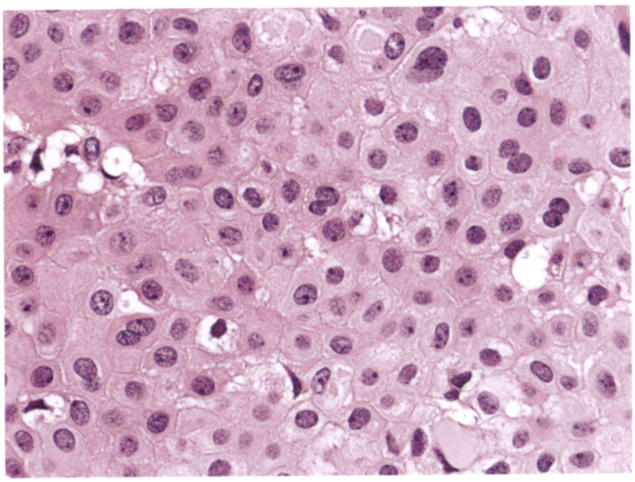

Fig. 21.10 Calcifying epithelial odontogenic tumour. Polyhedral epithelial cells with distinct outlines, nuclear variations, and eosinophilic cytoplasm

- *Non-neoplastic Component*: The vascular fibrous connective tissue is interspersed between the neoplastic odontogenic epithelial islands.

21.3.4 Adenomatoid Odontogenic Tumour

Key Features

- A benign epithelial odontogenic tumour originating either from an enamel organ, reduced enamel epithelium, epithelial cell rest of Malassez, or rest of the dental lamina.
- This neoplasm exhibits slow and self-limiting growth with extremely rare recurrence, even if partially removed. Hence, some investigators prefer to call it a hamartoma rather than a true neoplasm.

- The majority of patients are in the second decade of life (10–19 years of age), with a striking prevalence for the anterior maxilla. Females are affected more than males.
- A vast majority of lesions are intraosseous. However, they may be found peripherally on the maxillary facial gingiva as a small sessile mass. Intraosseous lesions are asymptomatic and often found during routine radiographic exams. A larger lesion results in an asymptomatic bony expansion. Neighbouring teeth may be displaced, but root resorption is rare.
- Radiographically, they present as well-defined unilocular radiolucent lesions. They are categorised as follicular and non-follicular adenomatoid odontogenic tumours. Follicular tumours involve a crown of an unerupted tooth, most commonly a canine. The non-follicular radiographic variant is present between roots of erupted teeth and may be completely radiolucent or may contain fine calcified structures (snow-flake calcifications).

- **Histologic Features**
- This epithelial odontogenic tumour may be solid or cystic.

Neoplastic Component: The neoplasm is composed of spindle-shaped and cuboidal or columnar cells. The spindle-shaped cells are arranged in sheets, strands, or whorled nodules with a central space which may be empty or contain eosinophilic amyloid. The columnar or cuboidal cells are arranged in a single layer to form duct-like structures. The nuclei of this single layer of cells is situated away from the lumen, These duct-like structures may or may not be present (Figs. 21.11 and 21.12).

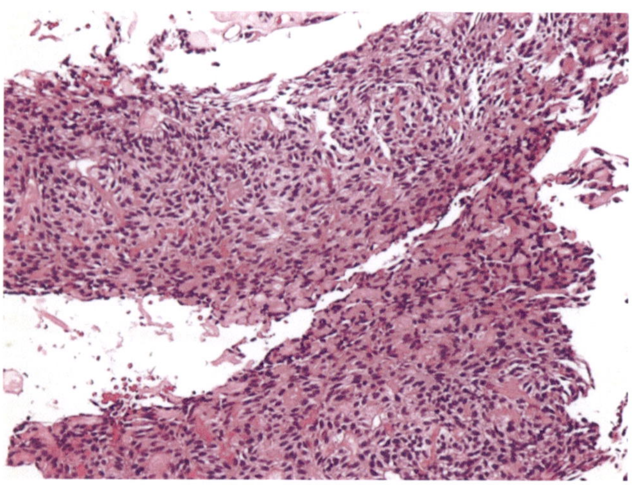

Fig. 21.11 Adenomatoid odontogenic tumour. The tumour is composed of spindle-shaped epithelial cells that form whorled masses

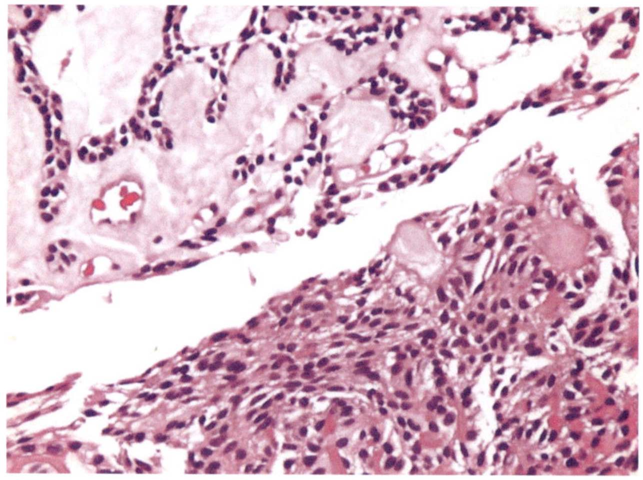

Fig. 21.12 Adenomatoid odontogenic tumour. Epithelial cells form rosette-like structures containing eosinophilic material. Dentinoid-like material is also seen

Non-neoplastic component: a thick fibrous capsule of connective tissue surrounds the tumour. Scanty fibrous connective stroma is present within the neoplastic spindle-shaped cells. Small foci of calcifications may be scattered within the neoplastic epithelium (Fig. 21.9).

21.4 Benign Mixed Epithelial and Mesenchymal Odontogenic Tumours

21.4.1 Ameloblastic Fibroma

- **Key Features**
- Ameloblastic fibroma is an uncommon true mixed odontogenic tumour. Both the epithelial and ectomesenchymal components are neoplastic.
- The average age of development is 15 years, with most patients diagnosed in the first two decades of life. They are frequently found in the posterior mandible and are often associated with an impacted tooth.
- Large lesions manifest as a painless bony swelling.
- Radiographically, they present as well-defined unilocular or multilocular radiolucent lesions with corticated margins. An unerupted tooth may be associated with the tumour in up to 75% of cases. These lesions can grow to large sizes and may involve the ascending ramus.

- **Histologic Features**
- *Neoplastic Epithelial Component*: There are two patterns of the epithelial component. The first pattern comprises proliferating columnar or cuboidal epi-

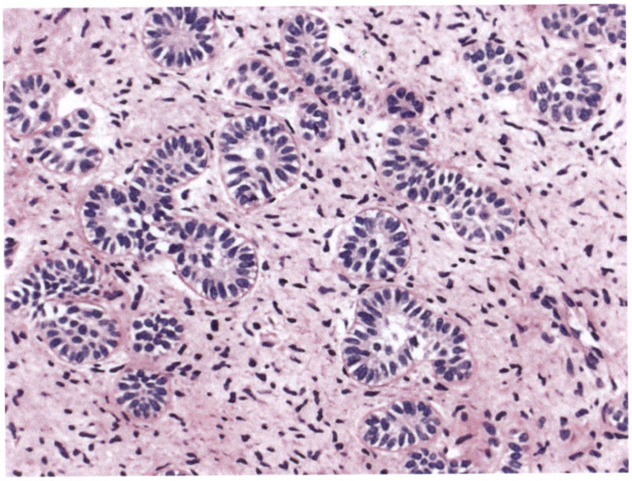

■ Fig. 21.13 Ameloblastic fibroma. Basophilic odontogenic epithelial islands with peripheral nuclear palisading supported by rich cellular primitive connective tissue

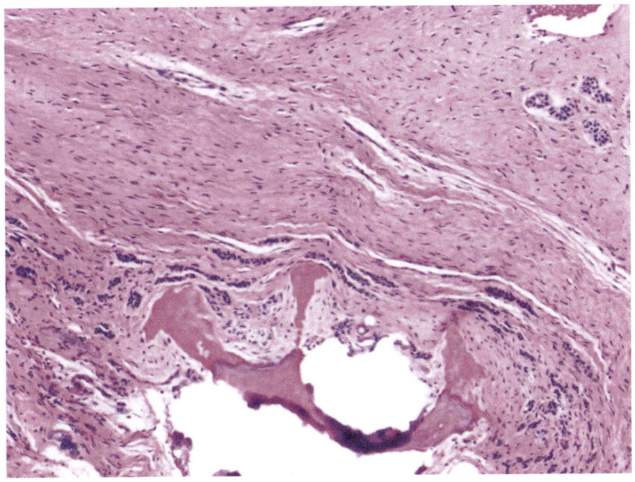

■ Fig. 21.14 Ameloblastic fibro-odontoma. Small islands of odontogenic epithelium in primitive appearing cellular connective tissue with calcifying elements

thelial cells forming anastomosing cords which are two cells thick. This is the most common pattern. The second pattern comprises islands of proliferating epithelial cells, formed by columnar peripheral cells surrounding loosely arranged central cells. These islands seldom show microcystic formation (■ Fig. 21.13).

- *Neoplastic Ectomesenchymal Component*: This component consists of a mildly collagenised cell-rich connective tissue stroma containing plump stellate and ovoid cells. It resembles the developing dental papilla. The portion of the mesenchyme adjacent to the epithelial islands or cords may be hyalinised and acellular.

21.4.2 Ameloblastic Fibro-odontoma

- **Key Features**

- Ameloblastic fibro-odontoma is an uncommon true mixed odontogenic tumour. Both the epithelial and ectomesenchymal components are neoplastic. It must be noted that the latest World Health Organization (WHO) classification had eliminated ameloblastic-fibro-odontoma from its classification; they consider it a developing odontoma. Other investigators propose that if the lesion is seen in patients younger than 13.5 years of age and the lesion exceeds 2.1 cm, it is a neoplasm rather than an odontoma.
- Average age of development is 10 years, with most patients diagnosed in the first two decades of life. They are frequently found in the posterior mandible.
- Manifests as an asymptomatic lesion often associated with an impacted tooth. They are discovered when a radiograph is taken to investigate the cause of a missing tooth.

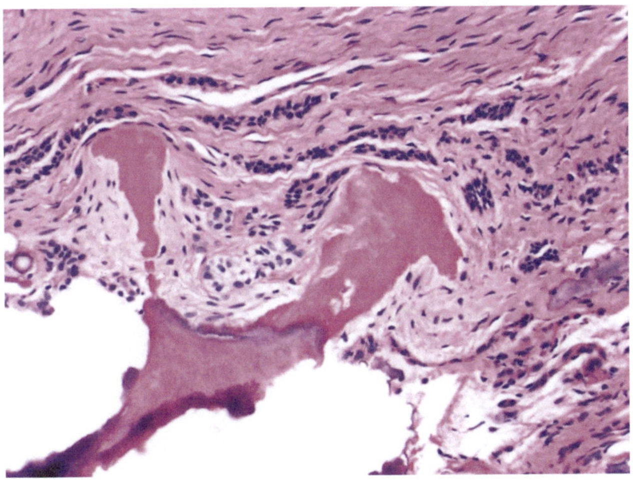

■ Fig. 21.15 Ameloblastic fibro-odontoma. Calcifying elements represent the formation of a disorganised tooth structure

- Radiographically, a well-defined unilocular or multilocular radiolucent with variable amounts, sizes, and shapes of radiopacities is seen. Margins are corticated.

- **Histologic Features**

- *Neoplastic Epithelial Component*: There are two patterns of the epithelial component. The first pattern comprises proliferating columnar or cuboidal epithelial cells forming anastomosing cords, which are two cells thick. This is the most common pattern. The second pattern comprises islands of proliferating epithelial cells formed by columnar peripheral cells surrounding loosely arranged central cells. These islands seldom show microcystic formation (■ Figs. 21.14 and 21.15).

- *Neoplastic Ectomesenchymal Component*: This component consists of a mildly collagenised cell-rich connective tissue stroma containing plump stellate and ovoid cells. It resembles the developing dental papilla. The portion of the mesenchyme adjacent to the epithelial islands or cords may be hyalinised and acellular. Variable amounts of enamel and dentine are closely associated with the neoplastic epithelial components. They may be present haphazardly or form rudimentary teeth.

21.4.3 Odontoma

▪ **Key Features**

Odontomas are the most common odontogenic tumour. They are considered hamartomas rather than true neoplasms composed of enamel, dentine, and variable amounts of pulp. They are further classified as compound (tooth-like) and complex (haphazard mass) odontomas. In rare cases, both complex and compound features may be seen in a single odontoma.

- The mean age at the time of diagnosis is 14 years. They may be found in any site of either jaw; however, they have a predilection for the maxilla. Commonly, compound odontomas are found in the anterior maxilla and complex odontomas are found in the posterior segment of either jaw. They may be seen peripherally in the gingival tissue as well.
- These are asymptomatic lesions discovered on radiographs taken for other reasons or because of a missing tooth. Most odontomas do not cause clinical expansion of the jawbones, but large odontomas causing bony expansions have been documented.
- Radiographic features are diagnostic, especially in the case of compound odontomas. They show a well-defined radiolucent lesion showing radiopaque tooth-like structures of various sizes. If a radiopaque mass is seen instead of tooth-like structures surrounded by a radiolucent rim, a diagnosis is that of complex odontoma.

▪ **Histologic Features**

- Compound odontomas show the histologic features of a normal tooth: an enamel matrix, mature tubular dentine cementum, and central pulp tissue (◘ Fig. 21.16).
- *Complex odontoma* shows the enamel matrix, tubular dentine, cementum, and pulp tissues arranged in a haphazard manner Ghost cells may be seen in a minority of cases.

21

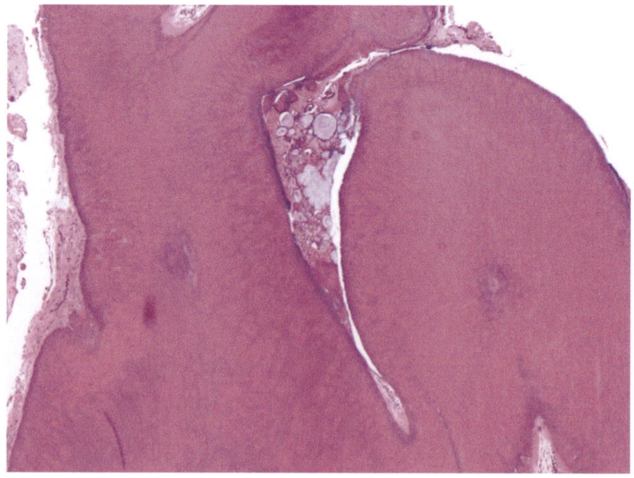

◘ **Fig. 21.16** Odontoma. The decalcified section shows a disorganised mass of dentine

21.4.4 Primordial Odontogenic Tumour

▪ **Key Features**

- These are benign mixed odontogenic tumours which microscopically resemble the early stages of tooth development. They were included in the WHO classification in 2017. Less than 25 cases have been reported so far. It has been suggested that its genesis starts between the 10th and 20th week of intrauterine life.
- This tumour has been primarily diagnosed in the first two decades of life. No gender predilection has been reported. The posterior mandible is the favoured site.
- The lesion initially manifests as an asymptomatic bony expansion. Over time the lesion becomes symptomatic.
- Radiographically, a well-defined radiolucent lesion is seen in association with the crown of a third molar tooth. Large, well-defined multilocular radiolucent lesions have also been reported.

▪ **Histologic Features**

- *Epithelial Component*: Thin layers of cuboidal or columnar epithelium line the periphery of the tumour. These epithelial cells show reverse polarity and subnuclear vacuolisation. Few cases have reported stellate reticulum-like loose cells adjacent to the tall or cuboidal cells (◘ Figs. 21.17 and 21.18).
- *Ectomesenchymal component* is myxoid and collagenous, resembling the primitive dental papillae, interspersed with spindle-shaped cells. The periphery of this component is lobulated. Few cases have demonstrated eosinophilic material or basophilic calcifications in the ectomesenchyme.

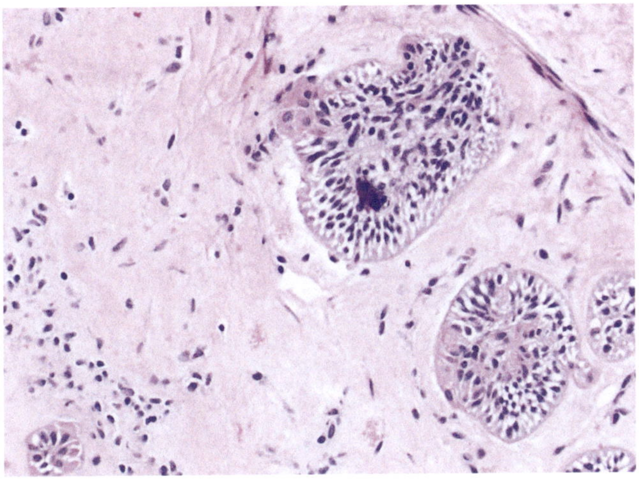

Fig. 21.17 Primordial odontogenic tumour. Odontogenic epithelium resembling inner enamel epithelium of a developing tooth within connective tissue resembling dental papillae

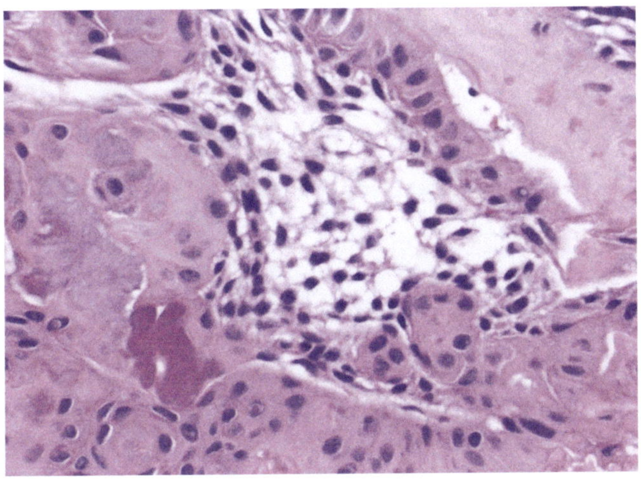

Fig. 21.18 Primordial odontogenic tumour. Edge of the epithelial tumour lined by a layer of cuboidal epithelium and centre has stellate reticulum-like differentiation. Eosinophilic "enameloid" material is present

21.4.5 Central Odontogenic Fibroma

- **Key Features**

- It is an uncommon benign odontogenic ectomesenchymal tumour. It arises from the periodontal ligament, dental follicle, or dental papillae. The lesion also develops peripherally on the gingiva. Peripheral variants are more common than central ones.
- The mean age of development is 33 years. Although most cases are seen between 20 and 30 years of age, they may be seen at any age. The mandible and maxilla are equally affected; however, the maxillary lesions have a predilection for the anterior maxilla, and the mandibular lesions are commonly seen in the posterior regions. Females are affected more than males.
- Small lesions are an incidental finding. Larger lesions can result in bony swelling accompanied by pain and loosening of adjacent teeth. Peripheral lesions are asymptomatic and present as a gingival bump.
- Radiographically, they present as well-defined unilocular or multilocular radiolucencies. A minority of cases show radiopaque flecks within the radiolucency. The resorption of adjacent teeth' roots is a common feature.

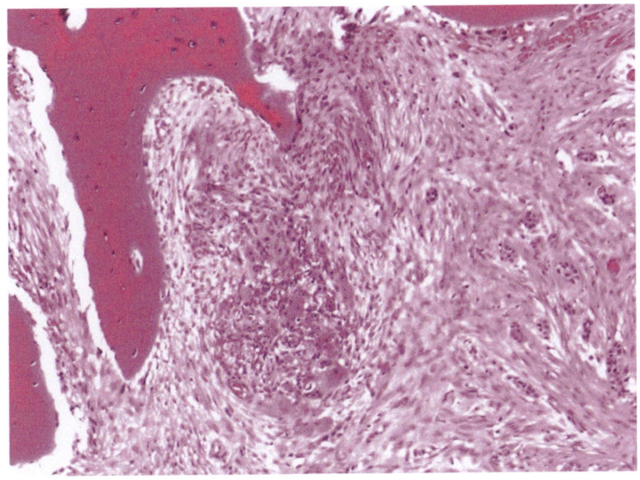

Fig. 21.19 Central odontogenic fibroma. Odontogenic epithelial islands within a fibrous background

- **Histologic Features**

- *Non-neoplastic Epithelium*: Odontogenic epithelium is inactive and bland and is arranged in the form of strands or small nests. In the "Simple type" of central odontogenic fibroma, the epithelial elements are scanty. In the "Epithelium-rich or WHO type", the epithelium component is abundant throughout the lesion and, in some cases, may even be the dominant component.
- *Neoplastic Ectomesenchyme*: The "Simple type" is composed of collagenous or myxoid stroma with a variable number of stellate fibroblasts, often arranged in a whorled pattern. In the "Epithelium-rich or WHO type", the ectomesenchyme may be collagenous or myxoid and highly cellular. Some lesions contain bone trabecular, cementum-like calcifications, amyloid, Langerhans cells, or giant cells within the stroma (Figs. 21.19 and 21.20).

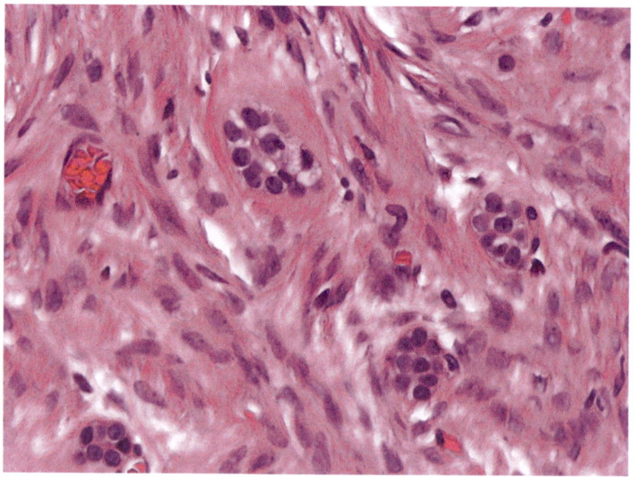

Fig. 21.20 Central odontogenic fibroma. Foci of odontogenic epithelium within cellular fibrous connective tissue

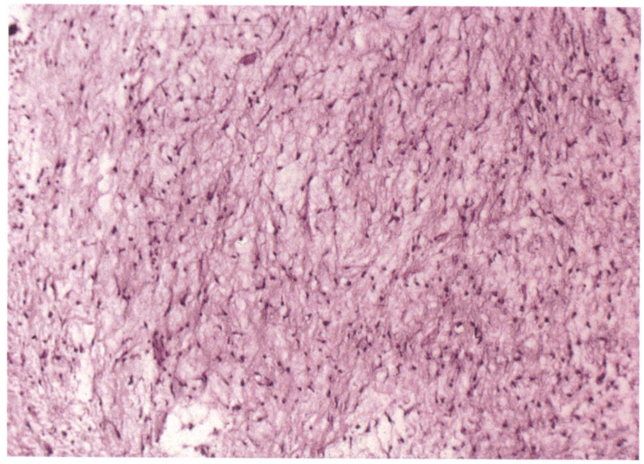

Fig. 21.21 Odontogenic myxoma. Loosely arranged spindle cells within fine collagen fibrils

21.4.6 Odontogenic Myxoma

- **Key Features**
- Odontogenic myxoma is an uncommon ectomesenchymal odontogenic tumour arising from the mesenchymal portion of the tooth germ. It is the third most common odontogenic tumour after odontoma and ameloblastoma. It has a recurrence rate of up to 25%.
- The mean age of manifestation is 26.5 years. Although most cases are seen between 25 and 30 years of age, it may be seen at any age. This lesion shows a mandibular predilection and can develop in any area of the jaw. A slight female predilection has been reported.
- Small lesions are incidental findings. A larger lesion can result in a bony swelling accompanied by pain and loosening of adjacent teeth.
- Radiographically, they present as well-defined unilocular or multilocular radiolucencies with irregular or scalloped margins. The radiolucency may show thin and wispy residual trabeculae arranged at right angles. The resorption of roots of adjacent teeth is a common feature. Lesions showing a sunburst periosteal reaction (osteosarcoma-like) have been reported. Cortical perforations may also be seen.

- **Histologic Features**
- *Non-neoplastic Epithelium*: Odontogenic epithelium is inactive and bland and arranged in small strands or nests throughout the lesion. These epithelial components are not required for the diagnosis (Fig. 21.21).
- *Neoplastic Ectomesenchyme*: tumour stroma is predominantly myxoid, containing a few collagen fibrils and variable amounts of spindle-shaped, stellate, or round activated fibroblasts. The myxoid ground substance is composed of glycosaminoglycans. Fibromyoma or myxofibroma is designated to lesions that contain a greater quantity of collagen fibres. Cementum-like calcifications within the myxoid stroma are an unusual feature.

21.4.7 Granular Cell Odontogenic Tumour

- **Key Features**
- Rare benign odontogenic ectomesenchymal tumour of neuroectodermal differentiation containing granular cells.
- The average age of manifestation is 45 years. Although most cases are seen between 50 and 70 years of age. This lesion shows a predilection for the premolar-molar mandibular areas. Peripheral lesions have also been reported. A strong female predilection has been reported.
- Small lesions are an incidental finding. Larger lesions can result in a bony swelling accompanied by pain and loosening of adjacent teeth. Cortical perforation and soft tissue extension have also been reported.
- Radiographically, they present as well-defined unilocular or multilocular radiolucencies with occasional calcifications.

- **Histologic Features**
- *Non-neoplastic Epithelium*: Odontogenic epithelium is inactive and bland and is arranged in the form of small strands or small nests throughout the lesion, scattered amongst the granular cells.

21

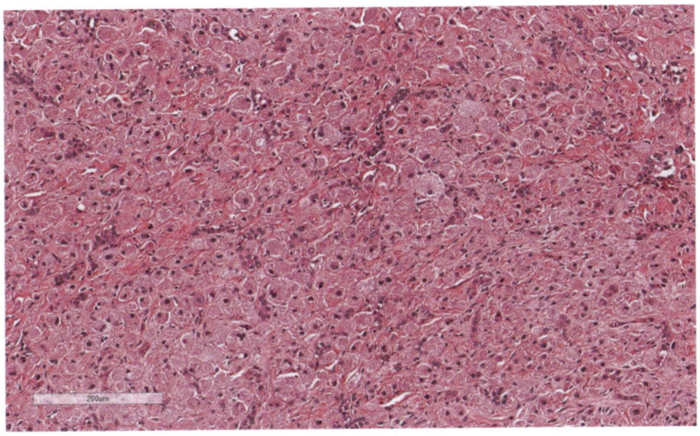

Fig. 21.22 Granular cell odontogenic tumour. Inactive odontogenic epithelial cell islands interspersed between granular cells

- *Neoplastic Ectomesenchyme*: Tumour stroma is composed predominantly of granular cells containing eosinophilic and granular cytoplasm and an eccentrically placed nucleus (Fig. 21.22). Cementum-like calcifications within the myxoid stroma are a feature of a minority of cases.

21.4.8 Cementoblastoma

Key Features

- An uncommon benign odontogenic ectomesenchymal tumour. They are seen on the root of an erupted permanent tooth and are formed by proliferating cementoblasts, producing cementum or cementum-like mineralisation. Primary teeth are very rarely involved.
- The mean age of manifestation is 24 years, and most cases are seen between the second and third decades of life. A large majority of cases are seen in relation to the mandibular permanent first molar tooth. Unusually impacted teeth, unerupted teeth or primary teeth may be involved.
- Swelling accompanied by pain is a common finding. The involved tooth is vital in 80% of cases. The mean lesional size is 2 cm. Most are slow-growing. Aggressive lesions causing cortical expansion, displacement of adjacent teeth, infiltration into the root canal and pulp chamber, or involvement of the maxillary sinus have been occasionally reported.
- Radiographically, the lesion presents as a radiopacity surrounded by a thin radiolucent rim. The lesion is fused to the root of the adjacent tooth, obscuring the root outline. The mandibular canal may be inferiorly displaced. Rarely, the lesion presents as a well-defined radiolucency.

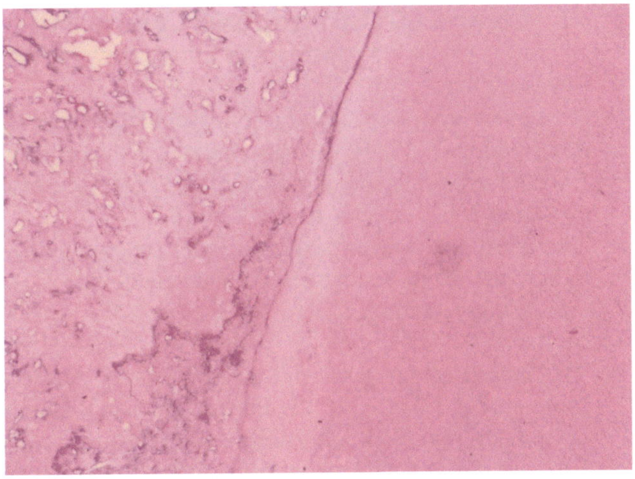

Fig. 21.23 Cementoblastoma. Mineralised tissue with basophilic reversal lines with uncalcified matrix at the periphery

Histology Features

- *Neoplastic Ectomesenchyme*: tumour stroma is composed predominantly of a well-defined mass of acellular sheets or trabeculae of cementum or cementum-like mineralisation entrapping cementoblasts supported by a fibrovascular stroma. This mineralised material shows prominent reversal lines (Fig. 21.23). The periphery of the lesion shows radiating trabeculae of the uncalcified matrix. Fusion with and resorption of the adjacent tooth root is characteristic. Pulp involvement is uncommon. An area of lace-like osteoid may also be seen.

21.5 Malignant Odontogenic Tumours

Malignant odontogenic tumours are rare. They arise either de novo from the tooth-forming tissues, their developmental residues or from existing odontogenic epithelial or mesenchymal neoplasms in the jaws and malignant transformation of benign odontogenic tumours. Due to their low incidence, these tumours remain poorly understood entities with respect to their cancer biology, clinical behaviour, management, and long-term prognosis. The most common microscopic diagnosis reported in a systematic study by Martin, Dave, and Hunter included ameloblastic carcinoma, followed by primary intraosseous squamous cell carcinoma, clear-cell odontogenic carcinoma, malignant ameloblastoma, and ameloblastic fibrosarcoma. Only clear-cell odontogenic carcinoma is included in this chapter.

21.5.1 Clear-Cell Odontogenic Carcinoma

- **Key Features**
- A rare malignant epithelial odontogenic tumour first described in 1985. Molecular studies have identified EWSR1-ATF1 gene translocation. This genetic mutation is not specific to this tumour.
- Though it is characterised as an odontogenic malignancy, the exact histogenesis is unknown. The clear cells are glycogen-rich, like the presecretory ameloblasts.
- The mean age at presentation is 58, and patients range in age from 17 to 89. Female predilection has been reported. The mandible is the favoured site. Patients present with or without pain, bony expansion, tooth mobility, and lower lip paresthesia. The tumour often penetrates the bone to present as a soft tissue swelling. Bleeding and ulcerations are uncommon presentations.
- It is very important to distinguish this odontogenic tumour from other entities with clear cells, namely, calcifying epithelial odontogenic tumour, hyalinising clear-cell carcinoma, intraosseous mucoepidermoid carcinoma, metastatic renal cell carcinoma, clear-cell breast carcinoma, and clear-cell melanoma.
- Radiographically, it presents as a poorly defined unilocular or multilocular radiolucency.

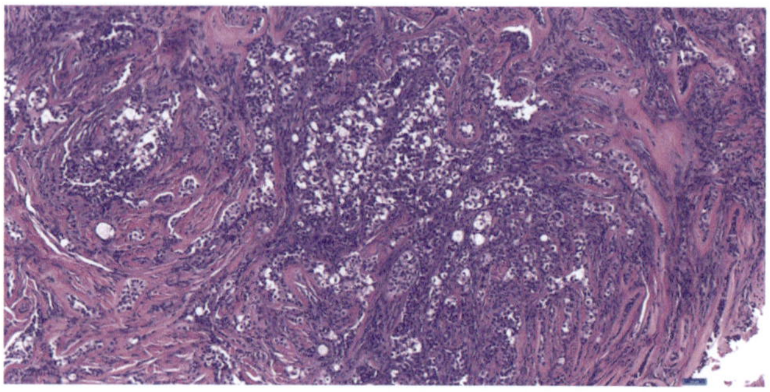

Fig. 21.24 Clear-cell odontogenic carcinoma. Epithelial cell nests showing hyperchromatic cells and clear cells

- **Histology Features**
- *Neoplastic Component*: This infiltrative tumour is composed of variously sized nests composed of either round or polygonal pale eosinophilic cells or cells with clear cytoplasm and a hyperchromatic nucleus with a small nucleolus. These lesional cells show sparse mitoses, atypia and pleomorphism. Necrosis is an uncommon feature. Three patterns are identified: (1) The biphasic pattern is composed of both the pale eosinophilic and clear cells. (2) Monophasic pattern composed of only clear cells. (3) An ameloblastoma-like pattern, composed of clear cells with the peripheral cells showing palisaded nuclei (Figs. 21.24 and 21.25).
- *Non-neoplastic Ectomesenchyme*: Thin strands of vascularised and hyalinised connective tissue are seen among the islands of neoplastic odontogenic epithelium.

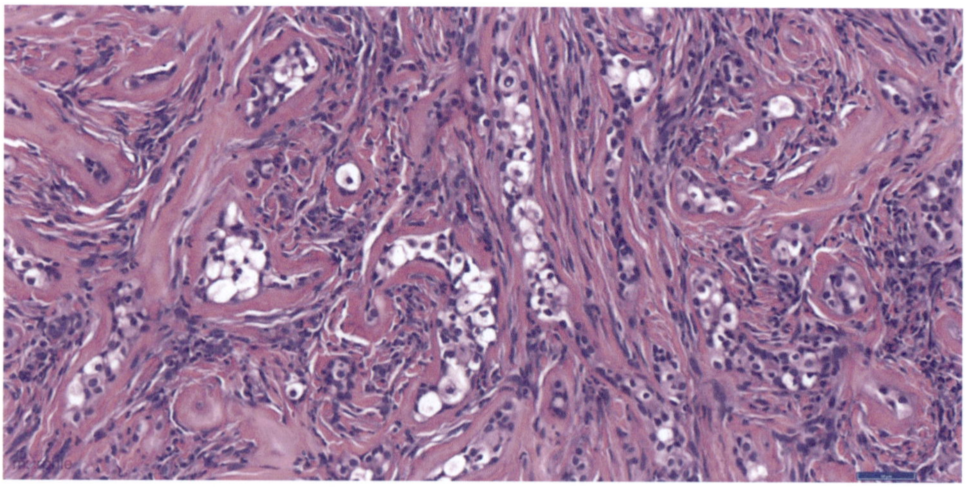

Fig. 21.25 Clear-cell odontogenic carcinoma. Tumour island cells have a clear cytoplasm

21.6 Summary

Odontogenic tumours are an uncommon group of lesions arising from remnants of odontogenic epithelium or ectomesenchyme. They show varied presentations both clinically and radiographically and are subdivided according to their neoplastic component. These tumours should be considered in the differential diagnosis when considering any jawbone lesion.

Further Reading

Bennabi S, Lescious P, Cloitre A. Central odontogenic fibroma: characteristics and management. J Oral Med Oral Surg. 2021;27(2):25. https://doi.org/10.1051/mbcb/2020066.

Bologna-Molina R, Pereira-Prado V, Sánchez-Romero C, González-González R, Mosqueda-Taylor A. Primordial odontogenic tumor: a systematic review. Med Oral Patol Oral Cir Bucal. 2020;25(3):e388–94. https://doi.org/10.4317/medoral.23432.

Borges DC, de Faria PR, Júnior HM, Pereira LB. Conservative treatment of a periapical cementoblastoma: a case report. J Oral Maxillofac Surg. 2019;77(2):272.e1–7. https://doi.org/10.1016/j.joms.2018.10.003.

Chrcanovic BR, Gomez RS. Odontogenic myxoma: an updated analysis of 1,692 cases reported in the literature. Oral Dis. 2019;25(3):676–83. https://doi.org/10.1111/odi.12875.

Cossiez M, Pin D. A rare case of maxillary ameloblastic fibro-odontoma and a review of the literature. J Oral Med Oral Surg. 2020;26:17. https://doi.org/10.1051/mbcb/2020010.

Labrador AJP, Marin NRG, Valdez LHM, Valentina MP, Sanchez KBT, Ibazetta KAR, Johan B, Cesar AV, Wright JM. Clear cell odontogenic carcinoma a systematic review. Head Neck Pathol. 2022;16(3):838–48. https://doi.org/10.1007/s12105-021-01383-9. Epub 2021 Oct 7.

Lakshmanan S, Lal B, Kumar RD, Mishra D, Bhutia O. Central granular cell odontogenic tumour of the mandible in a child. J Clin Pediatr Dent. 2022;46(6):54–7. https://doi.org/10.22514/jocpd.2022.027. Epub 2022 Nov 1.

Mamat Yusof MN, Ch'ng ES, Radhiah Abdul Rahman N. *BRAF* V600E mutation in ameloblastoma: a systematic review and meta-analysis. Cancers (Basel). 2022;14(22):5593. https://doi.org/10.3390/cancers14225593.

Marín C, Niklander SE, Martínez-Flores R. Genetic profile of adenomatoid odontogenic tumor and ameloblastoma. A systematic review. Front Oral Health. 2021;2:767474. https://doi.org/10.3389/froh.2021.767474.

Marin C, Dave M, Hunter KD. Malignant odontogenic tumours: a systematic review of cases reported in literature. Front Oral Health. 2021;2:775707. https://doi.org/10.3389/froh.2021.775707.

Nasir A, Khare A, Ali I, Khan MI. Ameloblastic fibroma: a case report. J Oral Maxillofac Pathol. 2023;27(Suppl 1):S60–3. https://doi.org/10.4103/jomfp.jomfp_337_22.

Ruddocks LA, Fitzpatrick SG, Bhattacharyya I, Cohen DM, Islam MN. Calcifying epithelial odontogenic tumor: a case series spanning 25 years and review of the literature. Oral Surg Oral Med Oral Pathol Oral Radiol. 2021;131(6):684–93. https://doi.org/10.1016/j.oooo.2021.01.007. Epub 2021 Jan 9.

Thompson LDR. Odontoma. Ear Nose Throat J. 2021;100(5_suppl):536S–7S. https://doi.org/10.1177/0145561319890175.

Upadhyaya JD, Banasser A, Cohen DM, Kashtwari D, Bhattacharyya I, Islam MN. Squamous odontogenic tumor: review of the literature and report of a new case. J Oral Maxillofac Surg. 2021;79(1):164–76. https://doi.org/10.1016/j.joms.2020.06.031.

Histopathology of Non-odontogenic Neoplasms of the Jaws

Radhika Manoj Bavle and Vinay K. Hazarey

Contents

S R Prabhu et al. (eds.), *Oral Histology and Oral Histopathology*, https://doi.org/10.1007/978-3-031-77481-2_22

Table 22.1 Classification: WHO (modified) Panlos and Portout

1. **Bone tumours forming bone**
– Benign—Osteoma, Osteoid osteoma, Osteoblastoma
– Malignant—Osteo sarcoma
2. **Bone tumours forming cartilaginous tissue**
– Benign—Chondroma, Osteochondroma, Chondroblastoma, Chondro-myxoid fibroma
– Malignant—Chondrosarcoma
3. **Giant cell Tumours**
4. **Bone marrow tumours**
Ewings sarcoma and reticular sarcoma
Lymphosarcoma
Myeloma
5. **Vascular tumours**
6. **Connective tissue tumours**
7. **Other bone tumours**
8. **Pseudo-tumoural lesions**
9. **Metastatic tumours**

22.1 Introduction

A plethora of tumours arise and manifest in gnathic jaw bones. The tumours that do not arise from the odontogenic apparatus and its derivatives are called and classified as the non-odontogenic neoplasms of the jaw. These tumours have no contribution from the odontogenic epithelium, odontogenic ectomesenchyme and its derivatives and/or rests. They commonly originate from ecto-mesenchymal or hemato-lymphoid and associated tissues. A spectrum of bone, cartilaginous tumours, hematogenous tumours, a variety of round cell tumours and reactive lesions are a part of non-odontogenic neoplasms of the jaw. These tumours have a fleeting spectrum from benign, aggressive to malignant behaviour, with variable histopathology and prognosis. The tumours arising in the gnathic skeleton are a small percentage and are considered quite uncommon.

The non-odontogenic neoplasms are classified by the World Health Organization (WHO) (2017). A modified WHO is advocated for use (Table 22.1).

22.2 Osteoma (Benign Osteoma)

Osteomas are benign bone lesions characterised by bony excrescences, usually arising in the intra-membranous bones.

Key Features

- Symptomatic to completely asymptomatic, incidental findings
- Age: one to seventh decade, 20–30 years common. 3:1 Female: Male ratio
- Histological types: compact and cancellous; common: compact followed by mixed
- Spongy osteomas: central (endosteal) or peripheral (sub-periosteal)
- Parosteal osteomas: head and gnathic jaws
- Skeletal osteomas involving skull and jaws: Gardner's syndrome
- Multiple osteomas are also seen in non-syndromic cases
- Associated with reactive lesions: trauma, infection/association with fibro-osseous dysplasia
- Classified based on location as peripheral, exophytic, periosteal, central (endosteal), and extraskeletal/soft tissue.
- Radiologically, well-circumscribed, compact, pedunculated/broad-based
- Osteomas are treated conservatively, using a surgical approach.

Histopathology

Well-circumscribed, well-delineated benign tumour with mature lamellar or woven bone. Smooth or lobulated (in large tumours) surface.

Compact Osteoma/Ivory or Ebony Osteomas: Consists of densely compact mature lamellar bone with an appearance similar to normal bone consisting of concentric lamellae around the Haversian canals. The periphery shows a compact layer of bone without remodelling. The core shows a compact, coarse mosaic pattern of lamellar bone with a few Haversian canals and vessels (Fig. 22.1).

Spongy/Trabecular Osteoma: Endosteal or sub-periosteal in location. Show predominantly cancellous trabecular bone, which is thin, irregular, and uneven in structure and thickness with occasional osteoblastic lining. The intertrabecular areas are made of medullary tissue with adipocytes and vessels. Merging trabeculae exhibit coral-like configuration completely enclosing fatty marrow on occasions. It may show fibrous tissue along with haemorrhage (Fig. 22.2).

Mixed Osteoma: Some of the osteomas show peripheral cortical bone with cancellous or trabecular bone at the core. Variable amounts of compact and trabecular bone may be seen.

22.3 Osteoid Osteoma

Osteoid osteoma is a benign osteoblastic bone tumour composed of osteoid and atypical bone. It is characterised by a well-demarcated, distinctive core (nidus),

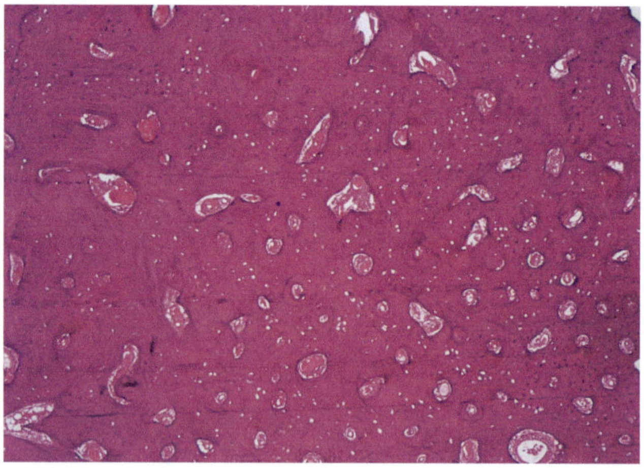

Fig. 22.1 Compact osteoma. This tumour shows compact bone with enclosed Haversian systems. Mature osteocytes are seen with resting and reversal mines

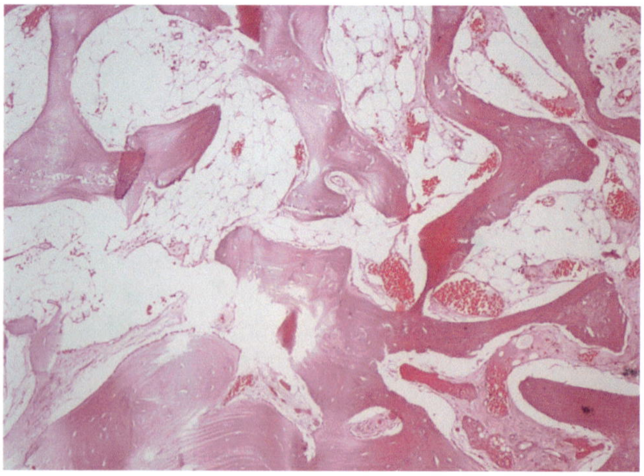

Fig. 22.2 Trabecular osteoma, which shows bony trabeculae enclosing the marrow spaces, rich blood vessels, and adipose tissue (fatty marrow)

usually less than 1 cm, surrounded by a zone of reactive bone.

Key Features

- Small-sized benign bone tumour creating a central nidus of osteoid
- Lesion painful, perceived at night, relieved by Aspirin
- Males > Females 2:1, second decade
- Common in the cortex or medulla of the bone
- Radiographically, well-circumscribed, cortical rim-opaque, central core-radiolucent
- Indolent/long-standing lesions exhibit a calcified central nidus
- Calcification/ossification: radio-opacity grows towards the outer rim
- Osteoid osteomas have limited growth potential but possess the potential to recur. Histopathological presentation is similar to osteoblastoma. Larger and more aggressive tumours are arbitrarily diagnosed as osteoblastomas.

Histopathology

Well-demarcated with central nidus. The nidus is surrounded by thickened cortical bone formation. The nidus is a rich vascular area of cellular stroma with varying components of osteoid and bone formation at different levels of maturation, ossification and/or calcification. The osseous tissue shows osteoblastic rimming. The osteoid can present as small pools/droplets surrounded by osteoblasts or in the form of mature, lace-like structures with osteoblastic rimming. Ossification is seen in a few areas of osteoid. Multiple vascular and capillary areas are seen in the vicinity. The surrounding bone appears more mature, spongy, or cancellous with merging bony trabeculae. Vascular marrow spaces, along with adipocytic tissue, are contained within them. An ageing lesion shows ossification, appearing like dense areas of osteosclerosis. A mosaic pattern is formed by lamellar bone, which is closely packed.

22.4 Osteoblastoma (Benign Osteoblastoma, Giant Osteoid Osteoma, Aggressive Osteoblastoma)

Osteoblastoma is a benign bone-forming tumour within the bone; by definition, it is greater than 1.5 cm.

Key Features

- Males > Females, 72% cases
- First to third decade of life, accounts for 80% cases
- Jawbone: 10% occurrence, maxilla < mandible
- Skull bones: temporal, frontal and ethmoidal bone
- Mostly asymptomatic, can manifest with pain, tenderness, and local swelling
- Average duration of growth >2 years
- Similar to osteoid osteoma but has a greater propensity for growth
- Osteoblastoma often exhibits aggressive behaviour
- Radiographically, size is 2–10 cm, expansile mass, predominantly well-defined border, variable areas of destruction, sclerosis, and well-mineralised masses at the base of teeth

Histopathology

Osteoblastoma is composed of woven bone spicules or trabeculae. Spicules are haphazardly arranged with a lining of a single layer of osteoblasts. The vascularity is rich, often with extravasated erythrocytes. The mitotic rate may be high. Diffusely scattered osteoclast-type, multi-nucleated giant cells are often present. Osteoblastomas are tumours of osteoblastic nature, circumscribed on the periphery, but may focally show trabeculae merging with the normal surrounding bone (◘ Fig. 22.3). They show variable amounts of calcified matrix ranging from non-mineralised osteoid/woven bone to well-mineralised bony trabeculae. The woven bone is lined by a prominent, single layer of osteoblasts that are compact and cuboidal with a central conspicuous nucleus—closed face or open face with nucleoli (◘ Fig. 22.4). In some variants, the osteoblasts are tall, columnar, cytoplasm-rich with prominent, polarised nuclei and few mitotic activities.

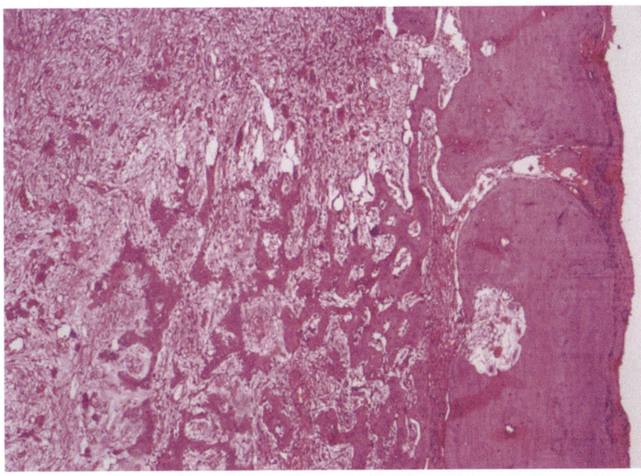

◘ **Fig. 22.3** Osteoblastoma. The periphery of the tumour is in the vicinity of normal bone. Some trabeculae are seen merging with normal bone

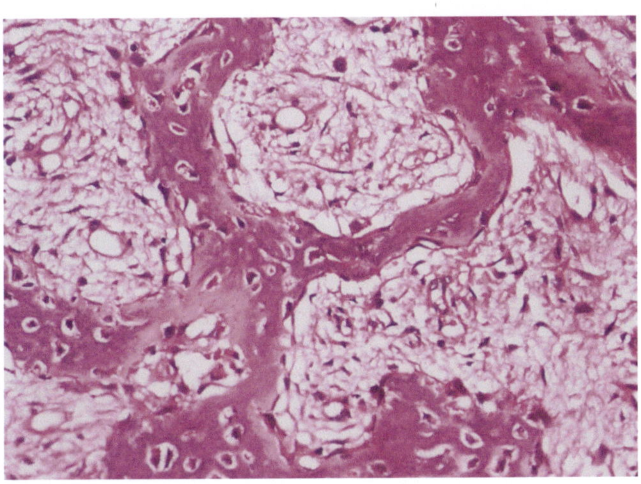

◘ **Fig. 22.4** Osteoblastoma. This high magnification shows woven bony trabeculae lined by osteoblasts and containing large osteocytes

Delicate thin/thick, well-formed trabeculae that are well-mineralised and woven bone with large, closely placed osteocytes can be noted. Mature-looking bone with resting/reversal lines is placed towards the periphery, depicting a pushing growth pattern rather than being destructive. A well-defined sharp tumour margin is seen. The background stroma is bland and well vascularised with loosely arranged spindle cells, capillaries, and vessels with multi-nucleated, osteoclastic giant cells. Areas of haemorrhage with giant cells around vascular spaces are seen. Necrosis is uncommon.

22.5 Osteochondroma

Osteochondroma is a "cartilage-capped bony projection arising on the external surface of bone containing a marrow cavity that is continuous with that of the underlying bone". There are two types: solitary osteochondroma (90% of cases) and hereditary multiple osteochondroma (HMO).

Key Features

- About 1% of osteochondroma occurs within the head and neck region
- Benign bone tumour
- 90% solitary tumours, common in second decade, around 20 years
- Account for 35% of primary bone tumours
- Seen in endochondral bones
- May undergo spontaneous regression and become quiescent
- 0–5% conversion to chondrosarcoma
- Radiographically, outward spur-like growth, a mushroom appearance
- Symptomatic osteochondromas need to be surgically removed

Histopathology

The tumour mass shows a mushroom-like cartilage cap with a bony stalk. The cartilaginous cap is covered by a thin periosteal layer and is made up of a mature chondroid matrix with chondrocytes in lacunae arranged in small clusters (◘ Fig. 22.5). The cartilaginous tissue cascades into regular bony trabeculae in the form of normal endochondral ossification. The bony trabeculae are discontinuous, with intervening tissue made of vascular components and adipose tissue.

22.6 Central Ossifying Fibroma

Central ossifying fibromas are fibro-osseous tumours of mesenchymal cells that ossify and calcify. They are well-circumscribed tumours that may be benign or aggressive in nature.

Key Features

- 75–95% of tumours arise in the mandible; the maxilla, paranasal sinus, and skull bones are other sites
- Variation with the presence of cementum can be noted (cementifying fibroma, cemento ossifying fibroma)
- Variant in the form of aggressive/juvenile ossifying fibroma
- Third to fourh decade
- Female > Male 5:1
- Radiographically, well-circumscribed, uni/multi-locular with well-demarcated periphery. Small/large, ossified opacities. With cortical expansion and teeth displacement.
- The tumours are treated by enucleation surgically and show good prognosis with low recurrence rate.

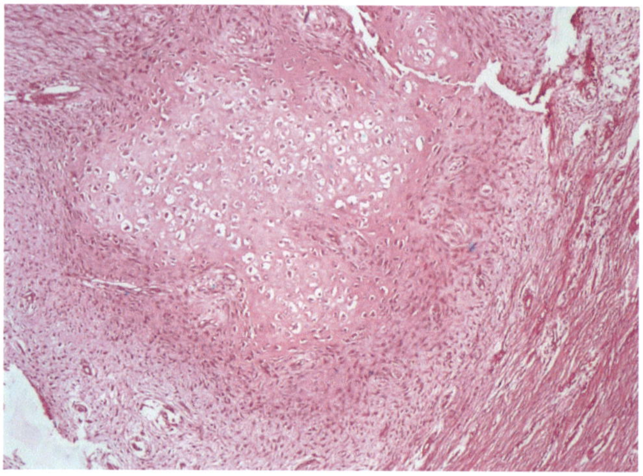

Fig. 22.5 Osteochondroma showing formation of cartilage surrounded by dense cellular stromal component

Histopathology

Tumours show varying amounts of fibrous tissue with mineralised areas of ossification &/or cementum. The connective tissue shows mature collagen fibres with areas of plump fibroblasts (Fig. 22.6a). Variable amounts of immature, stellate, and hypocellular areas can be noted. This stroma is intervened by mineralised areas of trabeculae of woven or lamellar metaplastic bone. The metaplastic bone displays a carpet end-like collagenisation very frequently (Fig. 22.6b). Basophilic deposits with a few cellular components and cementum-like areas can be seen in many instances with or without metaplastic bone. The tumours might show areas of cystic degeneration and secondary aneurysmal bone cyst (ABC) formation with haemorrhage.

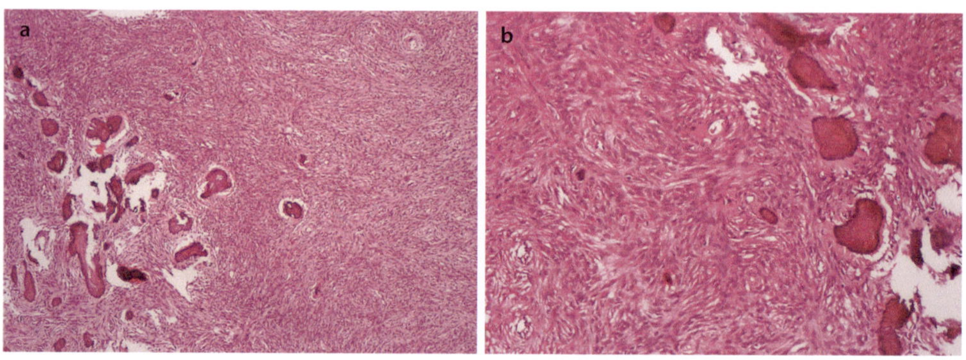

Fig. 22.6 **a** Central ossifying fibroma. Cellular stroma of spindle cells with areas of ossification and mineralisation. **b** The high-power view shows plump spindle cells with areas of ossification and metaplastic bone islands

22.7 Aggressive Ossifying Fibroma (Juvenile Ossifying Fibroma, Active Ossifying Fibroma) (WHO 2017)

Aggressive, ossifying fibroma, a rare tumour entity, occurs predominantly but not exclusively in children, with no gender predilection.

Key Features

- Rare variant of ossifying fibroma
- Two variants: trabecular and psammomatoid
- First to second decade of life, Male = Female
- Trabecular variant: common in mandible
- Psammomatoid variant: common in maxilla
- Radiographically, it shows an expansile growth, well delineated with foci of ossification and calcification. The periphery may show ill-delineated invasive areas.
- Aggressive and recurrent tumours (58%), demand a well-planned and assessed surgical therapy.

Histopathology

Aggressive ossifying fibroma consists of cellular fibrous stroma, plump fibroblasts, variable amounts of collagen and mineralised eosinophilic or basophilic deposits. These areas are intervened by eosinophilic immature bony trabeculae and/or basophilic small droplet-like psammomatous ossifications. The bone is metaplastic, immature, and woven with the collagenous rim. The psammomatous structures show inconspicuous cellular components with concentric lamination. The stroma is well vascularised with small vessels and capillaries and consists of a variable number of multi-nucleated giant cells in the cellular and vascular areas (Fig. 22.7). The cellular stroma shows few mitotic figures.

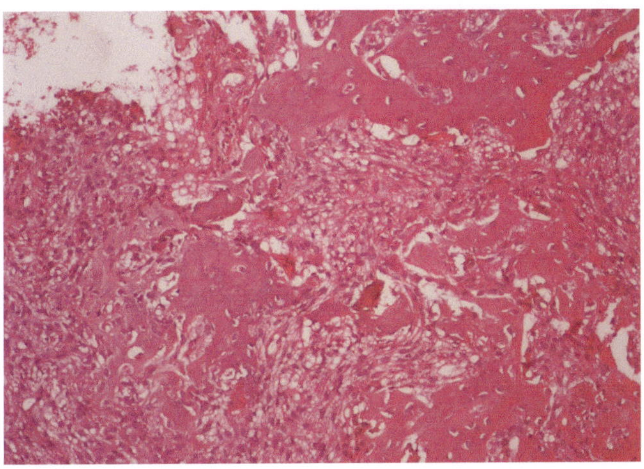

Fig. 22.7 Aggressive ossifying fibroma. Giant cells in the fibrous stroma and vascular channels along with irregular woven bone

22.8 Chondroma

A rare benign tumour in craniofacial bone composed of mature hyaline cartilage.

Classification

- Centrally located chondromas—enchondromas
- Periosteal involvement—periosteal chondromas
- Multiple chondromas (dysplasia of bone)—Ollier's Disease
- Multiple osteochondromas—skeletal osteochondromatosis. Example: Maffuci syndrome.

Key Features

- 15.6% of all benign tumours
- 4.7% of all tumours—gnathic skeleton
- Female > Male—solitary chondromas
- Female < Male—multiple chondromas
- 50% of the cases are in second, third, fourth decade
- Multiple lesions generally seen in first and second decade
- Radiographically, well-circumscribed, demarcated by the opaque rim
- Chondromas are benign tumours with good prognosis and rare recurrence. A recurrence might commonly point towards a missed anaplastic or dysplastic change.

Histopathology

A well-circumscribed lesson with lobular architecture. The peripheral rim of bone with intervening bony trabeculae may be seen in the lobular areas. The lobular/nodular growths show hypocellular pale blue areas of calcification of cartilaginous tissue with intervening myxoid areas. The cartilaginous matrix shows well-placed lacunae with chondrocytes that sometimes have large areas of glassy, well-calcified tissue (Fig. 22.8). Chondrocytes appear in two to three cells with inconspicuous small nuclei. Periosteal chondromas show clustering of chondrocytes with nuclear hyperchromasia. Multiple chondromas show hypercellular and myxoid areas. Permeation of surrounding bone/tissue is absent. Areas of fibrous dysplasia, when seen, are indicative of fibro-cartilaginous dysplasia or cases of multiple chondromas.

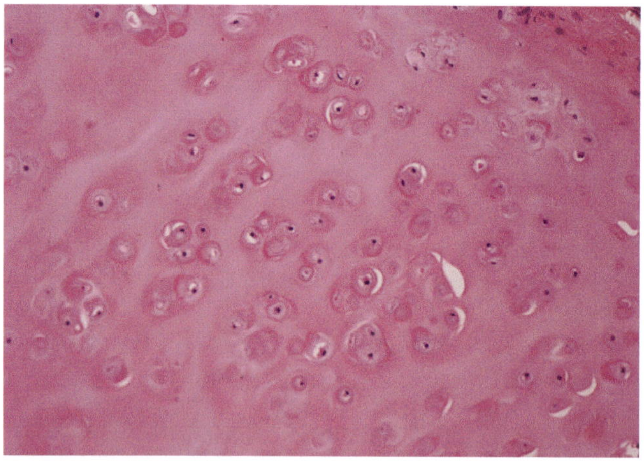

Fig. 22.8 Chondroma. Pale glassy areas of calcification of the cartilaginous tissue with lacunae containing chondrocytes

22.9 Chondroblastoma

Chondroblastoma are benign bone tumours with a chondroid matrix and abundant giant cells.

- **Key Features**
  - Incidence—4.79% of all benign tumours, 1.45% of all bone tumours
  - Common in temporal bone
  - Male > Female (2:1)
  - Older patients: third to fourth decade; second decade-60% cases
  - Symptoms—local pain
  - Radiographically, it is an expansile, round/oval cortical mass with/without mineralisation. A thin sclerotic rim of ossification, and a peri-tumoural area with a lucent border is seen.

- **Histopathology**

Chondroid differentiation of variable types is seen in almost 95% of cases. Chondroid areas are associated closely with ossified areas and calcific deposits in 4/5th of the tumours. Predominance of hyaline cartilage that is more eosinophilic than basophilic. Interspersed between the calcified areas are cellular areas of chondroblasts that are oval or epithelioid with a prominent, pink-stained cytoplasm. Closely packed cells lead to a syncytium pattern of sheets with an oval or coffee bean or open vesicular nucleus. Benign giant cells with 5–40 nuclei with chondroblasts are scattered in the stroma, that is well vascularised and scanty. Atypical cellular and nuclear morphology can be seen with very few mitotic figures but no atypical mitosis. The stroma might show cells and macrophages with brown/yellow pigment, positive for iron suggestive of hemosiderin.

22.10 Chondromyxoid Fibroma

A Rare cartilaginous, benign tumour seen in young adults, it is made of variable amounts of chondroid, myxoid, and fibrous components.

- **Key Features**
  - Second decade of life, 10–30 years
  - Male > Female
  - Skull bones—2% of the cases
  - Maxilla and mandible, sinus involvement, common
  - Radiographically, small (1–5 cm diameter), well-demarcated and scalloped, lytic lesions, occasionally with calcification, and rarely lobulated with irregular borders.
  - Tumours show a benign biological behaviour with a rare tendency to undergo malignant transformation and a 25% risk of recurrence.

- **Histopathology**

A biphasic tumour of a predominant histological pattern that completely replaces the other tissue but is well delineated from surrounding bone. Tumours with dominant fibrous tissue show collagenisation and myxoid areas with small or negligible areas of chondroid differentiation (Fig. 22.9). The tumour might show exuberant cartilage formation simulating chondroma or chondrosarcoma with lobular pattern. Myxoid car-

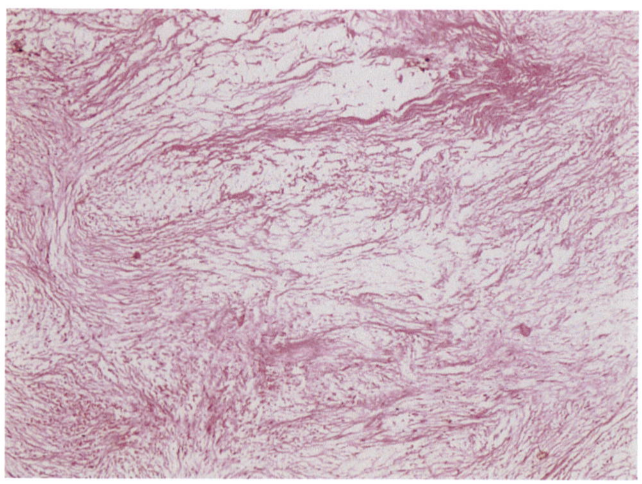

Fig. 22.9 Chondromyxoid fibroma. This photomicrograph shows dominating fibrous tissue with collagen and myxoid areas and a negligible amount of chondroid differentiation

tilaginous tissue shows pleomorphic and large cells at the periphery of the lobes. Generally, these tumours are rich in fibromyxoid stroma with small areas of cartilaginous differentiation with or without complete mineralisation. The stroma is well vascularised with small, inconspicuous capillary areas. Calcification foci in long-standing tumours and ABC-like features are seen.

22.11 Central Giant Cell Granulomas (CGCG)

Craniofacial, central giant cell granulomas (CGCG) are a non-neoplastic, solid tumour-like pathology with small tumefactions. They resemble giant cell tumours, predominantly showing fibrogenesis with new bone formation and benign giant cells. Craniofacial, central giant cell granulomas, previously considered as true tumours, are currently referred to as reactive lesions in the jaws and calvarium.

- **Key Features**
  - Adolescents and young adults
  - Female > Male, 2:1
  - Mandibular > maxillary, in the anterior quadrants of the jaw
  - Pronounced expansion of bony plates in the gnathic skeleton
  - Radiographically, radiolucent, destructive lesions with soft tissue extensions, well/poorly marginated, and uni-/multi-locular lesions with root resorption
  - Differentiating between the giant cell granuloma and giant cell tumour is vital as the latter has a higher recurrence rate and a low but possible tendency to undergo sarcomatous changes.

- **Histopathology**

The lesion shows peripheral osteoclastic activity with thin residual bone and patchy areas of reactive bone. The core tissue shows cellular fibrous stroma with plump spindle cells and uneven distribution of giant cells (Fig. 22.10). The multi-nucleated giant cells are small, located close to vascular spaces, appearing to be exiting from vessels. The stroma shows areas of haemorrhage, hemosiderin, and necrosis. Metaplastic bone formation is evident (Fig. 22.11), and myxoid differentiation is variable. The lesional tissue bears great resemblance to the giant cell tumours and the brown tumour of hyperparathyroidism.

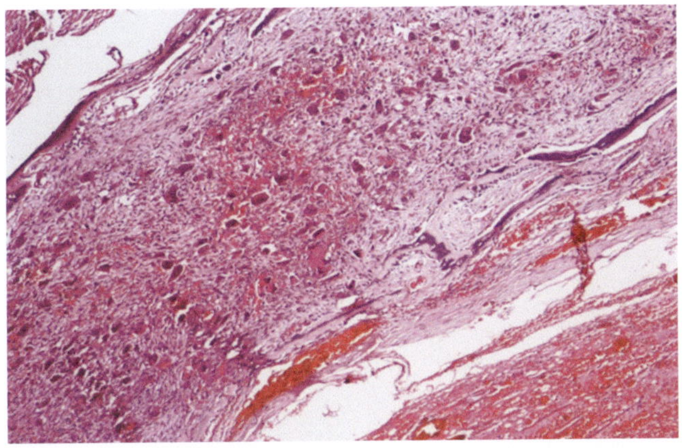

Fig. 22.10 Central giant cell granuloma. Lesional tissue showing stroma rich in giant cells and peripheral areas show reactive bone formation and a few areas of bone resorption

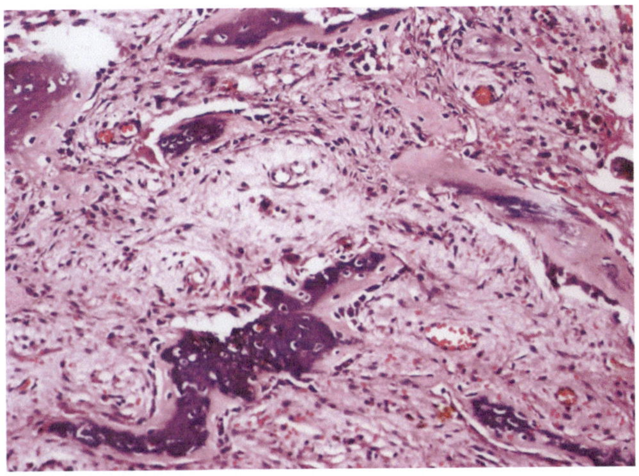

Fig. 22.11 Central giant cell granuloma shows areas of metaplastic bone formation with a few osteoblastic giant cells and congested capillaries

22.12 Giant Cell Tumour

Giant cell tumours are true, distinct tumours of undifferentiated cells that predominantly contain multi-nucleated giant cells and plump mononuclear stromal cells.

- **Key Features**
  - Osteoclastoma: true benign giant cell tumour
  - Giant cells of histiocytic origin, formed by fusion of mononuclear stromal cells
  - A malignant counterpart can metastasise
  - Female > Male, peak in third to fourth decade
  - Radiographically, radiolucent lesions are graded by Campanacci et al. as follows:

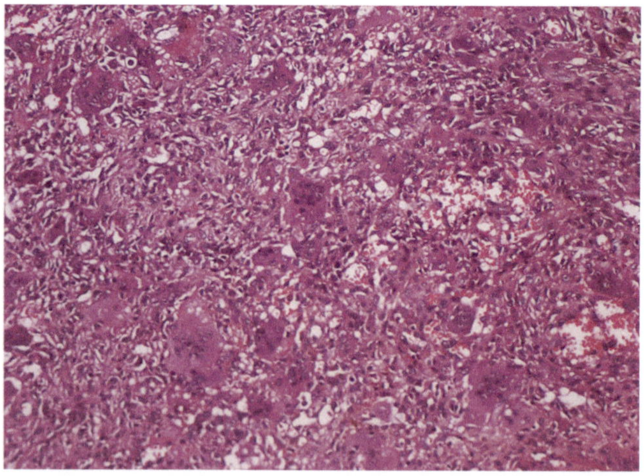

Fig. 22.12 Giant cell tumour with large giant cells showing variable size and number of nuclei; and plump mono/bi nucleated stroma cells

- Grade I—well-defined margin and a thin rim of mature bone. Intact cortex
- Grade II—well-defined tumour without a radio-opaque rim, thin limits, more expansile
- Grade III—fuzzy borders without bone limits, suggestive of aggressive tumour with invasion of soft tissues
- Occurrence: Grade I and Grade II tumours—52%, Grade III tumours—48%

Histopathology

Ill-demarcated periphery. Stromal cells are round to oval. Sometimes abundant background spindle cells are seen in between the giant cells. Cells with open-face nuclei with an ill-defined cytoplasmic border. Nuclear hyperchromasia or pleomorphism is generally absent. Mitotic activity of a varied spectrum is noted. The giant cells are evenly distributed throughout the stroma (Fig. 22.12) and contain 40–60 nuclei, which are open-faced or hyperchromatic. Small or large areas of stromal necrosis may be seen. Inflammatory cells are few, and clusters of foamy cells are common. Patches of metaplastic bone, foci of cystic change, and striking vascularity are evident in some instances. Variations in the giant cells are rare, but stromal variations are numerous. Conventionally, the stroma is cellular, prominent with oval plump cells.

22.13 Osteosarcoma

22

Osteosarcoma is a primary malignant primitive bone tumour in which the malignant cells produce osteoid or immature bone tissue ("Osteogenic"—derived from bone, producing bone).

Key Features

- Commonest primary bone malignancy next to multiple myeloma
- Aetiology: genetic, environmental factors
- Male:Female, slight male predilection, young and adolescents, spectrum: 14–80 years
- Primary tumour, younger patients
- Associated with Paget's disease, fibrous dysplasia, older patients
- During growth: common in long bones. Later, all bones equally affected
- Early symptoms—pain, insidious, transitory. Later, becomes persistent and severe
- Swelling: rubbery, firm to hard
- Cranial bones—7% cases. Rare, 6.5% arise in jaw, rarer in cranium

- Second to third decade, average 32 years
- Male > Female
- Mandible > maxilla: 1.6:1, frequent in posterior mandible and maxilla
- Destructive lesion with osteolytic/osteoblastic and sclerotic/mixed pattern
- X-ray features include periodontal ligament (PDL) widening, medullary origin with cortical destruction and periosteal reaction
- Ill-defined, radiolucent locular/non-locular destructive lesions
- Usually, mixed-radio-opaque and radiolucent. Rarely, dense opacity
- Moth-eaten/cloudy lesion with radio-opacity—very common
- Involved teeth—loss of lamina dura, periodontal destruction and tooth resorption
- Sunrise/sunburst appearance—bony spicules radiating at 90° angle from the expanded cortex
- Osteosarcoma forms the commonest primary skeletal sarcoma with 30–80% occurrence
- 20% of the tumours show lung metastasis and around 40% show distant metastasis at a later stage
- The 5-year survival rate for a local disease is around 65%, whereas for tumours with metastasis, it drops to 20%.

Histopathology

Conventional osteosarcoma is made up of oval or polygonal angular cells with prominent pleomorphic nuclei (Fig. 22.13). The tumour cells are seen to produce osteoid or bone, which is non or partially mineralised. Tumour osteoid lined by dysplastic osteogenic cells is characteristic for the diagnosis of osteosarcoma. The osteogenic cells are a part of the extracellular matrix rich in osseous, cartilaginous, or fibrous counterparts. Varying proportion of bone, cartilage formation and

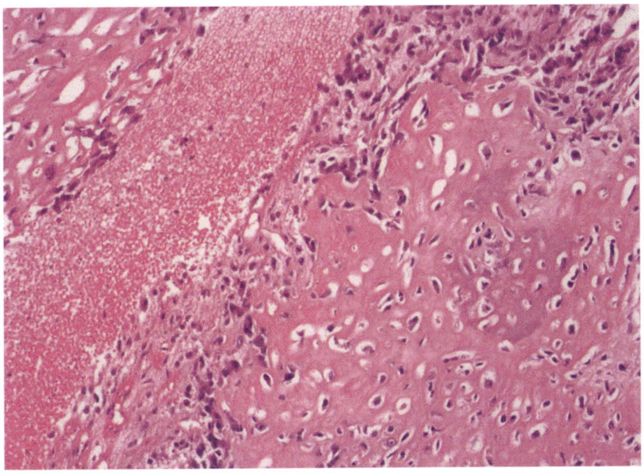

◘ Fig. 22.13 Osteosarcoma shows dysplastic bone, osteogenic cells, and tumour osteoid

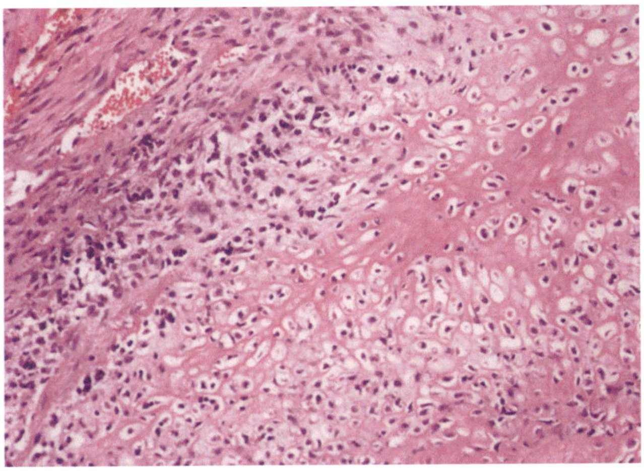

◘ Fig. 22.14 Osteogenic sarcoma shows areas of dysplastic hyaline cartilage formed by the dysplastic osteogenic cells and highly cellular hyaline cartilage with a partially mineralised matrix

rich vascularity is seen. Areas of necrosis and haemorrhage can be seen. Histological types are based on the predominant stromal differentiation. These include osteoblastic, chondroblastic (◘ Fig. 22.14), fibroblastic, mixed, and anaplastic.

22.14 Chondrosarcoma

A malignant tumour in which the basic neoplastic tissue is fully developed cartilage without tumour osteoid, formed directly by sarcomatous stroma. Myxoid changes, calcification, and ossification might be present, but no osteoid is seen.

Key Features

- Chondrosarcoma accounts for 17–22% of all primary bone tumours
- Occurs between
  - Second to sixth decade, average 40–45 years
  - Common in older age—sixth decade
- Craniofacial bones account for 9.4% of tumours: maxilla > mandible
  - Local recurrence, 20–35%
  - Radiographically, expansile large tumours with frequent calcification, multi-locular, destructive lesions with blotchy calcifications, and mottled bone
  - Core: lucent with patchy mineralisation
  - Low-grade tumours: large with surrounding bone destruction
  - High-grade tumours: more destructive with soft tissue extension
  - Teeth: periodontal widening and root resorption
  - Diagnosis relies on radiographic, clinical, and histopathological assessment, requiring the close cooperation of surgeons, radiologists, and pathologists. Evaluation of multiple sections is mandatory for confirmatory diagnosis.

Histopathology

Chondrosarcomas are large tumours with lobular/nodular arrangement. They lack a capsule but have a pseudopod appearance. The periphery of the lobular area has increased cellularity. The tumours show the presence of myxomatous areas, ossification, and cystic degeneration. Cytological evaluation of multi-nucleated tumour cells, pleomorphism and hyperchromasia are valuable for grading, but reduced cartilaginous areas and more fibro-sarcomatous areas depict high-grade variations. Myxoid chondrosarcoma shows myxoid, basophilic intercellular substance with irregular lacunae. Ossification in chondrosarcoma is generally metaplastic or endochondral ossification with the absence of malignant osteoid around the lobes at the periphery (◘ Fig. 22.15). The tumour chondrocytes have large hyperchromatic and pleomorphic nuclei with one, two or multi-nucleation. Rarely, large giant chondrocytes, ring cells with vacuolisation, and immature cartilage are seen.

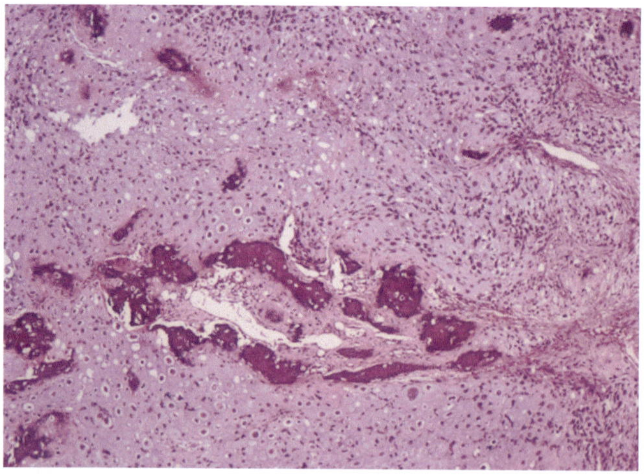

Fig. 22.15 Chondrosarcoma with abundant sheets of malignant cartilaginous tissue and foci of dysplastic bone formation. Chondrosarcoma showing large giant chondrocytes in an immature cartilaginous tissue

22.15 Ewing's Tumour

A malignant tumour of small round cells of undifferentiated mesenchymal cells-primitive neuroectodermal in origin.

Ewing's tumour is a primitive, malignant bone tumour characterised by uniform, densely packed small cells with round nuclei but without a distinct cytoplasmic border or prominent nucleoli.

- **Key Features**
- 8.64% of malignant bone tumours.
- 60–62% male predilection.
- First to second decade: account for 75% of cases.
- Mandible and skull bone involved more frequently, skull—2% and head and neck—18%.
- Radiographically, large destructive ill-defined radiolucent tumours, with resorption of involved teeth.

- **Histopathology**

An extremely cellular small round cell tumour of monotonous morphology. The cells have distinct round to oval hyperchromatic nuclei with a scanty, ill-defined cytoplasmic periphery. The cells are oval or polygonal in shape and are clustered closely in large aggregates or sheets with minimal intervening stroma (Fig. 22.16). The cell clusters or islands are separated by fibrous stroma of variable maturity. The tumour cells have an ill-defined granular cytoplasm with a prominent nucleus with a finely dispersed chromatin network. A closer look reveals a two-cell population. One population of cells is large cells with lightly stained cytoplasm and granular nucleus, whereas the other has a moderately defined cytoplasmic border with a small hyperchromatic nucleus.

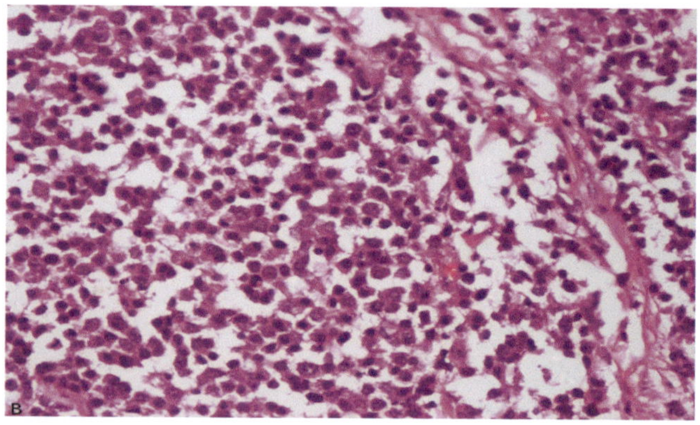

Fig. 22.16 Ewing's tumour shows aggregates of non-cohesive round cells with ill-defined cytoplasmic areas and minimal stroma

A small subset of cells might show spindling and pleomorphism. Mitotic figures are not frequent. A rich vascular stroma shows areas of necrosis and Azzopardi effect around the blood vessels. Peripheral reactive fibrosis and ossification are evident.

22.16 Malignant Lymphoma of Bone

This group of tumours encompasses a variety of non-Hodgkin's lymphomas and Hodgkin's Disease. Primary non-Hodgkin's Lymphoma occurs as a solitary bone lesion. It is a rare extra-nodal lymphoma with histopathology similar to the soft tissue counterparts.

- **Key Features**
- Primary malignant lymphomas of bone, 3.9–12.7%
- Male predominance, fifth to eighth decade common.
- Radiographically, solitary lesions are radiolucent, destructive, and ill-defined with ragged edges. Invasion into surrounding bone or soft tissue may be noted. Rarely, they are multi-locular. Core-radiolucent and lytic with patchy opacities may be present.
- The primary B-cell lymphomas encountered in the mandible have a better prognosis. All malignant lymphomas need a skeletal survey and a pertinent soft tissue evaluation. Staging is mandatory before treatment considerations.
- Myeloid sarcomas and leukaemic infiltration are more frequent in the posterior quadrant of the gnathic skeleton. Appropriate clinical, histopathological, and immunohistochemical evaluation is needed to distinguish them from lymphomas.

- **Histopathology**

The lymphomas of the jawbone are generally extranodal non-Hodgkin's lymphomas of B-cell type, diffuse

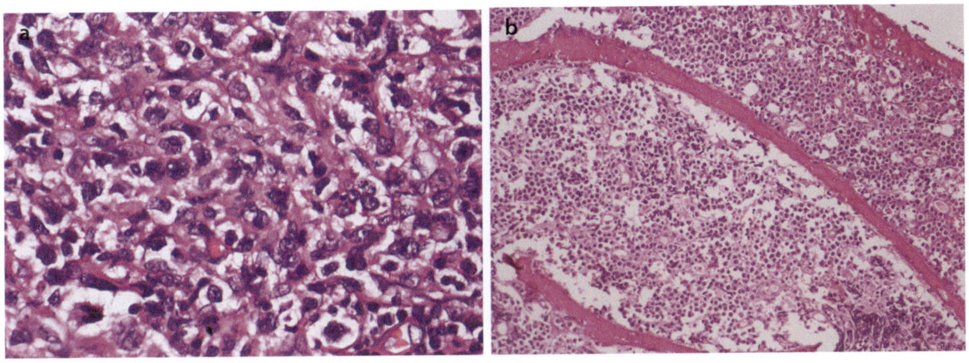

Fig. 22.17 **a** Lymphoma showing malignant lymphocytes with prominent nuclei and mitotic figures. Note large polygonal cells with hyperchromatic nuclei **b** Lymphoma showing intramedullary invasion with dysplastic lymphocytes

large B-cell lymphoma (DLBCL) being more common. Rarely they are T cell or plasmablastic. DLBCL consists of abundant cells in sheets or large clusters. The cells may be of similar morphology with well-defined nuclei and an ill-defined scanty cytoplasm. Variations in cell size, shape and nuclei with frequent multiple mitotic figures are evident (Fig. 22.17a, b). Centroblastic and immunoblastic cells are seen. The cells intend to permeate through the marrow fat, but the medullary trabeculae appear intact. Cellular areas may show crushed artefacts. Fine reticular fibrils may be seen clustering around cells where the tumour cells form small, large islands and strands simulating a filigree pattern. The dysplastic lymphoma cells permeate in a classical sieve-like pattern through adipocytes and show vascular and neural invasion.

Hodgkin's lymphomas are rare. They show the presence of classic Reed-Sternberg cells in a background of variable mixed inflammatory cell infiltrate consisting of eosinophils, histiocytes, neutrophilic mature granulocytes, and plasma cells.

Burkitt's tumour consists of large lymphocytic cells with a basophilic cytoplasm (pyroninophilic) of B-cell origin in the gnathic skeleton. These cells are intervened by large tangible body histiocytes, giving the tumour a starry sky appearance. The cells may show lipid droplets and display sudanophilic (lipid special stain) nature.

22.17 Multiple Myeloma

Multiple myeloma is a neoplasm of plasma cells disseminated in multiple intra-osseous sites. It is often associated with anaemia, hypercalcaemia, and renal dysfunction and is rarely associated with amyloid deposition, derangement of coagulation, cryo-globinemia and elevated serum viscosity.

Key Features

- Haematopoietic, primary neoplasm of bone with involvement of bone marrow by plasma cells like tumour cells of varying differentiation
- A multi-centric neoplasm
- 80% of solitary extra-medullary plasmacytoma occur in oral and upper airways
- 14.9% are malignant bone tumours
- Male > Female, sixth to seventh decade
- Radiographically, the tumour is noted in the skull, ribs, vertebrae and pelvis. Punched out, well-defined lucent areas. Destructive, osteoporotic areas of varying dimensions, but no sclerotic borders. 1/3rd of multiple myeloma patients have gnathic lesions, and 30% are initial pathological presentations. Solitary gnathic lesions are lytic, expanding cortical plates. Multiple lesions coalesce to form multi-locular areas.

Histopathology

Rich cellular patterns are made up of predominantly non-cohesive cells but are clustered together in small areas that finally form large, monotonous, sheet patterns with scanty intercellular stroma (Fig. 22.18a). The cells are classically non-cohesive myeloid cells, and their morphology is similar to plasma cells with clock-faced (or cartwheel morphology) arrangement (Fig. 22.18b). The cells are oval to round, with an indistinct cell outline and an eccentrically placed round or oval monotonous nucleus that appears granular and basophilic. The sparse investing stroma is delicate, consisting of reticulin meshwork, fibrous septa, thin-walled blood vessels, areas of haemorrhage and rare necrosis.

Well-differentiated cells unmistakably have similarities to plasma cells. Multiple nuclei or pleomorphic nuclei are seen in only a few instances. Most tumours are better differentiated, showing monotonous cells with

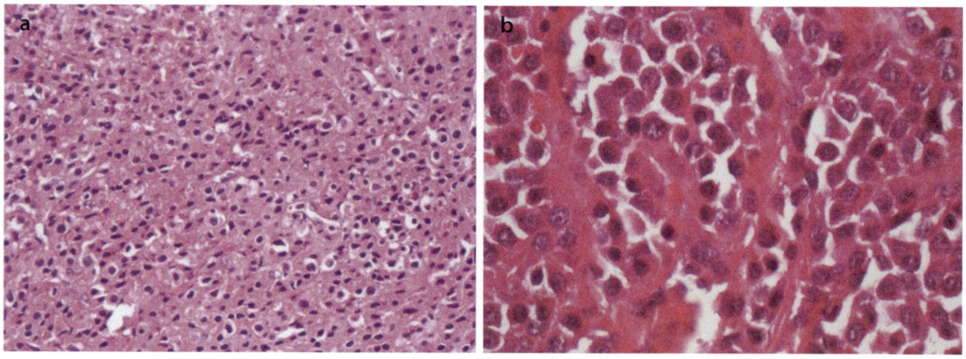

Fig. 22.18 **a** Multiple myeloma. Tumour cells show indistinct cell borders and round to oval distinct hyperchromatic nuclei. **b** Multiple myeloma. Non-cohesive myeloid tumour cells scattered with prominent nuclei show a clock-faced arrangement in some tumour cells similar to plasma cells

multiple nucleoli and clumped chromatin. Well-differentiated tumours have few mitotic figures and are well-vascularised. Poorly or undifferentiated tumours show bizarre anaplastic cells, giant cells, and cells with hyperchromatic large nuclei—may be grooved or lobulated, with the presence of mitotic figures. The mild pleomorphism of the plasma cells with few mitoses speaks of a moderate differentiation. Around 10% of cases show variable amyloid deposition. A monoclonal growth pattern with kappa or lambda light chains should be established for diagnosis. This disease needs detailed clinical and skeletal evaluation and follow-up to monitor treatment and prognosis.

22.18 Solitary Plasmacytoma (SP)

Solitary plasmacytoma (SP) is a rare disease characterised by a localised proliferation of neoplastic monoclonal plasma cells without evidence of systemic disease.

Key Features

- Solitary plasmacytoma of the jaw is rare.
- SP of the jawbone includes localised pain in the jaws and teeth, paresthesia, swelling, soft tissue masses, tooth mobility and migration, haemorrhage, and pathological fracture.
- Fatigue and fever are the most common systemic symptoms.
- A diagnosis of solitary plasmacytomas carries a threat of prelude to multiple myeloma in most cases. Hence, long-term follow-up and evaluation become significant to reign in the disease.

22

Histopathology

Plasmacytomas are histopathologically similar to multiple myelomas. Solitary lesions, ideally, show varying degrees of differentiation of plasma or myeloid cells. The amount of necrosis and amyloid formation mildly varies from multiple myeloma.

22.19 Melanotic Neuroectodermal Tumour of Infancy (MNTI)

Melanotic neuroectodermal tumour of infancy (MNTI) is a rapidly growing benign tumour arising from the neural crest cells.

Key Features

- A tumour in infancy and a small percentage of older children. Male > Female
- 90%—head and neck, 80%—maxilla
- Other sites: mandible < skull
- Metastasising tumours: 5%
- Rapidly growing blue-black or normal mucosal colour tumours in the maxilla
- Radiographically: large destructive, expansile, uni-/multi-locular lesions, cortical plate expansion, and displaced teeth with resorption in the jaw
- A benign but rapidly growing tumour which requires good evaluation for diagnosis and a detailed IHC evaluation for consideration of diagnosis and prognosis.

Histopathology

The tumour shows mature fibrous stroma with multiple small, medium-sized islands of tumour cells with few vessels. The islands are made of small, dark, round to oval cells (Fig. 22.19a), which may show a delicate eosinophilic neuropil or fibrils around the cells. Mature large polygonal cells with granular cytoplasm are seen. Some cells might show melanocytic differentiation with

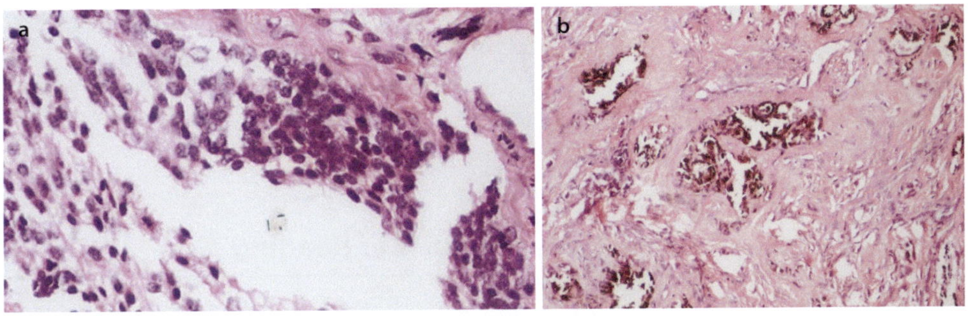

Fig. 22.19 **a** Melanotic neuroectodermal tumour of infancy showing round to oval tumour cells with dark hyperchromatic nucleus. **b** Melanotic neuroectodermal tumour of infancy showing tumour cells exhibiting melanotic differentiation and melanin pigment

the presence of melanin pigment of a variable quantity (Fig. 22.19b). Tumour cells may be in an alveolar or pseudo-glandular pattern. Melanin-rich tumours histopathologically show brown colour deposits and clinically appear as pigmented tumours. The small cells are taught to be of neuroblastic origin, and the larger cells are of melanocytic epithelioid origin. A variable number of mitotic figures are seen. Pleomorphic cells or necrosis are rare. Destruction of bone is noted at the periphery.

22.20 Metastatic Tumours

22.20.1 Metastatic Deposits

In the craniofacial skeleton, metastatic deposits from distant primary are not uncommon and account for 1% of all tumours. Around 30% of cases are the first presentation of the disease/tumour. 80%—posterior mandible. 5% cases—involvement of multiple sites.

Metastatic carcinomas may look very similar to a destructive primary malignant tumour of bone. They are frequently encountered in the posterior mandible and maxilla.

- **Key Features**

- Male = Female
- Fifth to eighth decade of life
- Early pain, expansion of bone, paresthesia
- Gender-specific tumours: Female: breast, adrenals, uterine, thyroid. Male: lung, prostate, kidney.
- Radiographically, lytic, destructive lesions with irregular, ragged borders, often with extension in soft tissue and indistinct radio-opacities: prostate and breast cancer
- The primary tumour types differ dramatically between the genders though carry the same message of widespread disease and dissemination. Frequently, they are in the form of carcinomas rather than sarcomas associated with mandibular posterior quadrants.

- **Histopathology**

In the gnathic skeleton, metastatic carcinomas are rare. They form an interesting spectrum of tumours of two sets. One set of metastatic carcinomas shows a classic picture of the primary tumour, the parent cell or organ type forming a common pattern as in the case of thyroid carcinoma, clear cell carcinoma, etc. The other set of metastatic deposits show anaplastic cells and unusual patterns. This suggests a possible primary tumour that needs definitive confirmation with newer techniques, as in the case of adenocarcinomas, frequently.

A small population of sarcoma/carcinoma can present as a spindle cell population, which is plump with a variety of dysplastic bone formations. Rarely, sarcomas are seen as metastatic deposits with a spectrum ranging from well-differentiated cells to pleomorphic cells. Good examples of mesenchymal well-differentiated spindle cell sarcoma are fibrosarcoma, synovial sarcoma, and leiomyosarcoma. Some sarcomas are seen as pleomorphic deposits of unknown origin.

22.21 Diagnostic Markers for Non-odontogenic Tumours of the Jaws: Immunohistochemistry (IHC)

The role of immunohistochemistry in the diagnosis of non-odontogenic tumours has a complete spectrum of relevance. On one end of the spectrum are the non-haematolymphoid bone tumours, where haematoxylin and eosin diagnosis give a much clearer picture, and the role of IHC remains meagre. On the other end are the hemato-lymphoid bone tumours like lymphomas, where IHC holds the mainstay of diagnosis.

22.22 Summary

Compilation of the various bone tumours with histopathology allows better correlation for diagnosis and for allotment of connotations of variants and variations. A detailed histopathologic presentation, along with molecular changes, depicts the tumour at the cellular level of differentiation to the pattern in the tissue it generates, elucidating tumour behaviour. This forms the basis of tumour pathology in bone and mesenchymal tumours arising in bone.

■■ Acknowledgements

The authors wish to thank the following colleagues for their advice and kind support during the preparation of this chapter.

1. Dr. Suchitra Gosavi, MDS, Retired Professor & HOD, Department of Oral Pathology, Government Dental College, Nagpur, India.
2. Dr. Abhay. Datarkar, MDS, DNB, Dean & Professor, Department of Oral & Maxillofacial Surgery, Government Dental College and Hospital, Nagpur, India.
3. Dr. Surya Narayan Das, MDS, Professor & HOD, Department of Oral and Maxillofacial Pathology, SCB Dental College, Cuttack, India.
4. Dr. Soumya Makarla, MDS, Diagnostic Pathologist, Care Oral Pathology Services (COPS), Bangalore, India.
5. Dr. Satyajit S Topajiche, MDS, Diagnostic Pathologist, Care Oral Pathology Services (COPS), Bangalore, India.
6. Dr. Naval Khan, MDS, Oral Pathologist, Srinagar, India.
7. Dr. Balasubramaniam Kumar, MDS, Oral & Maxillofacial Surgeon, Bangalore, India.
8. Dr. Anjan Shah, MDS, Oral & Maxillofacial Surgeon, Bangalore, India
9. Dr. Sanjiv Nair, MDS, Oral & Maxillofacial Surgeon, Bangalore, India.
10. Dr. Reshma V, MDS, Oral Pathologist, Bangalore, India.

Further Reading

Barnes L, editor. Surgical pathology of head and neck, vol. 2. 3rd ed. Informa Healthcare: Pittsburgh; 2009.

Bertin H, Gomez-Brouchet A, Rédini F. Osteosarcoma of the jaws: an overview of the pathophysiological mechanisms. Crit Rev. Oncol Hematol. 2020;156:1–9. https://doi.org/10.1016/j.critrevonc.2020.103126.

Czerniak B. Dorfman and Czernialis's bone tumours. 2nd ed. Amsterdam: Imprint: Elsevier Ltd; 2015.

Dyalram D, Aslam-Pervez N, Lubek JE. Nonodontogenic tumors of the jaws. Oral Maxillofac Surg Clin North Am. 2016;28(1):59–65. https://doi.org/10.1016/j.coms.2015.08.002.

Huvos AG. Bone tumours—diagnosis, treatment and prognosis. 2nd ed. Philadelphia: W.B. Saunders Company; 1991.

Klein MJ, Siegal GP. Osteosarcoma: anatomic and histologic variants. Am J Clin Pathol. 2006;125(4):555–81.

Lam SW, Ijzendoorn DGP, Cleton-Jansen AM, Szuhai K, Bovée JVMG. Molecular pathology of bone tumors. J Mol Diagn. 2019;21(2):171–82.

Lichtenstein L. Bone tumours. 4th ed. C.V. Saint Louis: Mosby Company; 1972.

Liu K, Gao Y, Han J, Han X, Shi Y, Liu C, et al. Diffuse large B-cell lymphoma of the mandible diagnosed by metagenomic sequencing: a case report. Front Med (Lausanne). 2021;23(8):1–5. https://doi.org/10.3389/fmed.2021.752523.

Paulos J, Poitout DG, Bone tumours. Diagnosis & therapy today. 1st ed. London: Springer Publications; 2021.

Rothzerg E, Xu J, Wood D. Different subtypes of osteosarcoma: histopathological patterns and clinical behaviour J. Mol Pathol. 2023;4(2):99–10.

Thompson LDR. Head and neck pathology—a volume in series foundations in diagnostic pathology. 2nd ed. Philadelphia: Elsevier; 2013.

Unni KK, Inwards CY, editors. Dahlin's bone tumours. 6th ed. Philadelphia: Wolters Kluwer, Lippincott Williams & Wilkins; 2010.

Histopathology of Non-Neoplastic Jawbone Lesions

Yeshwant Rawal

Contents

S R Prabhu et al. (eds.), *Oral Histology and Oral Histopathology*, https://doi.org/10.1007/978-3-031-77481-2_23

23.1 Introduction

Non-neoplastic lesions of the jawbones are a diverse group of conditions, including reactive lesions, infection of the bone and marrow, and jawbone manifestations of systemic disease such as hyperparathyroidism and fibro-osseous lesions. Many of these conditions are present near the teeth and mimic tooth-related pathologies. Suppurative osteomyelitis is a result of uncontrolled dental or periodontal infection. Lesions like cherubism and cemento-osseous dysplasia are unique to the jawbones. While in most cases, the diagnosis is based on clinical and radiographic findings; a biopsy may be required to arrive at a correct diagnosis in conditions such as brown tumour of hyperparathyroidism and aneurysmal bone cyst.

23.2 Classification

Non-neoplastic lesions of the jawbones may be classified as follows.

23.2.1 Reactive Lesions

- Condensing osteitis **(focal sclerosing osteomyelitis)**
- Idiopathic osteosclerosis

23.2.2 Osteomyelitis

- Acute suppurative osteomyelitis
- Chronic suppurative osteomyelitis
- Chronic non-bacterial osteomyelitis (CNO)

23.2.3 Giant Cell Lesions

- Brown Tumour of Hyperparathyroidism
- Cherubism
- Aneurysmal Bone Cyst

23.2.4 Fibro-Osseous Lesions

- Fibrous dysplasia
- Cemento-osseous dysplasia

23.3 Condensing Osteitis (Focal Sclerosing Osteomyelitis)

Condensing osteitis is a reactive bone condition intimately associated with the roots of a pulp inflamed or non-vital tooth.

- **Key Features**
- Condensing osteitis is mostly asymptomatic and an incidental finding.
- Dull pain related to pulpal inflammation may be present.
- Patients are young, and the affected mandibular molar teeth are not vital.
- On radiographs, condensing osteitis presents as an area of sclerotic bone surrounding and cupping the apex of the affected tooth root/s. The margins of the sclerotic bone are not well defined. The periodontal membrane space around the apex may show some widening.

- **Histopathology**

Usually, a biopsy is not required to establish a diagnosis. However, when biopsied, the tissue consists of dense, vital, lamellated bone with scant fibrofatty marrow and mild chronic inflammation.

23.4 Idiopathic Osteosclerosis

Idiopathic osteosclerosis is a non-neoplastic, reactive bone condition that is also referred to as a dense bone island, bone scar and enostosis. The aetiology is not known and therefore the term idiopathic.

- **Key Features**
- It is seen in the mandible in young adults.
- The teeth in the vicinity of the area of osteosclerosis are vital and the periodontal membrane space is unaffected.
- The bone condition is asymptomatic and is diagnosed as an incidental finding on radiographs with no associated jawbone enlargement.
- The area of bone sclerosis is encountered between and around the roots of molar and premolar teeth in the mandible. The area of sclerosis may or may not show defined boundaries.
- The size of the lesion can vary over time with physiologic remodelling of bone.

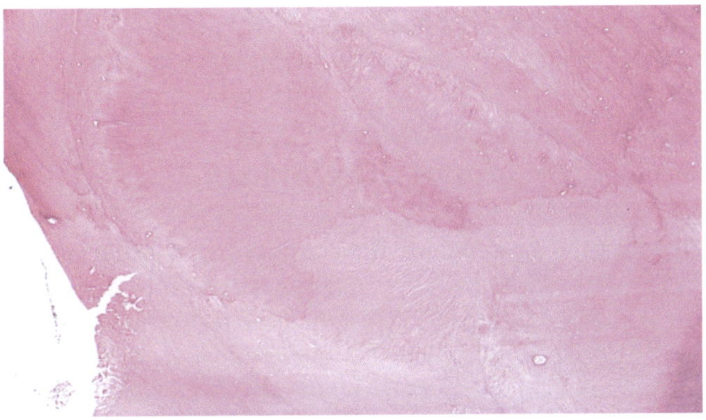

Fig. 23.1 A lesion of Idiopathic Osteosclerosis that shows dense bone encircling a fragment of dentin. H & E decalcified section, 10×

Histopathology

A diagnosis of idiopathic osteosclerosis is an incidental finding on radiographs. A biopsy is not required. However, if a biopsy is submitted, the tissue shows dense, vital, lamellated bone with scant fibrofatty marrow. In a handful of biopsies of idiopathic osteosclerosis reviewed by this author, the dense bone was seen fused with fragments of dentin (Fig. 23.1).

23.5 Osteomyelitis

23.5.1 Bacterial/Suppurative Osteomyelitis

Osteomyelitis is an inflammatory condition of the bone and marrow. While it may affect any bone, it is more common in the jawbones, with most cases affecting the mandible. In contrast to the maxilla, the mandible's bone is more compact and has a limited single blood supply, which lowers its resistance to infection. Most cases of jawbone osteomyelitis are bacterial infections with suppuration.

Key Features

- The anatomy of the jawbones with embedded tooth roots and the common occurrence of dental infections such as periapical abscesses and periodontal inflammation, infections from fracture lines, peri-implantitis, infections following surgical bone exposure, infections following medication, and radiation-associated bone necrosis are all reasons for the higher incidence of osteomyelitis in the jawbones.
- Other factors such as diabetes, sickle cell anaemia, malnutrition states, chronic systemic infectious diseases, tobacco, alcohol and drug use, and the local condition florid cemental dysplasia also contribute to a higher incidence of osteomyelitis in the jawbones.
- The causative organisms may include enteric rods, staphylococci, and oral anaerobes such as *Fusobacterium, Porphyromonas, Prevotella, Eikenella,* and actinomycetes.
- *Acute suppurative osteomyelitis* is the result of a rapidly spreading infection with little to no response from the host tissue to the inflammation in the bone and marrow spaces.
  - Patients present with severe pain, tenderness, swelling, fever, lymphadenopathy, and leukocytosis.
  - Early lesions may show no radiographic changes. This may progress to vague bone destruction, loss of lamina dura, and widened periodontal ligament space. Further bone involvement will result in the separation of fragments of necrotic bone, known as a sequestrum.
- *Chronic suppurative osteomyelitis* is the result of the persistence of the infection, or it may arise de novo.
  - Patients present with painful swelling, tenderness, sinus formation with purulent discharge, mobility and exfoliation of teeth, exposure and exfoliation of sequestra, pathological fractures, and paresthesia of the lower lip.
  - The bone shows a characteristic moth-eaten appearance with ragged, patchy radiolucencies mixed with radio-dense areas. Sequestrae of varying sizes surrounded by patchy osteolysis may be noted. Periosteal stimulation may trigger cortical duplication with new bone, resulting in an onion-peel-like appearance.

Histopathology

Acute Suppurative Osteomyelitis: Non-vital bone fragments with empty osteocytic lacuna are surrounded by dense neutrophilic infiltration and necrotic debris. The bone fragments show irregular peripheral resorption that may be colonised by bacteria.

Chronic Suppurative Osteomyelitis: The non-vital bone fragments are mixed with larger amounts of fibrocellular soft tissue. The bone fragments show an irregular periphery and empty osteocytic lacuna (Fig. 23.2). The fibrocellular soft tissue shows mixed acute and chronic inflammation with scattered neutrophilic abscesses.

23.5.2 Chronic Non-bacterial Osteomyelitis

Chronic non-bacterial osteomyelitis (CNO), also known as primary diffuse sclerosing osteomyelitis, is not associated with a bacterial infection. Most cases of this condition are seen in females less than 20 years of age.

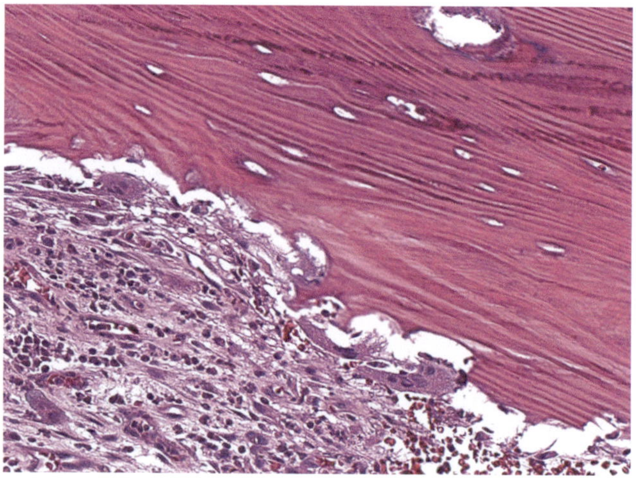

Fig. 23.2 Chronic suppurative osteomyelitis: The photomicrograph shows bone fragments with an irregular periphery and empty osteocytic lacuna

- **Key Features**

- Patients present with pain, trismus, swelling, and fever that is unresponsive to antibiotics.
- Mandibular involvement is also accompanied by clavicular, long bone, joint, and vertebral disease.
- Inflammatory bowel disease and cutaneous lesions such as pustules of the palms and soles of the feet, psoriasis, and acne may also be seen. These various clinical manifestations of CNO are closely related to the **S**ynovitis, **A**cne, **P**ustulosis, **H**yperostosis, and **O**steitis (SAPHO) syndrome.
- Radiographs show a diffuse expansion of the mandible with sclerosis to a ground-glass-like appearance. Focal radiolucencies secondary to bone loss may also be noted.
- Laboratory findings include elevated levels of the erythrocyte sedimentation rate (ESR) and the acute phase C-reactive protein. White blood cell counts are, however, within normal limits.

- **Histopathology**

These are best recognised in large bone samples and include parallel to intersecting trabeculae of bone with copious amounts of medullary fibrosis with little to no chronic inflammation. The trabeculae consist of woven bone lined by osteoblasts and contain plump osteocytes. Smaller biopsies with curvilinear bone and marrow fibrosis may be mistaken for fibrous dysplasia.

23.6 Giant Cell Lesions

23.6.1 Brown Tumour of Hyperparathyroidism

Brown tumour is one of the changes in the bone associated with primary hyperparathyroidism. The term derives its name from the brown appearance of the biopsied tissue because of the accumulation of copious amounts of haemoglobin and hemosiderin secondary to red cell exocytosis in the tissue.

- **Key Features**

- Brown tumours may present as either solitary unilocular, multi-locular, or multiple areas of radiolucency with variable degrees of painless cortical expansion.
- Many bones may be affected.

- **Histopathology**

Brown tumour of hyperparathyroidism is identical in its microscopic features to the central giant cell granuloma of bone. It is characterised by the presence of well-vascularised fibrocellular connective tissue with abundant foreign-body type multi-nucleated giant cells that resemble osteoclasts (Fig. 23.3). Red cell exocytosis is plentiful.

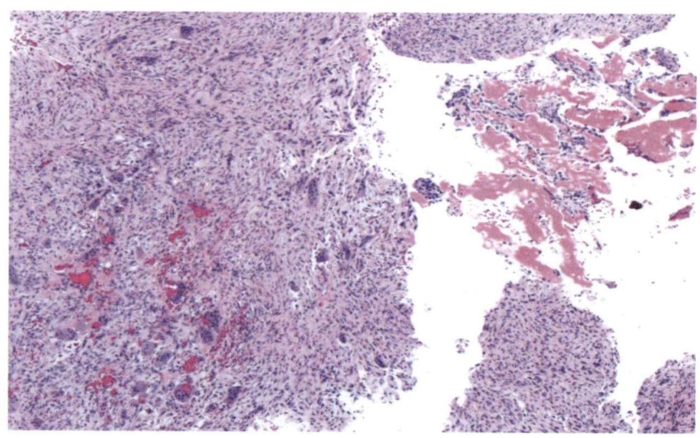

Fig. 23.3 Brown tumour of hyperthyroidism. Note well-vascularised fibrocellular connective tissue with abundant multi-nucleated giant cells

23.6.2 Cherubism

Cherubism is an inherited condition that selectively affects the jawbones. Rare cases with rib involvement have been reported. The name of the condition Cherubism refers to the facial appearance of patients, that resembles cherubs.

Key Features

- It is transmitted as an autosomal dominant condition with sporadic cases representing new mutations.
- The most common cause is a mutation of the *SH3BP2* gene on chromosome 4p16, the product of which increases osteoclastic function with resultant osteolytic lesions. Increased levels of macrophage tumour necrosis factor alpha (TNF-α) suggest a role of inflammation as well.
- Cases of cherubism are seen in the first two decades of life. There is a slight male predilection. A family history of the condition is present in over two-thirds of cases.
- Patients present with an expansile fullness of the face due to a painless swelling of the posterior mandible.
- The presentation is mostly bilateral, but sporadic unilateral cases have also been reported.
- Maxillary bone involvement results in some upward rotation of the eyeball.
- Jawbone involvement causes delayed eruption, migration, and loosening and premature loss of teeth.
- Patients have trouble in oral functions such as mastication and speech.
- Radiographic presentation is of multi-loculated radiolucencies of the body and ramus of the mandible. Involvement of the posterior maxilla is identical. Teeth appear to be displaced towards the anterior portions of the jawbones.
- Missing teeth, root resorption, taurodontism, and teeth with hypercementosis have all been reported.
- Serum alkaline phosphatase levels may be elevated during periods of active bone remodelling.
- The condition stabilises after the second decade of life and appears to regress.

Histopathology

A biopsy from the radiolucencies shows vascularised and haemorrhagic fibrous tissue with clusters of a foreign body or osteoclast-like multi-nucleated giant cells ◘ Fig. 23.4). Small blood vessels show a perivascular zone of hyalinisation (◘ Fig. 23.5).

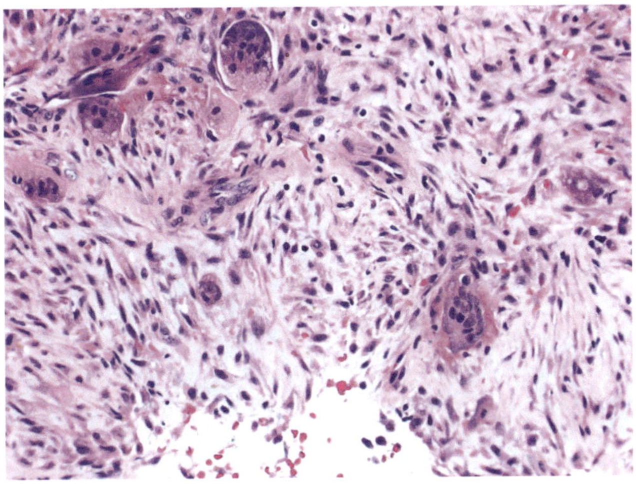

◘ **Fig. 23.4** Cherubism. Photomicrograph shows fibrous tissue with clusters of a foreign body or osteoclast-like multi-nucleated giant cells

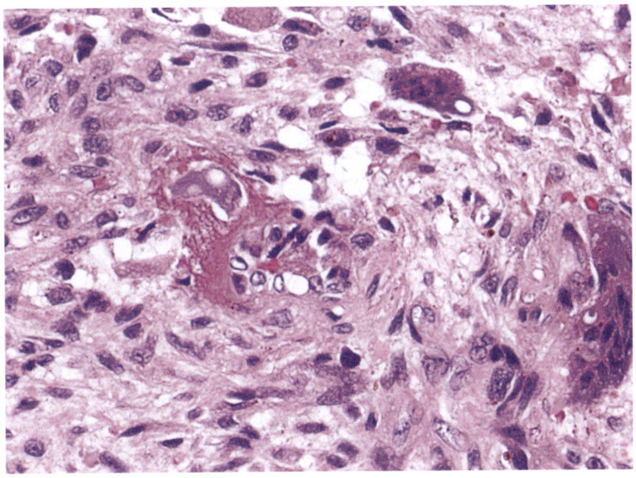

◘ **Fig. 23.5** Cherubism. Small blood vessels show a perivascular zone of hyalinisation

23.6.3 Aneurysmal Bone Cyst

This is a pseudo cystic locally destructive cavitation that affects the long bones. Up to 2% of cases are seen in the jawbones. Aneurysmal bone cysts of the jawbones may occur as primary lesions or may be associated with other conditions of the jawbones such as fibrous dysplasia, ossifying fibroma, osteoblastoma, and central giant cell granuloma.

Key Features

- Primary aneurysmal bone cysts have shown gene rearrangements with upregulation of the ubiquitin-

specific protease 6 (*USP6*) oncogene on chromosome 17p13 with the most common translocation t(16;17)(q22;p13) with the cadherin 11 gene (*CDH11*).
- Aneurysmal bone cysts associated with other jawbone conditions do not express such genetic abnormalities and are thought to arise due to altered haemodynamics within the lesional tissue.
- While long bone lesions are noted below 30 years of age, jawbone aneurysmal bone cysts present by the second decade of life. There is a slight female predilection.
- Patients present with a variably painful jawbone expansion that affects the mandible predominantly. The body, angle and ramus are affected more commonly.
- Maxillary lesions expand to affect the sinus, nose (obstruction) and eyes (proptosis and double vision).
- The aneurysmal bone cyst presents as a well-circumscribed, multi-locular expansile radiolucency with a sclerotic periphery and fine intralesional bony septa. Cortical thinning and perforation may be noted in larger lesions. Unilocular lesions may also be seen.
- Aneurysmal bone cysts in association with other jawbone lesions will show features of the associated pathology with areas of cavitation.

■ **Histopathology**

The biopsied tissue shows multiple cyst-like spaces surrounded by well-vascularised, loose connective tissue that resembles granulation tissue due to the presence of plump fibroblasts and foreign body type multi-nucleated giant cells. Intralesional haemorrhage is copious. The giant cells are seen approximating pseudocyst-like spaces. Reactive and fragments of residual host bone may also be seen. Immunohistochemical and gene rearrangement studies locate the genetic abnormality to the stromal fibroblasts.

23.7 Fibro-Osseous Lesions

Fibro-osseous lesions are a diverse group of bone-altering conditions. The term itself is non-specific and indicates any process that results in the destruction of host bone followed by its replacement with variably cellular fibrous connective tissue that eventually also demonstrates the formation of hard tissue. In this context, therefore, many authors include reactive, developmental, hamartomatous, metabolic, and neoplastic lesions. We will limit the scope of this chapter to fibrous dysplasia and cemento-osseous dysplasia.

23.7.1 Fibrous Dysplasia

Fibrous dysplasia is a bone condition resulting from a sporadic postzygotic mutation of the *GNAS* gene on chromosome 20. The GNAS gene helps stimulate the activity of an enzyme called adenylate cyclase, which is believed to play a key role in signalling pathways that help regulate the development of bone. Adenylate cyclase is also involved in controlling the production of several hormones that help regulate the activity of endocrine glands such as the thyroid, pituitary gland, ovaries, testes (gonads), and adrenal glands.

If the mutation occurs during the early postzygotic period, the effect is widespread due to the presence of pluripotent stem cells. This results in polyostotic disease with the involvement of multiple bones, endocrine glands, melanocytes, etc. If the mutation were to happen later, the result would be monostotic disease alone.

23.7.2 Monostotic Fibrous Dysplasia

■ **Key Features**

- Patients with monostotic fibrous dysplasia exhibit single-bone involvement in 80% of cases. The bone involved may be the jawbones, ribs, femur, or the tibia.
- Jawbone disease is more common in the maxilla.
- There is no gender predilection, and the condition presents itself in the second and third decades of life mostly.
- Jawbone expansion is slow and painless. Teeth may be displaced with resulting malocclusion.
- Lesions of the maxilla, by contiguity of structures may involve the zygoma, sphenoid, ethmoid, frontal, temporal and occipital bones. This extension is called **craniofacial fibrous dysplasia.**
- Facial asymmetry and disfigurement are proportionate to the bone involvement

23.7.3 Polyostotic Fibrous Dysplasia

■ **Key Features**

- Patients with polyostotic disease are younger than those with monostotic disease and mostly under 10 years of age. There is also a female predilection for this condition.
- Up to 75% of the bones of the skeleton may be affected, including the jawbones, craniofacial bones, long bones, and those of the pelvic girdle.

- Bone disease results in pain, pathological fractures, and growth abnormalities such as shortened and bowed limbs.
- Craniofacial features are like craniofacial fibrous dysplasia and include significant facial asymmetry, displaced teeth with malocclusion, altered vision and hearing, and progressive airway compromise.
- Patients with polyostotic fibrous dysplasia show involvement of other tissue and this clinical presentation is of two types: McCune-Albright syndrome and Mazabraud syndrome.

23.7.4 McCune–Albright Syndrome

- McCune-Albright syndrome is characterised by a complex of polyostotic fibrous dysplasia, *café au lait* macular pigmentation of the skin, and endocrinopathies.
- The most common of the endocrinopathies produce precocious puberty in females with early menstrual bleeding and breast and pubic hair development as early as 1 year of life.
- Other endocrinopathies include hyperfunction of the thyroid, parathyroid, adrenal, and pituitary glands.

23.7.5 Mazabraud Syndrome

- Mazabraud syndrome is a form of polyostotic fibrous dysplasia in which patients develop intramuscular myxomatous tumours, in addition to macular pigmentation and endocrine disturbances.
- Routine X-rays show bone expansion with a ground-glass-like appearance.
- Lesional bone appears to blend in with the surrounding bone.
- Progressive loss of lamina dura is noted.
- Some lesions may show a mixed radiolucent and radiopaque appearance.
- Computed tomography may show better delineation of lesional tissue and presence of simple bone cyst-like radiolucencies.
- Long bone radiographs of the femur may show the characteristic shepherd's crook deformity (coxa vara) of the proximal neck.
- The disease stabilises at skeletal maturity.

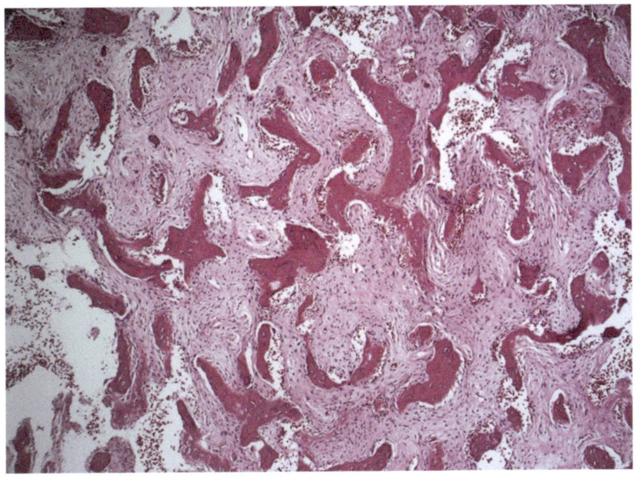

Fig. 23.6 Photomicrograph showing the delicate curvilinear woven bone of fibrous dysplasia. The trabeculae are set in a fibrocollagenous stroma that exhibits a retraction artefact from the bone

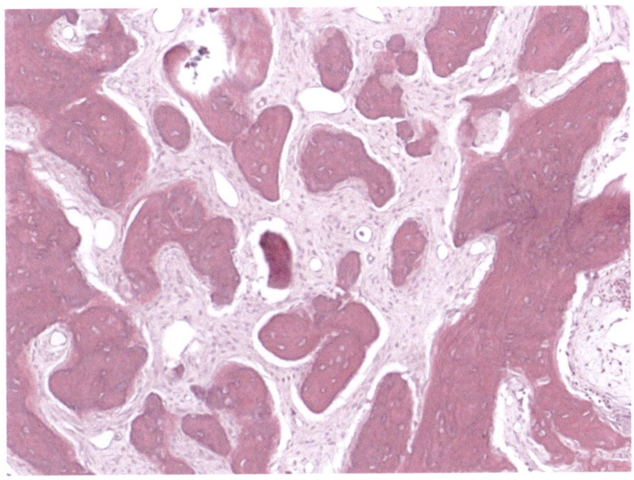

Fig. 23.7 As the lesion matures, the bone trabeculae broaden and exhibit lamellations. The cellularity reduces in the fibrocollagenous tissue. The interphase between the bone trabeculae and fibrocollagenous tissue is replaced by a retraction artifact. H & E decalcified section, 10X

Histopathology

Histopathological features of fibrous dysplasia can vary depending on the age of the lesion. The two tissues that comprise the lesion include fibrocellular connective tissue and bone. The former consists of spindle and plump cells within a collagenous stroma with little inflammation. In the early stages of the lesion, the mineralised component is in the form of irregular trabeculae of woven bone. These eventually exhibit a curvilinear outline resembling the alphabets C, U or Y (Figs. 23.6 and 23.7). While some areas may show osteoblastic rimming, this is not a uniform feature. As the lesion matures, the bone trabeculae broaden and exhibit lamellations. The cellularity reduces in the fibrocollagenous tissue. The interphase between the bone trabeculae and fibrocollagenous tissue is replaced by a retraction artefact. Occasional osteoclast-like giant cells and basophilic cementum-like masses may be seen. Lesional tissue merges with surrounding bone in the absence of a collagenous capsule.

23.7.6 Cemento-Osseous Dysplasia

Cemento-osseous dysplasia is the most common fibro-osseous lesion to affect the jawbones. The cause of cemento-osseous dysplasia is not known. Based on the extent and area of involvement, cemento-osseous dysplasia is classified into the following three categories. Focal cemento-osseous dysplasia, periapical cemento-osseous dysplasia, and florid cemento-osseous dysplasia.

Key Features

- All forms of cemento-osseous dysplasia share some common features. These bone conditions are most prevalent in middle-aged women of African and East Asian descent.
- Focal cemento-osseous dysplasia affects the posterior mandible.
  - It is asymptomatic and is diagnosed as an incidental finding.
- Periapical cemento-osseous dysplasia is mostly detected in the vicinity of the roots of the mandibular anterior teeth.
  - The teeth test is vital.
  - The lesions are asymptomatic and are identified as an incidental finding.
- Florid cemento-osseous dysplasia presents in multiple quadrants of the jaws including that of the maxilla.
  - Although most lesions are asymptomatic and diagnosed as an incidental finding, some cases may show bone expansion and present with dull pain.
  - Rarely, sequestration and exposure of the rough-surfaced, yellowish cemento-osseous masses may be encountered.
- Focal cemento-osseous dysplasia may present as an entirely radiolucent lesion of the mandibular posterior alveolar bone.
  - More commonly, the lesion is mixed with an opaque centre surrounded by a thin radiolucent rim that is surrounded by a sclerotic margin.
  - A focal lesion may be the first sign of florid disease.
- Periapical cemento-osseous dysplasia presents as multiple radiolucencies surrounding the apex of mandibular anterior teeth.
  - They may be from round to ovoid. Although there may be significant superimposition over the root tips, a continuous lamina dura and periodontal ligament space are noted around the roots.
  - Progressive mineralisation changes the radiographic appearance to radiopaque.
  - Round to oval foci of mineralisation are surrounded by a thin radiolucent rim.
  - Some lesions may superimpose over the roots to give a false impression of cementoblastoma or cemental hyperplasia.
- Florid cemento-osseous dysplasia may begin as a focal area of radiolucency. Eventually, multiple areas affecting more than one quadrant are noted.
  - The lesions present as radiolucencies that undergo mineralisation to form irregular mixed masses that may confluence with each other within the alveolar bone.
  - Cortical expansion and perforation may also be seen eventually, especially in the posterior segments.
  - Both dentate and edentulous areas may be affected.
  - Lesions would tend to lie more superficially in edentulous areas.
  - Superimposition with roots may give a hypercementosis-like appearance.
  - Radiolucencies may persist focally, and some may represent simple bone cysts in association with cemento-osseous dysplasia.

Histopathology

All forms of cemento-osseous dysplasia show similar histopathological features. When a biopsy is attempted, the bone is often described as rough and gritty with no lesional boundary. The harvested tissue's macroscopic appearance shows tiny pieces of hard tissue mixed with soft tissue fragments. Decalcified sections show fragments of variably inflamed fibrocellular connective tissue with tiny ginger root-like fragments of bone (Fig. 23.8). Basophilic cementicle-like globular droplets may also be seen focally. Mature lesions may show large sheets of cemental tissue.

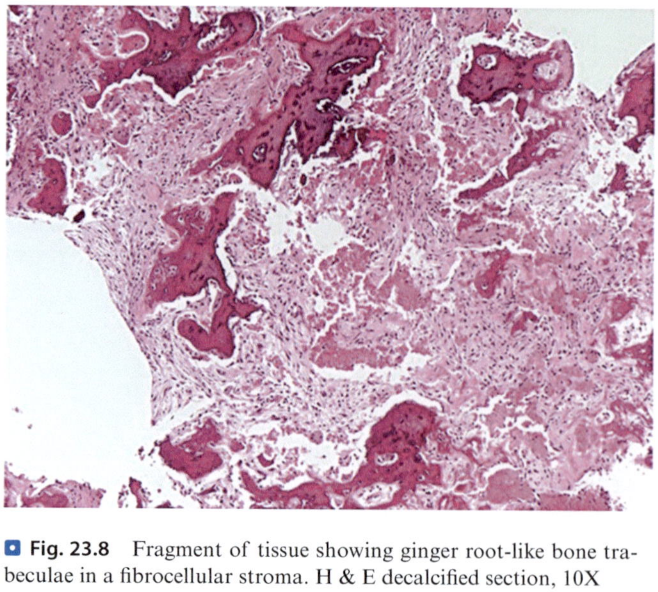

Fig. 23.8 Fragment of tissue showing ginger root-like bone trabeculae in a fibrocellular stroma. H & E decalcified section, 10X

Further Reading

Gaetti-Jardim E Jr, Landucci LF, de Oliveira KL, Costa I, Ranieri RV, Okamoto AC, Schweitzer CM. Microbiota associated with infections of the jaws. Int J Dent. 2012;2012:369751. https://doi.org/10.1155/2012/369751. Epub 2012 Jul 8. PMID: 22829824; PMCID: PMC3399405.

Lima Gde M, Almeida JD, Cabral LA. Cherubism: clinicoradiographic features and treatment. J Oral Maxillofac Res. 2010;1(2):e2. https://doi.org/10.5037/jomr.2010.1202. PMID: 24421967; PMCID: PMC3886048.

Nam I, Ryu J, Shin SH, Kim YD, Lee JY. Cemento-osseous dysplasia: clinical presentation and symptoms. J Korean Assoc Oral Maxillofac Surg. 2022;48(2):79–84. https://doi.org/10.5125/jkaoms.2022.48.2.79. PMID: 35491138; PMCID: PMC9065647.

Stevens KJ, Stevens JA. Aneurysmal bone cysts. [Updated 2023 Aug 14]. In: StatPearls [Internet]. Treasure Island, FL: StatPearls Publishing; 2024. https://www.ncbi.nlm.nih.gov/books/NBK546654/.

Tafti D, Cecava ND. Fibrous dysplasia. [Updated 2023 Jul 24]. In: StatPearls [Internet]. Treasure Island, FL: StatPearls Publishing; 2024. https://www.ncbi.nlm.nih.gov/books/NBK532947/.

Zhao DY, McCann L, Hahn G, Hedrich CM. Chronic nonbacterial osteomyelitis (CNO) and chronic recurrent multifocal osteomyelitis (CRMO). J Transl Autoimmun. 2021;4:100095. https://doi.org/10.1016/j.jtauto.2021.100095. PMID: 33870159; PMCID: PMC8040271.

Histopathology of Developmental Anomalies and Anatomical Variants of the Oral Mucosa

Ajith Polonowita

Contents

S R Prabhu et al. (eds.), *Oral Histology and Oral Histopathology*, https://doi.org/10.1007/978-3-031-77481-2_24

24.1 Introduction

Developmental anomalies and variants of normal oral mucosa may give rise to concerns for patients and they may seek treatment. A thorough knowledge of such lesions by clinicians can avert the need for further investigations and be reassuring for the patient. Notwithstanding, lesions may occasionally require biopsy due to a concerning appearance or because the lesion is symptomatic or interfering with function. This chapter deals with a few developmental oral mucosal lesions and their variants.

24.2 Fordyce Granules

Fordyce granules (Fordyce spots) are sebaceous glands that normally occur on hairless areas of the skin. They produce sebum, which includes cholesterol and fatty acids. John Fordyce first described them in 1896. Sebaceous glands are ectopic in the mouth. They occur commonly on the lips and the buccal mucosa.

Key Features

- Fordyce granules have a male-to-female ratio of 11:5, with the upper lip being the area of highest occurrence.
- They are typically 0.2–2 mm in diameter and creamy/yellow in colour. They may occur following puberty.
- They are diagnosed on clinical history and appearance.
- No treatment is usually required unless for cosmetic reasons. When indicated, electrodesiccation, pulsed dye laser, or micro punch technique are used for the removal of Fordyce granules.

24.2.1 Histopathological Features

Microscopically, the sebaceous glands are overlayed with stratified squamous epithelium (Fig. 24.1). The gland's excretory duct relates to this squamous epithelium and can directly open to the mucosa. The gland is usually a single lobule.

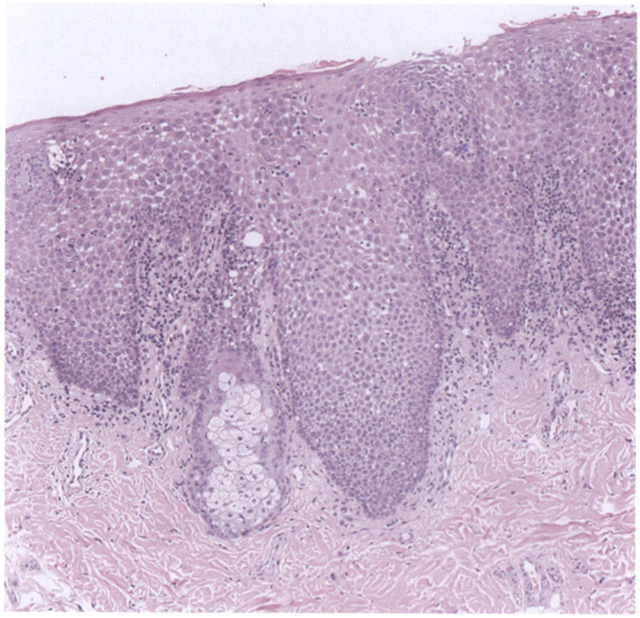

Fig. 24.1 Fordyce granules. Note a lobular glandular structure in one of the rete ridges of the epithelium

24.3 Leukoedema

Leukoedema is a mucosal greyish-white diffuse opaque area that cannot be rubbed off with gauze. Leukoedema is often seen bilaterally on the buccal mucosa.

Key Features

- The prevalence is difficult to assess from studies due to different clinical parameters used to make the diagnosis.
- Stretching the buccal mucosa will cause the altered appearance to disappear.
- The aetiology is unknown, but smoking may make the appearance more noticeable.
- Biopsy is seldom indicated unless other pathology is suspected.

Histopathology

Histologically, parakeratosis and acanthosis are seen with vacuolated cytoplasm and minimal inflammation (Fig. 24.2).

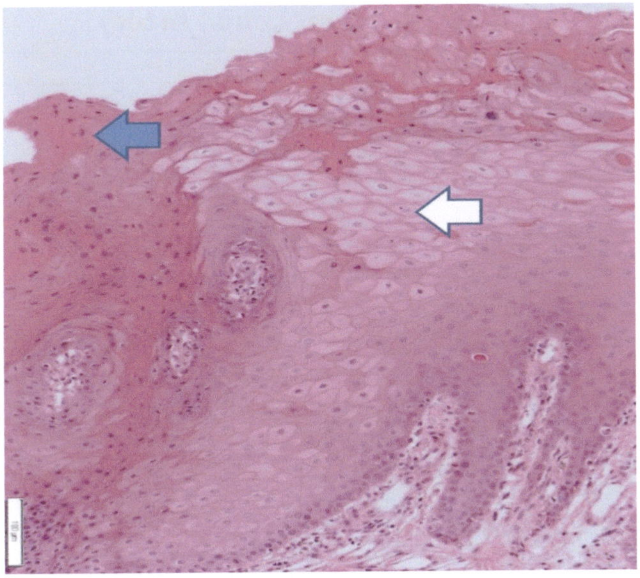

Fig. 24.2 Parakeratosis of the epithelium (blue arrow) and marked intracellular oedema of the cells of the spinous cell layer (white arrow). (Source: Hariri, F. (2023). Bilateral Whitish Patches on the Inner Cheek: Leukoedema. In: Tilakaratne, W.M., Kallarakkal, T.G. (eds) Clinicopathological Correlation of Oral Diseases. Springer, Cham. ► https://doi.org/10.1007/978-3-031-24408-7_30). (With permission from Springer Nature)

24.4 Geographic Tongue (Erythema Migrans)

The geographic tongue or benign migratory glossitis is also called erythema migrans (EM), as the condition is not restricted to the tongue.

▪ **Key Features**

- Also called benign migratory glossitis, erythema areata migrans, geographic stomatitis, and wandering rash of the tongue.
- The lesions commonly occur on the tongue, both dorsal and ventral; occasionally, the cheek mucosa, lips, and palate are affected.
- Aetiology is unknown.
- Clinically appears as an irregular erythematous centre with an irregular white/creamy border. The pattern changes and moves around, hence the term migrans. These are usually asymptomatic and diagnosed on history and clinical picture.
- Suggested to be the most common manifestation of Lyme disease.
- Management: Usually involves reassurance, but if pain is present, then management strategies for pain should be instituted (e.g. topical anaesthetic gels).

▪ **Histopathology**

Commonly non-specific superficial and deep perivascular lymphohistiocytic infiltrate with or without periadnexal involvement. Central eosinophils and peripheral plasma cells are typically present. Spongiosis, peripheral neutrophils, periadnexal without perivascular involvement, and absence of plasma cells may all be seen in certain cases.

Accompanied focal interface dermatitis may be suggestive. If other symptoms are present or if later stages of Lyme disease are suspected, the Centers for Disease Control and Prevention (CDC) recommends 2-step serologic testing consisting of (step 1) enzyme immunoassay followed by (step 2) western blot analysis if IgM/IgG result for *Borrelia burgdorferi* is positive or equivocal for step 1.

24.5 White Sponge Naevus

White sponge naevus is an inherited autosomal dominant rare condition with irregular penetrance and variable expressivity affecting predominantly oral mucosa.

▪ **Key Features**

- The lesions are white plaques with an irregular surface and ill-defined borders.
- Bilateral buccal mucosal involvement is the most common site, but any non-keratinised mucosa may be involved.
- The cause is a mutation in the genes for keratin intermediate filaments keratin 4 and 13.
- Lesions may be seen in children but become more readily visible with age.
- The clinical resemblance to other white lesions of the oral mucosa may be the reason for the biopsy. Biopsy is not essential, particularly if a family history is established. No treatment is required.

▪ **Histopathology**

Histopathological features are parakeratosis, epithelial hyperplasia with acanthosis, and vacuolisation of keratinocytes (Fig. 24.3.) with perinuclear eosinophilic condensation. There are no features of epithelial dysplasia and minimal inflammation.

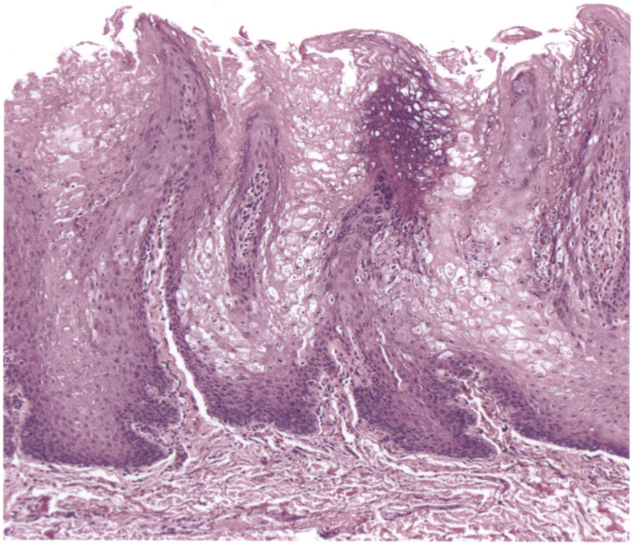

Fig. 24.3 Photomicrograph from hematoxylin and eosin (H&E) stained from the left buccal mucosa sample demonstrating acanthosis and vacuolisation. (Source: Belknap, A. N., Bhattacharyya, I., Islam, M. N., & Cohen, D. M. (2021). White Sponge Nevus, a Rare but Important Entity. *Oral*, *1*(4), 307–312. ► https://doi.org/10.3390/oral1040030). CC by Licence

24.6 Lingual Thyroid

Ectopic thyroid tissue results from the failure of the embryonic thyroid anlage to descend into the neck along the path of the thyroglossal tract. It is usually located at the base of the tongue but may present clinically on the dorsum of the tongue.

- **Key Features**
- Lingual thyroid is rare, so other causes of midline swelling of the tongue should be considered. Lesions may be asymptomatic, presenting as a purplish mass in the midline.
- Dysphagia may be a presenting symptom.
- Appropriate investigations, including establishing that the thyroid gland is present in the neck, are required prior to removing lingual thyroid tissue. Removing lingual thyroid tissue in the absence of other thyroid tissue will result in hypothyroidism and the need for life-long thyroxine supplementation.
- The diagnosis of lingual thyroid requires clinical examination, biochemical tests, and appropriate imaging methods, including ultrasonography, thyroid scintigraphy, computed tomography scan, and magnetic resonance imaging, followed by fine-needle aspiration cytology to confirm the diagnosis.

24.7 Calibre-Persistent Labial Artery

Calibre-persistent labial artery (CPLA) is a ► vascular anomaly in which the labial artery loops into the ► submucosa of the lip without reduction in diameter.

- **Key Features**
- CPLA commonly presents as a bluish or normal-coloured elevated mass and may be pulsatile on manual palpation.
- It can resemble a ► mucocele but is encountered in middle-aged to elderly patients.
- CPLA carries the risk of profuse bleeding if the artery is transected during the biopsy, so ideally, the condition is recognised clinically, possibly with ultrasound to confirm the arterial nature of the lesion to avoid biopsy.

- **Histopathology**

The histopathology shows a thick-walled vessel within the lamina propria covered by stratified squamous epithelium. Inflammation is usually not marked, and neural and vascular elements and minor salivary glands may be seen.

24.8 Dermoid and Epidermoid Cysts

Dermoid and epidermoid cysts are uncommon developmental cysts found in the sublingual region or, less commonly, tongue, lips, or buccal mucosa.

- **Key Features**
- Sublingual dermoid cysts may be in the midline or to one side and lie above the hyoid bone and mylohyoid muscle.
- If located above the geniohyoid muscle, the tongue is elevated.

- **Histopathology**

The cysts are lined by keratinising stratified squamous epithelium and are designated dermoid cysts if skin appendages (sebaceous glands and hair follicles) are in the cyst wall or epidermoid cyst if skin adnexal structures are not present. Sublingual lesions lack the blue coloration seen in the ranula. The size of lesions varies but may be over 10 cm with keratin in the lumen.

24.9 Lymphoid Aggregates

Lymphoid aggregates are collections of normal or hyperplastic lymphoid tissue occurring anywhere in the mouth, but most notably in regions of Waldeyer's ring, including the oropharynx, lateral tongue, soft palate, and the floor of the mouth.

Key Features

- They are considered normal and generally do not require treatment.
- Occasionally, they may resemble other lesions and warrant a biopsy. This is often related to inflammation due to an antigenic stimulus causing erythema and enlargement, and while self-limiting, it may appear suspicious for malignancy.
- Foliate papillae are vertical ridges of lingual papillae on the posterior lateral tongue and are normal anatomical structures, as are the lingual tonsils at the base of the tongue.
- These may become hyperplastic or tender due to local inflammation or infection but do not require treatment.
- Lymphoepithelial cysts may develop in association with foliate papillae or lingual tonsils appearing as a yellow ovoid mass and simple excision is curative.

Histopathology

Hyperplasia affects the normal architecture of lymphoid tissue, and occasionally, differentiating lymphoid hyperplasia from a neoplastic process may be difficult. The presence of an increased number of tingible body macrophages (unique, large phagocytic cells that reside in germinal centres (GCs) of secondary lymphoid tissues) is distinctive. However, a non-specific feature of hyperplasia and a polymorphic pattern of small "normal" lymphocytes is helpful in distinguishing lymphoid hyperplasia from lymphoid neoplasms.

Lymphoepithelial cysts are lined by stratified squamous epithelium surrounded by lymphoid tissue in the fibrous wall.

24.10 Physiological (Racial Pigmentation)

Physiologic pigmentation is the most common reason for oral mucosal pigmentation. Majority of the world's population can show different degrees of mucosal pigmentation. The reason for the pigmentation is increased melanocytic activity leading to an increased melanin pigment.

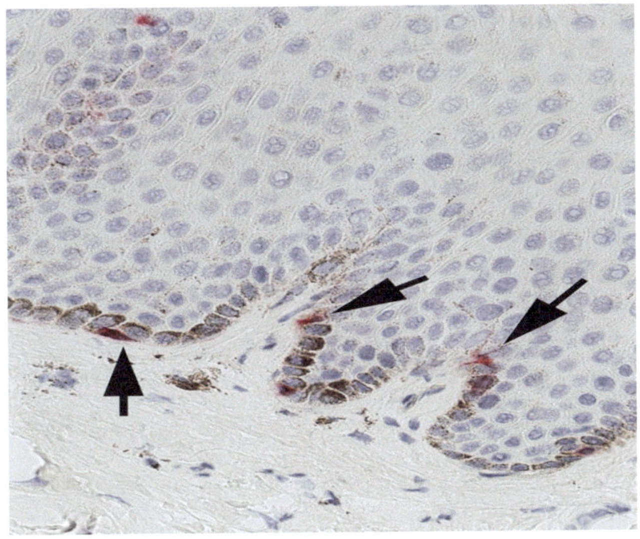

Fig. 24.4 Physiologic pigmentation. Anti-MART1 antibody was used to highlight normal melanocytes (*arrows*) residing in the basal epithelial layer. (Source: Stoopler, E.T., Alawi, F. (2019). Pigmented Lesions of the Oral Mucosa. In: Farah, C., Balasubramaniam, R., McCullough, M. (eds) Contemporary Oral Medicine. Springer, Cham. ▸ https://doi.org/10.1007/978-3-319-72303-7_17) (With permission from Springer Nature)

Key Features

- Can occur in African, Asian, and Mediterranean people amongst others.
- Typically affects the gingiva in a symmetrical manner.
- Can increase with age.
- Depending on the amount of pigment, the clinical appearance may be light brown to blue-black in appearance.
- Management involves reassurance and exclusion of other causes of mucosal discoloration.

Histopathology

Normal structure of the mucosa with an increased amount of melanin deposited in the basal cell layer (Fig. 24.4).

24.11 Summary

Developmental anomalies and anatomic variants of the oral mucosa are usually asymptomatic. However, patients are often concerned because of their altered morphology. Patient assurance is of importance in such circumstances.

Further Reading

Awni S, Conn B. Caliber-persistent labial artery: a rarely recognized cause of a lower lip swelling—report of 5 cases and review of the literature. J Oral MaxFac Surg. 2016;74(7):1391–5.

Belknap AN, Bhattacharyya I, Islam MN, Cohen DM. White sponge nevus, a rare but important entity. Oral. 2021;1(4):307–12. https://doi.org/10.3390/oral1040030.

Bezerra KT, Leite TC, Roza ALOC, Araújo R, Israel MS, Canedo NHS, Agostini M, Benevenuto de Andrade BA, Romañach MJ. White sponge nevus: a condition not always clinically suspected. J Cutan Pathol. 2020;47:22–6.

della Vella F, Lauritano D, Lajolo C, Lucchese A, Di Stasio D, Contaldo M, Serpico R, Petruzzi M. The pseudolesions of the oral mucosa: differential diagnosis and related systemic conditions. Appl Sci. 2019;9(12):2412. https://doi.org/10.3390/app9122412.

Eisen D. Disorders of pigmentation in the oral cavity. Clin Dermatol. 2000;18:579–87.

Elfatoiki FZ, Capatas S, Skali HD, Hali F, Attar H, Chiheb S. Oral white sponge nevus: an exceptional differential diagnosis in childhood. Case Rep Dermatol Med. 2020;2020:9296768. https://doi.org/10.1155/2020/9296768. PMID: 32908720; PMCID: PMC7471808.

Fordyce JA. A peculiar affection of the mucous membrane of the lips and oral cavity. J Cutan Dis. 1896;14:413–9.

Guiducci AA, Hyman AB. Ectopic sebaceous glands. A review of the literature regarding their occurrence, histology and embryonic relationships. Dermatologica. 1962;125:44–63.

Huang H, Lin Y-H. Lingual thyroid with severe hypothyroidism: a case report. Medicine. 2021;100(43):e27612. https://doi.org/10.1097/MD.0000000000027612.

Kumar LK, Kurien NM, Jacob MM, Menon PV, Khalam SA. Lingual thyroid. Ann Maxillofac Surg. 2015;5:104–7.

Lee JH, Hae LJ, Kwon NH, et al. Clinicopathologic manifestations of patients with fordyce's spots. Ann Dermatol. 2012;24(1):103–6.

Lee JH, Lee JH, Kwon NH, et al. Clinicopathologic manifestations of patients with fordyce's spots. Ann Dermatol. 2012;24(1):103–6.

Martelli H, Pereira SM, Rocha TM, Nogueira dos Santos PL, Batista de Paula AM, Bonan PR. White sponge nevus: Report of a three-generation family. Oral Surg Oral Med Oral Pathol Oral Radiol Endodontol. 2007;103:43–7.

Meleti M, Vescovi P, Mooi WJ, van der Waal I. Pigmented lesions of the oral mucosa and perioral tissues: a flow-chart for the diagnosis and some recommendations for the management. Oral Surg Oral Med Oral Pathol Oral Radiol Endod. 2008;105:606–16.

Noussios G, Anagnostis P, Goulis DG, Lappas D, Natsis K. Ectopic thyroid tissue: anatomical, clinical, and surgical implications of a rare entity. Eur J Endocrinol. 2011;165:375–82.

Pupić-Bakrač J, Pupić-Bakrač A, Bačić I, Kolega MŠ, Skitarelić N. Epidermoid and dermoid cysts of the head and neck. J Craniofac Surg. 2021;32(1):e25–7. https://doi.org/10.1097/SCS.0000000000006834.

Rosdy NM, Firth NA, Rich AM. Calibre-persistent labial artery: often misdiagnosed as a mucocoele. Int J Oral Maxillofac Surg. 2010;39:1230–3. https://doi.org/10.1016/j.ijom.2010.05.003.

Sanchez E, Vannier E, Wormser GP, et al. Diagnosis, treatment, and prevention of lyme disease, human granulocytic anaplasmosis, and babesiosis: a review. JAMA. 2016;315(16):1767–77. https://doi.org/10.1001/jama.2016.2884.

Santangelo G, Pellino G, De Falco N, et al. Prevalence, diagnosis and management of ectopic thyroid glands. Int J Surg. 2016;28:S1–6.

Taylor RS, Perone JB, Kaddu S, Kerl H. Appendage tumors and hamartomas of the skin. In: Wolff K, Goldsmith LA, Katz SI, Gilchrest BA, Paller AS, Leffell DJ, editors. Fitzpatrick's dermatology in general medicine. 7th ed. New York, NY: McGraw-Hill; 2007. p. 1085.

Taylor RS, Perone JB, Kaddu S, Kerl H, Wolff K, Goldsmith LA, Katz SI, Gilchrest BA, Paller AS, Leffell DJ, editors. Appendage tumors and hamartomas of the skin. Fitzpatrick's dermatology in general medicine. 7th ed. New York, NY: McGraw-Hill; 2007. p. 1085.

Wilson TC, Legler A, Madison KC, et al. Erythema migrans: a spectrum of histopathologic changes. Am J Dermatopathol. 2012;34(8):834–7.

Histopathology of Non-infective Stomatitis

Ajith Polonowita and Norman A Firth

Contents

S R Prabhu et al. (eds.), *Oral Histology and Oral Histopathology*, https://doi.org/10.1007/978-3-031-77481-2_25

25.1 Introduction and Classification

Non-infective stomatitis refers to inflammation of the oral mucosa caused by agents other than infections. It's classified based on specific causes, e.g. trauma, autoimmune conditions, or allergic reactions. Histopathologically, in addition to inflammation, it shows epithelial alterations, e.g. atrophy or hyperplasia, intra-epithelial separation or sub-epithelial-connective tissue separation, or ulceration.

25.2 Recurrent Aphthous Stomatitis (RAS)

Recurrent Aphthous ulceration, also known as recurrent aphthous stomatitis and commonly as "canker sores" is characterised by the recurrent development of painful aphthous ulcers on non-keratinised oral mucous membrane.

- **Key Features**

- The pathogenesis of RAS is multifactorial. Some suggested etiological factors include genetics, stress, dysfunction of the immune system, and deficiencies in nutrition/haematinics.
- RAS are common oral ulcerations (25% of the world population) present in three typical types: minor, major, and herpetiform.
- Diagnosis is made on history and clinical appearance.

Three classic clinical presentations recognised are as follows:

1. ***Minor Aphthous:*** Less than 1 cm in diameter and lasting typically 1–2 weeks and heals without scarring. These are by far the most common form and involve non-keratinised mucosal sites. Single or multiple lesions occur with a short or prolonged interval between episodes.
2. ***Major Aphthous:*** Larger than 1 cm diameter (by definition) and lasting more than 4 weeks and often heals with scar formation. Less than 10% of aphthous ulcers are major aphthae. They usually involve non-keratinised mucosa, but not exclusively.
3. ***Herpetiform:*** Clusters of up to 100 very small, i.e. 2 mm diameter ulcers that often coalesce to form larger ulcers and heal within 3 weeks. Lesions occur on the floor of the mouth, ventral tongue or soft palate and are usually yellow with a fibrinous ovoid centre surrounded by a red peripheral halo on a diffuse red background. They may often present in adolescents and young adults. Histopathology indicates a T-cell-mediated immune condition.

Association with Systemic Conditions. RAS may be associated with other underlying conditions, so it is important to exclude Behçet syndrome, including mouth and genital ulcers with inflamed cartilage (MAGIC) syndrome, systemic lupus erythematosus, gluten sensitivity, another inflammatory bowel disease**, p**eriodic **f**ever with **a**phthous stomatitis, **p**haryngitis, and **a**denitis **(PFAPA) syndrome,** and HIV infection.

Multiple aetiological factors may or have been proposed to contribute, but none are always implicated. These include genetic predisposition, an exaggerated response to minor trauma, immunological abnormalities, gastrointestinal disease, haematological deficiencies, hormonal factors, stress, and HIV infection. Interestingly, smoking cessation may lead to RAS in susceptible people.

Management involves supportive measures, pain relief (topical anaesthetics), topical steroids (especially for the major type), topical tetracycline, vitamins, and, as second-line therapy, colchicine, Dapsone, pentoxifylline, chemical, or laser cauterisation.

- **Histopathology**

A biopsy is not required for diagnosis. The surface of the ulcer is covered by a fibrinous exudate infiltrated by polymorphs. Beneath is a layer of granulation tissue with dilated capillaries and oedema. These features are non-specific and not diagnostic of RAS.

25.3 Oral Lichen Planus

Oral lichen planus (OLP) is an immune-mediated (T-cell) chronic inflammatory disease affecting the oral mucosa with a 1–2% prevalence, with a female predilection.

- **Key Features**

- Clinically OLP may have many presentations (white reticular, papular, atrophic, plaque-like, erythematous, erosive, and mixed white /red).
- The clinical significance of these different presentations is low except that the ulcerative and erythematous lesions perhaps may have a higher index of suspicion for malignant change.
- OLP is listed as an oral potentially malignant disorder with approximately 2% malignant transformation.
- OLP more commonly occurs in females 40 years of age and older. In some people with OLP, there may be extraoral lesions (skin, scalp, nails, genitals) or a history of extraoral lesions. OLP may be uni- or bilateral.

- Gingival involvement may cause desquamative gingivitis.
- Diagnosis is through biopsy leading to a classical histopathology (see below).
- The management of symptomatic OLP is with topical steroids as a first line. Regular review to control disease and monitoring for early diagnosis of possible malignant change.
- Recalcitrant lesions may require intralesional or systemic steroids or tacrolimus (controversial due to the potential increasing risk for malignancy).

Histopathology

Characteristic histopathological features include:

- Hyperkeratosis or parakeratosis.
- Band-like distribution of predominantly a T-lymphocytic infiltrate in the superficial lamina propria immediately beneath the epithelium (▫ Fig. 25.1).
- Basal cell "liquefactive degeneration" with Civatte bodies, which are apoptotic degenerative basal cells (▫ Fig. 25.2).
- Presence of fibrinogen in the basement membrane zone (detected with direct immunofluorescence staining with anti-fibrinogen)(▫ Fig. 25.3).
- Saw tooth rete ridges more commonly in skin LP rather than OLP.

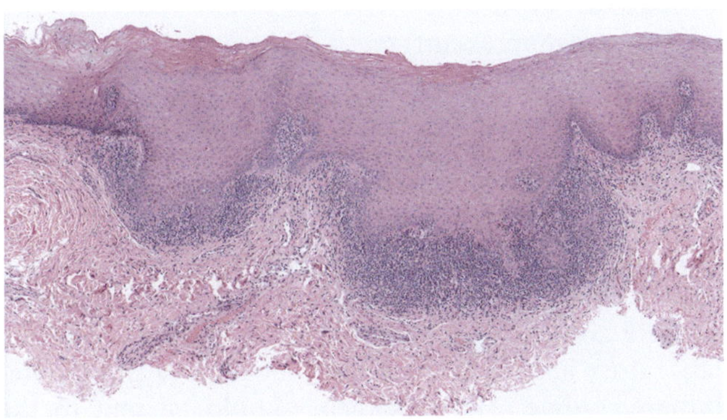

▫ Fig. 25.1 Lichen planus. A low-power photomicrograph showing a band-like chronic inflammatory cell infiltrate in the superficial lamina propria

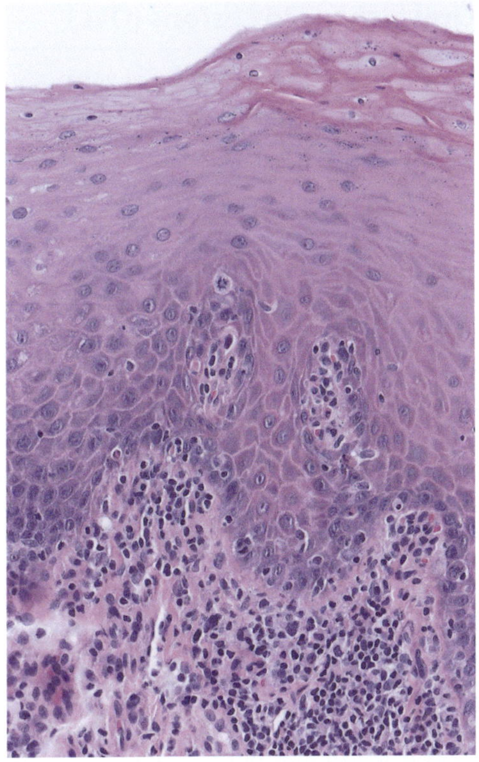

▫ Fig. 25.2 Lichen planus. A photomicrograph showing surface parakeratosis, an eosinophilic coagulum in the basement zone, Civatte bodies, and disruption to the basal layer of the epithelium

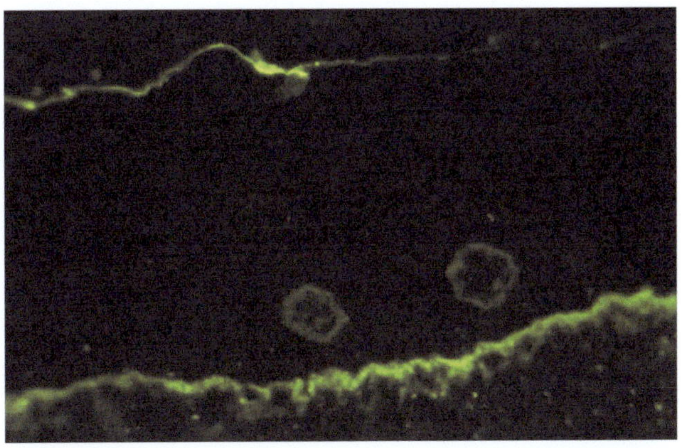

▫ Fig. 25.3 Lichen planus. This is a direct immunofluorescence photomicrograph showing anti-fibrinogen in the basement membrane zone. Although this may be considered non-specific, it can be helpful in distinguishing lichen planus from other conditions in which immunoglobulin and/or complement fluorescence is seen

25.4 Oral Lichenoid Lesions (OLL)

Clinically, OLL is the same entity as OLP but is suggested to occur in association with medications (antihypertensives, NSAIDS, hypoglycaemics, and numerous others), dental restoration contact, and graft versus host disease (a common complication of allogeneic stem cell transplantation).

Key Features

- The behaviour and management of OLL is similar to OLP.
- The adverse reactions on the oral mucosal tissues can be either due to the toxic or irritative nature of the material or allergic.
- OLL lesions are often unilateral.
- Management similar to OLP, but consideration may be given to removing the offending trigger.
- It should be noted that OLL is also listed as an OPMD.
- The treatment of OLL is the same as for OLP.
- If a systemic medication is implicated, withdrawal or change of such medication by the medical practitioner may result in resolution.
- Replacing dental restorations may result in resolution.

Histopathology

Characteristic histopathological features include:

- Histopathological features of OLL are similar or identical to OLP.
- The presence of eosinophils in the inflammatory cell infiltrate is considered by some to be indicative of OLL.
- Increased thickness of the basement membrane is not a feature in PAS-positive stained sections of OLL, nor is increased vascularity.
- The presence of perivascular lymphocytic infiltrates may be seen in restoration reactions.

25.5 Pemphigus Vulgaris (PV)

PV is an autoimmune mucocutaneous disorder characterised by blisters and erosions of the mucous membranes, especially of the mouth. 60–70% of pemphigus cases present with oral mucosal involvement before skin lesions develop.

Key Features

- The disease is more common in patients 40 years or older.
- PV has a female predilection and for people of Jewish and Indian descent.
- Vesicles and bullae form and rupture often without the patient being aware of the vesicles or bullae.
- The basal layer of the epithelium initially remains intact, and inflammation is not marked, resulting in limited healing, and frequently developing new lesions faster than old lesions heal.
- When a lesion is abrasion, the basal layer is lost, leaving an ulcer that can become secondarily infected. Protein, fluid, and electrolytes are lost.
- If untreated, the condition is fatal in those with extensive cutaneous involvement.
- PV may occur in the mouth, genitals, and skin with superficial blisters and erosions.
- A similar rare type of pemphigus may be associated with an underlying malignancy (lymphoma, leukaemia, Castleman's disease), in which case it is called paraneoplastic pemphigus.
- Management is with systemic steroids (e.g. prednisolone 80–100 mg/day are effective). Azathioprine is added to the regime as a steroid-sparing agent, and other systemic agents such as *Rituximab* (a monoclonal anti-CD20 antibody used to treat non-Hodgkin's lymphoma, chronic lymphocytic leukaemia, Wegener's granulomatosis, pemphigus vulgaris, and rheumatoid arthritis.). Mycophenolate mofetil (an immunosuppressant) may also be useful. Topical steroids are useful for localised oral lesions when overall control has occurred.

Histopathology

A biopsy is essential for diagnosis. Two specimens are essential: one for formalin fixation and routine processing and another fresh sample for transportation to the laboratory in Michel's transport medium or phosphate-buffered saline. The specimens should be sent to the laboratory promptly. This fresh specimen is used in the laboratory to prepare frozen sections for direct immunofluorescence (DIF) with a panel of antibodies. There may be circulating antibodies (anti-dsg1 and anti-dsg3 detected by a blood/saliva test) detected through indirect immunofluorescence).

Circulating autoantibodies permeating through the epithelium are directed against desmoglein 1 or 3 proteins in desmosomes, which hold the epithelial cells

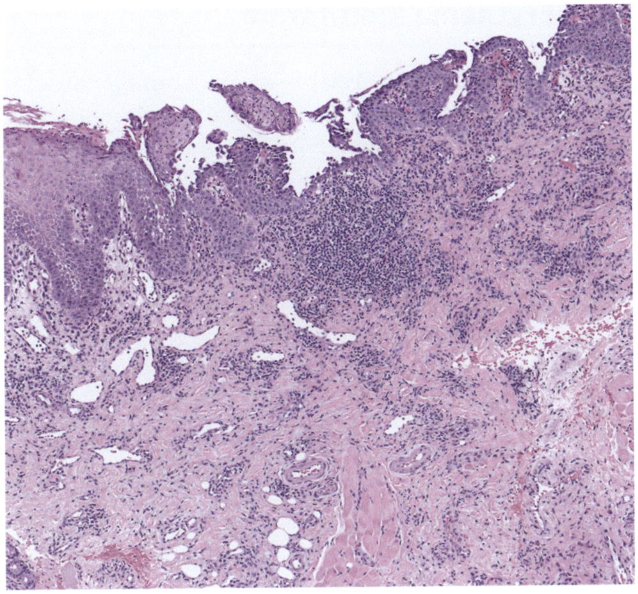

Fig. 25.4 Pemphigus vulgaris. A photomicrograph showing detachment of the epithelium above the still attached basal cell layer of the epithelium. Also, note the subepithelial intense inflammatory cell infiltrate

together. Cells lose their cohesion and detach from each other, causing the epithelium in the affected area to be totally detached, except for the basal cells, which remain attached to the underlying fibrous stroma.

Characteristic histopathological features include:

Suprabasal acantholysis with clefting (vesicle/bulla formation), acantholysis of the prickle cell layer, and subepithelial inflammatory cell infiltrate are typical features of PV (Fig. 25.4). Direct immunofluorescent testing on the fresh-frozen tissue shows autoantibodies (IgG and complement), targeting the junction between keratinocytes with a "chicken wire" pattern (Fig. 25.5).

MMP is an autoimmune disease involving the mucous membranes of the mouth and eyes (other areas include the oesophagus, nose, trachea, and genitals).

Key Features

- MMP mainly affects older females, with a peak incidence of around 70 years.
- In MMP, the epithelium lifts off from underlying connective tissue.
- Autoantibodies identified target the basement membrane mostly against the BP180 antigen, laminin or type VII collagen.
- MMP may lead to scarring in the ocular mucosa with adhesions and may lead to blindness.

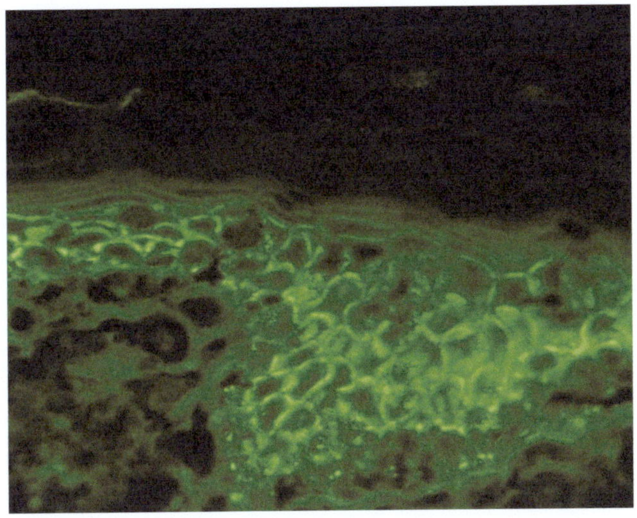

Fig. 25.5 Pemphigus vulgaris. Direct immunofluorescence demonstrating IgG antibodies targeting keratinocytes with a "chicken wire" pattern. (DermNet.Org. With permission)

- Oral lesions may present with bullae/vesicles or ulcerations.
- Desquamative gingivitis is frequently seen involving free and attached gingivae.
- Disease severity is variable and management for localised oral lesions is topical steroid.
- If lesions are refractive or extensive, then systemic steroids are used with Azathioprine added to allow steroid dose reduction.
- In cases of extensive involvement, other agents, including Rituximab or Mycophenolate mofetil, may be required.

Histopathology

Obtaining a good biopsy is difficult due to the friable nature of the affected tissue.

Characteristic histopathological features include:

Epithelial-connective tissue separation at the basement membrane level is a consistent feature. The specimen frequently shows a fragment of connective tissue with inflammation and a separate fragment of uninflamed stratified squamous epithelium (Fig. 25.6).

Direct immunofluorescence (DIF) reveals the autoantibody (usually IgG) binding at the basement membrane level and complement activation if present (Fig. 25.7). Unfortunately, if separation has occurred, the immunofluorescence staining is not diagnostic, so tissue immediately adjacent to a lesion without epithelial-connective tissue separation is preferred for the fresh-frozen direct immunofluorescence sample.

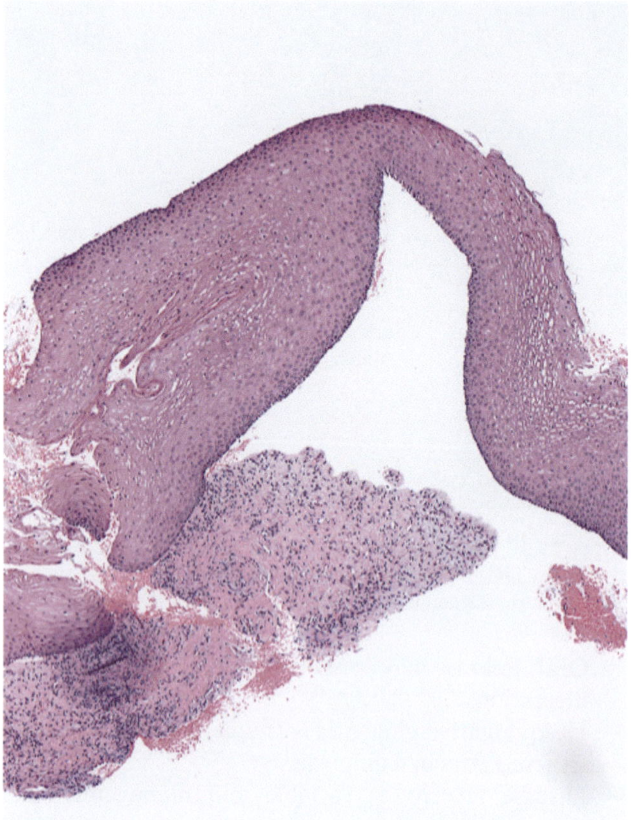

Fig. 25.6 Mucous membrane pemphigoid. This photomicrograph shows a clean separation between the epithelium and the connective tissue at the basement membrane level. Inflammation is in the connective tissue but not in the overlying epithelium

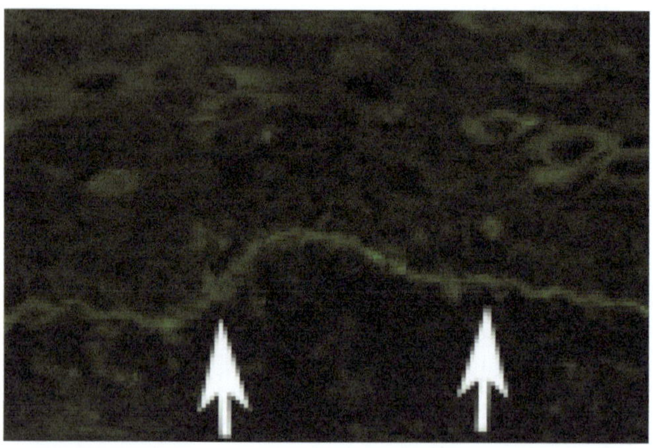

Fig. 25.7 Direct immunofluorescence of perilesional tissue from a patient with mucous membrane pemphigoid demonstrates a continuous linear band of IgG at the basement membrane zone (BMZ, arrows) (Source: Müller, S. Oral lichenoid lesions: distinguishing the benign from the deadly. Mod Pathol 30 (Suppl1), S54–S67 (2017)). ► https://doi.org/10.1038/modpathol.2016.121. (Creative Commons Attribution 4.0 International License)

25.6 Erythema Multiforme

Erythema multiforme (EM) is an uncommon cause of oral mucosal blisters and ulceration and is thought to be a cell-mediated hypersensitivity reaction.

- **Key Features**

- Established triggering factors include herpes simplex infection, mycoplasma pneumonia, varicella zoster, and medications including penicillin.
- The time delay between exposure to an identified triggering stimulus and the onset of lesions is often between 9 and 14 days.
- Triggering factors are not always identified.
- The age group most affected is 20–40 years of age, with a slight male predominance. Less commonly, children and adolescents may be affected.
- Clinically lesions of erythema multiforme show variation. Vague arthralgia with or without fever may precede lesion development.
- The classical "target lesion" of skin may be seen consisting of an erythematous macule with a central bullseye, but these lesions are variable in appearance and extent.
- The most conspicuous oral lesions are blood-crusted lips due to a continuous fibrin ooze.
- Intraoral blisters and large shallow ulcers are seen involving buccal, tongue, and labial mucosa.
- Pain is a feature, and oral examination may be difficult due to the extent of lesions and the inability to open the mouth comfortably.
- Skin and mild oral mucosal involvement may be relatively minor. Such patients may seek advice and management from a dental professional and may not link the skin lesions with the oral lesions, so specific questioning is important.
- Patients with more significant skin, oral, and other mucous membrane involvement may require hospitalisation.
- Stevens–Johnson syndrome, which is no longer considered as a severe form of erythema multiforme, is usually triggered by medication and requires hospitalisation. It may be fatal.
- Attacks of erythema multiforme are self-limiting, so minor cases may not require treatment.
- Frequently, a short tapering course of prednisone is helpful in reducing the time for resolution. Chlorhexidine may be useful in reducing secondary infection.
- Triggering factors should be identified and treated for patients with recurrent lesions (often up to 6 months apart).

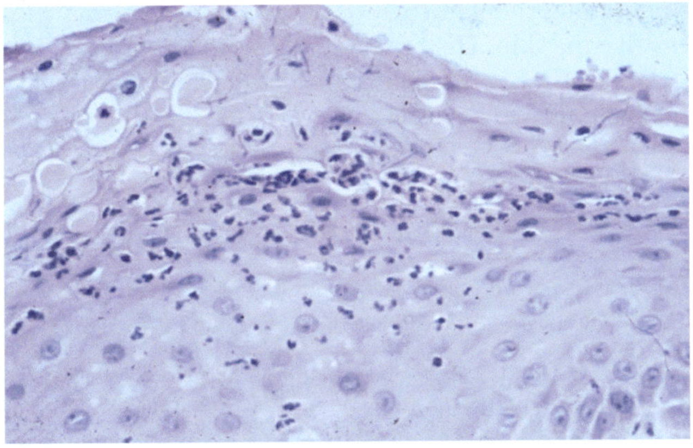

Fig. 25.8 Erythema multiforme. Histopathological features may be non-specific, but degenerative superficial keratinocytes and intra-epithelial vesicles may be seen

Histopathology

A biopsy may be indicated, but histopathological features are variable so the value of a biopsy may be to exclude other entities as pathognomonic features of EM are not present. Intra-epithelial and subepithelial vesicle formation with oedema may be seen, and subepithelial lymphocytic inflammation with basal cell degeneration and apoptosis similar to lichen planus are present (Fig. 25.8). Acute inflammation may be present and degenerate keratinocytes in the more superficial epithelium are prominent.

25.7 Lupus Erythematosus

Lupus Erythematosus (LE) is an autoimmune disease presenting with systemic LE (SLE) or cutaneous LE (CLE) lesions.

Key Features

- Oral mucosal involvement occurs in about 20% of cases and rarely may be the presenting lesion.
- In keeping with other autoimmune diseases, there is a female preponderance.
- Oral lesions often resemble lichen planus with white striae, erythema, and ulceration.
- Unilateral discrete lesions with surrounding erythema and radiating white striae on the buccal mucosa or uni- or bilateral palatal lesions should be viewed as suspicious for lupus erythematosus.
- Gingival lesions extending onto other adjacent mucosal sites may be seen.
- Diagnosis of systemic lupus erythematosus with positive antinuclear antibodies and/or double-stranded DNA is helpful, but a negative result does not exclude oral lupus erythematosus.
- Solitary oral lesions may respond to topical steroid treatment, but this is less effective in patients with systemic disease.

Histopathology

Histopathological features of LE are often very similar to those seen in lichen planus.

Characteristic histopathological features include:

- Due to fibrosis, the basement membrane zone and around blood vessels thicken, a feature highlighted by PAS staining. A chronic inflammatory cell infiltrate may extend into the overlying epithelium, and perivascular infiltrates may be seen. The epithelium may demonstrate both hyperplasia and atrophy. Direct immunofluorescence (DIF) with a band of immunoglobulin or complement is helpful. This is frequently negative in oral mucosal biopsies.

25.8 Traumatic Ulcers

Traumatic ulceration of the oral mucosa is common and may be caused by mechanical, thermal, or chemical injury. Depending on the duration of the trauma, trauma ulcers may be acute or chronic.

Key Features

- Occasionally, thermal, and chemical causes of injuries may be iatrogenic, with the former caused by the application of a hot instrument to anaesthetised mucosa and the latter due to chemical leakage under a rubber dam.
- Ulcers have a yellow fibrinous slough and often have erythematous margins. Induration is usually not a feature in acute ulcers.
- Healing may take several weeks following removal of the cause, so a biopsy is not indicated unless ulceration persists, and a chronic cause cannot be identified and managed.

Traumatic ulcerative granuloma with stromal eosinophilia (TUGSE) is a chronic ulcer in sites where skeletal muscle is present. Due to oedema and inflammation, ulcers have raised rolled margins and are often firm to palpation.

Ulcers are often present for some time, and a biopsy is indicated as the removal of possible causes of trauma does not result in healing. Clinicians are often suspicious that such solitary ulcers may be squamous cell carcinoma. Resolution usually occurs once a biopsy incisional or excisional is performed.

▪ **Histopathology**

The histopathological features of an ulcer show hyperplastic epithelium at the margins, often with cytological atypia and occasionally concomitant candidosis. A mixed acute and chronic inflammatory cell infiltrate is present in the region of ulceration. Eosinophils, macrophages, and endothelial cells are conspicuous in the lamina propria, and together with chronic inflammatory cells, they extend into the underlying muscle.

Factitious oral ulceration may be difficult to diagnose. Such lesions are usually solitary in readily accessible sites, e.g. the anterior part of the mouth. The history does not fit with the clinical features or pattern of injury, and another recognisable disease cannot be identified. Significant psychosocial factors may be difficult to confirm if the patient is reluctant to discuss. A biopsy may be required to exclude other causes of ulceration, but even then, a patient may not disclose a habit.

25.9 Summary

Non-infective stomatitis can present in different clinical forms. Some are ulcerative, and others may be vesicular. Causes of non-infective stomatitis range from trauma to immunological abnormalities. Some disorders may also involve the skin. Histopathological and immunofluorescent assessment is required to confirm some immunologically related disorders.

Further Reading

Becker J, Houben R, Vetter C. The carcinogenic potential of tacrolimus ointment beyond immune suppression: a hypothesis creating case report. BMC Cancer. 2006;6:7.

Khaleel Ahmed M, Jafer M, Nayeem M, et al. Low-level laser therapy and topical medications for treating aphthous ulcers: a systematic review. J Multidiscip Healthc. 2020;13:1595.

Marakoğlu K, Sezer RE, Toker HC, Marakoğlu I. The recurrent aphthous stomatitis frequency in the smoking cessation people. Clin Oral Investig. 2007;11:149.

Scully C, Porter S. Oral mucosal disease: recurrent aphthous stomatitis. Br J Oral Maxillofac Surg. 2008;46:198.

Warnakulasuriya S, Kujan O, Aguirre-Urizar J. Oral potentially malignant disorders: a consensus report from an international seminar on nomenclature and classification, convened by the WHO Collaborating Centre for Oral Cancer. Oral Dis. 2021;27(8):1862–80. https://doi.org/10.1111/odi.13704. Epub 2020 Nov 26

Histopathology of Infective Stomatitis

Janina Christoforou

Contents

S R Prabhu et al. (eds.), *Oral Histology and Oral Histopathology*, https://doi.org/10.1007/978-3-031-77481-2_26

26.1 Introduction

An infection occurs when a microorganism invades host tissues, multiplies and incites an immunological reaction to the microorganism or the pathogenic toxins.

Infections within the oral cavity can be bacterial, fungal, or viral in origin. They may be spread by physical contact, transfer of bodily fluids, or inhalation of airborne particles, and individuals may have increased susceptibility due to an immune compromise. Each of the infections presented has specific clinical and histopathological characteristics that aid in obtaining a diagnosis. Furthermore, each of these conditions is managed in different ways, ranging from pharmacological to surgical management modalities.

26.2 Classification

Below is a classification of infective stomatitis:

Bacterial infections	Fungal infections	Viral infections
Necrotising periodontal diseases • Necrotising gingivitis • Necrotising periodontitis • Necrotising stomatitis **Actinomycosis** **Gonorrhoea** **Oral tuberculous ulcer** **Oral syphilitic ulcer**	**Candidosis** • Pseudomembranous candidosis • Erythematous candidosis • Hyperplastic candidosis **Candida-associated lesions** • Angular cheilitis • Denture stomatitis • Median rhomboid glossitis **Mucocutaneous candidosis** • Histoplasmosis • Aspergillosis	Primary herpetic gingival stomatitis Herpes labialis Herpes zoster Herpangina Hand, foot, and mouth disease Oral hairy leukoplakia Squamous papilloma Condyloma acuminatum Multi-focal epithelial hyperplasia Verruca vulgaris

26.3 Bacterial Infective Stomatitis

26.3.1 Necrotising Periodontal Diseases

- Necrotising periodontal diseases (NPD) include a spectrum of infectious diseases caused by mixed bacterial flora that affect the periodontium, leading to necrosis and ulceration. Three clinical types of NPD include necrotising ulcerative gingivitis (NUG), necrotising ulcerative periodontitis (NUP) and necrotising ulcerative stomatitis (NUP).

26.3.1.1 Necrotising Gingivitis/Necrotising Periodontitis/Necrotising Stomatitis

▪ **Key Features**

- Necrotising ulcerative gingivitis is limited to the gingiva. Crater-like "punched out" ulcers appear on the interdental gingiva, which is covered with pseudomembrane.
- Necrotising ulcerative periodontitis is an extension of NUG and is characterised by the destruction of the periodontal ligament without forming a periodontal pocket.
- Necrotising ulcerative stomatitis occurs when tissue destruction occurs beyond the mucogingival junction and affects the mucosa.
- Pain and intense halitosis are characteristic. Systemic symptoms may include fever.
- Microorganisms involved include *Fusobacterium nucleatum, Borrelia vincentii, and Porphyromonas gingivalis.*
- The disease is prevalent among malnourished children in developing countries.
- Some predisposing factors include malnutrition and immune defects such as HIV and leukaemia.
- Diagnosis is on clinical grounds. Management includes debridement of necrotic debris, chlorhexidine mouth rinses, and Metronidazole antibiotic for anaerobic organisms.

▪ **Histopathology**

Biopsy is generally not required for confirmation of diagnosis. However, the ulcer of NUG shows a zone comprising fibrous mesh composed of degenerated epithelial cells, the neutrophil-rich zone, the necrotic zone, and the bacterial (spirochetal) zone.

26.3.2 Actinomycosis

Actinomycosis is a chronic suppurative infection of the jaw caused by Gram-positive anaerobic filamentous bacteria called Actinomyces.

▪ **Key Features**

- Relatively uncommon infection caused by an oral commensal organism, *Actinomyces Israeli.*
- Predisposing and risk factors include trauma from tooth extraction, jaw fracture, immunocompromised status, or poor oral hygiene.
- Clinical features include trismus, minimal pain, multiple abscesses and pus-discharging sinuses, "Sulfur granules" in the pus, and low-grade fever.

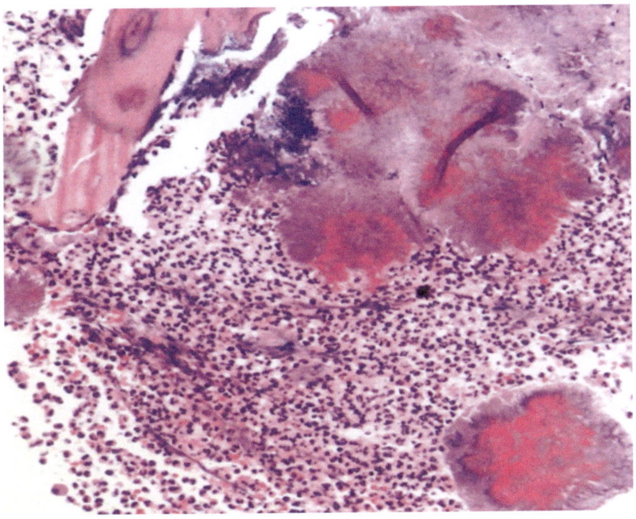

■ **Fig. 26.1** Actinomycosis. Histopathology exhibits filamentous organisms ("sulfur" granules) in the centre, surrounded by an infiltrate of neutrophils and dead bone (top left corner). (Courtesy of Professor Narayan Nagamani, UNMC Nebraska, USA)

- **Histopathology**
  - A biopsy of the abscess reveals numerous filaments with peripheral radially arranged club-shaped thickenings, neutrophils, chronic inflammatory cells and a fibrous wall of the abscess (■ Fig. 26.1).

26.3.3 Gonorrhoea

26.3.3.1 Gonococcal Stomatitis

Gonorrhoea is a sexually transmitted infection caused by Gram-negative diplococcus *Neisseria gonorrhoeae.*

- **Key Features**
  - Oral and pharyngeal lesions of gonorrhoea may rarely occur from oral sex with an infected partner.
  - Most lesions occur in the genital area with purulent discharge.
  - Oral involvement of gonorrhoea can cause mucosal inflammation with erythematous, pustular, or erosive lesions (gonococcal stomatitis). An atrophic lesion (central papillary atrophy) on the dorsum can occur when the tongue is involved.
  - Clinical history and Gram-negative diplococci shown in urethral discharge by direct examination and microbial culture.

- **Histopathology/Cytopathology**

Biopsy of the oral lesion in gonococcal stomatitis is generally not required. Bacterioscopic examination of urethral discharge, fixed and stained by the Gram method (■ Fig. 26.2), is useful.

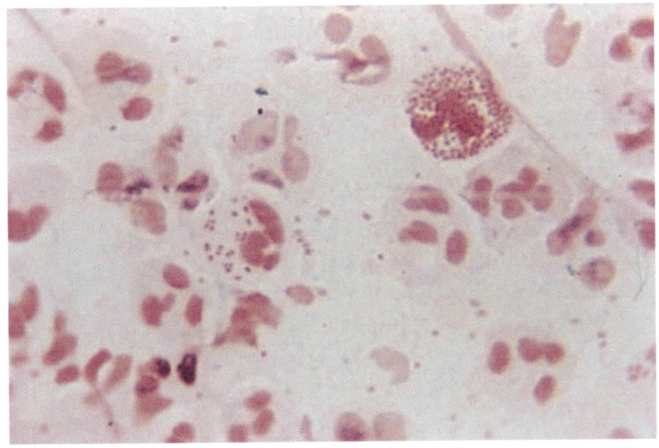

■ **Fig. 26.2** Gonorrhoea. The presence of intracellular Gram-negative diplococcus is shown in urethral discharge by direct examination, fixed and stained by the Gram method. (Source: Belda, W. (2023). Sexually Transmitted Diseases. In: Rangel Bon amigo, R. (eds) Dermatology in Public Health Environments. Springer, Cham. ► https://doi.org/10.1007/978-3-031-13505-7_8. (Reproduced with permission from Springer)

26.3.4 Oral Tuberculous Ulcer

Tuberculosis is a chronic granulomatous disease caused by *Mycobacterium Tuberculosis.* Oral manifestations of tuberculosis are rare.

- **Key Features**
  - Oral tuberculous lesions may occur as primary (rare) or secondary ulcers in patients with pulmonary tuberculosis.
  - Mycobacteria are usually secondarily inoculated with infected sputum or due to hematogenous spread.
  - The ulcer is painful with a granulomatous centre and presents a whitish, well-defined border with slight elevation, undermined edges, and induration.
  - Diagnosis involves a good history and clinical examination. A biopsy of the ulcer is performed for histopathological evaluation.
  - Acid-fast bacilli cultures and polymerase chain reaction (PCR) of sputum will show positive Mycobacterium Tuberculosis. Also, an Interferon Gamma Release Assay (IGRA) using QuantiFERON-TB Gold would be positive.
  - A radiological examination of the chest and a Mantoux skin test is mandatory to rule out systemic TB.
  - Treatment for a patient with oral TB has to be multidisciplinary and should include a respiratory physician.
  - The oral lesions are relieved after pharmacological management of systemic tuberculosis with a combination of antibiotics.

26

- Topical application of anti-inflammatory ointments and protective agents is useful for the symptomatic management of ulcers.

▪ **Histopathology**

The ulceration histopathologically presents with granulomatous inflammation (mediated by a type IV hypersensitivity reaction). Langhans' giant cells are formed by the fusion of macrophages with nuclei arranged in a horseshoe-shaped pattern in the cell periphery (◘ Fig. 26.3). There is central caseous necrosis, with surrounding lymphocytes, plasma cells, and fibroblasts with collagen. Ziehl–Neelsen staining shows acid-fast bacilli of the mycobacterial organisms.

26.3.5 Oral Syphilitic Ulcer

Syphilis is a sexually transmitted infection caused by the spirochete *Treponema pallidum.* If left untreated, syphilis can progress through four stages: primary, secondary, latent, and tertiary.

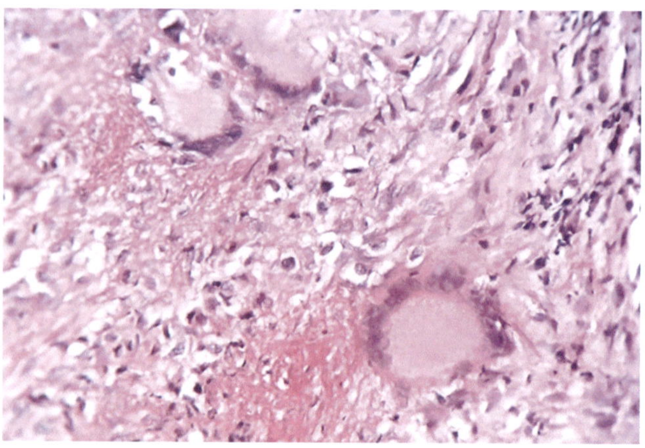

◘ **Fig. 26.3** Oral tuberculous ulcer. Granuloma is composed of epithelioid cells, Langhans' giant cells, and small foci of caseous necrosis. (Source: Kadar N, Namboodiripad A, Haris M, Divya R. Tuberculous Ulcer of Oral Cavity. Oral Maxillofac Pathol J 2017;8(2):105–107. (Reproduced with permission)

▪ **Key Features**

- Oral manifestations can occur in primary, secondary and tertiary stages of the disease. In primary syphilis, a solitary, indurated, painless ulcer called a chancre can occur at the sites of inoculation, which commonly include the lip or tip of the tongue.
- Chancre generally resolves spontaneously in 3–8 weeks.
- In secondary syphilis, skin rash, macules, fever, and generalised lymphadenopathy are common. Oral lesions include greyish membrane-covered ulcers (snail track ulcers) on the tongue, tonsils, and lips.
- Oral lesions of tertiary syphilis include interstitial glossitis, syphilitic leukoplakia and a necrotic palatal lesion called gumma.
- History of sex with an infected partner, clinical findings, dark-ground illumination of the smear from the lesion, serology, polymerase chain reaction (PCR) results, and histological and immunohistochemical staining of the biopsied lesional tissue confirm the diagnosis.
- Serological tests include *T. pallidum* particle agglutination assay (TP-PA), which can be utilised for additional diagnostic confirmation. This will show positive *T. pallidum* IgG and IgM.
- Syphilis is treated by a sexually transmitted disease expert with antibiotics from the penicillin family. If there is a penicillin allergy, azithromycin or doxycycline are used.

▪ **Histopathology**

The primary syphilitic lesion (chancre) histopathologically presents with focal ulceration, extensive neutrophilic exocytosis, and a dense plasmacytic/lymphocytic infiltrate in the superficial lamina propria and occasionally in the deeper stroma. This infiltrate characteristically surrounds blood vessels (◘ Fig. 26.4a) and nerves. Immunohistochemical staining with anti-*T. pallidum* reveals the presence of numerous spirochetes that infiltrate the epithelium (◘ Fig. 26.4b). Of note, cross-reactivity of anti-*T. pallidum* has been reported with other bacterial organisms. Hence, clinical correlation is of major significance.

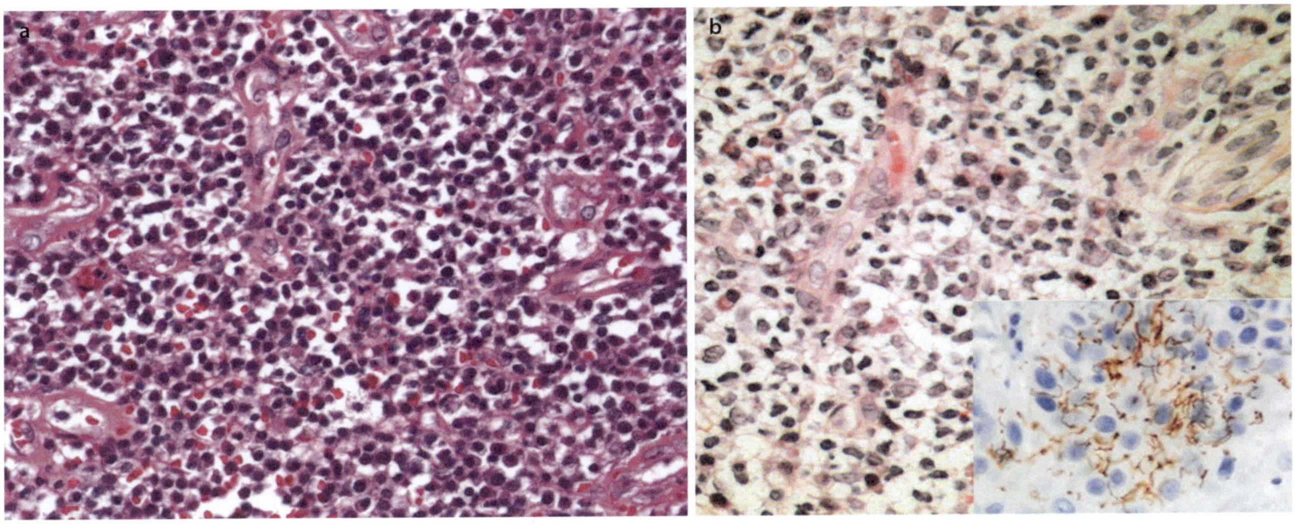

▣ **Fig. 26.4** **a** Syphilitic chancre. This higher magnification shows an infiltrate composed of plasma cells, histiocytes, and lymphocytes. The findings are non-specific; however, a combination of endarteritis and plasma cell infiltrate should point to the diagnosis. (Courtesy of Dr. Dharam Ramnani, USA. ► Webpathology.com). **b** Immunohistochemistry of primary chancre. Numerous organisms are seen using immunohistochemistry directed against *Treponema pallidum* (inset). (► Courtesy DermnetNZ.com)

26.4 Fungal Infective Stomatitis

26.4.1 Oral Candidosis (Oral Candidiasis)

Oral candidosis is a fungal infection caused by pathogenic candidal species, of which *Candida albicans* is common. The fungus is a commensal non-pathogenic opportunistic organism which becomes pathogenic in those with local or systemic predisposing factors. Oral candidosis includes a spectrum of presentations, including pseudomembranous candidosis (thrush), erythematous candidosis, chronic hyperplastic candidosis (candidal leukoplakia), angular cheilitis, denture stomatitis, median rhomboid glossitis, and chronic mucocutaneous candidosis.

Pseudomembranous candidosis (thrush) clinically presents as loosely adherent white curd-like plaques or flakes predominantly on the buccal mucosa and the dorsum of the tongue. Plaques can be wiped off with a gauge, exposing the underlying erythematous mucosa.

Erythematous candidosis is common in the dorsum of the tongue in those with a history of using broad-spectrum antibiotics. Loss of papillae resulting in "bald" patches is common.

Chronic hyperplastic candidosis presents as a white patch that cannot be wiped off by a gauge located on the anterior buccal mucosa, commonly seen in heavy smokers. In a small percentage of patients, this is a potentially malignant disorder.

Angular cheilitis is painful fissuring and inflammation of one or both labial commissures in individuals who are complete denture wearers, immunocompromised and malnourished.

Denture stomatitis is a candida-associated condition which presents as palatal erythema and pinpointed diffuse or nodular lesions in those who continuously wear maxillary removable dentures.

Median rhomboid glossitis is a candida-associated lesion which occurs as central atrophy of the tongue around the midline. It presents as a well-demarcated, symmetric, depapillated area, which can be smooth or lobulated, arising anterior to the circumvallate papillae.

Mucocutaneous candidosis is a rare primary immunodeficiency disease characterised by persistent or recurrent *C. albicans* infections of the skin, nails, and mucous membranes.

A detailed history, including predisposing conditions, clinical findings, microbiological examinations of scrapings/smears stained with periodic acid-Schiff (PAS) reagents, fungal culture, and histopathological examination of biopsied samples of lesions, are the methods available for diagnosing candidosis.

Treatment includes administration of (where appropriate) topical/systemic antifungal agents and elimination of predisposing factors.

▪ Histopathology

Pseudomembranous candidosis: Periodic acid-Schiff-stained scrapings show masses of tangled fungal hyphae, exfoliated epithelial cells and neutrophils. Erythematous candidosis and rhomboid glossitis scrapings may not show candidal hyphae. Hyperplastic candidosis shows mildly parakeratotic epithelium, scanty candidal hyphae

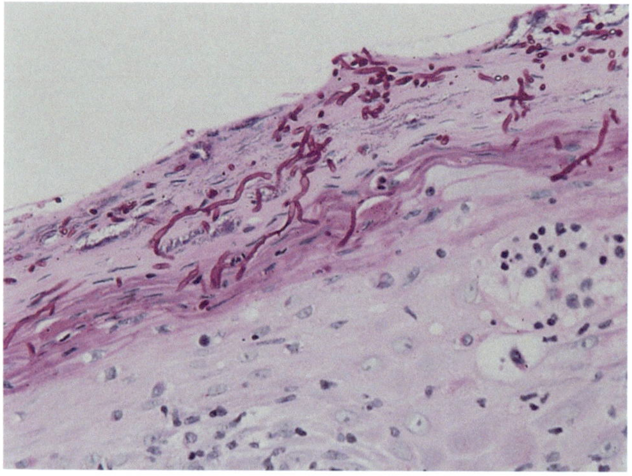

Fig. 26.5 Candidal hyphae in the superficial layers of epithelium in hyperplastic candidosis (PASD stain). (Courtesy of Professor David F Wilson, Adelaide)

in the superficial layers (Fig. 26.5), hyperplastic rete ridges, and rarely mild epithelial dysplasia. Connective tissue shows chronic inflammatory cell infiltration. Median rhomboid glossitis presents with the atrophic stratified squamous epithelium of the filiform papillae overlying a moderately fibrotic stroma with chronic inflammation. Candida species are noted superficially as well as a pseudoepitheliomatous hyperplasia. Mucocutaneous candidosis shows an increased thickness of parakeratin, elongation of the epithelial rete ridges, collections of neutrophils (microabscesses) in the parakeratin layer and the superficial spinous cell layer, some lymphocytes, and macrophages in the superficial connective tissue. Special stains include Grocott and Gomori methenamine silver (GMS), which highlight the fungal cell wall, and Periodic acid-Schiff (PAS) stains, which detect glycogen in fungal walls.

Histoplasmosis

An infectious disease caused by the fungus Histoplasma capsulatum. It is a deep fungal infection that affects pulmonary tissue or mucocutaneous areas. It is acquired by inhalation of infectious microconidia in soil contaminated by bird or bat droppings.

Key Features

- Three forms of histoplasmosis are acute (self-limiting pulmonary infection), chronic (primarily affecting the lungs), and disseminated (may affect multiple organ systems, including the oral mucosa).
- Regarding the oral mucosa, the lesions are noted on the tongue, palate, and buccal mucosa.
- Oral ulcerations typically present with firm, rolled borders and last several weeks, mimicking a malignant neoplasm.
- A diagnosis is made when the pathogen is isolated by culture, histopathology of a lesion or cytopathology of aspirates.
- Chest radiographs should also be considered.
- The severity of the infection and the patient's underlying health problems will often direct treatment.
- Antifungal medication, such as Amphotericin B and Itraconazole, is generally indicated.

Histopathology

- Histopathologically presents with granulomatous inflammation (both caseating or non-caseating granulomas) with multi-nucleated giant cells and macrophages in the stroma. Fungal elements (small yeasts [2–4 um] with ovoid, narrow-based budding) are mainly detected within the cytoplasm of macrophages. The yeasts appear clustered since they are initially ingested by macrophages. With hematoxylin and eosin (H&E) stain, the basophilic yeast cytoplasm is separated from the surrounding tissue by the cell wall (clear zone), and this is highlighted with the special stains such as Grocott and Gomori's methenamine silver (GMS) and periodic acid-Schiff (PAS).

26.5 Viral Infective Stomatitis

26.5.1 Primary Herpetic Gingivostomatitis

An acute herpes simplex virus-1 (HSV-1) infection affecting the oral cavity is transmitted by direct contact with a lesion or infected body fluids (saliva).

Key Features

- It typically has a prodrome of 3–4 days and consists of fever, irritability, malaise, headaches, and cervical lymphadenopathy before generalised gingival inflammation and numerous vesicles and ulcers on the oral mucosa.
- It is self-limiting and resolves in 10–14 days.
- Diagnosis is generally made based on clinical presentation.
- If additional testing is required, primary herpetic gingivostomatitis can be confirmed using a swab or Tzanck smear from the vesicle for cytology and PCR testing to determine the presence of HSV DNA.
- Management is generally supportive care with fluid maintenance, paracetamol to reduce fever and the potential use of topical lidocaine preparations, i.e. Magic mouthwash.
- If an individual presents within 24–48 hours of the onset of vesicle eruption, antiviral medication may accelerate healing by inhibiting DNA replication in HSV-infected cells.

■ **Histopathology/Cytopathology**

The virus exerts its main effects on the epithelial cells and shows degeneration of stratified squamous epithelial cells. The infected epithelial cells from the Tzanck smear exhibit acantholysis, nuclear margination of chromatin, eosinophilic cytoplasm and occasional multi-nucleation of infected epithelial cells (◘ Fig. 26.6). Intercellular oedema develops and leads to the formation of an intraepithelial vesicle with Tzanck cells. There are intranuclear inclusion bodies (Cowdry type A), which are found on electron microscopy and show arrays of viral capsids and electron-dense glycoproteins. There is a mixed inflammatory cell infiltrate (lymphocytes, neutrophils).

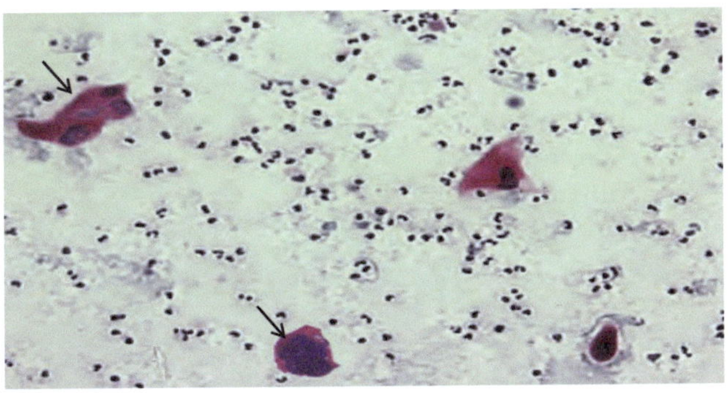

◘ **Fig. 26.6** Cytology of Tzanck smear: multi-nucleated giant cells with pink viral inclusions (arrows). (Source: Pramod KJ, Nandini DB, Mohan Kumar KP, Madhushankari GS. A case report of recurrent herpetic gingivostomatitis with special reference to the role of cytology in diagnosis, CODS J Dent 2014;6;56–60 (With permission)

26.5.2 Recurrent Herpetic Stomatitis (Herpes Labialis)

Recurrent herpetic stomatitis (herpes labialis/cold sore) is a secondary infection of HS-1 characterised by multiple vesicular lesions on the vermilion border of lips and adjacent skin.

■ **Key Features**

- Reactivation of the latent virus in the trigeminal nerve ganglion and travels along the nerve to a new site.
- Triggering factors include ultraviolet radiation, stress, cold and immunosuppression.
- Prodromal sensations such as tingling, itching and paraesthesia at the site are common symptoms.
- Clusters of multiple vesicles appear on the mucocutaneous junction of the lips.
- Vesicles rupture shortly after they appear, and crust or scab forms in about 2 days.
- History and clinical findings offer diagnosis; viral culture and PCR test of vesicular fluid and cytology of the smear are confirmatory.
- Usually a self-limiting infection.
- In some cases, with severe symptoms, antiviral topical treatment is required.

■ **Histopathology/Cytopathology**

Histopathological (◘ Fig. 26.7) and cytopathological features are the same as for herpesvirus infections (see herpetic gingivostomatitis above).

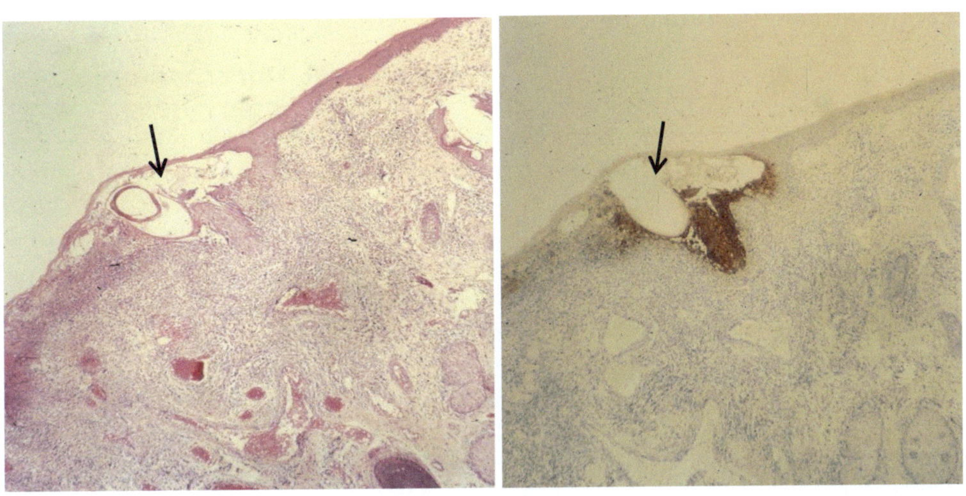

◘ **Fig. 26.7** Low-power light microscope sections illustrating an intraepithelial vesicle (arrows) in an H&E-stained section and an adjacent section immunolabelled for (HSV-1) from a biopsy of a herpes labialis lesion of the lip. (Courtesy of Professor David F Wilson, Adelaide)

26.5.3 Herpes Zoster (Shingles)

Herpes zoster (shingles) is a secondary/recurrent varicella-zoster virus (human herpesvirus-3 or HHV-3) infection due to the reactivation of the latent virus in neurons of the cranial nerve ganglia. The primary infection is varicella (chickenpox).

- **Key Features**
  - Risk/predisposing factors include old age, immunosuppressive drugs, HIV infection, radiation, malignancy, stress, and trauma during dental treatment.
  - Reactivation of varicella-zoster virus (VZV) in the trigeminal ganglion with subsequent travelling of the viruses along the sensory nerve that supplies the oral mucosae causes vesicles and ulcerations on the oral mucosae.
  - Lesions do not cross the midline.
  - Herpes zoster is diagnosed from characteristic clinical presentation.
  - Laboratory tests, such as viral culture, immunofluorescence staining of cytologic smears with fluorescent monoclonal VZV antibodies, dot-blot hybridisation, and polymerase chain reaction (PCR), help identify VZV as the causal virus of the disease.
  - Patients with pain require analgesics and need those with severe symptoms to be treated with topical or systemic antiviral drugs.

- **Histopathology/Cytology**

Histopathological and cytopathological features are the same as for herpes virus infections (see herpetic gingivostomatitis above).

26.5.4 Herpangina

Herpangina is a highly contagious enterovirus infection caused by Coxsackie group virus A (1–16) or group B (1–5).

- **Key Features**
  - Soft palate or tonsillar region shows macular erythematous areas followed by vesicles and ulcers.
  - Pharyngitis, dysphagia, fever, and cough are common symptoms.
  - Children commonly affected.
  - Self-limiting infection.
  - Diagnosis by history, clinical findings, culture, and PCR test.
  - Symptomatic treatment is adequate.

- **Histopathology/Cytopathology**

Biopsy of an ulcer does not show any specific features. Non-specific acute inflammatory are seen. Polymerase chain reaction (PCR) testing is fast and highly sensitive for enteroviruses. Samples may be obtained from mucocutaneous ulcers or vesicular fluid.

26.5.5 Hand-Foot and Mouth Disease (HFMD)

Hand-foot and mouth disease is a childhood Coxsackie (A10 or A16) virus infection characterised by erythematous and ulcerative lesions on the hands, feet, and mouth.

- **Key Features**
  - A common childhood infection.
  - Vesicles on palms, soles, feet, and mouth appear with mild systemic symptoms such as pharyngitis and mild fever.
  - Usually resolves within a week.
  - Symptomatic treatment may be necessary for some patients.

- **Histopathology/Cytopathology**

Histopathologic findings of HFMD include an intraepidermal/epithelial vesicle containing neutrophils and eosinophilic cellular debris. The adjacent epithelium/epidermis has reticular degeneration, which is intercellular and intracellular oedema. The dermis has a mixed infiltrate. Histopathology features are similar to those of viral infections, which cause acantholysis.

26.5.6 Oral Hairy Leukoplakia

Oral hairy leukoplakia (OHL) is a benign lesion that presents most often as an opportunistic infection in immune-suppressed patients. It is associated with the Epstein–Barr virus (EBV). This is not an inflammatory lesion. However, some inflammatory changes may occur in the connective tissue, hence its inclusion in this chapter.

- **Key Features**
  - This is not a predominantly inflammatory lesion that causes stomatitis.
  - OHL manifests as unilateral or bilateral, white or grey patches on the lateral margins and dorsal or ventral surfaces of the tongue that cannot be wiped off.

- It exhibits a range of appearances from faintly visible white streaks to deep furrowed, "shaggy"-surfaced leukoplakia.
- The clinical appearance is due to the productive replication of EBV in the oral mucosa.
- A diagnosis is generally made on a clinical basis.
- Demonstration of EBV in the koilocyte-like cells by immunocytochemistry or DNA in situ hybridisation can also be undertaken.
- Oral hairy leukoplakia itself doesn't usually need treatment, but it means investigations are required to determine reasons for immunocompromised status.
- Subsequent management to improve immunity will be required.

Histopathology

Histopathologically, the epithelium is acanthotic and hyperparakeratinised. Sometimes, candida hyphae may be present in the parakeratin. A band of EBV-infected, koilocyte-like cells is present in the upper part of the prickle cell layers. These cells are swollen and pale-stained, with prominent cell borders and perinuclear vacuoles (Fig. 26.8). There is sparse inflammation in the epithelium and lamina propria.

26.5.7 Squamous Papilloma

Squamous papilloma is a common benign neoplasm of the oral cavity, which appears to be mainly related to the human papillomavirus (HPV) types 6 and 11. This is not an inflammatory lesion. However, some inflammatory changes may occur in the connective tissue, hence its inclusion in this chapter.

Key Features

- Squamous papilloma is a proliferation of stratified squamous epithelium that usually presents with a verrucous or cauliflower-like appearance with a sessile or pedunculated base.
- There is low transmissibility with direct contact.
- Squamous papilloma is a slow-growing lesion commonly found on the tongue, gingiva, vermilion, and palate and appears as clinically isolated lesions.
- Diagnosis is generally made in combination with clinical manifestations and histopathological appearances.
- Management generally requires excision of the lesion.
- Recurrences are rare.

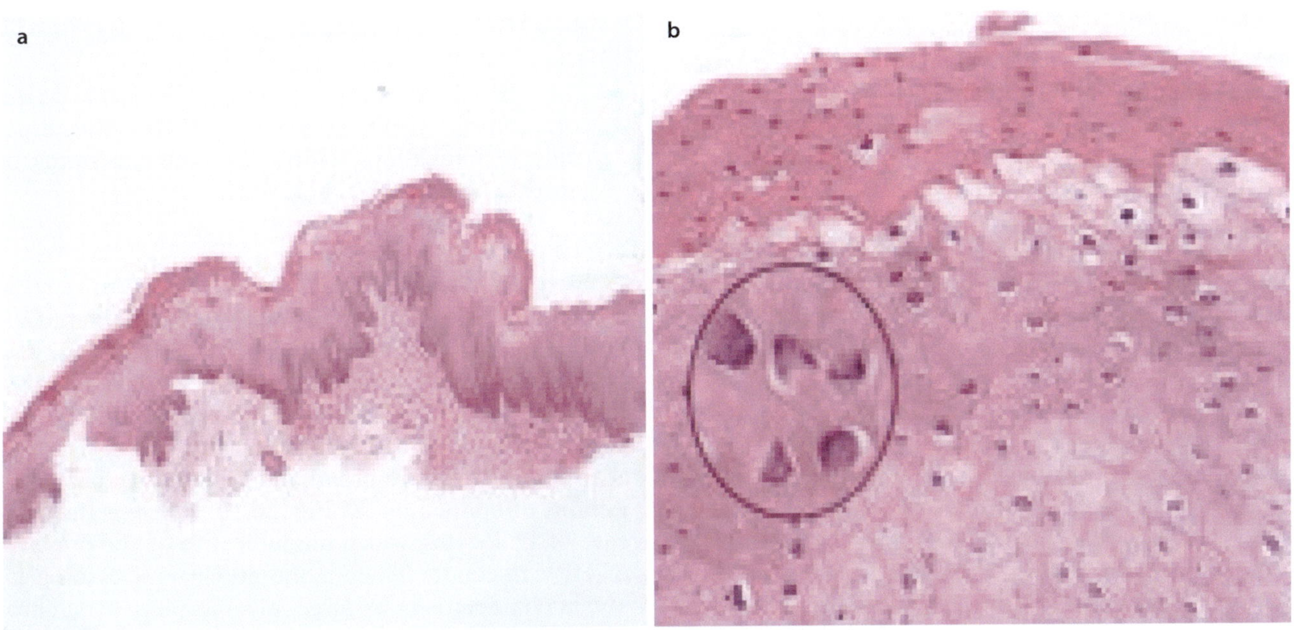

Fig. 26.8 Oral hairy leukoplakia. **a** Hyperkeratosis and acanthosis, with prominent intracellular oedema, are noted at low power. **b** Peripheral "beading" of the chromatin is noted in superficial keratinocytes. (Source: Alramadhan, S.A., Bhattacharyya, I., Cohen, D.M. et al. Oral Hairy Leukoplakia in Immunocompetent Patients Revisited with Literature Review. *Head and Neck Pathol* **15**, 989–993 (2021). ► https://doi.org/10.1007/s12105-021-01287-8. (With permission from Springer Nature))

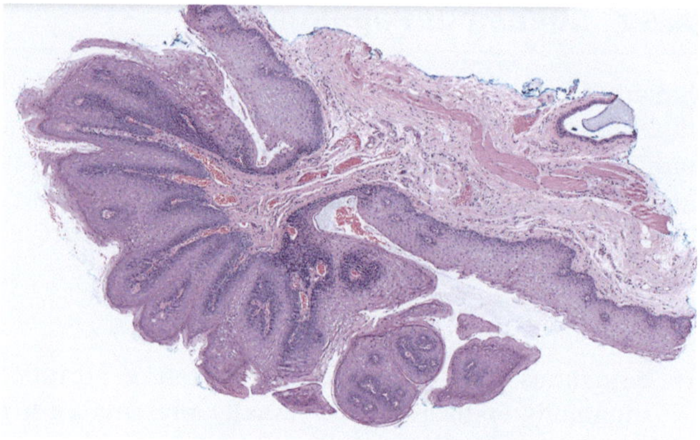

■ **Fig. 26.9** The sections show mature fibrous connective tissue covered by parakeratinised hyperplastic stratified squamous epithelium with no features of epithelial dysplasia or malignancy. The epithelium is arranged as multiple exophytic blunt-ended projections. Oedema is seen in the epithelium. Viral cytopathic changes are not present. A sparse chronic inflammatory cell infiltrate is in the fibrovascular core. No PASD positive fungal elements are seen. (Courtesy of A/Prof Norman Firth)

■ **Histopathology**

Histopathologically, they present with a hyperkeratinised surface of stratified squamous epithelium, with epithelial hyperplasia forming finger-like projections with fibrovascular connective tissue cores (■ Fig. 26.9). Koilocyte-like cells may be present in the spinous layer of the epithelium. Multiple mitoses may be present, but these are limited to the basal layer. The lamina propria often contain a chronic inflammatory cell infiltrate.

26.5.8 Condyloma Acuminatum

Condyloma acuminatum is induced by the human papillomavirus (HPV). HPV subtypes 6 and 11 are commonly associated with this lesion. HPV 2, 53, and 54 have also been detected in some cases.

■ **Key Features**

- Condyloma acuminatum is a sexually transmitted disease commonly found in the genital and anal areas.
- This DNA virus is highly transmissible. It penetrates the outer epithelial surface and infects the nucleus of squamous cells, resulting in a proliferation that is recognised as condyloma acuminatum.
- The clinical appearance may vary from solitary or multiple, pinkish, sessile papules/plaques with a pebbled surface texture or as pedunculated lesions with finger-like projections.

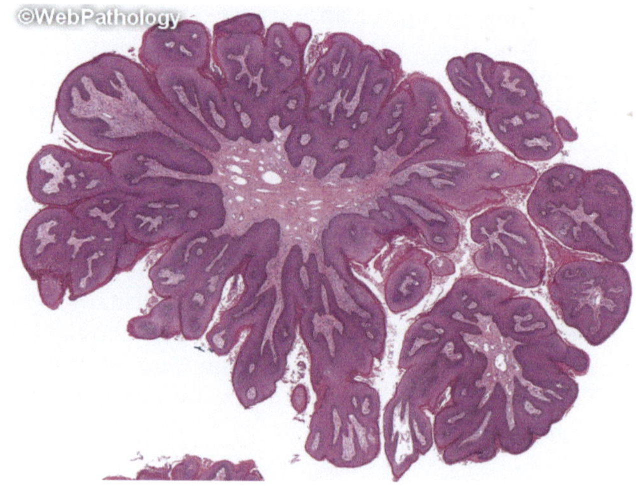

■ **Fig. 26.10** Condylomas show marked acanthosis, papillomatosis, hyperkeratosis, and parakeratosis. Superficial layers show vacuolated keratinocytes (koilocytes) and prominent coarse keratohyalin granules. Binucleated cells, dyskeratocytes, and wrinkled nuclei (resinoid appearance) may also be seen. Cytologic atypia is minimal, and mitotic figures are confined to the basal region. (Courtesy of Dr. Dharam Ramnani, ► Webpathology.com)

- Oral lesions commonly affect the lips, oral mucosa and rarely the gingiva.
- Diagnosis is generally made in combination with clinical manifestations and histopathological appearances.
- These lesions are surgically excised. Recurrences are common due to the persistence of the virus, especially in individuals with a low immune status or untreated genital or anal lesions.

■ **Histopathology**

Histopathologically presents with non-keratinised or hyperkeratinised stratified squamous epithelium supported by connective tissue cores with marked acanthosis and pseudoepitheliomatous hyperplasia with moderate-to-marked degrees of basilar hyperplasia and acanthosis. There are broad and blunted papillary projections of epithelium (■ Fig. 26.10). There is the presence of koilocytes, which are indicative of the presence of HPV infection. There is the presence of cytological atypia characterised by large, pleomorphic, hyperchromatic, and angular nuclei predominately in the superficial layers of the epithelium, and the basal layers are least affected. There is also the presence of intense chronic inflammatory cell infiltrate in the connective tissue stroma.

26.5.9 Multi-Focal Epithelial Hyperplasia (Heck's Disease)

Multi-focal epithelial hyperplasia (MEH) is a benign, rare familial disorder. The main aetiological factor is the presence of the human papillomavirus, primarily HPV 13 and 32.

- **Key Features**
- It is characterised by multiple circumscribed, discrete, sessile, soft, flattened or elevated, and round papulonodular lesions of the oral mucosa, with a colour similar to the adjoining oral mucosa.
- Geographically, it is more prevalent in North, South, and Central American Indians and less common in Caucasians.
- Generally, younger individuals with MEH exhibit multiple nodular lesions, whereas single or fewer lesions are seen in elderly individuals.
- It predominantly affects children and individuals in the first and second decades of life, with the lower lip being the most commonly involved site.
- Diagnosis is generally made in combination with clinical manifestations and histopathological appearances.
- The management of MEH is not always necessary since the lesions are asymptomatic and often tend to regress spontaneously.
- If there is an aesthetic concern, treatment generally involves surgical or laser excision or cryotherapy.

- **Histopathology**
- Histopathological features consist of extensive acanthosis, parakeratin layering, degeneration of koilocytes, mitosoid cells, and elongated rete ridges, some of which form horizontal anastomosing and other rete ridges form clubbing.

26.5.10 Verruca Vulgaris

Verruca vulgaris (VV) is a viral-induced neoplasm of the skin caused by the human papillomavirus (HPV) and is associated with HPV types 2 and 4.

- **Key Features**
- Clinically, VV are sessile, circumscribed, exophytic growths with a papillomatous surface.
- The lesion can occur at any age, with a preference for children, and involves the vermilion and mucous membranes of the oral cavity.
- VV may rapidly enlarge to a maximal size and then remain constant unless the lesion is irritated.

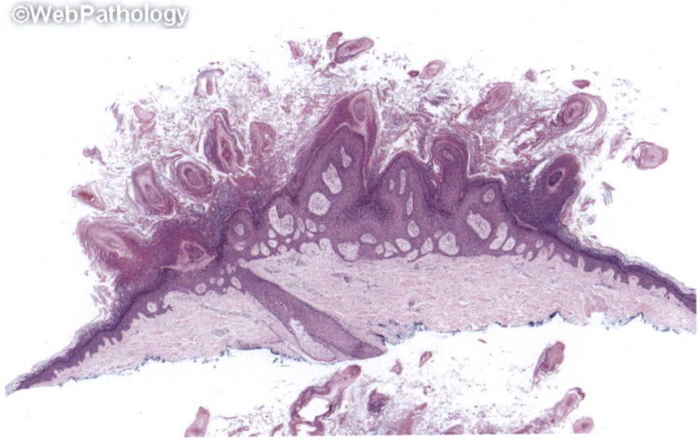

Fig. 26.11 Verruca vulgaris is an exophytic lesion that shows epidermal/epithelial hyperplasia manifesting as papillomatosis, acanthosis, and hyperkeratosis. Filiform papillae with parakeratosis over the tips are present. (Courtesy of Dr. Dharam Ramnani, ▶ Webpathology.com)

- Multiple or clustered lesions are common.
- Diagnosis is generally made based on clinical features and confirmed with histopathological evaluation.
- These lesions are surgically excised.

- **Histopathology**

The VV is histopathologically characterised by a proliferation of hyperkeratotic stratified squamous epithelium arranged into finger-like or pointed projections with connective tissue cores. Chronic Inflammatory cells often infiltrate the supporting connective tissue (Fig. 26.11). Elongated rete ridges tend to converge toward the centre of the lesion, producing a "cupping" effect. A prominent granular cell layer (hypergranulosis) exhibits coarse, clumped keratohyalin granules. Abundant koilocytes are often seen in the superficial spinous layer. Eosinophilic intranuclear viral inclusions are often noted within the cells of the granular layer.

26.6 Summary

Infective stomatitis is predominantly inflammatory and caused by a variety of infections of bacterial, fungal, or viral origin. Several of these oral lesions are secondary to systemic diseases, and some result because of the individuals' immunocompromised status. Investigative techniques are required to arrive at a diagnosis so that effective management can be undertaken. In most cases, histopathological examination of the oral lesions is essential in arriving at a diagnosis.

26

Further Reading

Borgstrom E, Edvinsson SA, Perez M, et al. Three adult cases of STAT1 gain-of-function with chronic mucocutaneous candidiasis treated with JAK inhibitors. J Clin Immunol. 2023;43(1):136–50.

Carneiro TE, Marinho SA, Verli FD, Mesquita AT, Lima NL, Miranda JL. Oral squamous papilloma: clinical, histologic and immunohistochemical analyses. J Oral Sci. 2009;51(3):367–72.

Deng F, Thompson LDR, Lai J. Unexpected Reason for Non-healing Oral Ulcers: Syphilis. Head Neck Pathol. 2022;16(2):544–9.

Fatahzadeh M, Schwartz RA. Human Herpes Simplex Virus Infections: epidemiology, pathogenesis, symptomatology, diagnosis and management. J Am Acad Dermatol. 2007;57(5):737–63.

Goregen M, Miloglu O, Buyokkurt MC, Caglayan F, Aktas AE. Median Rhomboid Glossitis: A Clinical and Microbiological Study. Eur J Dent. 2011;5(4):367–72.

Guarner J, Brandt ME. Histopathologic Diagnosis of Fungal infections in the 21st Century. Clin Microbiol Rev. 2011a;24(2):247–80.

Guarner J, Brandt ME. Histopathologic Diagnosis of Fungal infections in the 21st Century. Clin Microbiol Rev. 2011b;24(2):247–80.

Heliotis I, Whatling R, Desai S, Visavadia M. Primary herpetic gingivostomatitis in children. BMJ. 2021;375:e065540.

Housley Smith M, Vargo RJ, Bilodeau EA, Anderson KM, Trzcinska A, Canterbury CR, Fantasia JE, Rawal YB. Oral manifestations of Syphilis: a Review of the Clinical and Histopathologic Characteristics of a Reemerging Entity with Report of 19 New Cases. Head Neck Pathol. 2021;15(3):787–95.

Kauffman CA. Histoplasmosis. Clin Chest Med. 2009;30:217–25.

Kiykim C, Charbonnier A, Akcay LM, et al. Hematopoietic stem cell transplantation in patients with heterozygous STAT1 gain-of-function mutation. J Clin Immunol. 2019;39(1):37–44.

Leinweber B, Kerl H, Cerroni L. Histopathological features of cutaneous herpes virus infections (herpes simplex, varicella/zoster): a broad spectrum of presentations with common pseudolymphomatous aspects. Am J Surg Pathol. 2006;30(1):50–8.

Nagaraj M. Verruca vulgaris of the tongue. J Maxillofac Oral Surg. 2013;12(3):329–32.

Patil K, Guledgud MV, Sanjay CJ, Penumatsa B. Oral Multifocal Epithelial Hyperplasia: An Unusual Entity. Int J Appl Basic Med Res. 2019;9(4):253–5.

Sen R, Shah N, Sheikh MA, Chatterjee RP. Oral condyloma acuminatum in a 75-year-old geriatric patient. BMJ Case Rep. 2018;1(2018):bcr2017222905.

Southam JC, Felix DH, Wray D, Cubie HA. Hairy Leukoplakia- a histological study. Histopathology. 1991;19(1):63–7.

Wang W, Chen J, Chen Y, Lin L. Tuberculosis of the head and neck; a review of 20 cases. Oral Surg Oral Med Oral Pathol Oral Radiol Endod. 2009;107(3):381–6.

Wang Z, Zhang Y, Ma W. Chronic Mucocutaneous Candidiasis: A Case Report. Clin Cosmet Investig Dermatol. 2023 Jan;25(16):231–6.

Histopathology of Reactive Hyperplastic Lesions of the Oral Mucosa

H. M. Hussaini

Contents

S R Prabhu et al. (eds.), *Oral Histology and Oral Histopathology*, https://doi.org/10.1007/978-3-031-77481-2_27

27

27.1 Introduction

A reactive lesion is a response of the oral mucosa to a low-grade irritation or injury, such as broken teeth, chewing, food impaction, calculus, overhanging dental restorations and denture flanges. These long-standing and chronic low-grade irritations commonly induce exophytic reactive proliferation in the oral cavity. Clinically, these proliferations are usually painless and may present as pedunculated or sessile masses. Sometimes, the surface can be ulcerated and will normally appear reddish or fiery red, and other lesions would have yellow slough (ulceration) with white (surface keratinisation). In most instances, the surface would be smooth pink with no obvious ulceration. These reactive lesions can vary from a few millimetres to several centimetres in size, and most tend to appear on the gingival or the alveolar ridge. Other sites of occurrence are the lip, tongue, and buccal mucosa. Histologically, these lesions commonly consist of fibrous connective tissue proliferation covered by mucosa. Each lesion will have its unique features, as mentioned in each category. All lesions have a good prognosis and do not tend to recur unless the irritation or trauma is not sufficiently removed.

27.2 Frictional Keratosis

Frictional keratosis presents as a white, keratotic lesion found within the oral mucosa, stemming from persistent mechanical friction caused by different irritation factors or habits.

Key Features

- Clinically, these lesions can emerge on keratinised and non-keratinised tissues, appearing as broad white patches or plaques ranging from faintly translucent to notably dense white, often exhibiting irregular shapes.
- Examples of frictional keratosis include 'linea alba' presenting along both buccal mucosa where the occlusal line of the teeth meets with the mucosa.
- Frictional keratosis usually begins to disappear once the causative factor is removed. Sometimes, excisional biopsy becomes necessary due to failure to reverse the condition, or it is cosmetically preferred by the patients.
- Frictional keratosis lesions do not carry malignant potential.

Histopathology

Microscopically, frictional keratosis will appear with a thickened surface keratin layer with or without corresponding acanthosis in the spinous layer. The epithelium shows epithelial hyperplasia with intracellular oedema featuring ballooned cells (Fig. 27.1a, b). There is a general lack of inflammatory cells within the superficial connective tissue unless the trauma results in an ulceration, whereby granulation tissue will dominate around the ulcer base. The surface keratin may show parakeratosis or orthokeratosis. Sometimes, both histological features can present in the same lesion. Frictional Keratoses do not show epithelial dysplastic features, although some normal mitotic figures may be present in the basal cell layer.

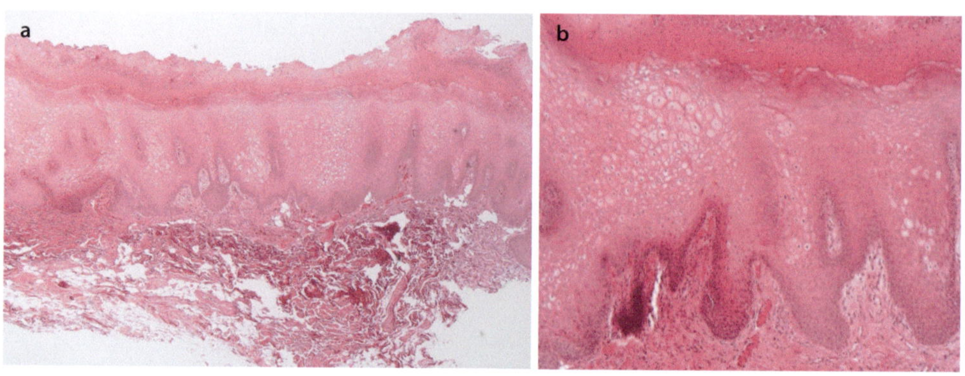

Fig. 27.1 **a** and **b** The histological appearance of frictional keratosis shows acanthosis and intracellular oedema in the epithelium's prickle cell layer **a** and ballooning of prickle cells

27.3 Denture-Induced Hyperplasia (Denture-Induced Granuloma, Epulis Fissuratum)

Denture-induced hyperplasia refers to a reactive oral mucosal response to excessive mechanical irritation or pressure from an ill-fitting prosthesis.

Key Features

- This lesion normally occurs adjacent to the flanges of complete or partial ill-fitting prosthesis.
- Virchoff introduced the term 'epulis,' meaning 'over the gums'; however, it was later replaced by 'denture-induced hyperplasia' based on the prevalence of occurrence of the lesion in the vestibular sulcus rather than the gingiva.
- It normally affects the anterior part of the jaw rather than the posterior region, and the size varies from 1 cm to much more extensive lesions.
- Clinically, denture-induced hyperplasia will appear as hyperplastic tissue arising from the alveolar vestibule with a polypoid appearance. The surface architecture is normally smooth and pink, and the lesion is firm. However, if there is trauma, it can be ulcerated and erythematous, which may also bleed from time to time.
- Apart from being polypoid, it can take a 'leaf-like' appearance, which can have several folds or 'several leaves' between the ill-fitting prosthesis as the flanges impinge on the mucosa.
- The treatment of denture-induced hyperplasia includes removing surgically the hyperplastic tissue. After complete resolution and healing, a new denture should be made, or the existing denture should be re-lined to prevent the lesion from recurring.

Histopathology

Microscopically, denture-induced hyperplasia will reveal hyperplasia of the fibrous connective tissue as well as the overlying epithelium (Fig. 27.2). Hyperkeratosis of the epithelium is frequently followed by elongated or cascading epithelial rete ridges. The underlying connective tissue is normally dense with coarse fibrous collagen bundle and almost avascular with very minimal blood vessels. The deeper area will often have other connective tissue appendages such as neural tissue, collection of adipose tissue, skeletal muscle and sometimes minor salivary gland acini. If it is traumatised, the surface presents with an area of ulceration with inflammatory exudate and an intense inflammatory cell infiltrate with granulation tissue. With inflammation settling in, this can resemble the histological features of pyogenic granuloma. Often, in long-standing lesions, there is a formation of calcified tissues or an osteoid mass termed osseous metaplasia, and this should not be mistaken for a malignant process.

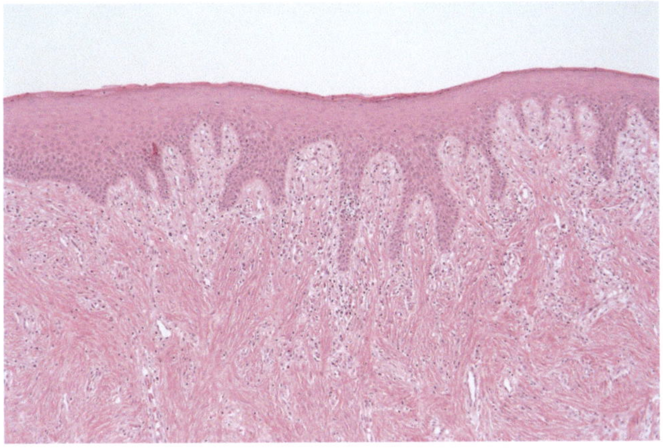

Fig. 27.2 The histological appearance of denture-induced hyperplasia shows dense fibrous connective tissue covered by hyperplastic stratified squamous epithelium. Inflammation within the dense fibrous connective tissue and vasculature are minimal

27.4 Pyogenic Granuloma

Pyogenic granuloma, also known as lobular capillary haemangioma, is a benign, non-neoplastic vascular growth found in the oral mucosa in response to chronic local irritation.

Key Features

- Pyogenic granuloma is commonly seen in children, young adults, and occasionally in pregnant women.
- Previously thought to be caused by organisms hence the term 'pyogenic', it is rarely related to an infection.
- Clinically, it manifests as a protruding or flat mass of tissue, either smooth or ulcerated.
- Initially, it appears bright red with ulcers but eventually organises and fills with fibrous collagen, taking on a pinkish hue. The frequent bleeding of this lesion, along with its redness and ulceration, can cause concern for patients, leading them to fear it might be a neoplastic lesion.
- Pyogenic granuloma typically presents as a painless lesion, most commonly on the gingiva, resulting from poor oral hygiene or irritation from an overhanging margin of a poorly constructed tooth restoration.
- Less commonly, the tongue, lip, and buccal mucosa are sites of occurrence.
- Pyogenic granulomas are more common in the anterior maxilla than in other regions of the oral cavity.

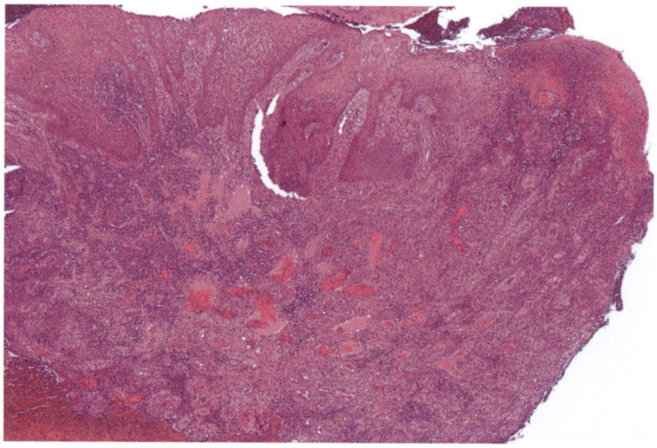

Fig. 27.3 Microscopically, a pyogenic granuloma shows a large mass of granulation tissue that is partly ulcerated and partly covered by hyperplastic stratified squamous epithelium

- Pyogenic granulomas can occur in pregnant women, commonly thought to be due to hormonal imbalance during pregnancy. The terms pregnancy epulis, pregnancy tumour, or granuloma gravidarum are commonly used to describe gingival pyogenic granuloma in pregnant women.
- The usual treatment of pyogenic granuloma is a surgical intervention that needs a deeper excision down to the periosteum to avoid the lesional recurrence.
- Proper scaling and polishing with the investigation of the tooth-filling margin should be performed to eliminate the source of irritation.
- For pregnancy epulis or granuloma, the lesion tends to regress postpartum. However, if it is a significant aesthetic problem, it can be surgically removed during pregnancy.

Histopathology

Microscopically, pyogenic granuloma will reveal a high vascularity and cellularity of connective tissue with an ulcerated surface covered by a fibrinopurulent exudate (Fig. 27.3). The base of the ulceration is mostly granulation tissue with a mixed acute and chronic inflammatory cell infiltrate consisting of neutrophils, lymphocytes, and plasma cells. The most striking feature is the presence of numerous newly formed endothelial-lined vascular channels of various sizes, filled with erythrocytes. The stroma is immature and filled with acute and chronic inflammatory cells. These histological features are diffuse throughout the connective tissue or can sometimes be arranged in a lobulated fashion, hence the term lobular capillary haemangioma. Older lesions sometimes become organised and filled with collagen bundles or fibrous maturation, leading to the formation of fibroepithelial polyps (see below).

27.5 Fibroepithelial Polyp (Traumatic Fibroma, Irritation Fibroma)

A fibroepithelial polyp represents a reactive hyperplasia of the fibrous connective tissue in response to local irritation. The synonyms such as traumatic/irritation fibroma, fibroepithelial hyperplasia, and fibrous nodule are used interchangeably.

Key Features

- Fibroepithelial polyp often results as the healed outcome of an inflammatory hyperplastic lesion.
- Clinically, fibroepithelial polyps develop at any oral soft tissue location, especially around the tongue, gingiva, and buccal mucosa, in various age groups.
- A fibroepithelial polyp on the gingiva is called fibrous epulis and is generally thought to be the fibrous maturation counterpart of the pyogenic granuloma.
- In most cases clinical presentation of a fibroepithelial polyp is a polypoid lesion with a smooth pinkish surface and a sessile or pedunculated base. It is often a small nodule but can grow up to 1.5 cm in diameter if left untreated. The nodule does not produce any pain or other symptoms, but if it is ulcerated, it can be slightly uncomfortable.
- The usual treatment of fibroepithelial polyp is conservative surgical excision.

Histopathology

Microscopically, fibroepithelial polyp shows a pedunculated nodular mass of relatively uninflamed fibrous connective tissue covered by stratified squamous epithelium (Fig. 27.4a). The surface epithelium can be keratotic if the lesion is constantly traumatised. The underlying connective is filled with dense and coarse fibrous collagen bundles with minimal blood vessels (Fig. 27.4b). The fibrous connective tissue is not encapsulated but shows a diffuse and haphazard arrangement of the connective tissue. The deeper connective tissue often has other soft tissue appendages such as nerve bundles, occasional adipose tissue, or minor salivary gland acini. An inflammatory cell infiltrate is not present unless there is surface ulceration or infection such as Candida.

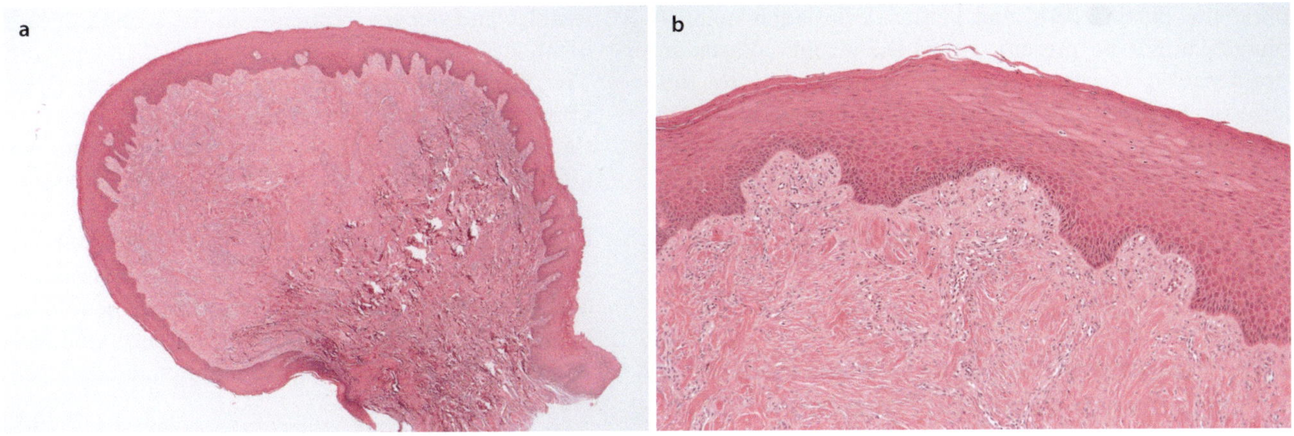

Fig. 27.4 **a** Histological appearance of fibroepithelial polyp on low magnification showing a sessile pedunculated mass of minimally inflamed connective tissue covered by hyperplastic epithelium. **b** Fibroepithelial polyp shows dense and coarse minimally inflamed connective tissue

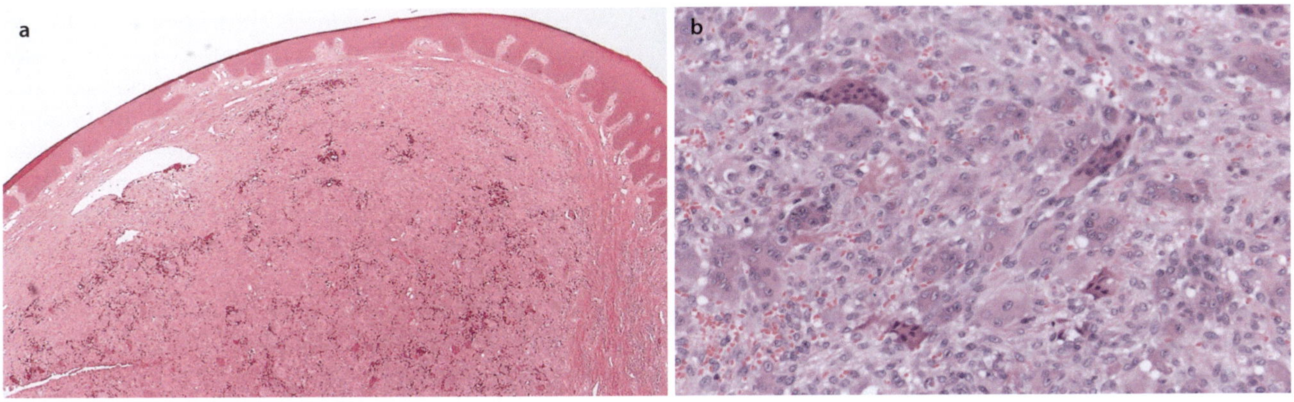

Fig. 27.5 **a** Low magnification histological appearance of peripheral giant cell granuloma showing areas of haemosiderin pigmentation. **b** Peripheral giant cell granuloma showing abundant giant cells within the stroma. (Courtesy of Associate Professor Norman Firth, Perth, Australia)

27.6 Peripheral Giant Cell Granuloma

The peripheral giant cell granuloma (PGCG), also known as reparative giant cell granuloma, is a non-neoplastic, reactive gingival growth characterised by large, multi-nucleated cells within the oral mucosa.

Key Features

- PGCG arises due to local irritation or trauma, often near the affected area. Most studies indicate that these multi-nucleated cells likely originate from osteoclasts.
- Clinically, peripheral giant cell granulomas typically appear as a nodular mass on the gingiva or alveolar ridge.
- PGCG can occur in any age group, with women slightly affected more than men, with the mandible more commonly involved than the maxilla.
- PGCG has a distinct red-blue or purple coloration, and the nodular mass can be pedunculated or sessile. As it occurs on the gingiva, it is sometimes mistaken for a pyogenic granuloma, given the almost similar clinical appearance.
- Treatment for oral peripheral giant cell granuloma involves surgical excision. Surgical removal often includes underlying bone and periosteum to ensure complete removal of causative irritation. Following excision, careful monitoring and regular follow-ups are essential to detect any signs of recurrence. Other treatment modalities, including cryotherapy or laser ablation, may be considered.

Histopathology

Microscopically, PGCG shows a fibrovascular stroma interlaced with numerous multi-nucleated giant cells, often found scattered or clustered throughout the tissue (Fig. 27.5). These giant cells possess multiple nuclei and are bordered by spindle-shaped mesenchymal cells. Additionally, a mix of inflammatory cells, such as lym-

27

phocytes, plasma cells, and hemosiderin-laden macrophages, might be present within the stroma. Vascular proliferation is often observed, contributing to the lesion's vascularity. It must be noted that these histological features are typical of any giant cell lesion. Therefore, if any indication that the lesion could be a central giant cell granuloma or hyperparathyroidism, further clinical investigations (such as imaging, etc.) are warranted to assist the definitive diagnosis.

27.7 Peripheral Ossifying Fibrous Epulis (Cemento-Ossifying Fibroma)

Peripheral ossifying fibrous epulis, also known as cemento-ossifying fibroma or peripheral ossifying fibroma, is a common reactive soft tissue lesion occurring around the gingiva.

Key Features

- Peripheral ossifying fibrous epulis is believed to arise from the periodontal ligament, particularly the mineralising tissue counterpart and its formation is reactive in nature rather than neoplastic.
- Clinically, peripheral ossifying fibroma occurs commonly on the gingiva and interdental papilla.
- It appears as a pedunculated mass or broad-based with a smooth surface and the colour ranges from pale pink to red. Often but not always.
- The nodular mass is less than 2.5 cm and may have been present for months or years before it is detected by patients.
- Peripheral ossifying fibrous epulis mainly occurring in the anterior maxilla, has a higher predilection for females and occurs frequently in the second decade of life.
- The common treatment for peripheral ossifying fibroma is surgical intervention. Surgical excision of the lesion must extend down to the periosteum and affected periodontal ligament to avoid recurrence of the lesion.
- Comprehensive root scaling of the affected teeth and removal of subsequent sources of irritant should be completed. In cases where periodontal health has been compromised, periodontic surgery and cosmetic repair with appropriate maintenance are generally needed.

Histopathology

Microscopically, peripheral ossifying fibroma shows a pedunculated nodular mass of fibrous connective tissue covered by stratified squamous epithelium with the formation of mineralised foci in the connective tissue area (◘ Fig. 27.6a, b). If it is ulcerated, the surface is often covered by fibrinous exudate with an area of granulation tissue underneath. The connective tissue often shows the proliferation of fibrous collagen bundles with less vascularity and high cellularity. The mineralised tissue in the connective tissue can be one or more types: (1) trabecular or woven bone, (2) cementum-like material, and (3) dystrophic calcification. In most cases, all three mineralised tissue types are formed and are seen within the connective tissue. In more mature lesions, the bone can be organised and show a mature lamellar architecture. Dystrophic calcifications are commonly seen in ulcerated lesions and cementum-like lesion is often seen in less than one-fifth of the lesions.

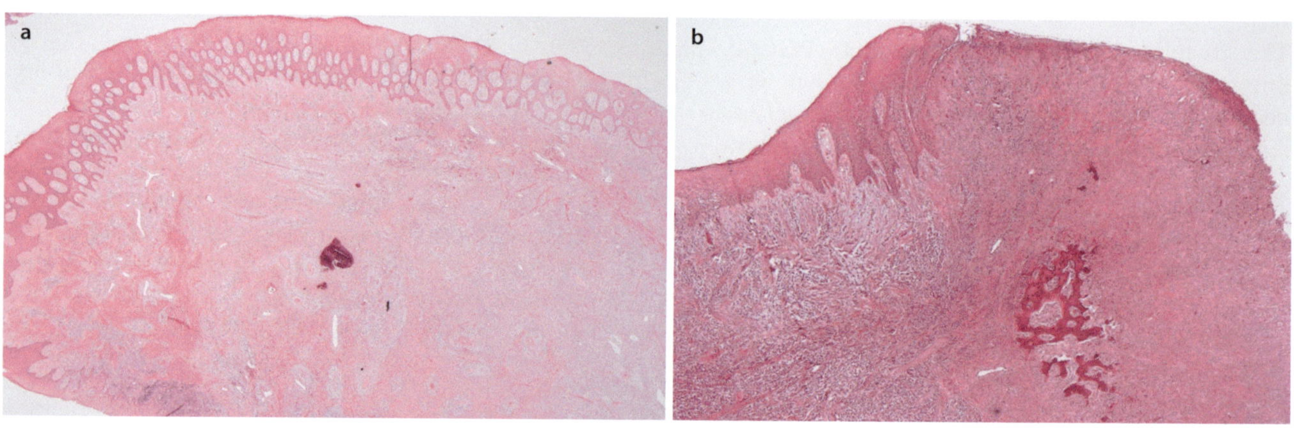

◘ **Fig. 27.6** **a** Low-power magnification of peripheral ossifying fibroma showing proliferation of fibrous collagen bundles with area of mineralised tissue formation within the deeper connective tissue. **b** Histology showing ulcerated peripheral ossifying fibroma with areas of mineralised tissue formation in the fibrous connective tissue

27.8 Inflammatory Papillary Hyperplasia

Inflammatory papillary hyperplasia is a reactive lesion of the oral mucosa, normally characterised as small papillary multiple lesions under a maxillary denture in those with poor denture hygiene.

Key Features

- Inflammatory papillary hyperplasia is known to occur in patients with an old, ill-fitting denture and/or patients with poor denture hygiene.
- In most patients, fungal infections such as Candida sp. are thought to be the main cause of inflammatory papillary hyperplasia.
- Clinically, inflammatory papillary hyperplasia is predominantly on the hard palate under the base of a prosthesis, but in some cases, it has been reported to occur in the mandible.
- The lesion is mostly asymptomatic, and the colour of the oral mucosa ranges from pink to erythematous. It has a distinct nodulous or papillary pattern of growth and occurs mainly in the palatal vault.
- The treatment for inflammatory papillary hyperplasia varies depending on the stages of the lesion. For early lesions, abstaining from wearing the prosthesis may allow the lesion to heal and subside.
- Adjunct therapy with mouth rinse such as Chlorhexidine or topical antifungal may accelerate the healing process.
- For a more advanced and recalcitrant lesion, clinicians have advocated surgical excision with cryotherapy, electrosurgery, and laser.
- After the surgery, the prosthesis is usually re-made or re-lined depending on denture assessment. Denture hygiene should be encouraged to reduce the likelihood of recurrence.

Histopathology

Microscopically, the lesion shows multiple papillary projections on the surface covered by hyperplastic stratified squamous epithelium with or without chronic inflammation. The connective tissue may vary from loose and vascularised to highly dense fibrous collagen bundles. In most cases, there is an intense and diffuse chronic inflammatory cell infiltrate consisting predominantly of lymphocytes and plasma cells. The surface epithelium can exhibit areas of neutrophil aggregation if there is apparent Candida colonisation. In this case, the epithelium will show pseudoepitheliomatous hyperplasia with broad rete ridges responding to the Candida irritation (Fig. 27.7).

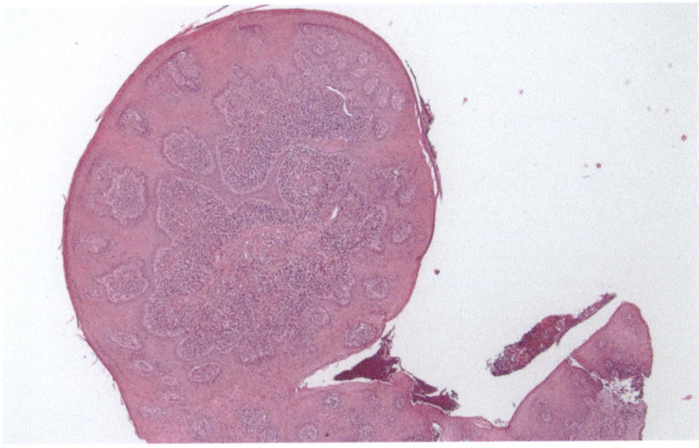

Fig. 27.7 Histological appearance of the papillary projections on the surface. It is normally covered by hyperplastic stratified squamous epithelium with intense and diffuse chronic inflammatory cells in the connective tissue

27.9 Summary

Oral mucosa reactive hyperplastic lesions encompass a spectrum of benign lumps and growths. These arise from the oral mucosa in response to various stimuli. Common examples include fibrous hyperplasia, pyogenic granuloma, and irritation fibroma. These lesions often manifest as painless, exophytic masses, requiring clinical and histopathological examination for diagnosis. Understanding their aetiology, histopathology, and management is crucial for diagnosis and appropriate treatment planning.

Further Reading

Anisa MK, Nayana VG, Somayaji KSG, Saimanohar S, Sheetal R. Fibroepithelial polyp from retromolar trigone. Arch Med Health Sci. 2019;7(1):87–9.

Dutra KL, Longo L, Grando LJ, Rivero ERC. Incidence of reactive hyperplastic lesions in the oral cavity: a 10 year retrospective study in Santa Catarina. Brazil Braz J Otorhinolaryngol. 2019;85:399–407.

Gual-Vaqués P, Jané-Salas E, Egido-Moreno S, Ayuso-Montero R, Marí-Roig A, López-López J. Inflammatory papillary hyperplasia: a systematic review. Med Oral Patol Oral Cir Bucal. 2017;22(1):e36–42.

Kamal R, Dahiya P, Puri A. Oral pyogenic granuloma: various concepts of etiopathogenesis. J Oral Maxillofac Pathol. 2012;16(1):79–82.

Nair BM, Basavaraju SM, Pachipulusu B. Reactive hyperplastic lesions of oral cavity: a review of literature. J Health Sci Res. 2019;10(2):42–6.

Parveen R, Patil VA, et al. A case report on epulis fissuratum. J Oral Health Comm Dent. 2019;13(2):59–61.

Poonacha KS, Shigli AL, Shirol D. Peripheral ossifying fibroma: a clinical report. Contemp Clin Dent. 2010;1(1):54–6.

Histopathology of the Benign Neoplasms of the Oral Mucosa

Benedict Seo

Contents

S R Prabhu et al. (eds.), *Oral Histology and Oral Histopathology*, https://doi.org/10.1007/978-3-031-77481-2_28

28

Table 28.1 Types of mesenchymal lesions that may affect the oral cavity

	Developmental/uncertain	Reactive	Neoplastic
Fibrous	Giant cell fibroma, orofacial mucinosis	Fibromas, fibrous epulis with ossification	True fibromas, fibromatosis, myofibroma
Lymphovascular	Vascular malformations (lymphovascular anomalies, haemangioma)	Pyogenic granuloma, Kaposi's sarcoma	
Neural		Traumatic neuroma	Neurilemmoma, neurofibroma, solitary encapsulated neuroma, granular cell tumour
Muscle			Leiomyoma, rhabdomyoma,
Adipose		Fat herniation	Lipoma
Bone	Tori, bony exostosis, osseous, and cartilaginous choriostoma	Osteosclerosis, periostitis ossificans, reactive osseous and chondromatous metaplasia	Osteoma, osteoblastoma/osteoid osteoma
Cartilage	Osseous and cartilaginous choriostoma	Osseous and cartilaginous metaplasia	Chondroma
Others	Congenital epulis	Peripheral giant cell lesions	

28.1 Introduction

Mucosal benign tumours (neoplasms) may arise from a range of different tissues and may be developmental, reactive, hamartomatous, or neoplastic in origin. Most of these mucosal lesions are mesenchymal in origin, deriving from the mesoderm, and include pathologies arising from the fibrous, lymphovascular, neural, muscular, adipose, bone, and cartilaginous tissues (Table 28.1). In this chapter, the focus will be on the soft tissue lesions that originate from the mesenchymal connective tissues.

28.2 Fibroma

Fibroma is a term used to describe common hyperplastic growths in the mouth. In most cases, these lesions are reactive and arise in response to local stimuli such as low-grade chronic trauma and plaque accumulation. Thus, it is recommended to use alternate terms, such as fibro-epithelial polyp/hyperplasia or fibrous epulis (if on the gum), in place of 'fibroma,' which may imply it is a true fibroblastic neoplasm. The term 'peripheral ossifying fibroma' has also been used to describe fibrous epulis with ossification (or ossifying fibrous epulis). As this may be confused with ossifying fibroma (cemento-ossifying fibroma), which is a true neoplasm, the use of such nomenclatures should be discouraged.

Key Features

- Fibro-epithelial polyps are common and may occur in any part of the oral cavity, but buccal/labial mucosa, gingiva and tongue are the common sites affected.
- Although these lesions may occur across a wide age range, they are typically diagnosed in adults.
- They present as asymptomatic pale-to-normal mucosa-coloured smooth surfaced nodules or polyps, which may be sessile or pedunculated. Subsequent surface ulceration or (hyper)keratotic changes may be present.
- Patient history and intraoral examination will usually reveal a local precipitating factor or a history of trauma to the site.
- Conservative excision is diagnostic and curative.
- Most fibro-epithelial polyps/hyperplasia are biopsied for aesthetic or functional purposes and histopathology confirms the reactive hyperplastic nature of the lesion.
- It is important to address local precipitating factors, such that, if the stimuli persist, the lesion may recur *de novo*.

Histopathology

Histopathologically, there is evidence of generalised fibroplasia or hyperplasia of the fibrous connective tissue (Fig. 28.1). The fibrous connective tissue is dense,

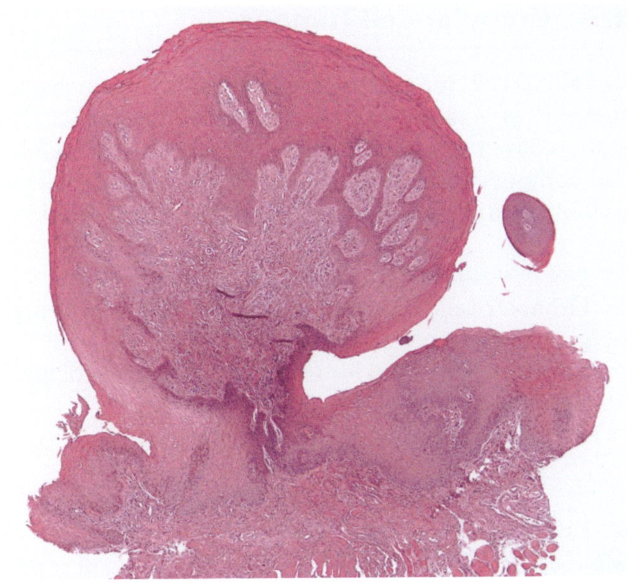

Fig. 28.1 Photomicrograph showing a polypoid fibrous lump. Note the lesional tissue is connected to the underlying normal mucosal tissue by a stalk. The epithelium shows keratosis and acanthosis. The fibrous connective tissue component is dense, mature, and relatively acellular and avascular

relatively acellular, and avascular with limited active inflammation in most cases. The surface epithelium is usually condensed but may show acanthosis or (hyper) keratosis. Depending on the stage of development, the lesion may be more inflamed, vascular, and immature with plump fibroblasts. Indeed, preexisting lesions such as pyogenic granuloma and mucocoele may 'mature' into a fibro-epithelial polyp over time.

28.3 Lipoma

Lipoma is a benign neoplasm of adipocytes and one of the most common true mesenchymal neoplasms. It represents around 30% of all connective tissue tumours diagnosed. Lipomas occur mostly in the adult population and are more commonly found in obese people, although the precise mechanism and direct correlation between bodily metabolism and the evolution of lipoma have not been established.

Key Features

- Lipoma presents as an asymptomatic, smooth-surfaced, mucosal-coloured-to-yellowish elevation in the mouth.
- In most cases, lipomas are solitary, and involve a discrete area as a polypoid to sessile movable soft tissue mass.
- The buccal mucosa is the most common site. There is no evident sex predilection for oral lesions.

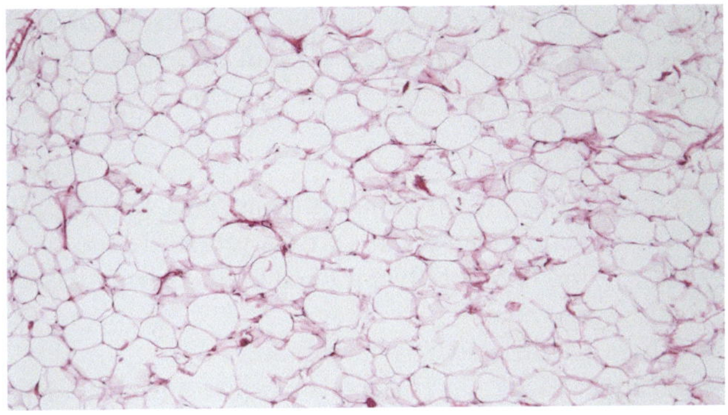

Fig. 28.2 An example of lipoma. Note the lesional tissue consists of adipocytes with completely normal and mature cytonuclear characteristics. The fat tissue is in excess but there is no atypia or mitotic activity

- Given the nature of the tissue composition, upon biopsy, the specimen readily floats in formalin.
- Lipomas are slow-growing benign tumours that are best treated with conservative surgical excision, except for intramuscular lesions which are best removed in total.

Histopathology

Histopathologically, lipomas present as well-circumscribed but incompletely encapsulated proliferation of fat. Lobulation of lesional adipose tissue with well-developed fibrous septae is often observed. The individual fat cells are mature and do not show signs of atypia. There is also no evidence of multi-vacuolation (Fig. 28.2). Secondary osseous and cartilaginous metaplastic changes may be seen, and where prominent, these become known as osteolipomas and chondrolipomas. Fibrolipoma is used when there is a significant fibrous/fibrotic change within the lesion. Exuberant vasculature encompassed within the boundaries of the tumour may lead to the use of the term angiolipoma. Sialolipoma denotes a phenomenon where lipomatous changes occur within the salivary glands. Still, these may be difficult to distinguish from age-related fatty degeneration, especially in the context of confounding factors such as chronic alcoholism and salivary gland agenesis. If lipoma extends through and between skeletal muscle bundles, this should be noted as intramuscular lipomas, which are known to exhibit more infiltrative behaviour.

28.4 Neurilemmoma

Neurilemmoma, also known as schwannoma, is a benign neoplasm of Schwann cell origin. Whilst uncommon, the head and neck region is a relatively common site. Intraorally, the tongue is the most commonly affected site, followed by the palate. Neurilemmomas occur in the adult population without evident sex predilection.

Key Features

- Clinically, neurolemmoma presents as a solitary, relatively firm mucosal mass with a yellowish hue.
- The lesion is generally not fixed to underlying tissues and is movable.
- There are no associated symptoms.
- Conservative total excision is curative and diagnostic as this lesion cannot be distinguished from other soft tissue tumours on the clinical grounds alone.
- Recurrence is unlikely following complete excision.

Histopathology

Histology is quite characteristic, and diagnosis requires the identification of so-called Antoni A and Antoni B regions within the tumour. Antoni A areas show the pathognomonic Verocay bodies, which comprise rows of palisaded Schwann cell nuclei separated by a hyalinised anucleate acellular zone (Fig. 28.3). The surrounding regions will show streaming fascicles of spindle-shaped cells with blunt-ended nuclei. Mitosis is generally not conspicuous. Antoni B regions are less cellular, and there is no distinct architectural arrangement. A thin zone of normal, slightly vascular fibrous connective tissue separates the lesion from the surface epithelium. Neurilemmoma is well-circumscribed and usually encapsulated.

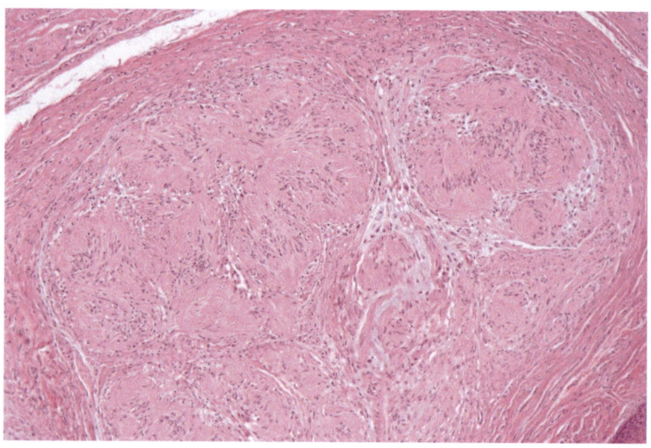

Fig. 28.3 Well-circumscribed neural proliferation with distinct transitional pattern. Note numerous Verocay bodies with palisaded nuclei with intervening acellular zones

28.5 Granular Cell Tumour

Granular cell tumour is a rare benign mesenchymal tumour of unclear aetiology. Immunohistochemical studies have supported its likely neural origin. Granular cell tumours emerge in the adult population, with a notable predilection for the tongue and female gender.

Key Features

- Granular cell tumours are slow-growing and benign in nature.
- Excision is required for the determination of diagnosis and cure.
- There is little probability of recurrence.

Histopathology

Microscopically granular cell tumour consists of a proliferation of round to ovoid cells with centrally located nuclei, pale granular cytoplasm, and distinct cell boundaries (Fig. 28.4). The lesion is usually not well delineated and may appear to merge or permeate through underlying skeletal muscle bundles. This phenomenon has previously led to the misbelief that granular cell tumours originate from the skeletal muscle. The overlying surface epithelium has been reported to show pseudo-epithelial hyperplasia (also known as pseudocarcinomatous hyperplasia) where tangential sectioning of the irregularly proliferating rete ridges results in the observation of apparent 'islands' likened to that seen in carcinomatous invasion of the underlying fibrous connective tissue.

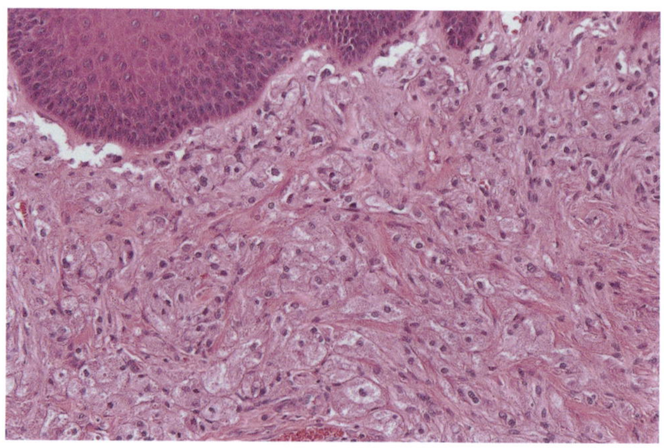

Fig. 28.4 Granular cell tumour. The lesional cells show granular eosinophilic cytoplasm with distinct round nuclei. In this example, the lesional cells directly abut the surface stratified squamous epithelium

28.6 Haemangioma/Lymphangioma/ Vascular Developmental Malformations

The term haemangioma has indiscriminately been used conventionally and historically to describe proliferative vascular lesions irrespective of their pathogenesis and disease behaviour. In a similar manner, lymphangioma has been used to describe developmental anomalies of lymphatic vessels. Both terms imply neoplastic pathogenesis. In recent times, efforts have been made to rationally classify vascular lesions and tumours using nomenclature reflective of individual lesions' pathogenesis and behaviour (◘ Table 28.2). This chapter will focus on developmental vascular malformations of the oral cavity.

Most developmental vascular malformations in the oral cavity are low-flow lesions involving the capillaries, but venous and arterial involvement may be seen.

▪ Key Features

- Clinically, a vascular malformation presents as an asymptomatic solitary movable soft tissue lesion.
- Owing to its vascular nature, the lesion has a deep red/purplish colouration and may blanch on palpation. Depending on the type and calibre of the vessels involved, pulselessness may also be noted.
- As these are developmental malformations, there is no concern about malignant transformation or continued growth. However, trauma to the area may lead to haemorrhage, at times serious, so determination to actively treat should be made on a case-to-case basis.
- Where surgical treatment is indicated, vascular malformations are best managed in a controlled surgical environment with careful presurgical planning and the aid of imaging, especially if the lesion is thought to be infiltrating into/originating from the underlying tissues.
- The use of oral or intralesional beta blockers and steroid and sclerotherapy have been advocated as the preferred mode of treatment for larger problematic lesions with increased risk of significant haemorrhage.

▪ Histopathology

Histologically vascular malformations may show several widely dilated endothelial-lined blood vessels and vascular channels, in which case the term cavernous (cave-like) haemangioma has been used (◘ Fig. 28.5). Alternately, there may be clusters and proliferation of numerous small capillaries, sometimes organised in lobules. The vessels often have indistinct lumina and these types of malformations have been referred to as capil-

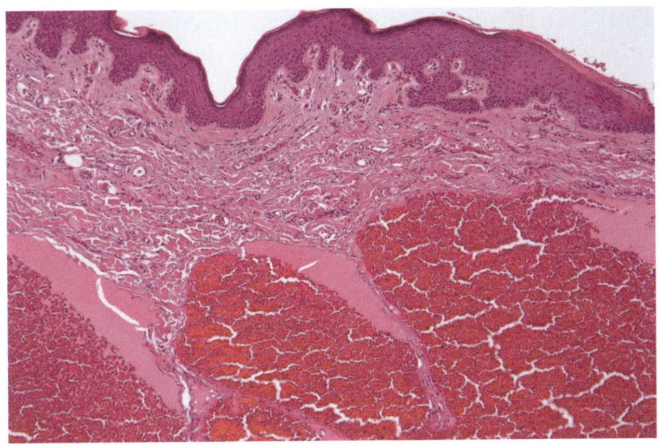

◘ **Fig. 28.5** An example of a vascular malformation with numerous widely dilated endothelial-lined, almost completely engorged blood vessels; these lesions are commonly referred to as cavernous haemangiomas

◘ **Table 28.2** International Society for the Study of Vascular Anomalies classification

Vascular tumours	Vascular malformations			
Benign • Infantile haemangioma • Congenital haemangioma pyogenic granuloma and others	**Simple** • Capillary • Lymphatic • Venous • Arteriovenous malformation • Arteriovenous fistula	**Combined** • Combination of the simple types	**Of major named vessel** • Lymphatics, veins, and arteries and include various anomalies	**Associated with other anomalies** • Sturge Weber • Others

28

lary haemangiomas. In many cases, there may be an admixture of different types of vessels and architectural patterns within the same lesion. Intramuscular infiltration of the lesional vascular tissue should noted as this may lead to adverse clinical complications and higher rates of recurrence.

Lymphatic malformations show dilation of thin-walled vessels of varying degrees. Histologically, lymphatic malformations may be capillary, cavernous or cystic (macro- or microcystic). The lymphatic vessels will not contain red blood cells present in other forms of vascular malformations but surgical haemorrhage may make the distinction difficult. Immunohistochemical markers (e.g. D2–40, podoplanin) have been used successfully to help distinguish lymph vessels from blood vessels.

28.7 Summary

Oral soft tissue benign neoplasms of connective tissue origin are common. Although these do not pose major problems in diagnosis, microscopic assessment of these lesions is essential. Mucosal benign neoplasms discussed in this chapter do not carry any malignant potential.

Further Reading

1. Dalal KM, Antonescu CR, Singer S. Diagnosis and management of lipomatous tumors. J Surg Oncol. 2008;97:298-313.
2. Pires FR, Souza L, Arruda R, et al. Intraoral soft tissue lipomas: clinicopathological features from 91 cases diagnosed in a single Oral Pathology service. Med Oral Patol Oral Cir Bucal. 2021;26:e90–e96.
3. Thompson LDR, Koh SS, Lau SK. Tongue Schwannoma: A Clinicopathologic Study of 19 Cases. Head Neck Pathol. 2020;14:571–76.
4. Lafuente Ibanez de Mendoza I, Lopez Ortega K, Trierveiler M, et al. Oral granular cell tumour: A multicentric study of 56 cases and a systematic review. Oral Dis. 2020;26:573–89.
5. Kunimoto K, Yamamoto Y, Jinnin M. ISSVA Classification of Vascular Anomalies and Molecular Biology. Int J Mol Sci. 2022;23.
6. Buckmiller LM, Richter GT, Suen JY. Diagnosis and management of hemangiomas and vascular malformations of the head and neck. Oral Dis. 2010;16:405–18.

Histopathology of the Mucosal Potentially Malignant (Dysplastic) Disorders

Muhammed Yakin and Omar Kujan

Contents

S R Prabhu et al. (eds.), *Oral Histology and Oral Histopathology*, https://doi.org/10.1007/978-3-031-77481-2_29

29

29.1 Introduction and Classification

The World Health Organization (WHO) Collaborating Centre for Oral Cancer defined oral potentially malignant disorders (OPMD) as: "any oral mucosal abnormality that is associated with a statistically increased risk of developing oral cancer" [1]. OPMD is a group of lesions and conditions that show variable clinical and histopathological presentations (Box 29.1). Hence, stratifying the risk for progressing to carcinoma is paramount [2]. Once an OPMD is detected, primarily through a thorough and systematic diagnostic process involving complete dental and medical history and rigorous examination of the mouth for any local contributing factors, the mainstay of investigation is biopsy with the aims of obtaining a definitive diagnosis and assessing the presence of dysplasia or carcinoma to guide clinical management. Therefore, knowledge of the histological features of oral epithelial dysplasia (OED) is essential to the practising healthcare professional in managing patients with OPMD. Similarly, diagnostic histopathologists must be familiar with the clinical correlation and its importance in the diagnosis, risk assessment, and management of patients with OPMD [2].

This chapter discusses the latest 2020 WHO classification covering OPMDs in general with a focus on oral epithelial dysplasia under the following headings:

- Oral potentially malignant disorders
- Oral epithelial dysplasia
- Proliferative verrucous leukoplakia
- Oral submucous fibrosis
- HPV-associated oral epithelial dysplasia

The clinical spectrum of leukoplakia, speckled leukoplakia, and erythroplakia are addressed together, followed by proliferative verrucous leukoplakia (PVL). Oral lichenoid lesions (OLLs), including those of graft vs. host disease (GvHD), are recognised as OPMD. Perhaps the most obvious omission from the list in this chapter is actinic cheilitis, which is relevant to oral and maxillofacial pathology practice.

Box 29.1: 2020 Classification of OPMD. (Adopted from Warnakulasuriya et al. (2021) [1])

Disorders included in the 2020 OPMD classification
Leukoplakia Proliferative verrucous leukoplakia Erythroplakia Oral submucous fibrosis Oral lichen planus Actinic keratosis (actinic cheilitis) Palatal lesions in reverse smokers Oral lupus erythematosus Dyskeratosis congenita
New disorders included in the 2020 OPMD classification
Oral lichenoid lesion Oral graft vs. host disease
Disorders removed from the 2020 OPMD classification due to limited evidence
Oral epidermolysis bullosa
Disorders with insufficient epidemiological evidence
Chronic hyperplastic candidosis Exophytic verrucous hyperplasia/verrucous hyperplasia

29.2 Leukoplakia

The WHO Collaborating Centre of Oral Cancer, in their latest 2020 classification update, kept the definition of leukoplakia as "A predominantly white plaque of questionable risk having excluded (other) known diseases or disorders that carry no increased risk for cancer" [1]. In practice, this term is a clinical diagnosis by exclusion. It carries a specific significance, indicating that dysplasia or neoplasia is suspected and needs to be ruled out or confirmed through biopsy [1].

Key Features

- The clinical spectrum of leukoplakia with an increasing risk of malignant transformation includes thin homogenous leukoplakia and non-homogenous leukoplakia, which includes thick leukoplakia with deep fissures and nodular, granular or verrucous leukoplakia.
- Common differential diagnoses or diseases to exclude include frictional keratosis, smoker's keratosis, chronic hyperplastic candidosis, leukoedema, chemical injury, white sponge nevus and -in specific situations, lichen planus, and related lesions [1].
- Leukoplakias tend to be sharply demarcated from adjacent clinically normal-appearing oral mucosa. Frictional keratosis, most commonly of edentulous alveolar ridges, is more diffuse and may have ill-defined borders. However, it may have some clinical features of nodular or granular leukoplakia.
- The critical point is to thoroughly examine the mouth for any friction or mechanical irritation, remove the possible causative factor, and conduct a clinical review to ensure the lesion disappears.
- The white appearance of the oral mucosa in leukoplakia is due to the increase in the thickness of the epithelium and the increase in the thickness of the keratin layer. In non-keratinised mucosa, this would result from developing a keratin layer in addition to epithelial hyperplasia.

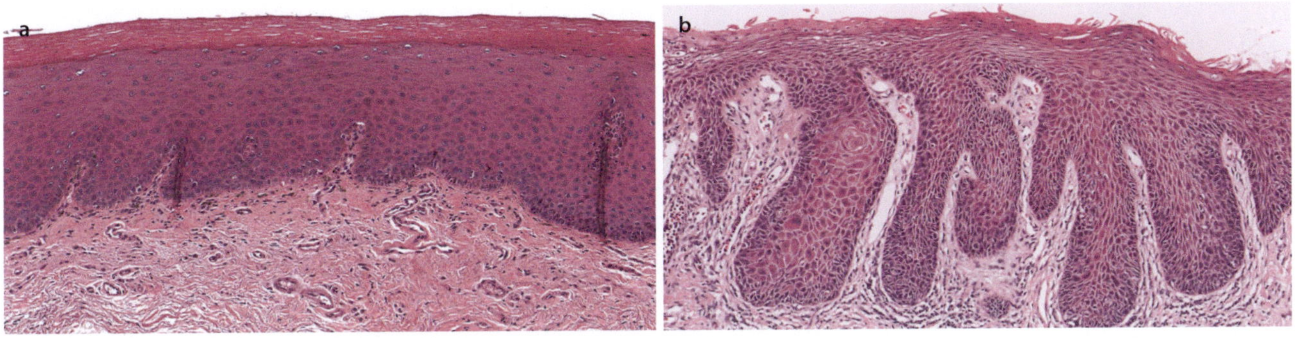

Fig. 29.1 **a** A biopsy of a leukoplakia lesion shows hyperkeratosis with no dysplasia. Note that the epithelium shows parakeratosis, basal cell hyperplasia, and acanthosis. **b** A biopsy of a leukoplakia lesion shows severe epithelial dysplasia. Note irregular epithelial stratification, hyperchromasia, abnormal variations in nuclear and cell size and shape, increased number of mitotic figures, and individual cell keratinisation

Histopathology

Histopathology of leukoplakia is described as keratosis with or without epithelial dysplasia (Fig. 29.1). The grade of oral epithelial dysplasia (OED) is critical to stratify the risk of malignant transformation for better management.

29.3 Proliferative Verrucous Leukoplakia

Proliferative verrucous leukoplakia (PVL) is a rare, distinct, and aggressive type of leukoplakia characterised by the presence of verrucous (wart-like) leukoplakia involving two or more sub-sites, a high rate of recurrence, and malignant transformation.

Key Features

- Proliferative verrucous leukoplakia (PVL) is perhaps the most challenging entity of OPMD in terms of histopathological diagnosis and management [3].
- PVL has a propensity to present in the attached gingiva as thick white patches, usually with a verrucous surface texture, that may encompass the whole gingiva and the free gingival margin [4].
- PVL presents changes affecting several sites in the oral cavity. However, it has to be distinguished from multifocal leukoplakia.
- Once removed and wholly excised, it usually recurs at the same site or a different one, covering a wide area of oral mucosa.
- The rate of malignant transformation of PVL is around 55% [5]. It may transform into verrucous or squamous cell carcinoma.
- Thompson et al., (2023) developed consensus guidelines with the support and endorsement of the American Academy of Oral and Maxillofacial Pathology and the North American Society of Head and Neck Pathologists, recommending the use of standardised histopathologic criteria and descriptive terminology to indicate three categories of lesions within PVL: (1) "corrugated ortho(para)hyperkeratotic lesion, not reactive," (2) "bulky hyperkeratotic epithelial proliferation, not reactive," and (3) "suspicious for" or "squamous cell carcinoma" [3].
- A diagnosis can be made confidently with sufficient clinical-pathological correlation and liaison between the clinician and histopathologist.
- A sufficiently deep and long incisional biopsy is a must to exclude verrucous carcinoma, which, unlike squamous cell carcinoma, shows broad phases of invasion. Therefore, an adequate amount of adjacent normal-appearing tissue must assess the presence of invasive carcinoma by comparing the most profound front of the rete ridges in the lesional tissue compared to the normal-appearing mucosa. This can be challenging with gingiva biopsies.
- In addition to wide surgical excision, treatment can involve laser ablation, preferably following initial diagnosis with incisional biopsy. Photodynamic therapy has also shown promising results.

Histopathology

Biopsy of PVL may reveal no more than ortho(para) hyperkeratosis with or without a verrucous surface, with broadly enlarged rete pegs (Fig. 29.2a) with little space for connective tissue papillae. Cellular atypia is minimal, where only occasional suprabasal mitoses are seen. A lichenoid pattern of inflammation may be seen, usually lacking the typical feature for prominent basal cell liquefaction but should not be confused with lichen planus and lichenoid lesions [1, 3, 6] (Fig. 29.2b).

29

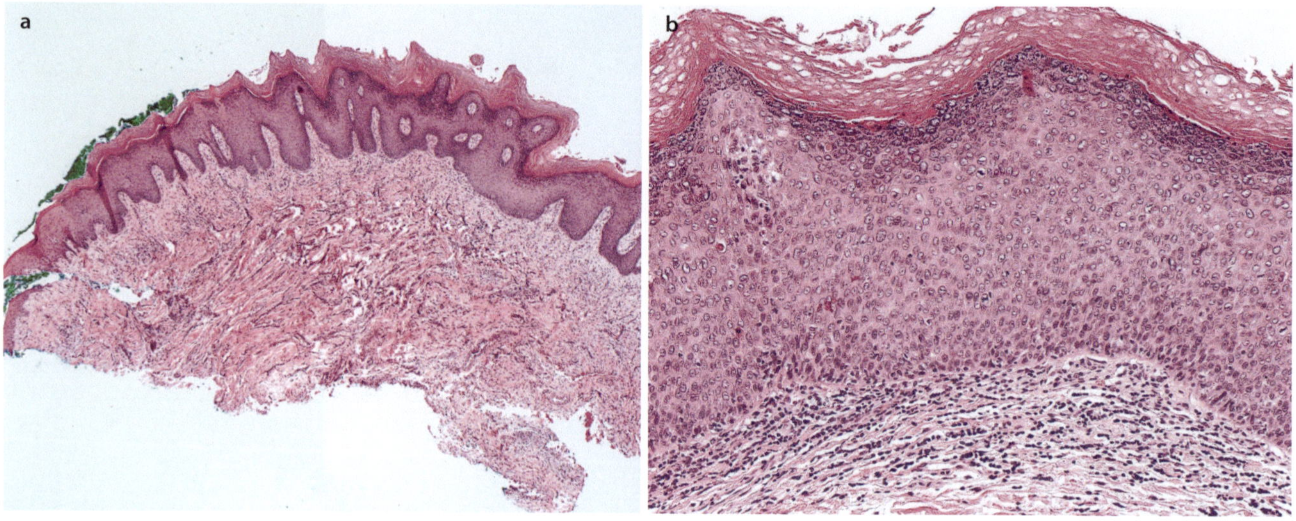

Fig. 29.2 **a** Proliferative verrucous leukoplakia exhibiting orthokeratin and forms of prominent crests/spikes. (Courtesy of Molly Housley Smith DMD, Pathology outlines .com). **b** Proliferative verrucous leukoplakia. Cytologic epithelial dysplasia arising in a patient with PVL. In addition to the corrugated layer of orthokeratin and prominent granular cell layer, atypical cytologic features (e.g. increased nuclear size, hypercellulariy, hyperchromasia, and increased mitotic figures) are seen throughout the epithelium. (Courtesy of Molly Housley Smith DMD, Pathology outlines .com)

29.4 Erythroplakia

Erythroplakia is a clinical term, which refers to a potentially malignant velvety red lesion with small nodules or granules, having excluded common red lesions such as those related to trauma, erosions, and erythematous candidosis.

Key Features

- Erythroplakia may clinically be accompanied by a variable degree of induration.
- The term carries special significance in that it indicates that the lesion should be biopsied and that invasive carcinoma is very likely.
- More than 90% of erythroplakia are invasive SCC or carcinoma in situ when biopsied [7].

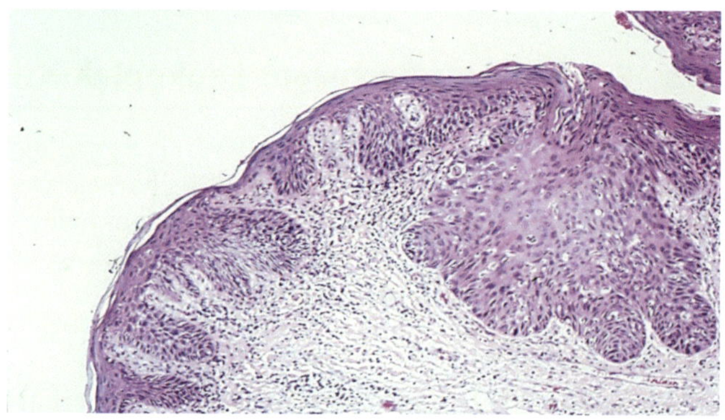

Fig. 29.3 The greatest majority of clinical erythroplakias exhibit severe OED- carcinoma in situ with or without evidence of frank invasive carcinoma. As illustrated in this lesion showing a focus on microinvasion. (Courtesy Professor David F Wilson, Adelaide, Australia)

Histopathology

There are no histological features which are specific to a microscopic diagnosis of erythroplakia. The epithelium is usually non-keratinised. At the time of microscopic examination, the lesion may show mild, moderate epithelial, severe OED (Fig. 29.3) or carcinoma in situ. Carcinoma in situ is characterised by a complete disorganisation of cells throughout all layers of the epithelium, with no keratin pearls. Increased vascularity of the lamina propria is usually seen, which may account for the clinical appearance.

29.5 Oral Submucous Fibrosis

Oral submucous fibrosis (OSF) is an OPMD that is associated with betel chewing habits common in the Indian subcontinent.

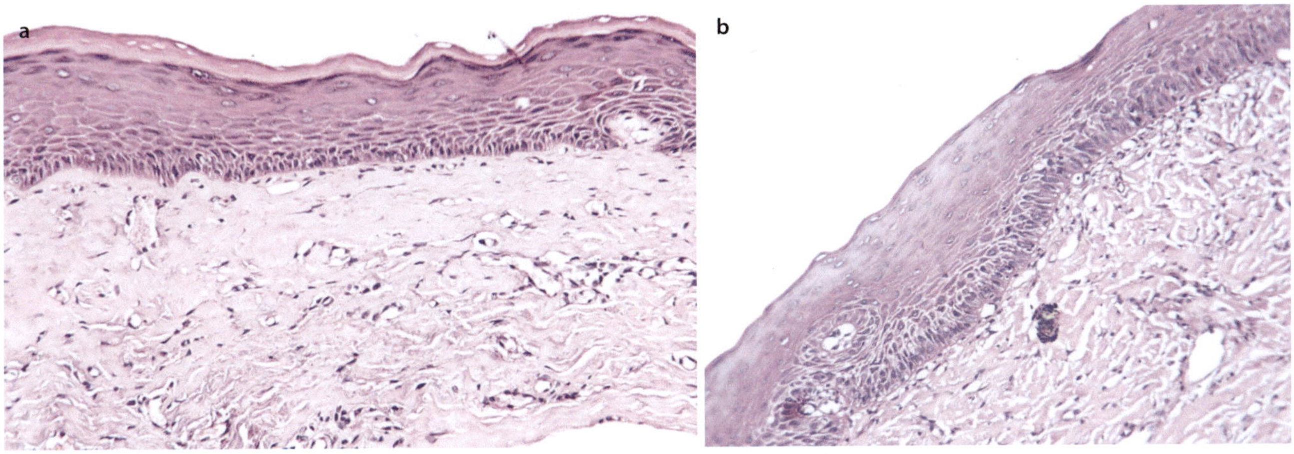

Fig. 29.4 **a** Oral submucous fibrosis exhibiting epithelial atrophy. (Source: Ranganathan, K., Loganathan, K. (2023). Pathology of Oral Submucous Fibrosis. In: Warnakulasuriya, S., Ranganathan, K. (eds) Oral Submucous Fibrosis. Textbooks in Contemporary Dentistry. Springer, Cham. ► https://doi.org/10.1007/978-3-031-12855-4_14). (With permission). **b** Oral submucous fibrosis exhibiting mild epithelial dysplasia. (Source: Ranganathan, K., Loganathan, K. (2023). Pathology of Oral Submucous Fibrosis. In: Warnakulasuriya, S., Ranganathan, K. (eds) Oral Submucous Fibrosis. Textbooks in Contemporary Dentistry. Springer, Cham. ► https://doi.org/10.1007/978-3-031-12855-4_14). (With permission)

- **Key Features**

- The active ingredient is areca nut, which is wrapped in a betel leaf with tobacco and slaked lime, and then placed in the buccal sulcus [1].
- The disorder is characterised by progressive loss of elasticity of the oral epithelium, eventually leading to limited mouth opening, and development of OED and then carcinoma.
- Clinically, the oral mucosa is leathery, pale, and inelastic with or without discrete white or red patches, or areas of ulceration.
- As with other OPMD, management is aimed at controlling modifiable lifestyle risk factors and regular monitoring for, and detection and removal of clinically visible changes indicative of progression to malignancy.

- **Histopathology**

Histopathological changes in oral submucous fibrosis involve both the epithelium and underlying connective tissue, including muscles in advanced stages. The epithelial changes involve hyperplasia progressing to atrophy, with varying degrees of dysplasia (Fig. 29.4a, b). The connective tissue changes include fibrosis of lamina propria initially progressing to hyalinisation and increasing fibrosis and lack of vascularity extending to and replacing muscle in advanced stages.

29.6 Actinic Keratosis

Actinic keratosis or actinic cheilitis involves the lip vermilion and part of the labial mucosa, particularly of the lower lip. It arises from sun damage and is mostly dysplastic [1, 8].

- **Key Features**

- Actinic keratosis is common in areas where ultraviolet radiation is high and in individuals with lighter skin complexion due to the lower protection imparted by the relative lack of melanin.
- Clinical features include loss of elasticity, white patches and nodules, a decrease in the delineation between the lip vermilion and skin of the lip, and a degree of induration of the lip vermilion.
- Features suggestive of carcinoma include crusting, lumps, and ulcers.
- Management includes patient education in terms of seeking shade, wearing sun-protective headwear, and use of sunscreens or lip balms with SPF50 or above.
- Any visible changes suggestive of malignancy can be excised or ablated by laser. Topical 5-fluorouracil is also used as a chemoablative treatment option.

- **Histopathology**

Histologically, dysplastic epithelium could be seen, accompanied by telangiectasia in the laminated pro-

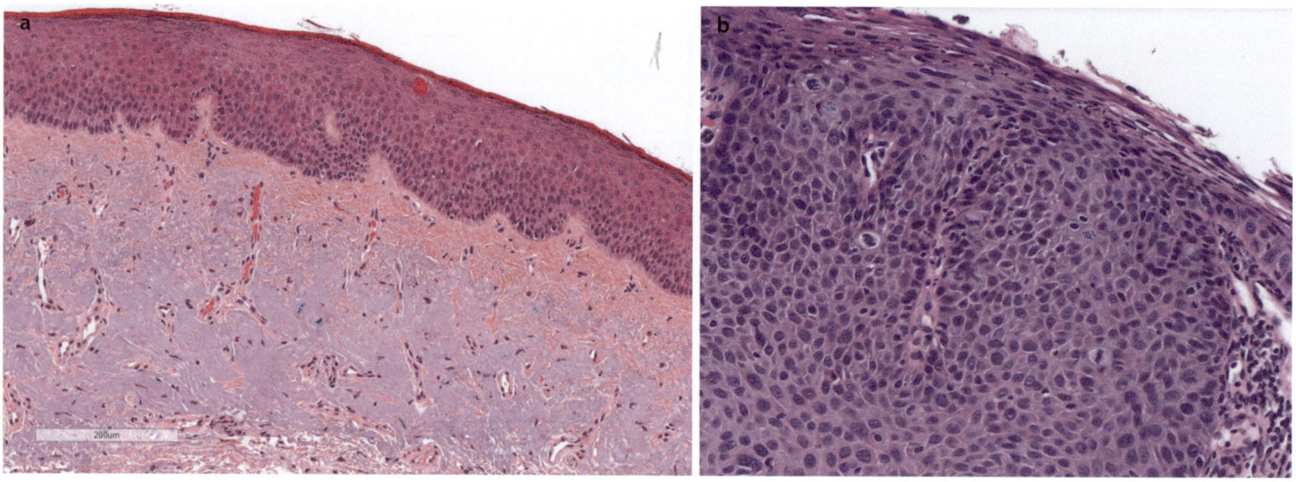

Fig. 29.5 **a** Photomicrograph of actinic cheilitis showing hyperkeratosis, acanthosis, dyskeratosis, and moderate dysplasia, with a dense chronic inflammatory infiltrate and basophilic degeneration of the lamina propria. **b** Severe dysplasia. Photomicrograph showing cytological atypia, architectural changes and mitoses, including abnormal mitoses in rete ridges above the basal layer

pria within a background of solar elastosis, which appears as an amorphous light purple background (Fig. 29.5) [6]. Mild, moderate, or severe dysplasia (Fig. 29.5) points to potential malignant nature of OSF.

29.7 Oral Lichen Planus and Oral Lichenoid Lesions

Oral lichen planus (OLP), lichenoid drug eruptions, and lichenoid contact hypersensitivity reactions are recognised as OPMDs. Lichen planus is a chronic mucocutaneous inflammatory disorder with oral lichen planus as its oral counterpart. Oral lichenoid lesion (OLL) is a term used to describe oral lesions that have clinical and/or histopathological features similar to oral lichen planus [9].

Key Features

- Oral lichen planus is seen clinically as reticular, papular, plaque-like, erosive, atrophic, or bullous types.
- Commonly involved intraoral sites include the buccal mucosa, tongue, and gingiva.
- Oral mucosal lesions present alone or concomitantly with violaceous, papular skin lesions. Characteristically the facial skin is spared.
- Oral lichenoid lesions clinically present as mucosal grey-white streaks, reticulated and plaque-like keratotic papules, often accompanied by erosion, ulceration, atrophy, and blistering.
- Diagnosis requires a thorough clinical history to ensure that diseases with similar presentation are excluded.
- Biopsy is mandatory for diagnosis, preferably both routine and fresh tissue biopsy for immunofluorescence against fibrinogen, C3, IgG, and IgA.
- The fresh tissue is best taken from perilesional tissue, and punch biopsy is best avoided to prevent artefactual epithelial separation which may complicate histopathological interpretation.

Histopathology

The histological features of lichen planus are detailed in Chap. 25: Histopathology of diseases of the oral mucosa. However, once epithelial dysplasia is identified on a biopsy sample, the lesion is dealt with as a dysplastic lesion and the presence of lichenoid inflammation would be of less relevance to management [6, 10] (Fig. 29.6a, b).

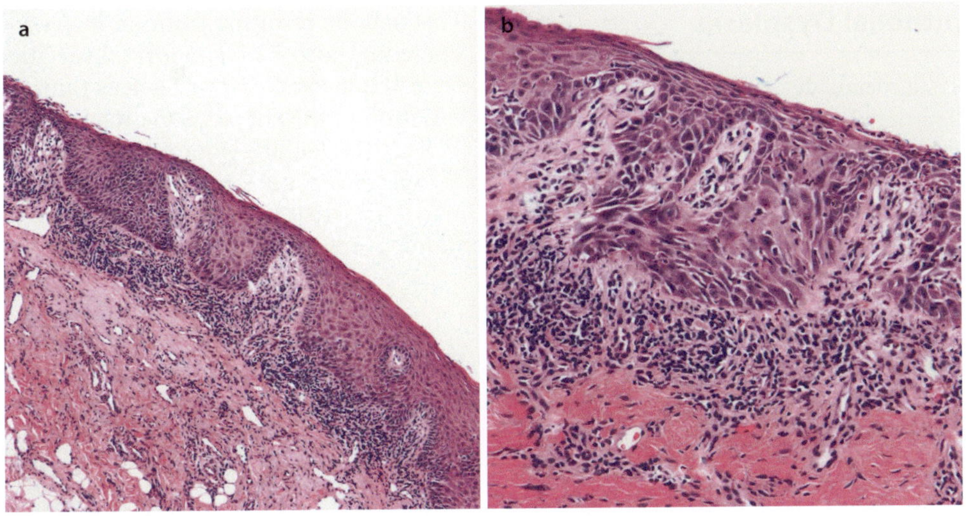

Fig. 29.6 **a** and **b** Dysplasia with lichenoid pattern of inflammation. **a** Low-power photomicrograph illustrating a lichen planus-like lymphoid infiltrate subjacent dysplastic oral epithelium. **b** Photomicrograph illustrating the markedly dysplastic epithelium. (Courtesy Professor David F Wilson, Adelaide, Australia)

29.8 Chronic Hyperplastic Candidosis (Candidal Leukoplakia)

In the most recent WHO classification, chronic hyperplastic candidosis (CHC), or candidal leukoplakia is listed as one of the diseases with insufficient evidence of having potential for malignant transformation [1]. However, in vitro studies have shown that candidal infection does promote malignant transformation [11], with evidence of correlation with dysplasia [12, 13].

Key Features

- CHC is most common in the buccal mucosa near the commissure.
- Clinically, CHC presents as a white lesion, often asymptomatic, which cannot be removed by gently scraping.
- Most frequent intraoral sites of CHC include the commissural angles, the anterior ▶ buccal mucosa, and on the dorsum or lateral of the ▶ tongue.
- CHC can be initially investigated with an oral smear followed by a course of anti-fungal therapy prior to biopsy.
- Should the lesion fail to resolve, biopsy is needed to exclude dysplasia and early invasive carcinoma.

Histopathology

The histopathological picture is that of epithelial hyperplasia and pseudoepitheliomatous hyperplasia, in which there are elongated rete ridges and seemingly separate islands of squamous epithelium when cut in cross-section mimicking invasive carcinoma. This results from a reaction of the epithelium to the candidal hyphae which can be highlighted in the superficial layers of the epithelium by Periodic Acid Schiff (PAS) staining (Fig. 29.7). However, the picture usually lacks prominent cellular atypia. The identification of candidal hyphae through PAS staining and also presence of neutrophilic exocytosis within the epithelium supports a diagnosis of CHC. Careful examination is required to exclude dysplasia changes and invasive carcinoma. When epithelial atypia or dysplasia is seen, the lesion should be managed as a dysplastic lesion with concurrent anti-fungal therapy.

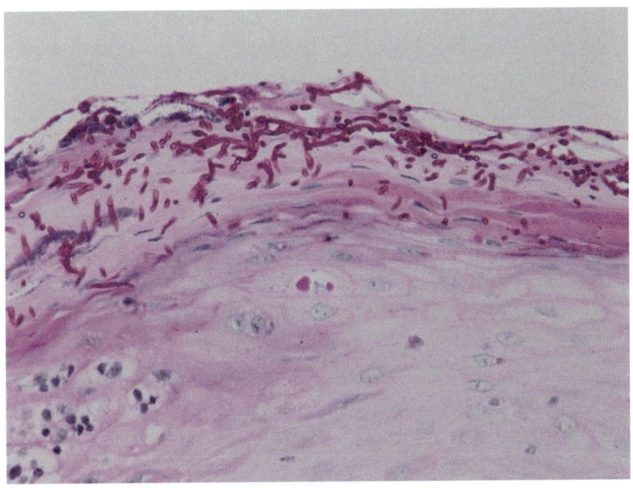

Fig. 29.7 Photomicrograph showing brightly staining fungal organisms in the superficial epithelium in a case of chronic hyperplastic candidosis (PASD stain). (Courtesy Professor David F Wilson, Adelaide, Australia)

29.9 Oral Epithelial Dysplasia

The term dysplasia means disordered tissue formation, *dys*-meaning disordered in Latin and *plasia* meaning formation of tissue [14]. The normal maturation of the oral epithelium follows a specific pattern, starting with proliferation in the basal layer where stem cells give rise to two daughter cells, one of which continues to differentiate into polygonal squamous cells in the prickle cell layers, then mature into intermediate cell layers and finally become superficial squamous cells or plates of keratin which then shed into the oral cavity. In dysplasia, this ordered maturation process is disrupted resulting in a combination of any of the cellular and architectural features of dysplasia [6].

The histological features seen in oral epithelial dysplasia is the same in other stratified epithelia and are categorised into cellular atypia pertaining to the changes on a cellular level, and architectural dysplasia pertaining to changes in the arrangement of the tissue architecture [6]. The WHO Blue Book of Head and Neck Tumour Classification has provided a new set of criteria for recognising epithelial dysplasia (◘ Table 29.1) [15].

The cellular features of dysplasia include a range of changes to the normal size and shape of the nucleus and the cell. There may be an increase in the nuclear to cytoplasmic ratio, which in prickle cells is approximately 1:3. This may be resulting from an increase in nuclear size. There may also be an abnormal variation in the size of the cell (anisocytosis) or nucleus (anisonucleosis) and a variation in the shape of the nucleus or the cell termed nuclear or cellular pleomorphism (◘ Fig. 29.8).

Specific to nuclear changes, nuclear hyperchromatism refers to the increase in the intensity of nuclear staining resulting from higher nuclear activity. An

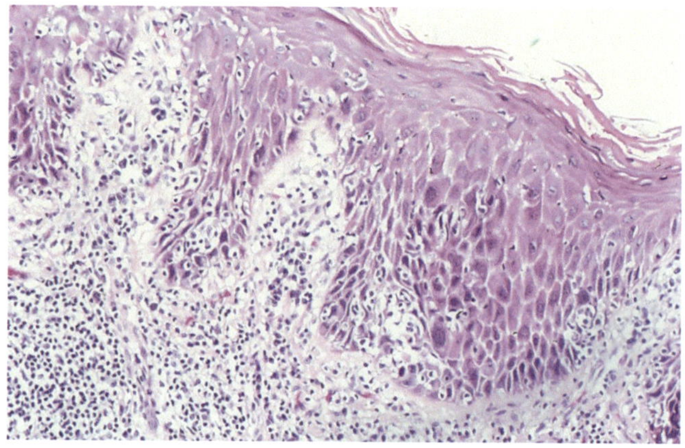

◘ **Fig. 29.8** Photomicrograph of dysplastic oral mucosal epithelium showing variation in the size of cells and nuclei and variation in the shape of cells and nuclei. (Courtesy of Professor David F Wilson, Adelaide, Australia)

◘ **Table 29.1** The architectural and cytological features of oral epithelial dysplasia. (Adopted from Odell et al. (2021) [6])

Architectural features	Cytological features
Irregular stratification	Abnormal variation in nuclear size
Loss of polarity or disorganisation of basal cells	Abnormal variation in nuclear shape
Drop-shaped rete processes	Abnormal variation in cell size
Basal cell clustering/nesting	Abnormal variation in cell shape
Expanded proliferative compartment	Increased mitotic activity
Mitoses high in epithelium	Increased nuclear size
Mitoses in maturing cells	Increased nucleus: Cytoplasm ratio
Generalised premature keratinisation	Atypical mitotic figures
Keratin pearls in rete processes	Increased number and size of nucleoli
Reduced keratinocyte cohesion	Single-cell keratinisation
Altered keratin pattern for oral sub-site	Nuclear hyperchromasia
Verrucous or papillary architecture	Apoptotic mitoses
Extension of changes along minor gland ducts	
Sharply defined margin to changes	
Multiple different patterns of dysplasia	
Multifocal or skip lesions	

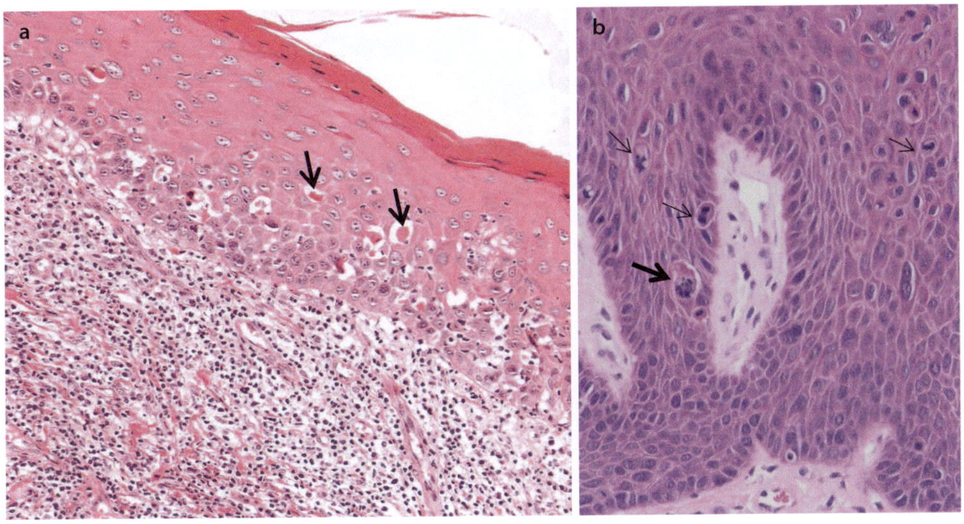

Fig. 29.9 **a** and **b** Dysplastic oral epithelium showing individual cell keratinisation (dyskeratosis) (arrows) in the prickle cell layer. **b** Dysplastic oral epithelium showing an abnormal mitotic figure (large arrow) and other mitotic figures (small arrows). (Courtesy Professor David F Wilson, Adelaide, Australia)

increase in the number and size of nucleoli is another nuclear feature that is seen in dysplasia. On an individual cell level, the cells close to the basal cell layer or in the prickle cell layer may undergo premature keratinisation (dyskeratosis), which can also be considered an architectural feature when it is seen in more than just individual cells. There may also be increased mitotic activity and abnormal mitotic figures (Fig. 29.9a, b).

On a tissue level, the architectural features of dysplasia involve disordered organisation of the epithelium. The basal cells may show loss of polarity which manifests by the loss of the palisaded appearance of the basal cell layer. Disordered epithelial stratification results from the loss of the ability of cells to undergo their normal process of proliferation, differentiation, and then maturation. An example is the individual cell keratinisation mentioned above, and the formation of keratin pearls within the rete ridges. Conversely, mitotic figures may be seen in the suprabasal and superficial layers of the epithelium. As a result of increased mitotic activity, the rete ridges become bulbous, with secondary budding extensions into the lamina propria. Reduced or loss of cohesion between keratinocytes is another feature. As mentioned in the section on PVL, a verrucous or papillary surface architecture is also a feature of architectural dysplasia [6].

It is worth noting that dysplasia may also be accompanied by hyperplasia, which can sometimes be profound, in the form of the increased thickness of the prickle cell layer called acanthosis. Similarly, an otherwise non-keratinised oral epithelium such as that of the floor of mouth, may become keratinised. This is called keratosis. Also, an already keratinised epithelial surface may become hyper-para or hyper-orthokeratinised, resulting in a whiter clinical appearance resulting from a combination of acanthosis and an increase in the thickness of the keratin layer termed hyperkeratosis, which presents as a white patch. In the absence of any triggering factors, and when the white patch is not characterised by any other known disease, it is termed leukoplakia. While keratosis and hyperkeratosis are not features specific to dysplasia, a sharp demarcation between lesional tissue and clinically and histologically normal mucosa is a feature of dysplasia [6].

There are two main systems for dysplasia grading, the first one is the WHO three-tier system which includes mild, moderate, and severe dysplasia. The assessment is mainly dependent on the thickness of epithelium that shows dysplastic features. Mild dysplasia shows up to one-third, moderate up to two-thirds, and severe more than two-thirds. However, in practice, this is usually modified according to the biopsy site and cellular and architectural features, and the pathologist may upgrade the degree of dysplasia accordingly. For example, a biopsy of leukoplakia of the floor of mouth that shows dysplastic features only up to one-third of the epithelium, can be upgraded to moderate due to the relatively thin epithelium of the floor of mouth, few pronounced cellular features of dysplasia, and keratosis imparting the white appearance [6, 16, 17]. The second system first presented by Kujan et al. [18], uses a two-tiered or binary method of low- vs. high-risk dysplasia, depending on how many cellular and architectural features of dysplasia are seen. The proposed cut-off with prognostic value is set at a minimum of four architectural and five cytological features [18] Both systems have shown comparative value and consistency [19].

In clinical practice, dysplasia grading is considered along with a number of patient and lesion-related factors, such as age, sex, lifestyle risk factors, size, site, type of lesion, and then dysplasia grading [2]. The management of dysplastic lesions involves patient education to control modifiable lifestyle risk factors, removal of the lesions by scalpel surgery or laser ablation, with continued follow-up including photographs taken on a regular basis in order to detect and promptly manage any lesions that arise in the oral mucosa [20].

29.10 Summary

OPMD are clinical mucosal changes associated with an increased risk of mouth cancer development and they are histopathologically recognised by the presence of epithelial dysplasia. Notably, disorders in epithelial proliferation and differentiation are the hallmark of epithelial dysplasia. It comprises alterations in the tissue architecture and cells that comprise the oral epithelium as a result of exposure to risk factors. Epithelial dysplasia can lead to malignancies and range in severity from low grade to severe. Hence, recognition and grading of oral epithelial dysplasia is paramount for better management of OPMD.

Further Reading

1. Warnakulasuriya S, et al. Oral potentially malignant disorders: a consensus report from an international seminar on nomenclature and classification, convened by the WHO Collaborating Centre for Oral Cancer. Oral Dis. 2021;27(8):1862–80.
2. Speight PM, Khurram SA, Kujan O. Oral potentially malignant disorders: risk of progression to malignancy. Oral Surg Oral Med Oral Pathol Oral Radiol. 2018;125(6):612–27.
3. Thompson LDR, et al. Proliferative verrucous leukoplakia: an expert consensus guideline for standardized assessment and reporting. Head Neck Pathol. 2021;15(2):572–87.
4. Eisenberg E, Fitzpatrick S, Kallarakkal TG, Warnakulasuriya S. Proliferative verrucous leukoplakia. Muller S, Odell EW, Tilakaratne WM, editors. In: WHO classification of tumours—head and neck tumours. Lyon: WHO; 2022.
5. Ramos-García P, et al. Malignant transformation of oral proliferative verrucous leukoplakia: a systematic review and meta-analysis. Oral Dis. 2021;27(8):1896–907.
6. Odell E, et al. Oral epithelial dysplasia: recognition, grading and clinical significance. Oral Dis. 2021;27(8):1947–76.
7. Muller S, Tilakaratne WM. Oral potentially malignant disorders. In: Odell EW, editor. WHO classification of tumours—head and neck tumours. Lyon: WHO; 2022.
8. Warnakulasuriya S. Oral potentially malignant disorders: a comprehensive review on clinical aspects and management. Oral Oncol. 2020;102:104550.
9. Cheng YS, et al. Diagnosis of oral lichen planus: a position paper of the American Academy of Oral and Maxillofacial Pathology. Oral Surg Oral Med Oral Pathol Oral Radiol. 2016;122(3):332–54.
10. Idrees M, et al. Observer agreement in the diagnosis of oral lichen planus using the proposed criteria of the American Academy of Oral and Maxillofacial Pathology. J Oral Pathol Med. 2021;50(5):520–7.
11. Mohd Bakri M, et al. Revisiting the association between candidal infection and carcinoma, particularly oral squamous cell carcinoma. J Oral Microbiol. 2010;2(1):5780.
12. McCullough M, et al. Oral yeast carriage correlates with presence of oral epithelial dysplasia. Oral Oncol. 2002;38(4):391–3.
13. Bakri MM, et al. Detection of Candida albicans ADH1 and ADH2 mRNAs in human archival oral biopsy samples. J Oral Pathol Med. 2014;43(9):704–10.
14. Ranganathan K, Kavitha L. Oral epithelial dysplasia: classifications and clinical relevance in risk assessment of oral potentially malignant disorders. J Oral Maxillofac Pathol. 2019;23(1):19–27.
15. Muller S, Tilakaratne WM. Update from the 5th edition of the World Health Organization classification of head and neck tumors: tumours of the oral cavity and mobile tongue. Head Neck Pathol. 2022;16(1):54–62.
16. Bouquot JE, Speight PM, Farthing PM. Epithelial dysplasia of the oral mucosa—diagnostic problems and prognostic features. Curr Diagn Pathol. 2006;12(1):11–21.
17. Speight PM. Update on oral epithelial dysplasia and progression to cancer. Head Neck Pathol. 2007;1(1):61–6.
18. Kujan O, et al. Evaluation of a new binary system of grading oral epithelial dysplasia for prediction of malignant transformation. Oral Oncol. 2006;42(10):987–93.
19. Sathasivam HP, et al. The clinical utility of contemporary oral epithelial dysplasia grading systems. J Oral Pathol Med. 2022;51(2):180–7.
20. Awadallah M, et al. Management update of potentially premalignant oral epithelial lesions. Oral Surg Oral Med Oral Pathol Oral Radiol. 2018;125(6):628–36.

Histopathology of Malignant Neoplasms of the Oral Mucosa-1

Benedict Seo

Contents

S R Prabhu et al. (eds.), *Oral Histology and Oral Histopathology*, https://doi.org/10.1007/978-3-031-77481-2_30

30.1 Introduction

Oral malignant neoplasms form a heterogeneous group of tumours. Over 90% of oral malignancies are squamous cell carcinomas (SCC), which arise from the squamous epithelium. The remaining 10% consist of malignant melanomas, carcinomas of the intraoral salivary glands, sarcomas of the soft tissues and bones, malignant odontogenic tumours, non-Hodgkin's lymphomas, and metastatic neoplasms from primary tumour sites located elsewhere in the body. This chapter will discuss the key features and histopathology of oral squamous cell carcinoma, verrucous carcinoma, and carcinoma cuniculatum. Malignant melanoma and non-epithelial malignant neoplasms are discussed in Chap. 31.

30.1.1 Oral Squamous Cell Carcinoma

Oral squamous cell carcinoma (OSCC) is a malignant tumour that arises from the squamous epithelial cells lining the oral cavity. It is the most common type of oral cancer and can occur in various areas, such as the lips, tongue, floor of the mouth, and gums. Risk factors include tobacco use, excessive alcohol consumption, poor oral hygiene, and human papillomavirus (HPV) infection.

▪ **Key Features**

- Oral squamous cell carcinoma (OSCC) includes squamous malignant neoplasms of the oral mucosa proper and vermillion aspect of the lip.
- Globally, OSCC, including the SCC of the oral cavity proper and lip, ranks as the 16th most common form of cancer, with more than 300,000 diagnoses made each year.
- OSCC accounts singularly for more than 90% of all cancers diagnosed in the head and neck region.
- OSCC should be differentiated from the oropharyngeal squamous cell carcinoma (OPSCC), which involves the oropharynx (including the soft palate and base of the tongue), many of which are caused by high-risk type human papillomavirus (HPV16).
- However, there are some significant regional variations in the epidemiology of OSCC dependent on geography and socioeconomic variations.
- Males are typically affected at a higher rate than females, and OSCC more commonly evolves in middle-aged adults.
- The use of tobacco remains the main etiological factor in the development of OSCC, often synergistically confounded by alcohol use. Betel nut use in Southeast Asia and adjacent regions is also an established risk factor.
- OSCC can manifest anywhere in the oral cavity. However, certain anatomical areas are more at risk, including the posterior, lateral, and ventral tongue, the floor of the mouth, and, to a lesser extent, gingiva/alveolar mucosa, and buccal mucosa.
- OSCC can present as an exophytic or endophytic proliferative growth with variable surface colouration and texture. Typical signs include raised rolled margins, induration, and fixation to underlying structures.
- OSCC may also present as asymptomatic mucosal chronic white or red patches.
- OSCC may also present as asymptomatic mucosal chronic white (leukoplakia) or red patches (erythroplakia) and chronic non-healing ulcers.
- Pain tends to be a late presentation. Once the malignancy has invaded through the alveolar/maxillary and mandibular bones, radiography reveals irregular radiolucency, often showing ill-defined uni- or multilocular appearance with a direct spatial relationship to the original site of the primary mucosal lesion.
- The TNM system of classification is important for planning the treatment, estimating recurrence risk, and overall survival assessment. TNM system reflects the extent of tumour growth and is based on an assessment of the size of the primary tumour (T), involvement of locoregional lymph nodes (N), and ▶ distant metastases (M).
- SCC is treated in a stage-dependent manner, but the main mode of treatment includes wide local excision (resection) with or without adjunct radiotherapy/chemotherapy. Neck dissection to examine sentinel lymph nodes may be warranted.
- Novel treatment modalities include brachytherapy. Prognosis is also stage-dependent, with a 5-year survival ranging from 85% to 10% from stage 1 to stage 4. Greater emphasis is placed on palliative care for stage 4 cancers.

▪ **Histopathology**

The essential histopathologic criteria for diagnosing OSCC are the demonstration of dissociated island invasion into the underlying fibrous connective tissue and the establishment of its association with surface dysplastic stratified squamous oral epithelium. The degree of adjacent epithelial dysplasia may vary. The tumour may also exhibit a range of micromorphological differentiation ranging from well to moderate and poor differentiation depending on the extent to which the lesional cells resemble the parental tissue of origin, i.e., stratified squamous surface epithelium (◘ Fig. 30.1a–c). Atypical cytonuclear changes within OSCC include features in common with oral epithelial dysplasia. Mitoses may be numerous and include abnormal mitotic figures. The pattern of invasion is an important prognostic factor. Squamous cell carcinoma infiltrates deep into the connective tissues in the form of islands,, as opposed to the pushing front, as seen in verrucous carcinoma. The infiltrating front may be cohesive or non-cohesive. The non-cohesive infiltrative front may comprise individual cells or small clusters of cells. A diffuse or focal effacement of normal structures occurs once the tumour has invaded the underlying fibrous connective tissue. Features to note include lymphovascular invasion, neurotropism/perineural invasion, and invasion into skeletal muscle, salivary glands, and bone (◘ Fig. 30.2a–c). Several histopathologic features are known adverse prognosticators and are summarised in ◘ Table 30.1.

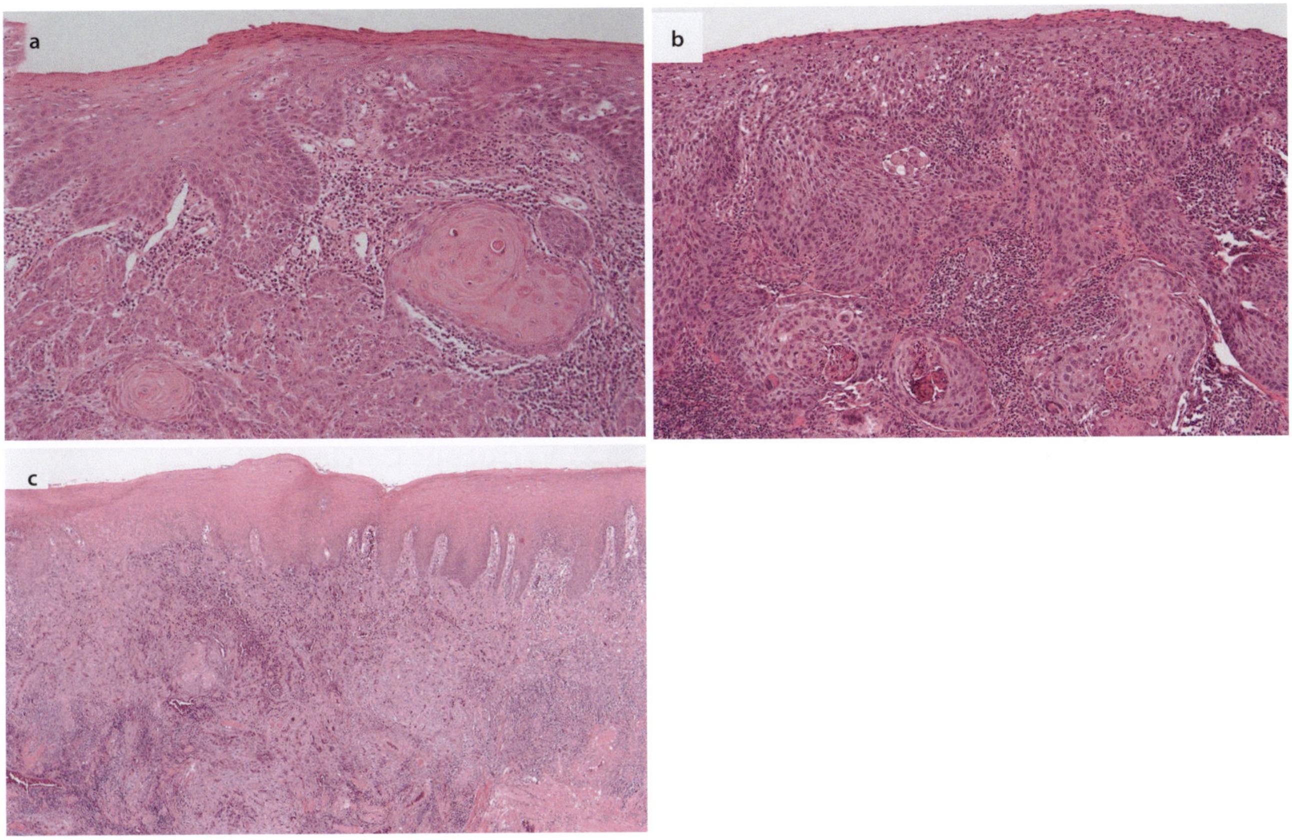

◘ **Fig. 30.1** **a** A well-differentiated squamous cell carcinoma. Note the islands of neoplastic in the connective tissue which resembles the parental tissue of origin. **b** SCC showing moderately differentiated neoplasm. **c** Poorly differentiated SCCs showing increasing degrees of cytonuclear atypia and mitotic activity

30

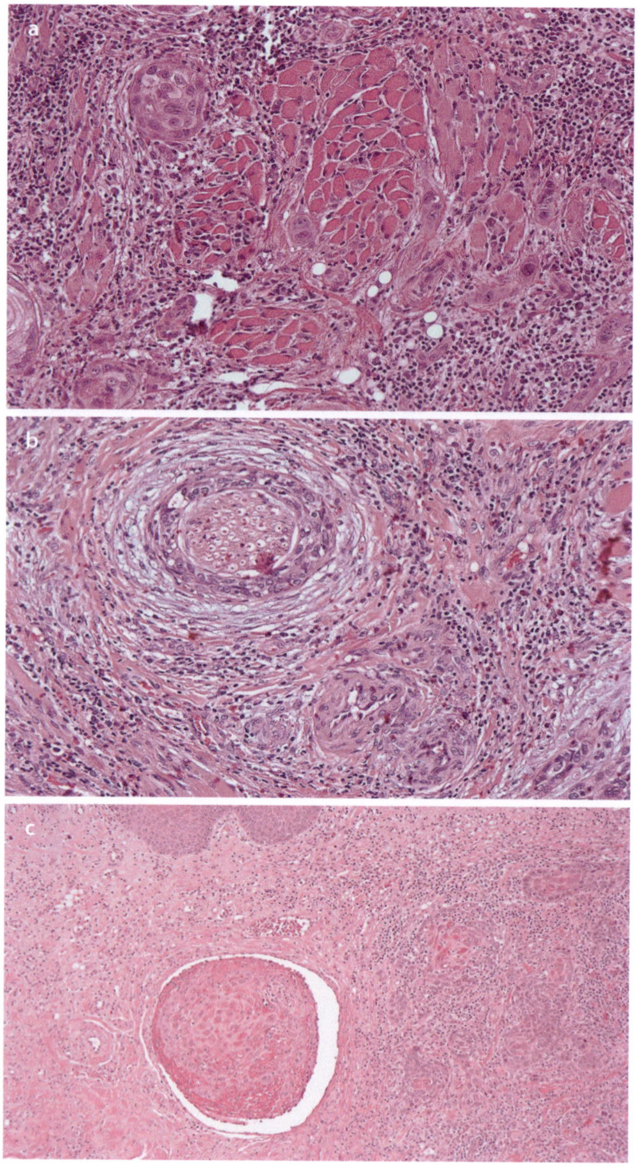

Fig. 30.2 **a–c** OSCC can invade and infiltrate through underlying tissues and anatomical structures. Examples of intramuscular invasion **a**, perineural invasion **b**, and tumour embolus **c** are shown

Table 30.1 Histopathological features associated with OSCC prognosis

Histopathological features	**Notes**
Tumour type	Acantholytic, adenosquamous, basaloid, carcinoma cuniculatum, lymphoepithelial, papillary, spindle cell, verrucous
Histological grade	Well, moderately and poorly differentiated
Depth of invasion	From the basement membrane to the deepest point of invasion
Pattern of invasion	At the most biologically active front. Cohesive (>15 cells) or non-cohesive (<15 cells)
Lymphovascular invasion	Within endothelial lines, vascular spaces
Perineural invasion	Perineural, endoneurial, and intraneural invasion
Invasion of bone and adjacent structure	Cortical/medullary bone, muscles, salivary gland, skin, etc.
Margin	>5 mm clear, 1–5 mm close, <1 mm involved. Also, the presence or absence of epithelial dysplasia

30.2 Verrucous Carcinoma

Verrucous carcinoma (VC) is a well-differentiated variant of OSCC characterised by a prominent verrucous surface architecture and exophytic-endophytic tumour invasion. The oral cavity is a common site for VC in the head and neck region.

Key Features

- Clinically, verrucous carcinoma presents as a solitary exophytic lesion, which may involve more diffuse contiguous areas within the oral cavity.
- With the notable exophytic surface configuration, white kerato-papillary, sometimes a fungating appearance may be evident.
- Classic signs of malignancy, such as fixation, raised border, and induration of malignancy, should be assessed and noted.

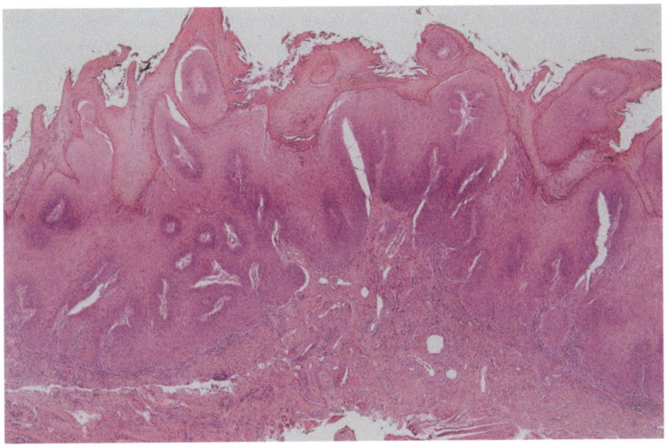

Fig. 30.3 Verrucous carcinoma, showing a prominent verrucopapillary surface architecture and broad and deep invasive front approximating underlying skeletal muscle bundles

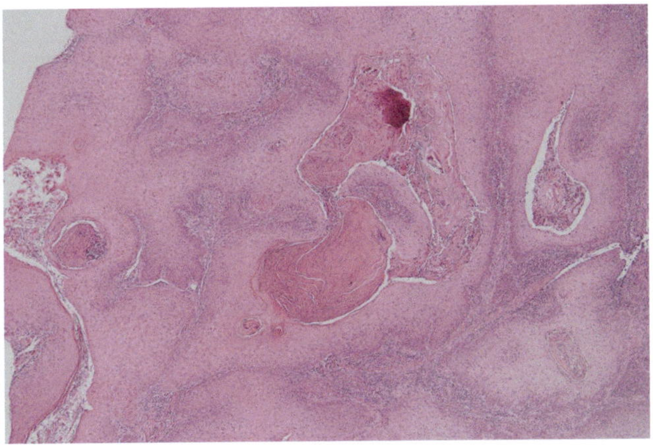

Fig. 30.4 Carcinoma cuniculatum showing an extensive labyrinth-like network of invading tumour epithelial proliferation with keratin-filled crypts. Note the lesion itself is well differentiated

- Verrucous carcinoma is a low-grade variant of SCC with low rates of lymph node metastasis.
- Whilst significant local destruction is possible, the mortality rate is low, and the lesion should not recur after complete excision.
- Verrucous carcinoma may develop into a conventional SCC or arise adjacent to it, especially in a patient who is considered to have preexisting lesion(s) judged to be on the spectrum of proliferative verrucous leukoplakia. In such cases, management strategies for SCC would apply.

Histopathology

At low power, verrucous carcinoma invades the underlying fibrous connective tissue in a broad pushing front (often described as an 'elephant feet' appearance) (Fig. 30.3). With both exophytic and endophytic epithelial proliferation, it is often difficult to ascertain whether there may be true pushing invasion into the underlying fibrous connective tissue, which is the cornerstone of verrucous carcinoma diagnosis. Therefore, it is important to assess (1) the lateral seemingly unaffected mucosa to judge the depth and laterality of the lesion and (2) the anatomical (e.g. skeletal muscle and fat layers) landmarks. Verrucous carcinoma is a well-differentiated variant of squamous cell carcinoma. Thus, significant cytonuclear atypia may not be present. When dissociated island invasion is present or suspected, the diagnosis of SCC, rather than verrucous carcinoma, should be considered. VC should also be distinguished from carcinoma cuniculatum, another example of a low-grade, well-differentiated, non-metastasizing variant of OSCC (see below).

30.3 Carcinoma Cuniculatum

Carcinoma cuniculatum (CC) is an uncommon variant of oral squamous cell carcinoma.

Key Features

- CC is a well-differentiated tumour which is locally destructive but is unlikely to metastasise.
- CC is a disease of the elderly with a predilection for gingiva and alveolar mucosa.
- Excision is curative and diagnostic. Incomplete excision may result in lesional recurrence.

Histopathology

Carcinoma cuniculatum shows prominent endophytic proliferation (Fig. 30.4) with extensive proliferation of the contiguous tumour cells in the associated stroma and adjacent fibrous connective tissue. This pattern of invasion has been described as 'labyrinthine' or likened to rabbit burrowing holes.

30.4 Summary

OSCC is the most important malignancy of the oral and maxillofacial regions in terms of the morbidity and mortality it causes. To arrive at an appropriate diagnosis, it is essential to recognise the histological features of malignancy in correlation with clinical presentation. The pattern of invasion and the degree of differentiation are important aspects to consider when distinguishing conventional SCC from its variants.

Further Reading

Asthana S, Labani S, Kailash U, et al. Association of smokeless tobacco use and oral cancer: a systematic global review and meta-analysis. Nicotine Tob Res. 2019;21:1162–71.

Gupta B, Johnson NW. Systematic review and meta-analysis of association of smokeless tobacco and of betel quid without tobacco with incidence of oral cancer in South Asia and the Pacific. PLoS One. 2014;9:e113385.

Koch BB, Trask DK, Hoffman HT, et al. National survey of head and neck verrucous carcinoma: patterns of presentation, care, and outcome. Cancer. 2001;92:110–20.

Kuruvilla J, Nayar KR. Distribution pattern and its correlation for oral cancer rate and human development rank for countries: an ecological approach. Contemp Clin Dent. 2021;12:9–13.

Mashiana SS, Navale P, Khandakar B, et al. Human papillomavirus genotype distribution in head and neck cancer: Informing developing strategies for cancer prevention, diagnosis, treatment and surveillance. Oral Oncol. 2021;113:105109.

Sung H, Ferlay J, Siegel RL, et al. Global cancer statistics 2020: GLOBOCAN estimates of incidence and mortality worldwide for 36 cancers in 185 countries. CA Cancer J Clin. 2021;71:209–49.

Histopathology of Malignant Neoplasms of the Oral Mucosa-2

S R Prabhu

Contents

S R Prabhu et al. (eds.), *Oral Histology and Oral Histopathology*, https://doi.org/10.1007/978-3-031-77481-2_31

31.1 Introduction

Oral malignant neoplasms form a heterogeneous group of tumours. Over 90% of oral malignancies are squamous cell carcinomas (SCC) arising from the squamous epithelium (► Chap. 30). This chapter deals with key features and histopathology of oral malignant melanoma, oral Kaposi sarcoma, oral fibrosarcoma, oral liposarcoma, and oral non-Hodkin's lymphoma.

31.2 Oral Malignant Melanoma

Malignant melanoma is characterised by uncontrolled proliferation of melanin-producing melanocytes. Oral melanoma is rare.

Key Features

- Intraoral sites of melanoma include the palate and the gingivae.
- The cause is unknown; intraoral melanomas are unrelated to UV exposure (unlike skin counterparts).
- Melanoma may present as an asymptomatic brown-to-black patch with irregular borders or a rapidly growing black mass with ulceration, bleeding, bone destruction and pain.
- Regional lymph node metastasis is a common feature.
- Diagnosis involves histopathology and immunohistochemistry.
- Wide surgical excision with simultaneous neck dissection followed by radiotherapy/chemotherapy.
- Prognosis is generally poor (30% node-negative, 10% node-positive).

Histopathology

The characteristic histopathological features of malignant melanoma include hyperchromatism and nuclear pleomorphism of melanocytes in the epithelium and connective tissue junction. The intracytoplasmic pigment is present in the cytoplasm of the melanocytes (◘ Fig. 31.1). This feature combined with positive S-100 and HMB-45 markers is confirmatory of mucosal melanoma. Melan A stain is also used to diagnose melanomas (◘ Fig. 31.2). Regional lymph node metastasis reveals the replacement of the lymph node architecture by the neoplastic cells (◘ Fig. 31.3).

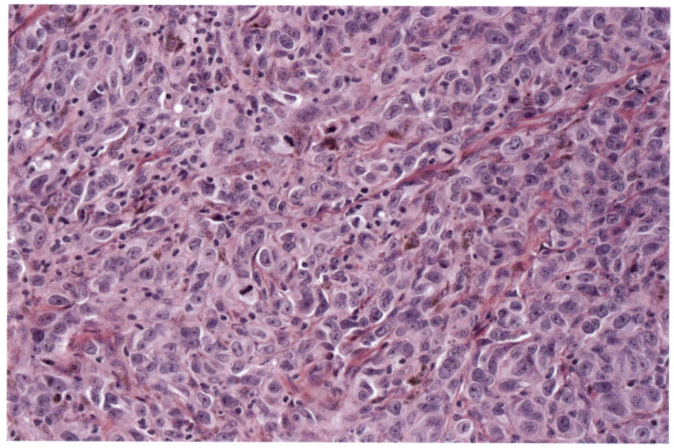

◘ **Fig. 31.1** Malignant melanoma. Fine intracytoplasmic pigment within the cytoplasm of neoplastic cells. Mitotic figures are prominent (hematoxylin and ► eosin stain). (Source: Yeshwant B. Rawal, Thomas B. Dodson, Harbinder S. Bal, Oral melanoma: Relevance to the dental team members, The Journal of the American Dental Association, Volume 148, Issue 2, 2017, Pages 113–119. (With permission from Elsevier)

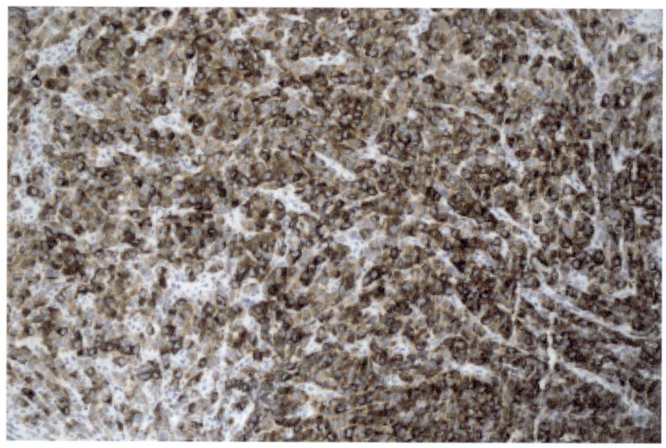

◘ **Fig. 31.2** Malignant melanoma. ► Melanocyte tumour cells express uniformly strong reactivity to cytoplasmic melan immunostaining. (Source: Yeshwant B. Rawal, Thomas B. Dodson, Harbinder S. Bal, Oral melanoma: Relevance to the dental team members, The Journal of the American Dental Association, Volume 148, Issue 2, 2017, Pages 113–119. (With permission from Elsevier)

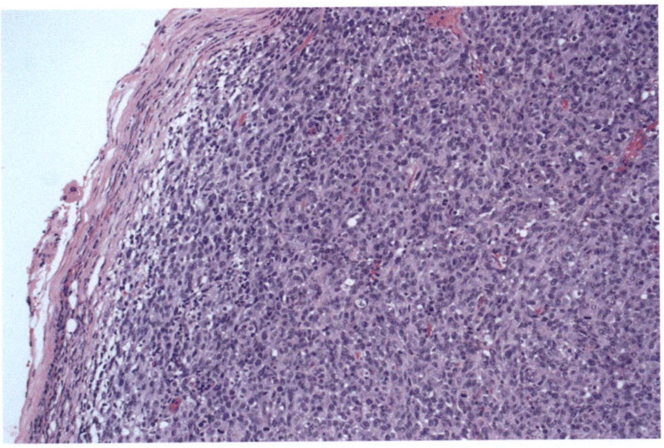

Fig. 31.3 Lymph node metastasis of malignant melanoma. Tumour cells replacing lymph node architecture and occupying the entire lymph node except the nodal capsule (hematoxylin and eosin stain). (Source: Yeshwant B. Rawal, Thomas B. Dodson, Harbinder S. Bal, Oral melanoma: Relevance to the dental team members, The Journal of the American Dental Association, Volume 148, Issue 2, 2017, Pages 113–119. (With permission from Elsevier)

31.3 Kaposi Sarcoma

Kaposi sarcoma (KS) is a multi-focal proliferative malignant condition of the blood vessels or lymphatics caused by human herpes virus 8 (HHV8) infection. KS can be subdivided into four clinical presentations: classic KS, endemic KS (African), iatrogenic KS (immunosuppression–/transplant-associated), and epidemic KS (HIV-related).

Key Features

- 70% of individuals with AIDS-related KS develop oral lesions.
- Oral presentation starts as a flat purple lesion, which enlarges into a nodular mass, ulcerates, and bleeds.
- Intraoral sites include hard palate, gingivae, and tongue.
- Diagnosis is based on history, histopathology, and immunohistochemical staining for HHV8 virus.
- Management includes surgical excision, chemotherapy, and treatment for opportunistic infections.
- Prognosis is variable.

Histopathology

Histopathological features of Kaposi's sarcoma include atypical vascular channels (in early lesions), a prominent spindle cell component, extravasated red blood cells, deposits of hemosiderin, the presence of eosinophilic bodies, and mitotic figures. In early lesions, chronic inflammatory cells are present. Slit-like vascular spaces are common, and some tumour cells contain intracytoplasmic eosinophilic hyaline globules (Fig. 31.4a, b).

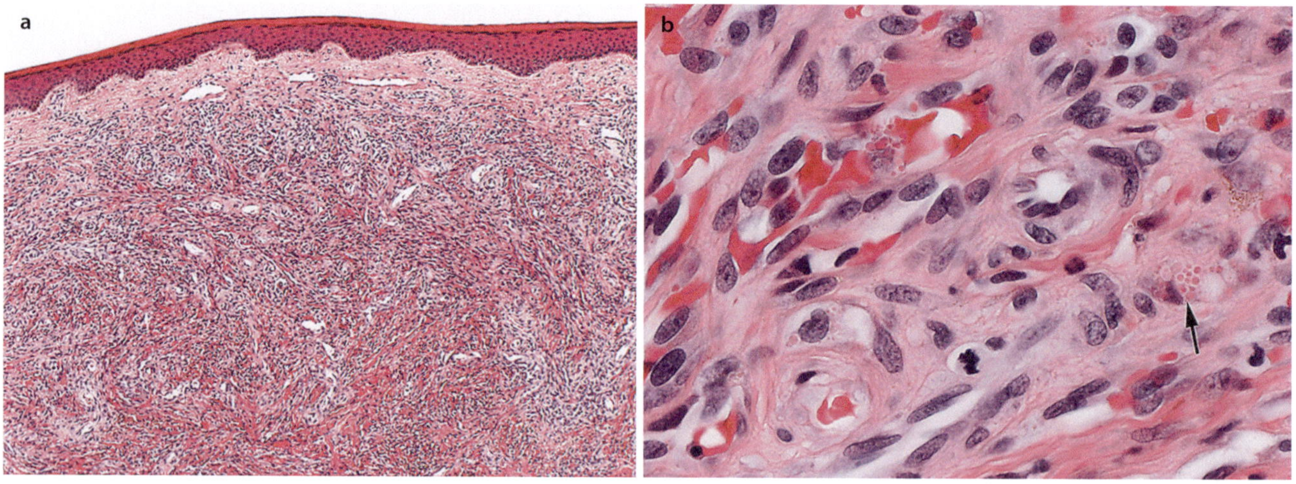

Fig. 31.4 a and b Kaposi sarcoma. a Microscopic features of the intraoral tumour mass show a densely cellular subepithelial tumour consisting of spindle cells with numerous slit-like spaces containing erythrocytes and some ectatic vessels at the edge of the lesion. b Spindle-shaped tumour cells with mild cytologic atypia form slit-like vascular spaces filled with erythrocytes; some tumour cells contain intracytoplasmic eosinophilic hyaline globules (arrow) characteristic of KS. The globules most likely represent phagocytosed erythrocyte fragments. (Source: Thieringer FM, Cede J, Glatz K, Roehling S, Stoeckle M, Leiggener CS. Oral Kaposi's Sarcoma: A Case Report and Literature Review on Treatment Management. *Craniomaxillofacial Trauma & Reconstruction Open*. 2021;6. doi:► https://doi.org/10.1177/24727512211036328. Open access. (► https://creativecommons.org/licenses/by-nc/4.0/).

31.4 Oral Fibrosarcoma

In 2002, the World Health Organization (WHO) defined fibrosarcoma as a malignant tumour composed of fibroblasts with variable collagen and, in classical cases, a herringbone architecture. Oral mucosal fibrosarcoma is rare.

Key Features

- Fibrosarcoma of the oral cavity clinically exhibits painless, lobulated sessile, non-haemorrhage mucosal mass and sometimes loosening of teeth, pain, and ulceration of overlying mucosa.
- The aetiology of fibrosarcoma remains obscure. Radiation exposure is an important etiological factor, followed by trauma. Underlying Paget's disease, fibrous dysplasia, or chronic osteomyelitis may also contribute as an etiological/risk factor.
- Fibrosarcoma may occur in the soft tissue or as a primary intraosseous tumour.
- Clinically, oral mucosal fibrosarcoma presents as a lobulated, sessile, painless submucosal mass or erythematous ulcerated lesion.
- Fibrosarcoma destroys the underlying bone and is associated with pain and numbness in the affected area.
- Histopathology and immunohistochemical tests are essential for diagnosis.
- Radical surgery is the common modality of treatment.

Histopathology

Neoplastic cells of fibrosarcoma are uniform, spindle-shaped with a large, elongated, hyperchromatic nucleus arranged in a typical herringbone pattern (fascicular pattern), which is characterised by parallel sheets of cells arranged in a streaming fashion or interlocking bands going in different directions (Fig. 31.5a, b). In addition to the abnormal proliferation of fibroblasts, there are variable amounts of collagen and reticulin fibre formation. Histopathologically, fibrosarcoma is graded into two forms: low and high grades. This grading is based on the degree of cellular differentiation, degree of cellularity, mitotic activity, amount of collagen produced by the tumour and the presence of necrosis. Low-grade fibrosarcoma shows spindle cells arranged in fascicles with low to moderate cellularity and a herringbone appearance. This type of fibrosarcoma has a mild degree of nuclear pleomorphism, rare mitosis and collagenous stroma. High-grade lesions show a higher degree of nuclear pleomorphism, greater cellularity and atypical mitosis. Immunohistochemical tests, such as MIB-1, vimentin, CD68, CD34, HMB45, S-100, desmin, and cytokeratins, are helpful in the diagnosis, particularly in distinguishing them from fibromyxosarcoma.

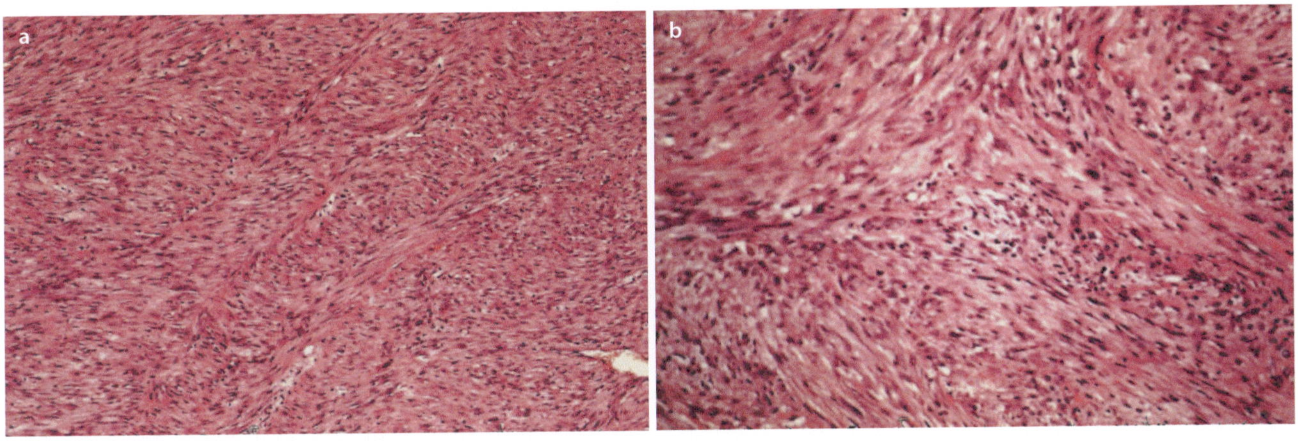

Fig. 31.5 **a** and **b** Fibrosarcoma. **a** low-power view, **b** high-power view with typical histological features of fibrosarcoma with fascicles of spindle-shaped cells distributed in interlacing fascicles with a 'herringbone' growth pattern. The tumour cells show mitotic activity and pleomorphism (haematoxylin and eosin stain). (Source: Francesca Angiero, Tommaso Rizzuti, Rolando Crippa and Michele Stefani. Fibrosarcoma of the Jaws: Two cases of primary tumors With Intraosseous Growth. Anticancer Research. 27: 2573–2582 (2007). (Courtesy of Michele Stephani)

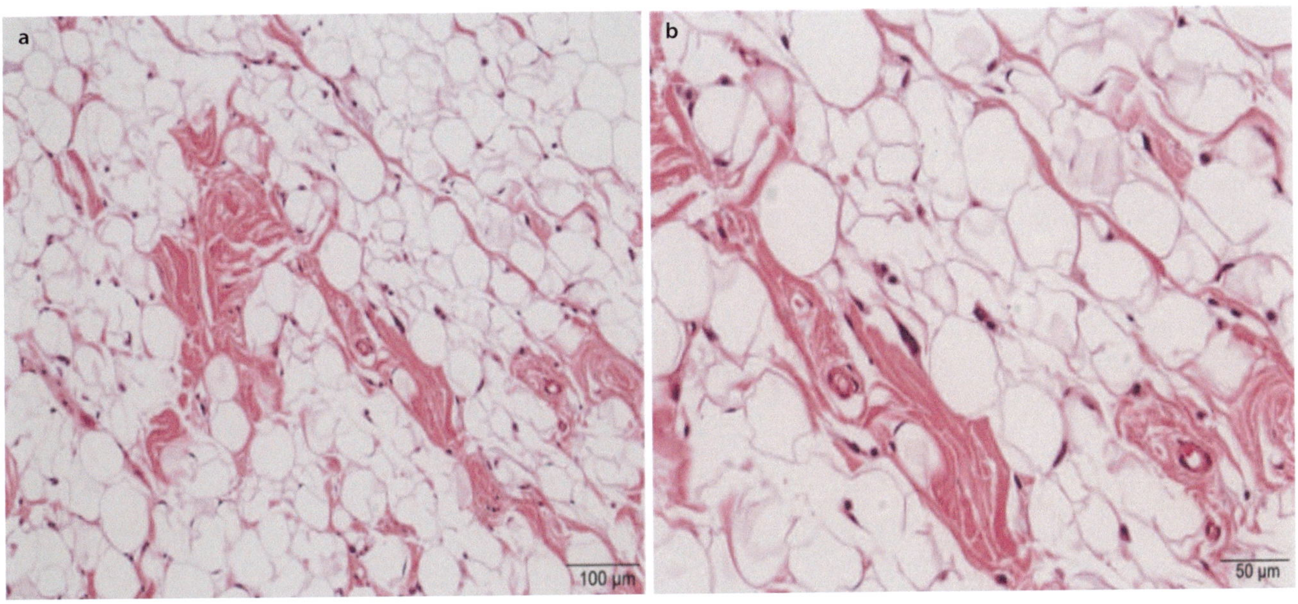

Fig. 31.6 **a** and **b** Liposarcoma. Histopathological findings show proliferation of adipocytes with hyperchromatic stromal cells in the fibrous connective tissue (hematoxylin and eosin stain). (Source: Ohta, Keiichi DDS; Yoshimura, Hitoshi DDS, PhD; Matsuda, Shinpei DDS, PhD; Imamura, Yoshiaki MD, PhD; Sano, Kazuo DDS, PhD. Oral liposarcoma in elderly: Case report and literature analysis. Medicine 99(6): p e18985, February 2020. ► https://doi.org/10.1097/MD.0000000000018985). Open Access

31.5 Oral Liposarcoma

Liposarcoma is a malignant mesenchymal neoplasm that arises from adipose tissue.

Key Features

- Liposarcoma of the oral cavity is rare. Common in lower extremities and retroperitoneum.
- Intraoral sites include cheek, the floor of the mouth, palate, gingiva, mandible, and the tongue.
- Tumour presents as a painless, slowly enlarging mass.
- Liposarcoma, unlike lipoma, is less yellow, firm, and more fixed.
- Histopathology is required for diagnosis.
- Wide surgical excision is the treatment of choice for liposarcoma.

Histopathology

Histologic features include the presence of lipoblasts, cellular pleomorphism, vascular proliferation, and mitotic activity (Fig. 31.6a, b). Histological variants include well-differentiated, myxoid, round-cell, and pleomorphic types.

31.6 Oral Non-Hodgkin's Lymphoma

Lymphomas are a group of heterogenous malignant diseases of the lymphatic system, characterised by a proliferation of lymphoid cells or their precursors. They occur in two forms: Hodgkin's lymphoma (HL) and non-Hodgkin's lymphoma (NHL). NHL originates from B-cell precursors, mature B cells, T-cell precursors, and mature T cells. Non-Hodgkin's lymphomas (NHLs) usually involve lymph nodes and occasionally in extra-nodal sites.

▪ **Key Features**

- Non-Hodgkin lymphomas (NHL) may be associated with various factors, including Epstein-Barr virus (EBV), human T-cell leukaemia virus type 1 (HTLV-1), hepatitis C virus (HCV), human herpesvirus 8, drugs (e.g. Phenytoin), autoimmune disorders like Sjögren syndrome, rheumatoid arthritis, and Hashimoto thyroiditis.
- Oral lesions of NHL can manifest centrally within the jawbone or in soft tissues such as the gingiva, palate, or buccal vestibule.
- Patients often present tooth mobility, localised swelling with an ulcer, unexplained dental pain, or ill-defined radiolucencies.
- The incidence of NHL is higher in immunodeficient conditions such as HIV patients.
- Most of the oropharyngeal NHL are B-cell type rather than T-cell type.
- The diagnosis is through histological examination of biopsy tissue, coupled with immuno-histochemical phenotyping.
- Chemotherapy, radiotherapy, or both are used for treating head and neck NHL.

▪ **Histopathology**

The common histological findings of non-Hodgkin lymphoma include follicular and diffuse patterns. In a follicular pattern, uniform nodularity is seen throughout the lymph node, and there is little variation in the size and shape of the follicle. The diffuse pattern, on the other hand, shows the normal architecture of the lymph node effaced by the infiltration of small lymphocytes (◘ Fig. 31.7a). Immunohistochemical stained sections are positive for CD3 (◘ Fig. 31.7b). The neoplastic lymphocytes show varying degrees of differentiation. These neoplasms are sometimes reported as Mycosis fugoides.

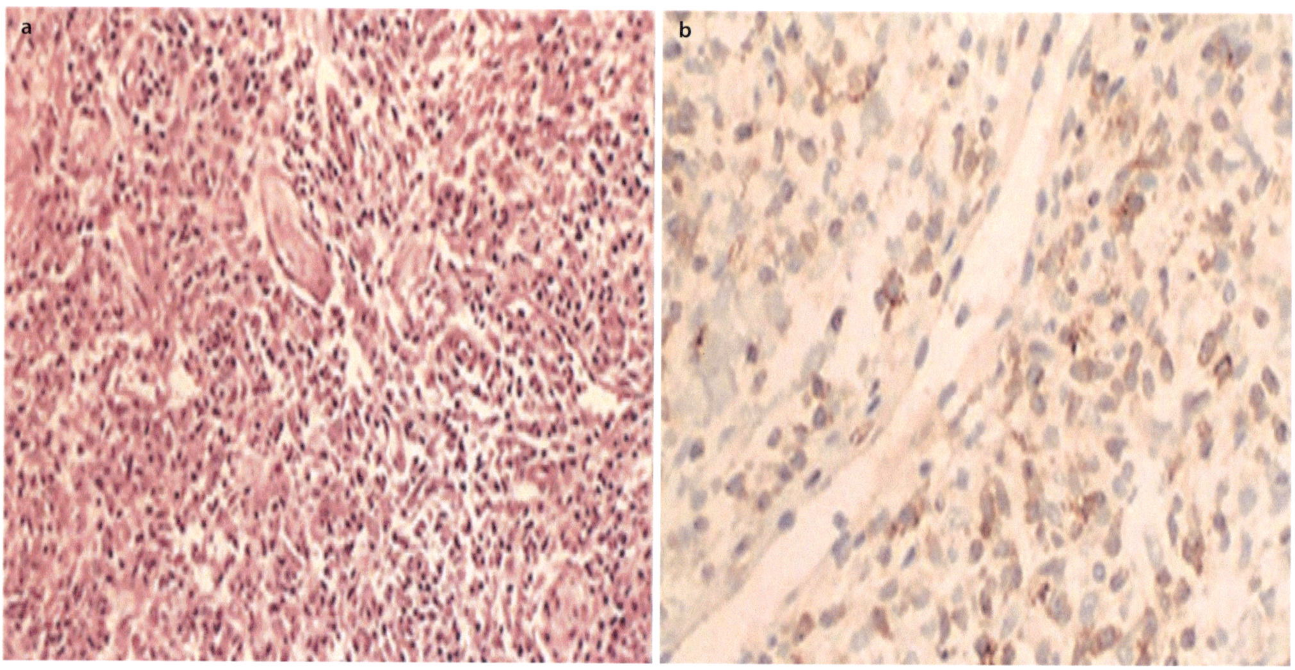

◘ **Fig. 31.7** **a** and **b** Non-Hodgkin's lymphoma. H&E is stained histopathological images showing medium-sized neoplastic cells with abundant cytoplasm, invading some of the epithelial area (**a**) The neoplastic cells are positive for CD3 (**b**) on IHC. *IHC* immunohistochemical. (Source: Deng, Da MD; Wang, Ying MD; Liu, Weisong MD, PhD; Qian, Yong MD, PhD. Oral and maxillofacial non-Hodgkin lymphomas: Case report with review of literature. Medicine 96(35): p e7890, September 2017. ▶ https://doi.org/10.1097/MD.0000000000007890. Open Access.

31.7 Summary

Malignant melanoma is characterised by uncontrolled proliferation of melanin-producing melanocytes. This is a rare neoplasm in the oral cavity. Oral malignant melanomas have a poor prognosis. Kaposi sarcoma (KS) is a multi-focal proliferative malignant condition of the blood vessels or lymphatics caused by human herpes 8 (HHV8) infection. 70% of individuals with AIDS-related KS develop oral lesions. Oral mucosal fibrosarcoma arises from the abnormal and uncontrolled proliferation of fibroblasts and is rare in the mouth. Liposarcoma is a malignant mesenchymal neoplasm that arises from adipose tissue. This is a rare intraoral neoplasm. NHL originates from B-cell precursors, mature B cells, T-cell precursors, and mature T cells. Non-Hodgkin's lymphomas (NHLs)usually involve lymph nodes and occasionally in extranodal sites such as gingivae.

Further Reading

Angiero F, Rizzuti T, Crippa R, Stefani M. Fibrosarcoma of the Jaws: two cases of primary tumors With Intraosseous Growth. Anticancer Res. 2007;27:2573–82.

Deng D, Wang Y, Liu W, Qian Y. Oral and maxillofacial non-Hodgkin lymphomas: case report with review of literature. Medicine. 2017;96(35):e7890. https://doi.org/10.1097/MD.0000000000007890. Open Access.

Ohta K, Yoshimura H, Matsuda S, Imamura Y, Sano K. Oral liposarcoma in elderly: case report and literature analysis. Medicine. 2020;99(6):e18985. https://doi.org/10.1097/MD.0000000000018985.

Rawal YB, Dodson TB, Bal HS. Oral melanoma: relevance to the dental team members. J Am Dent Assoc. 2017;148(2):113–9.

Thieringer FM, Cede J, Glatz K, Roehling S, Stoeckle M, Leiggener CS. Oral Kaposi's sarcoma: a case report and literature review on treatment management. Craniomaxillofac Trauma Reconstr Open. 2021:6. https://doi.org/10.1177/24727512211036328. Open access. (https://creativecommons.org/licenses/by-nc/4.0/).

Histopathology of Non-neoplastic Salivary Gland Disorders

Benedict Seo and Norman A Firth

Contents

S R Prabhu et al. (eds.), *Oral Histology and Oral Histopathology*, https://doi.org/10.1007/978-3-031-77481-2_32

32.1 Introduction

There are three pairs of major salivary glands (parotid, submandibular, and sublingual) and hundreds of minor salivary glands scattered throughout the mouth. Whilst differences do exist, the salivary glands consist of the acini (mucous, serous, or mixed) and the associated ductal system, which includes the intercalated, striated, and excretory ducts. Naturally, pathology may arise from any components that make up the salivary gland network and range from benign, malignant, developmental, infective, or reactive lesions. This chapter will focus on the non-neoplastic lesions of the salivary glands.

32.2 Mucocoele

32

The most common non-neoplastic lesion of salivary gland tissue is the mucocoele (pooling of mucin in a pseudocystic cavity). Two types of mucocoeles are recognised: (1) the extravasation type, in which mucin is spilt into the connective tissues from a ruptured or traumatised salivary gland duct and (2) the retention type, in which the mucin pooling is confined within a dilated excretory duct.

32.2.1 Mucocoele (Mucous Extravasation)

Mucocoele (mucous extravasation) is primarily a reactive lesion that follows mechanical disruption (trauma) of the salivary gland ducts, leading to the extravasation of mucin into the surrounding soft tissues.

- **Key Features**
- Mucocoele is the most common form of salivary gland pathology.
- Mucocoeles are most common in sites exposed to the potential for trauma, and the lower lip is by far the most common site affected.
- Mucocoeles are particularly prevalent in the paediatric population and young adults.
- Clinically, mucocoeles are present as a solitary translucent to light blue lump, usually fluctuant but may become more tense during active salivation.
- Mucocoeles are movable and not fixed to the underlying tissues. Over time, some lesions may undergo fibrotic healing and become a fibrous lump (fibroepithelial polyp or hyperplasia). When mucocoeles occur on the floor of the mouth (involving the sublingual glands), the term ranula may be used. (The term *ranula* is used since it looks like a frog's underbelly.)
- Clinically, mucocoeles are difficult to distinguish from mucous retention cysts (see below).

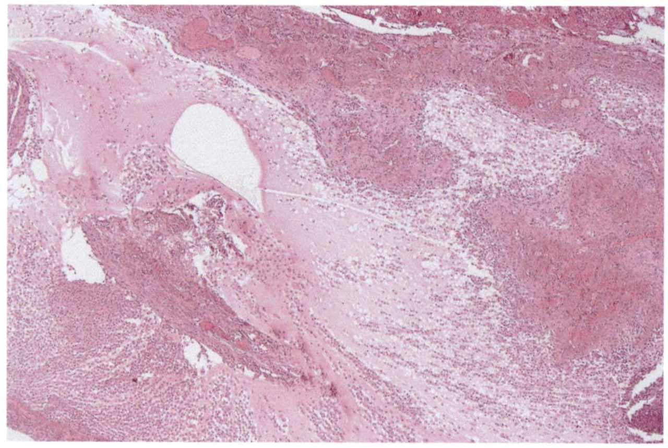

Fig. 32.1 Histological appearance of mucous extravasation. Note the large central area of mucin spillage with numerous mucinophages, 'walled off' by lightly inflamed granulation tissue

- Mucocoeles are self-limiting benign lesions; they may self-resolve whilst others may persist.
- The more persistent lesions and the associated damaged duct and feeding glands are best removed.

- **Histopathology**

Microscopically, there is evidence of mucin extravasation in the form of mucin pools of variable sizes surrounded by layers of granulation tissue (Fig. 32.1). This arrangement is pseudocystic in appearance but does not qualify as a true cyst due to the lack of lining epithelium. Mucin-laden foamy macrophages (mucinophages) are seen intermixed with the mucin, and the surrounding fibrous connective tissue will contain a variable degree of inflammation (acute, chronic, or mixed). A residual duct may be identified in some cases, and these ducts may show dilation and hyperplastic changes. Associated salivary glands in the vicinity show acinar atrophy and chronic inflammation (sialadenitis) with or without fibrosis. Depending on the stage of healing and the duration of the lesion, histology may show maturing granulation tissue, lack of active mucin extravasation, and fibrosis. Clinico-pathologic correlation with the positive history of trauma and clinical presentation usually leads to the correct interpretation of the histopathological findings.

32.2.2 Mucous Retention Cyst (Salivary Duct Cyst)

Mucous retention cysts are true cysts and may occur primarily as a developmental lesion (i.e. those present at birth and persist throughout life) or secondarily as a dilation of the duct in response to obstructions within the duct.

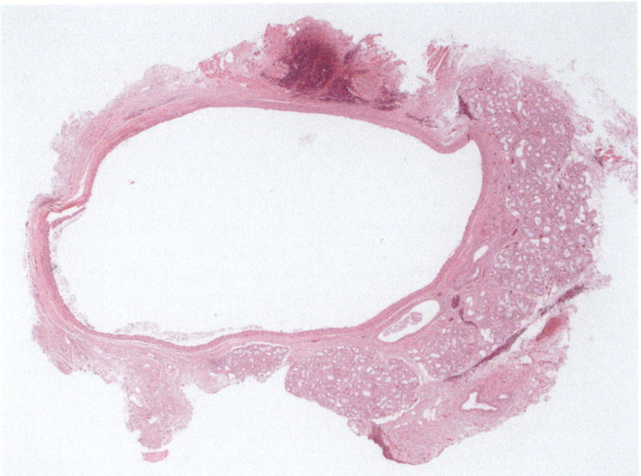

Fig. 32.2 Mucous retention cyst. There is a distinct layer of ductal epithelium lining, unlike in mucous extravasation (mucocoele)

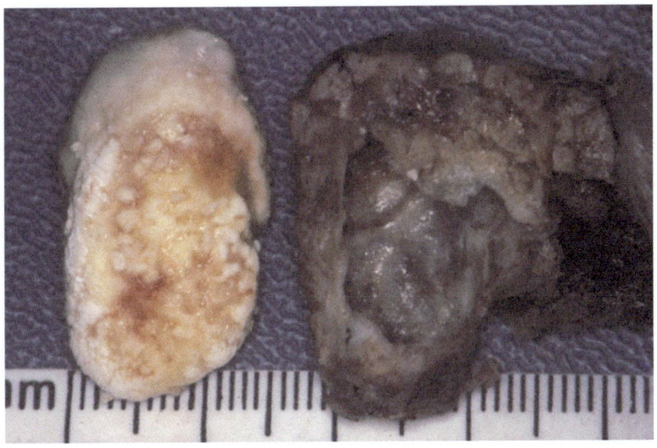

Fig. 32.3 Macroscopic photograph of a sialolith (left) and the associated submandibular gland duct

- **Key Features**
- Mucus retention cyst can occur in any site of the oral cavity.
- Clinical features of mucus retention cyst are similar to those of mucus extravasation phenomenon.

- **Histopathology**

The main histological distinguishing feature between mucocoeles (mucus extravasation) and mucous retention cysts is that the latter essentially represents a widely dilated duct (Fig. 32.2), not a pseudocyst with active mucin extravasation. The epithelium may be low cuboidal to stratified squamous in nature and vary in thickness. Mucous and oncocytic changes may be observed. At times, the surrounding fibrous connective tissue and the glands in the vicinity may show inflammatory changes (sialadenitis). Conservative surgical excision (considering removal of the feeding gland where indicated) is curative.

32.3 Sialolithiasis

Sialolithiasis represents the formation of a salivary calculus (calcified salivary stone) and accompanying changes within the duct and the original feeding gland.

- **Key Features**
- Proteinaceous debris (mucin, cell debris, bacteria, etc.) present in ducts, particularly those affected by salivary stasis, ductal obstruction, reduced salivary flow, or infection, may act as a nidus or focus for concentric growth and subsequent calcification.
- As the calcified mass increases in size, it may cause partial or total obstruction of the duct.
- The submandibular duct is most affected due largely to its tortuous path, but a sialolith may occur in association with any gland (Fig. 32.3).
- The position, size, and degree of mineralisation also have clinical implications for diagnosis and management. Radiographs may detect some larger, highly mineralised calculi. More specialised tests (CT, sialography) may be needed for more deeply seated or smaller lesions.
- Smaller, superficially located sialolith may be exuded through the duct orifices with ease. Larger, deeply seated chronic lesions often accompany damage to the feeding gland, in which case the gland will need to be removed.

- **Histopathology**

Microscopically, infiltration of mixed chronic inflammatory cells in the surrounding fibrous connective tissue and salivary gland is present (Fig. 32.4.). The sialolith shows variable staining characteristics depending on the constitution and the degree of mineralisation, but concentric lamellations are often observed (Fig. 32.5.). The affected duct is usually widely dilated and shows hyperplastic changes.

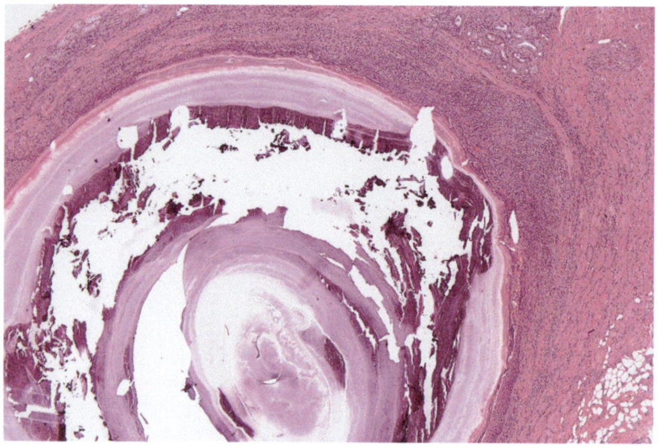

■ **Fig. 32.4** Sialolith within a dilated duct. There is an intense infiltration of mixed chronic inflammatory cells in the surrounding fibrous connective tissue and salivary gland

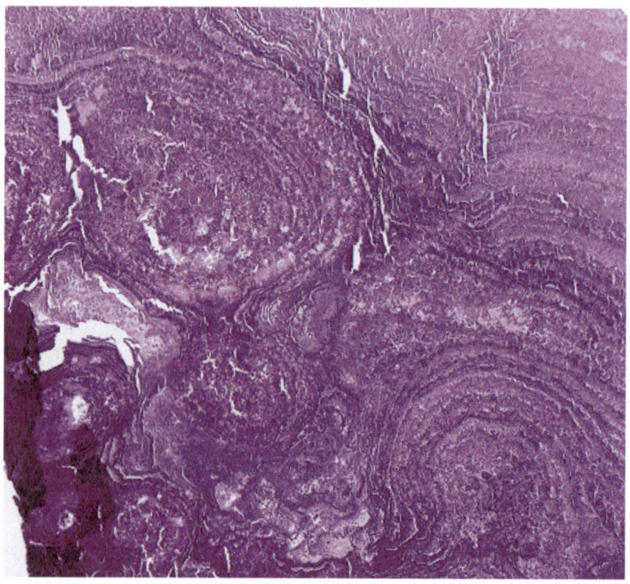

■ **Fig. 32.5** Sialolith. This photomicrograph shows the concentric lamellations commonly seen in a sialolith. This 5 × 4 × 6 mm sialolith was removed from a duct

32.4 Sjögren's Syndrome (Sjögren's Disease)

Sjögren's syndrome (SS) is an autoimmune condition characterised by the immunologic infiltration of the exocrine glands, notably the salivary and lacrimal glands.

Key Features

Two types: primary and secondary.

- Primary Sjögren's syndrome leads to dry mouth (xerostomia) and keratoconjunctivitis (sicca syndrome).

■ **Table 32.1** Diagnostic criteria for Sjögren's syndrome adapted by the American College of Rheumatology and the European League Against Rheumatism

Item	Weight/score
Labial salivary gland with focal lymphocytic sialadenitis and focus score of ≥1 foci/4 mm^2	3
Anti-SSA/Ro-positive	3
Ocular staining score ≥5 in at least one eye	1
Schirmer's test ≤5 mm/5 min in at least one eye	1
Unstimulated whole saliva flow rate ≤0.1 mL/min	1

- Secondary Sjögren's syndrome is frequently associated with other autoimmune disorders, including rheumatoid arthritis (RA) and systemic lupus erythematosus (SLE).
- Diagnosis of Sjögren's syndrome requires positive signs and symptoms (inclusion criteria) and exclusion of conditions with overlapping clinical features. A scoring system has been developed to aid in the diagnosis of those who meet the inclusion and exclusion criteria (■ Table 32.1).
- A biopsy of the minor salivary glands is the ideal test to confirm the diagnosis of Sjögren's syndrome.
- Sjögren's syndrome is a chronic condition and patients require symptomatic and supportive care in relation to the effects of dry mouth. There is an increased risk of developing lymphoma, and this should be discussed with the patients.

Histopathology

Histopathologic examination of labial salivary gland biopsy requires an adequate amount of glandular tissue included. Within the glandular tissue, features of focal lymphocytic sialadenitis (FLS), defined as a focal lymphocytic infiltration (≥50) with concomitant inflammatory destruction or replacement of the acini, should be identified (■ Fig. 32.6). These immunologic infiltrates are adjacent to normal-appearing acini. The focus score is calculated per 4 mm^2 of glandular tissue included. Where inflammation is coupled with prominent acinar atrophy, fibrosis, or ductal dilation, the changes are considered consistent with non-specific chronic sialadenitis and/or sclerosing chronic sialadenitis and these 'foci' are not counted (■ Fig. 32.7).

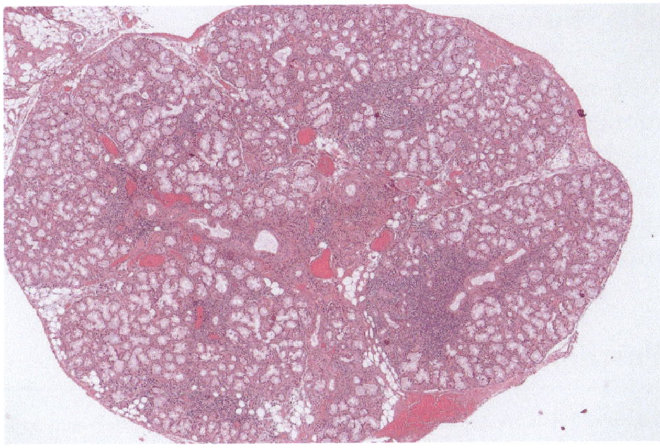

◘ Fig. 32.6 A minor labial salivary gland showing multiple foci of intense lymphocytic infiltration with seemingly normal adjacent acini.

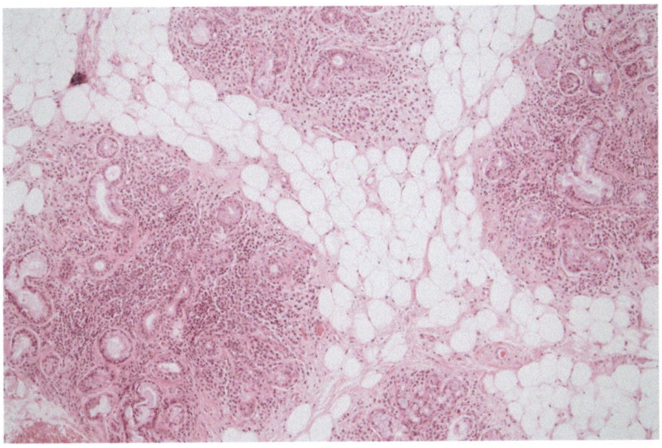

◘ Fig. 32.7 An example of non-specific chronic sialadenitis. There is clear evidence of acinar atrophy, and the inflammatory cell infiltrate is more diffusely distributed

32.5 Necrotising Sialometaplasia

Necrotising sialometaplasia is an inflammatory destruction of the minor salivary glands commonly occurring in the palate.

▪ Key Features

- Necrotising sialometaplasia is thought to be a secondary event to trauma or localised ischemic injury, which results in the necrosis of the glandular tissue and adaptive changes in the associated ducts.
- Necrotising sialometaplasia arises as a symptomatic erythematous swelling of the palate that evolves into a deep crater-like ulcer with time.
- As the clinical evolution of the lesion is striking, differential diagnoses often include neoplasms, particularly salivary gland malignancies.

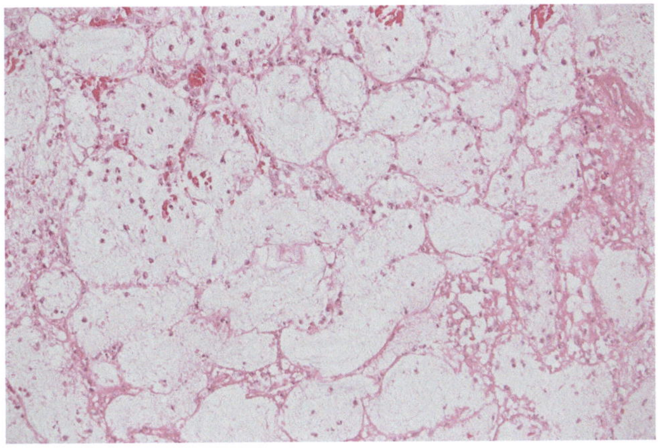

◘ Fig. 32.8 A mucous gland affected by necrotising sialometaplasia. The residual acini are necrotic, and no cytological detail can be discerned at this stage

- Biopsy is often indicated to exclude malignancies but most lesions self-resolve in due course without active treatment.

▪ Histopathology

Histopathological features include necrotic degeneration of the minor salivary gland acini with or without inflammation and extravasation of mucin. While individual acinar cell definition is lost, the overall lobular architecture remains intact (◘ Fig. 32.8). The associated ducts show a varying degree of squamous metaplasia. Prominent squamous metaplasia and hyperplasia, coupled with pseudoepithelial hyperplasia of the overlying epithelium, may give a confusing histologic impression.

32.6 Adenomatoid Hyperplasia

Adenomatoid hyperplasia is an idiopathic swelling of the oral mucosa with unclear aetiology.

▪ Key Features

- Adenomatoid hyperplasia is a completely benign process.
- There is a localised hyperplasia of the salivary gland involved, elevating the lesion so that it appears as a smooth surface lump clinically.
- This condition is most prevalent in the palate.
- Conservative local excision is the treatment of choice with little to no chance of recurrence. However, some reports suggest that adenomatoid hyperplasia may be a surrogate sign of an underlying lesion.
- The clinical appearance mimics salivary gland tumours, so an investigative biopsy is warranted.

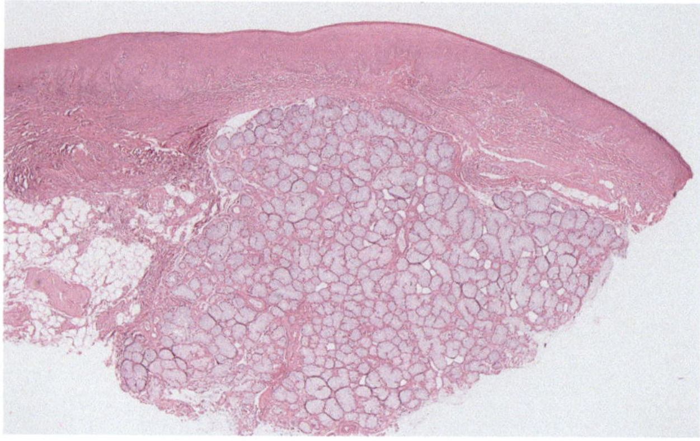

■ **Fig. 32.9** This is an example of adenomatoid hyperplasia of the palate. Note the excessive mucous gland, which presents as a nodular proliferation and has elevated surface mucosa

▪ **Histopathology**

Histopathology shows essentially normal but excessive glandular tissue for the anatomical site (■ Fig. 32.9). When the surface mucosa becomes traumatised, it may show a range of changes, including hyperplasia or atrophy/ulceration. Adenomatoid hyperplasia is a benign process.

32.7 Summary

Non-neoplastic salivary gland lesions include commonly encountered lesions, e.g. mucoceles, and rarely encountered lesions, such as necrotising sialometaplasia, which is important to be aware of so as not to misdiagnose clinically or histopathologically as a neoplastic process.

Further Reading

Daniels TE, Cox D, Shiboski CH, et al. Associations between salivary gland histopathologic diagnoses and phenotypic features of Sjögren's syndrome among 1726 registry participants. Arthritis Rheum. 2011;63:2021–30.

Shiboski CH, Shiboski SC, Seror R, et al. 2016 American College of Rheumatology/European League Against Rheumatism classification criteria for primary Sjögren's syndrome: A consensus and data-driven methodology involving three international patient cohorts. Ann Rheum Dis. 2017;76:9–16.

Histopathology of Salivary Gland Neoplasms

Norman A Firth

Contents

S R Prabhu et al. (eds.), *Oral Histology and Oral Histopathology*, https://doi.org/10.1007/978-3-031-77481-2_33

33.1 Introduction

The most common presentation of salivary gland tumours is a slow-growing mass in the parotid gland, submandibular gland or rarely sublingual gland or, in the case of minor salivary gland neoplasms, the palate (often near the junction of the hard and soft palate), the lip (frequently the upper lip) or buccal mucosa. Lesions are usually asymptomatic; however, if ductal obstruction occurs, symptoms may result, or if nerve involvement occurs, there may be associated symptoms, e.g. facial palsy or facial pain. Nerve involvement is usually indicative of a malignant salivary gland neoplasm. For example, adenoid cystic carcinoma (ACC) is commonly associated with perineural invasion. There is considerable variation in incidence rates across the world, and accurate information is difficult as benign neoplasms are not included in cancer registry data. Most salivary gland neoplasms are slightly more common in females. Neoplasms can occur at any age, with a mean age for most types in the fifth decade.

The current World Health Organization (WHO) classification was published in 2022 and has significantly evolved from the first classification of 1972. The fifth edition includes four categories of lesions. The two main categories are benign and malignant epithelial tumours, and the other two categories are non-neoplastic epithelial lesions and mesenchymal tumours specific to the salivary glands. Changes in the classification are important as treatment modalities of malignant salivary gland neoplasms now and in future will include specific targeted therapies reliant on correct diagnosis which in turn is reliant on correct classification. It is beyond the scope of this chapter to include all benign and malignant salivary gland neoplasms (39 salivary gland pathologies are included in the WHO 2022 classification), so this chapter is limited to the more common benign and malignant neoplasm.

33.2 Pleomorphic Adenoma

Pleomorphic adenoma (PA) is the most common benign salivary gland neoplasm in the major and minor glands. It comprises epithelial, myoepithelial, and stromal/mesenchymal cells.

Key Features

- About 75% of parotid tumours and approximately 40% of minor salivary gland tumours are PA.
- PA can occur at any age but is most frequently seen in middle age.
- The lesion is slow-growing with a slight female predilection.
- The superficial lobe of the parotid gland in front of the ear is the most common site.
- Bilateral lesions are rarely encountered.
- Genetic alterations in PA include the PLAG1 and HMGA2 fusions or amplification.
- Based on the history and clinical features, a diagnosis of PA may be suspected, leading to investigations including ultrasound, computed tomography, and magnetic resonance imaging to assess the extent of the tumour.
- A fine needle/core needle biopsy or incisional biopsy precedes definitive surgical removal.
- A small incisional biopsy may be misdiagnosed as it may not be representative of the whole lesion.
- PA is treated by excision. If left untreated, lesions continue to grow slowly and may attain a large size. These are at risk of malignant transformation, particularly in older patients with long-standing untreated lesions. Other risk factors for malignant transformation include the presence of multiple recurrences and the site of the primary lesion, the submandibular gland.
- Multi-focal recurrences may be difficult to remove surgically, and radiotherapy is occasionally employed. Intraoral lesions have a much lower recurrence rate even if lesional tissue extends to surgical margins.

Histopathology

PA is circumscribed but frequently is multi-lobular and microscopically has an incomplete capsule. The lesion consists of a mixture of glandular epithelium and myoepithelial cells in a background of variable stromal tissues (mucous, myxomatous, and cartilaginous) (◘ Fig. 33.1a). The ratio of epithelial and myoepithelial cellular areas compared with stroma is greater in intraoral lesions in contrast to parotid lesions. Mucin-filled duct-like structures may be conspicuous or barely detectable. Myoepithelial cells frequently take on the structure and function of connective tissue cells and may be spindle or stellate in shape or resemble plasma cells (plasmacytoid cells) (◘ Fig. 33.1b). The latter is a strong indicator of a diagnosis of PA. Parotid lesions have a propensity for recurrence (15–25%), which may be related to several factors. These include the lack of complete encapsulation and the presence of lobules extending through the capsule, the relationship with branches of the facial nerve, and myxomatous lesions, which may be disrupted during excision, possibly leading to the widespread seeding of residual neoplastic tissue. Pleomorphic adenomas in minor salivary glands are usually not encapsulated but are well-demarcated (◘ Fig. 33.1c).

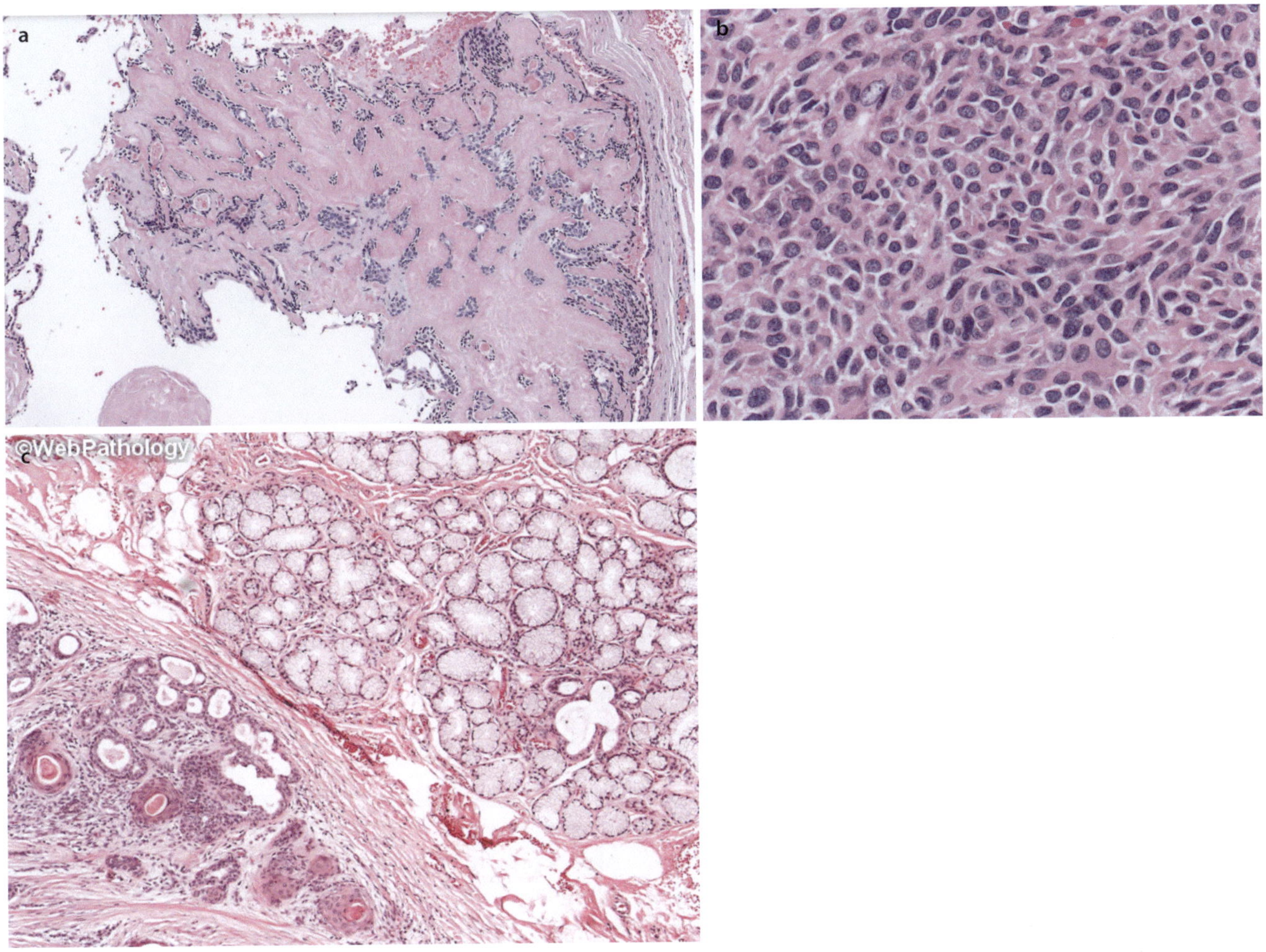

Fig. 33.1 **a** Pleomorphic adenoma. This photomicrograph shows a portion of a lesion with hyalinised stroma, epithelial and myoepithelial cell nests, and a fibrous capsule. **b** Pleomorphic adenoma. This photomicrograph shows a prominent plasmacytoid cell component. **c** Pleomorphic adenomas in minor salivary gland. This image shows a minor salivary gland (mucous glands in the right upper half of the slide) and a well-defined pleomorphic adenoma without encapsulation (left lower half of the slide). Foci of squamous metaplasia are seen. (Courtesy: Dr. Dharam Ramnani, USA ► Webpathology.com)

33.3 Warthin's Tumour

Warthin's tumour is characterised by the presence of lymphoid tissue and cystic/ductal structures lined by columnar epithelial cells exhibiting oncocytic changes associated with the inflammatory infiltrate.

Key Features

- Warthin's tumour is a benign neoplasm of the parotid gland. Involvement of the other major salivary glands or minor glands is extremely rare.
- Tumours develop from heterotopic salivary ducts trapped within intraparotid or paraparotid, e.g. deep cervical chain lymph nodes.
- Warthin's tumour is the second most common salivary gland tumour, accounting for approximately 10% of all parotid tumours.
- Lesions present as a slow-growing, painless, firm, or fluctuant mass usually located near the tail of the parotid gland. Up to 17% may be bilateral. The majority of patients are smokers over 40 years of age, and it has been reported that males are affected more than females; however, current data does not support the earlier reported epidemiological data.
- Multi-focal lesions in the ipsilateral gland or contralaterally are reported in up to 15% of cases. Presentation is a slow-growing, painless lump or lumps.
- Diagnosis relies on accurate history and assessment of clinical findings, and fine needle aspiration (FNA) is usually accurate in confirming the diagnosis with both lymphocytes and columnar epithelial cells making up the bulk of the aspirate.
- Lesions are treated by surgical removal, and recurrence is rare (5%), although new unrelated lesions may develop. Malignant change is extremely rare.

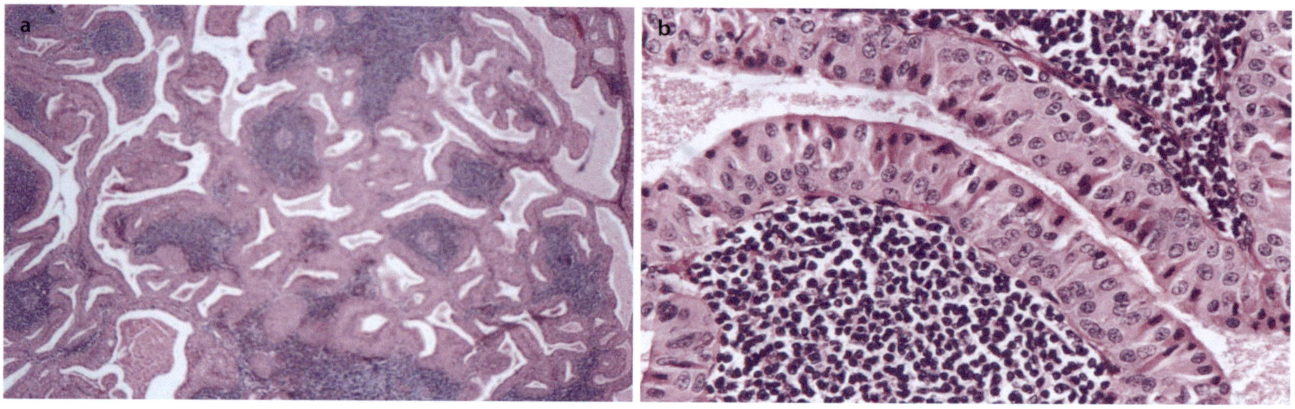

Fig. 33.2 a Low-power photomicrograph of a Warthin's tumour showing many irregular and convoluted spaces lined by pale-staining cells associated with dense lymphoid cell aggregates. (Courtesy Professor David F Wilson, Adelaide, Australia). b High-power photomicrograph of Warthin's tumour showing the pale, space-lining epithelial cells and the dense lymphoid cell aggregate. (Courtesy Professor David F Wilson, Adelaide, Australia)

Histopathology

The tumours have a thin capsule, are frequently partially solid, and have varying numbers of cystic structures. They have both a lymphoid and ductal epithelial component. The lymphoid tissue contains lymphoid follicles with germinal centres. The epithelial cells are columnar cells with eosinophilic cytoplasm and form multi-folded epithelial-lined cystic structures with papillary projections into the cystic spaces. The eosinophilic cytoplasm represents oncocytic change (Fig. 33.2a, b).

33.4 Other Benign Salivary Gland Neoplasms

Other benign salivary gland neoplasms include, among others, canalicular adenoma, basal cell adenoma, and oncocytoma. Canalicular adenomas are encountered in the minor salivary glands, occurring in the upper lip or buccal mucosa. Occasionally, multi-focal lesions are encountered. Histologically, lesions are circumscribed and consist of strands, trabeculae, or duct-like structures of basaloid epithelial cells with a uniform cytological appearance. Myoepithelial cells and stromal changes seen in PA are not encountered. Lesions do not recur following simple excision. Parotid gland basil cell adenomas occur in elderly patients and consist of an encapsulated lesion composed of basaloid cells arranged in solid sheets, strands, or trabeculae. Stromal changes (as seen in PA) are not encountered. Lesions do not recur following excision. FNA may prove difficult to differentiate basal cell adenoma from PA, and often, the diagnosis is confirmed after examination of the entire lesion following superficial parotidectomy. Oncocytomas are rare tumours of the parotid gland seen in the elderly. The lesion consists of solid cords, nests, or sheets of oncocytes (large eosinophilic cells with small compact nuclei). These cells are like the eosinophilic cells seen in Warthin's tumour; however, the extensive lymphoid component required for that diagnosis is not seen in oncocytoma.

33.5 Mucoepidermoid Carcinoma

Mucoepidermoid carcinomas (MECs) is a salivary gland tumour that comprises mucin-secreting cells, squamous cells, and intermediate-type cells.

Key Features

- Mucoepidermoid carcinoma (MEC) is the most common malignant salivary gland neoplasm, accounting for 10–15% of all salivary gland tumours and 12–29% of malignant salivary gland tumours. It occurs in both children and adults, with a female predilection.
- The parotid gland is most commonly affected, accounting for about 50% of all MEC, followed by the submandibular and sublingual glands. Facial nerve involvement may occur. The palate is the most frequent intraoral site.
- Lesions are often slow-growing and asymptomatic. Intraoral lesions may have an extensive cystic component and appear as a fluctuant blueish mass and, therefore, clinically resemble a mucocele.
- The majority of MECs have a t(11;19)(q21;p13) translocation and CRTC3-MAML2 gene fusion.
- Fine needle aspiration (FNA) followed by biopsy is essential for diagnosis.
- Treatment involves surgical removal of the tumour. Radiotherapy is used in selected cases, and chemotherapy is used in cases that are not amenable to sur-

gery or radiotherapy. Approximately 40% of high-grade lesions metastasise and carry a 30% mortality rate. Targeted gene therapy is being investigated as a promising future treatment modality.

Histopathology

Histopathological features of MEC are variable, and the neoplasm is graded as low intermediate and high-grade types (◘ Fig. 33.3a–d). Lesions consist of a mixture of mucous-secreting cells, squamous epithelial cells, intermediate cells, and clear cells. Keratinisation is usually not a feature in the epithelial component. The greater the cystic component, the lower the tumour grade. MEC is unencapsulated and shows an infiltrative growth pattern. Higher-grade lesions demonstrate cytological atypia and a higher mitotic rate. Low-grade lesions with an extensive cystic component and mucin production are difficult to diagnose on FNA and/or incisional biopsy. In some instances, diagnosis of MEC is aided by detecting the translocation.

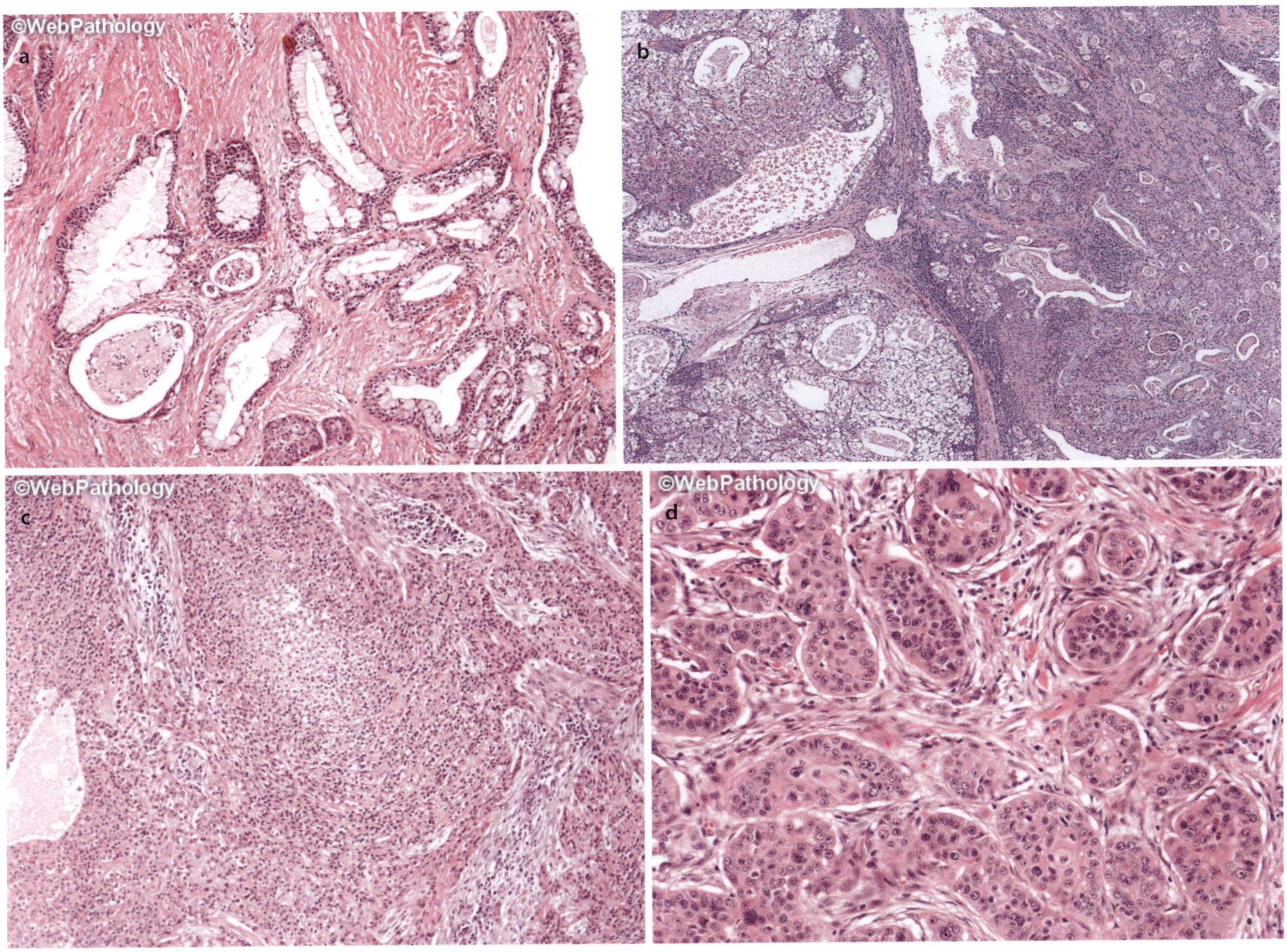

◘ **Fig. 33.3** **a** Mucoepidermoid carcinoma (Low-grade). Low-grade tumours are composed of cystic or gland-like spaces lined by mucinous cells admixed with epidermoid cells. The mucinous cells are goblet or balloon-shaped, with abundant foamy cytoplasm and small, dark, peripherally placed nuclei. In some foci, they may be just admixed with solid clusters and nests of epidermoid cells. The cyst lining may be simple, with one or more layers of cells, or it may show complex cribriform and papillary architecture. (Courtesy: Dr. Dharam Ramnani, USA ► Webpathology.com). **b** Mucoepidermoid carcinoma. This photomicrograph shows sheets and trabeculated arrangements of predominantly intermediate and squamous cells, some with clear cytoplasm; these are punctuated by glandular lumina and glands lined by mucinous epithelium. **c** Mucoepidermoid carcinoma (intermediate grade). The tumour is solid and does not show any prominent cystic areas (unlike the low-grade mucoepidermoid carcinomas). The tumour is composed predominantly of intermediate cells, which are intermediate in size and appearance is between the small basal cells and the larger epidermoid cells. The intermediate cells are mixed with epidermoid cells, forming solid sheets and tumour islands. There are only scattered mucinous cells. Nuclear atypia and prominent nucleoli are seen only focally. (Courtesy: Dr. Dharam Ramnani, USA ► Webpathology.com). **d** Mucoepidermoid carcinoma (high grade). High-grade mucoepidermoid carcinomas are solid tumours with no cyst formation. They are predominantly composed of solid sheets and clusters of epidermoid and intermediate cells with cytologic atypia. They have prominent nucleoli and show brisk mitotic activity. (Courtesy: Dr. Dharam Ramnani, USA ► Webpathology.com)

33.6 Adenoid Cystic Carcinoma

Adenoid cystic carcinoma (ACC) is an uncommon form of malignant neoplasm that arises within secretory glands, most commonly the major and minor salivary glands of the head and neck.

Key Features

- Adenoid cystic carcinoma (ACC) is nearly as common as MEC, occurring in any salivary gland, including about a third of malignant salivary glands in the minor salivary glands.
- ACC has a deceptively benign histological appearance and is composed of cells with bland cytology, but the lesion is locally invasive with a high propensity for local recurrence and distant metastasis.
- ACC, in most cases, is caused by activation of the oncogenic transcription factor gene MYB, and overexpression of MYB may be detected by fluorescence in situ hybridisation (FISH) as an adjunct to diagnosis.
- ACC is most commonly seen in the fifth and sixth decades of life. There is a slightly increased female: male ratio.
- The lesion presents as a slow-growing mass, and pain may be a presenting feature. Swelling is often, but not always present, and the surface may be ulcerated.
- Radiographic evidence of bone destruction may be seen.
- The lesion has a propensity for neural involvement (perineural spread). Parotid lesions may present with facial nerve involvement or other unusual sensory changes rather than a clearly discernible mass, and MRI features may be indicative of neural involvement.
- The most common genetic alterations are a t(6;9) chromosomal translocation or, less commonly, a t(8;9) translocation which results in fusions involving the MYB or MYBL1 oncogenes and the transcription factor gene NFIB.
- More than 80% of ACC have MYB/MYBL1 activations and this may offer a useful potential role for targeted gene therapy in future.
- Treatment is surgery or surgery in combination with radiotherapy. Unfortunately, radiotherapy cannot always kill these radioresistant neoplastic cells.
- The five-year survival rate is fair however the long-term survival rate is very poor. Lymph node metastasis is uncommon; however, a third of patients develop blood-borne metastasis in the lung, liver, or bone.

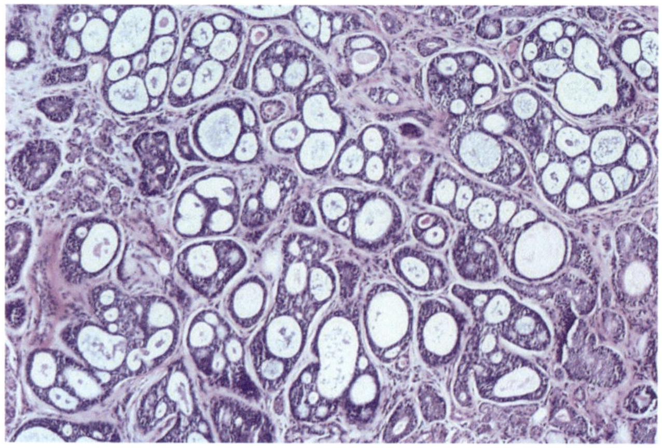

Fig. 33.4 Adenoid cystic carcinoma. The tumour cells are arranged in variously sized and irregularly shaped islands, which exhibit a "punched out" (Swiss cheese pattern) appearance. (Courtesy of Professor David F Wilson, Adelaide, Australia)

Histopathology

Histopathologically, ACC is composed of groups of myoepithelial and ductal cells with three distinct patterns: cribriform, tubular and solid. Multiple cystic spaces surrounded by darkly staining cells without cytological atypia are seen and form a characteristic cribriform or "Swiss cheese" pattern (Fig. 33.4). The solid or trabecular pattern may, however, predominate. Perineural invasion is helpful in diagnosis. The lesion is unencapsulated with an infiltrative destructive growth pattern through the surrounding soft tissue stroma or bone.

33.7 Summary

Salivary gland neoplasms frequently present as a lump, and patients may initially present to a dentist or a dentist may pick up a lesion in either the major salivary glands or intraorally as part of a routine dental examination. The classification has evolved over the years and continues to do so with advances in molecular testing. Advances in targeted gene therapy and other treatment modalities also continue to evolve.

Further Reading

Dillon PM, Chakraborty S, Moskaluk CA, Joshi PJ, Thomas CY. Adenoid cystic carcinoma: A review of recent advances, molecular targets, and clinical trials. Head Neck. 2016;38(4):620–7. https://doi.org/10.1002/hed.23925.

Mendenhall WM, Mendenhall CM, Werning JW, Malyapa RS, Mendenhall NP. Salivary gland pleomorphic adenoma. Am J Clin Oncol. 2008;31(1):95–9. https://doi.org/10.1097/COC.0b013e3181595ae0.

Quer M, Hernandez-Prera JC, Silver CE, Casasayas M, Simo R, Vander Poorten V, Guntinas-Lichius O, Bradley PJ, Tong-Ng W, Rodrigo JP, et al. Current trends and controversies in the management of warthin tumor of the parotid gland. Diagnostics. 2021;11:1467. https://doi.org/10.3390/diagnostics11081467.

Rapidis AD, Givalos N, Gakiopoulou H, Stavrianos SD, Faratzis G, Lagogiannis GA, Katsilieris I, Patsouris E. Mucoepidermoid carcinoma of the salivary glands. Review of the literature and clinicopathological analysis of 18 patients. Oral Oncol. 2007;43(2):130–6. https://doi.org/10.1016/j.oraloncology.2006.03.001. Epub 2006 Jul 20

Skalova A, Hyrcza MD, Leivo I. Update from the 5th Edition of the World Health Organization classification of head and neck tumors: salivary glands. Head Neck Pathol. 2022;16(1):40–53.

Skálová A, Stenman G, Simpson RHW, Hellquist H, Slouka D, Svoboda T, Bishop JA, Hunt JL, Nibu KI, Rinaldo A, Vander Poorten V, Devaney KO, Steiner P, Ferlito A. The role of molecular testing in the differential diagnosis of salivary gland carcinomas. Am J Surg Pathol. 2018;42(2):e11–27. https://doi.org/10.1097/PAS.0000000000000980.

Weaver AN, Lakritz S, Mandair D, Ulanja MB, Bowles DW. (2023) A molecular guide to systemic therapy in salivary gland carcinoma. Head Neck. 2023;45(5):1315–26. https://doi.org/10.1002/hed.27307.

WHO Classififcation of Tumours Editorial Board. Head and Neck tumours. WHO classification of tumours series. 5th ed. Lyon: IARC; 2022.

Żurek M, Fus Ł, Niemczyk K, Rzepakowska A. Salivary gland pathologies: evolution in classification and association with unique genetic alterations. Eur Arch Otorhinolaryngol. 2023;280(11):4739–50. https://doi.org/10.1007/s00405-023-08110-w. Epub 2023 Jul 13. PMID: 37439929; PMCID: PMC10562281.

Histopathology of Oral Granulomatous Diseases

Nidhi Handoo

Contents

S R Prabhu et al. (eds.), *Oral Histology and Oral Histopathology*, https://doi.org/10.1007/978-3-031-77481-2_34

34.1 Introduction

Oral granulomatous diseases are a diverse group of conditions which present as a chronic inflammatory response to a variety of stimuli. This reaction could be due to infectious or non-infectious agents, maybe localised or part of a systemic disseminated disease process. In the orofacial region, a limited number of conditions, namely, foreign body reactions, infections, sarcoidosis, Crohn's disease, and orofacial granulomatosis, are the main causes.

Granulomatous inflammation is a host defence mechanism to limit infections or foreign antigens, which makes macrophages and monocytes integral to this inflammatory process.

Microscopically, granulomas are distinct and consist of epithelioid-shaped macrophages (which, upon activation, coalesce, producing multi-nucleated giant cells), surrounded by lymphocytes (predominantly CD4+ T lymphocytes), collagen and fibroblasts.

The multi-nucleated giant cells may be foreign body-type (haphazard arrangement of nuclei), Langhans type (horseshoe-shaped arrangement of nuclei), or have clustered peripherally located nuclei. This inflammation may be necrotising (with or without evidence of caseous necrosis on gross examination) or non-necrotising in nature. In the absence of recognisable foreign material, periodic acid Schiff (PAS), Gomori methenamine–silver nitrate (GMS), and Ziehl–Neelsen (ZN) special stains should be obtained as a matter of routine to rule out infectious disease aetiology. Furthermore, diagnosis of the cause of this type of inflammation may be challenging in the absence of identifiable foreign material or infectious agents. In such cases, a comprehensive medical work-up with additional testing is recommended.

34.2 Foreign Body Granuloma

Foreign body granulomatous inflammation is typically non-necrotising and caused by endogenous or exogenous foreign material that is not readily absorbable. It is considered the most common cause of granulomatous inflammation in the oral cavity. Though the causative particles or crystals are quite varied, the reactions occasioned by them show common features.

▪ **Key Features**

- Dental material, cosmetic fillers and graft material are some of the offending agents.
- Granulomatous inflammation associated with temporary, long-term, and permanent cosmetic fillers is considered a late complication and is on the rise.
- Clinically, non-descript, painless, or painful papule/nodular enlargement at the site of trauma or iatrogenically introduced material. Rarely ulcerations/ridges.
- Dermal/cosmetic fillers may migrate to sites distant from the original injection.
- Common sites are lips, vestibule, gingiva, or graft material seen as radiolucent/mixed radiolucent and radio-opaque appearance on radiographs.
- May present months to years from time to exposure, so patients may not recall exposure.

▪ **Histopathology**

Even though the histopathological features are variable, the presence of the foreign material, introduced accidentally, therapeutically or for cosmetic purposes, is typically evident. Evaluation of foreign material under visible and through polarised light to identify potentially birefringent substances is helpful. Depending on the material, inflammatory reactions may be minimal. However, well-formed granulomas composed of lymphocytes, foreign body-type giant cells and histiocytes may be seen with dental material and cosmetic fillers. Dental amalgam eliciting a foreign body reaction with scattered small to large aggregates of black pigmented granular material may be seen (◘ Figs. 34.1, 34.2, 34.3, 34.4, and 34.5).

Granulomas associated with poly-L-lactic acid show polarisable fusiform or ovoid 10–50 microns in diameter foreign material similar to cholesterol clefts (◘ Fig. 34.6a–c). The spiky, elongated particles are within and surrounded by multi-nucleated giant cells, epithelioid histiocytes, and lymphocytic inflammation (◘ Fig. 34.6b). In long-standing lesions, fibrosis can be present. Inclusion within the giant cells, such as asteroid bodies, may be seen in multiple granulomatous conditions, including foreign body granulomas (◘ Fig. 34.7).

Granulomas associated with calcium hydroxyapatite show non-polarisable, uniformly sized, 25–40 μm in diameter tan-grey fine granular material within microspheres surrounded by epithelioid histiocytes, foreign body giant cells and lymphocytes (◘ Fig. 34.8). This biodegradable filler sometimes shows a cracked appearance with amorphous material of dark/black staining accompanied by foreign body giant cells (◘ Fig. 34.9).

Granulomatous reaction associated with biodegradable polyacrylamide hydrogel filler shows a collection of multiple pools of amorphous basophilic gel surrounded by macrophages and multi-nucleated giant cells (◘ Figs. 34.10 and 34.11). This filler is used largely outside of the United States.

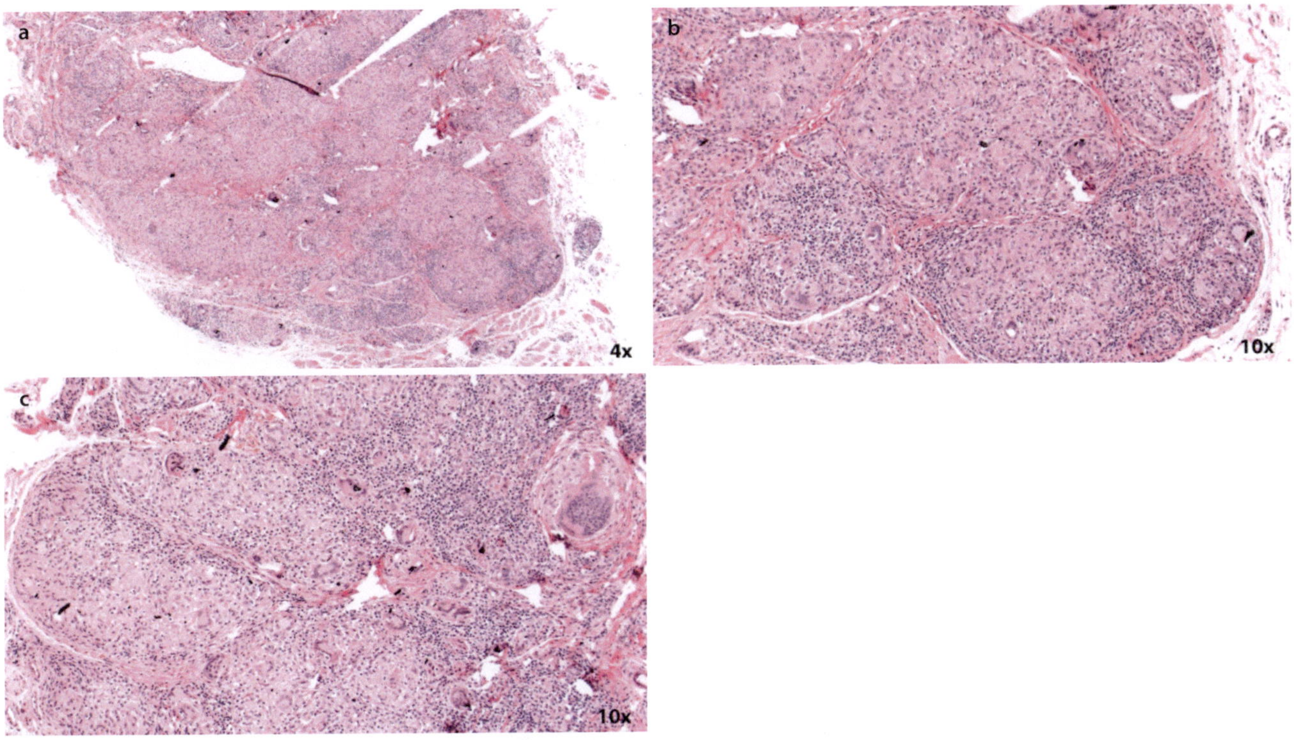

■ **Fig. 34.1** Foreign body granuloma. **a** Multiple granulomas with scattered non-birefringent, black foreign material (amalgam) (magnification 40×). **b** and **c** Higher magnification showing the granulomas consisting of dense epithelioid histiocytes with scattered multi-nucleated giant cells and the foreign material (amalgam) (magnification 100×)

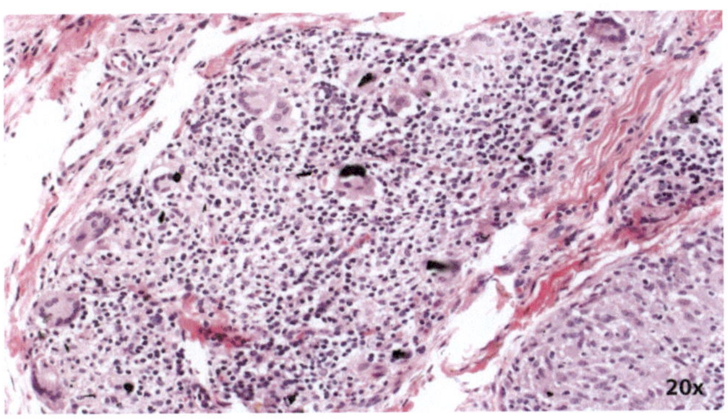

■ **Fig. 34.2** Foreign body granuloma. Granulomas consisting of dense epithelioid histiocytes with some multi-nucleated giant cells associated with non-birefringent, black foreign material (amalgam). Some lymphocytic infiltration (magnification 200×)

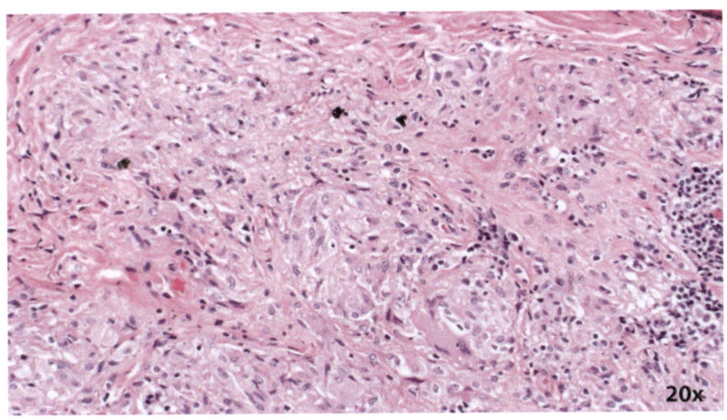

■ **Fig. 34.3** Foreign body granuloma. Granulomas consisting of dense epithelioid histiocytes with some multi-nucleated giant cells associated with non-birefringent, black foreign material (amalgam) (magnification 200×)

Some surgical adjuncts like suture material and polyvinyl alcohol (PVA) sponge may elicit a similar foreign body response (■ Figs. 34.12 and 34.13).

Deproteinised sterilised bovine bone used as bone graft material may show loss of osteointegration and large defects with loose connective tissue around the non-polarisable, amphophilic graft material interspersed within vital bone tissue (■ Figs. 34.14 and 34.15). Resorbable bone graft material composed of bioactive glass particles shows clear spaces with amorphous, acellular, eosinophilic to basophilic material within a connective tissue matrix (■ Fig. 34.16).

Some foreign substances (e.g., food matter—■ Fig. 34.17) may not exhibit an overt granulomatous reaction, but an attempt to identify diagnostic, medicolegal, and therapeutic reasons should be made.

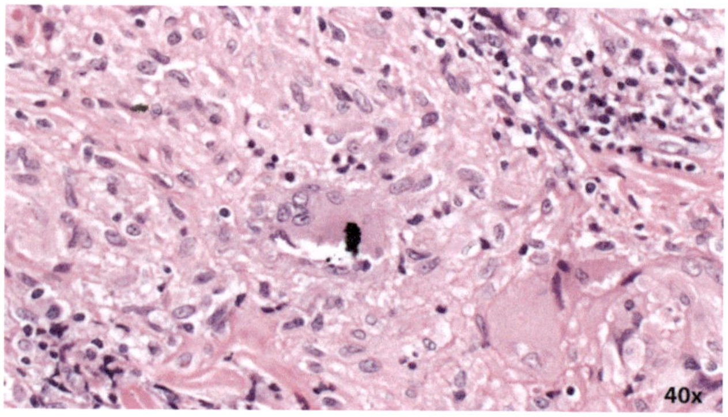

Fig. 34.4 Foreign body granuloma. Dense epithelioid histiocytes with some multi-nucleated giant cells associated with non-birefringent, black foreign material (amalgam) (magnification 400×)

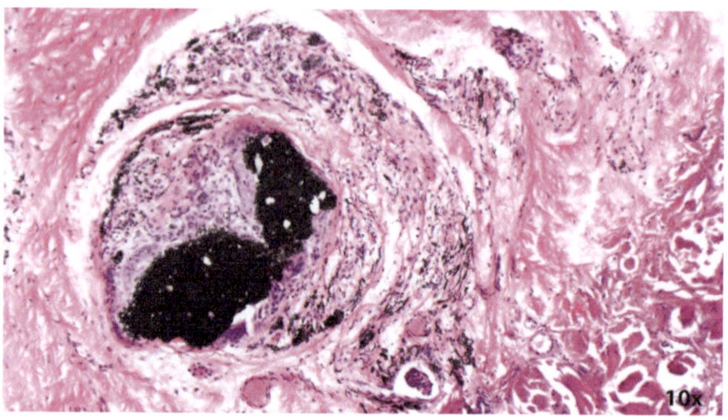

Fig. 34.5 Foreign body granuloma. A granuloma consisting of dense epithelioid histiocytes associated with some multi-nucleated giant cells associated with non-birefringent, black foreign material (amalgam). Cautery artefact at the right periphery (magnification 100×)

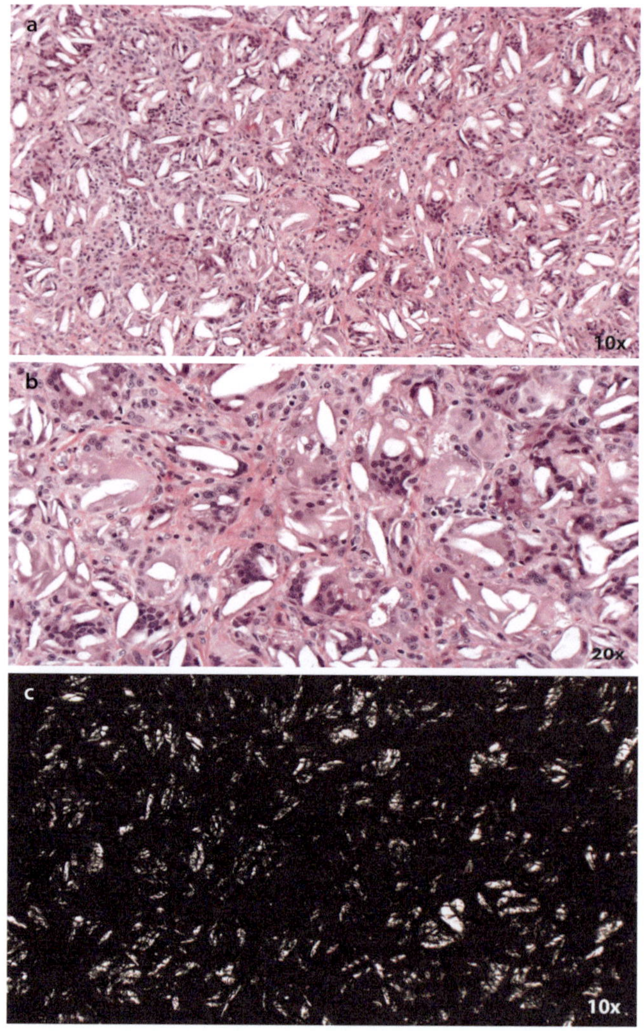

Fig. 34.6 **a–c** Foreign body granuloma. **a** Multiple ovoid, rice-shaped pseudomicrocystic spaces of foreign material (cosmetic material: poly-L-lactic acid (Sculptra)) (magnification 100×). **b** Higher magnification showing the foreign material associated with dense epithelioid histiocytes and multi-nucleated giant cells, some of which contain asteroid bodies (magnification 200×). **c** The foreign material showing birefringence under polarised microscope (magnification 100×)

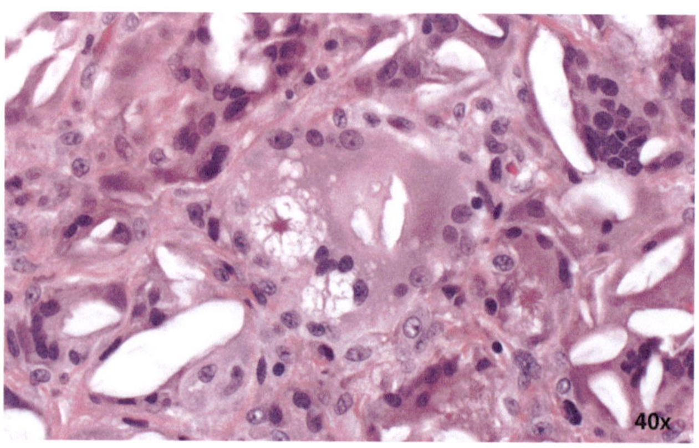

Fig. 34.7 Foreign body granuloma. Some multi-nucleated giant cells containing asteroid bodies and associated with birefringent, ovoid, rice-shaped pseudomicrocystic spaces of foreign material (cosmetic material: poly-L-lactic acid (Sculptra)) (magnification 400×)

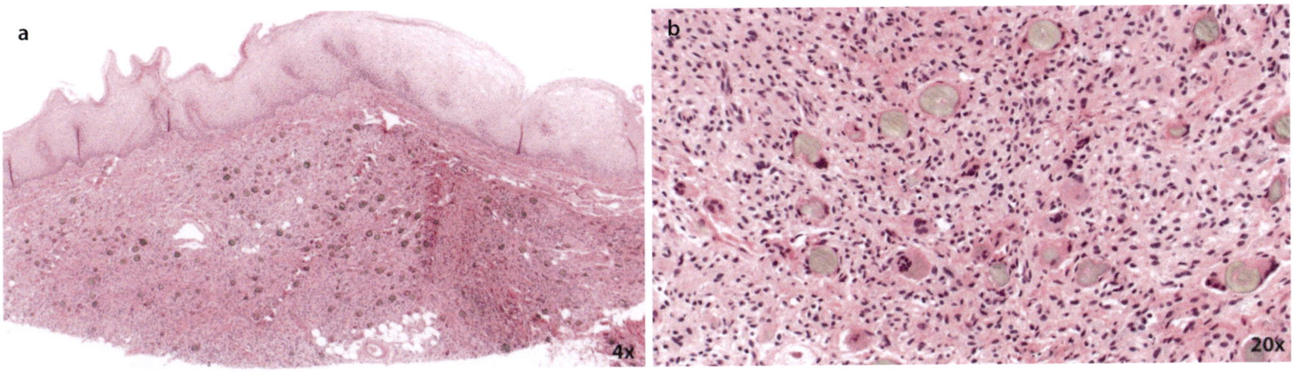

Fig. 34.8 **a** and **b** Foreign body granuloma. **a** Oral mucosal mass with granulomas associated with non-birefringent, beige foreign material (cosmetic material: calcium hydroxyapatite (Radiesse)) (magnification 40×). **b** Higher magnification showing dense epithelioid histiocytes with multi-nucleated giant cells associated with microspherules of the foreign material (magnification 200×)

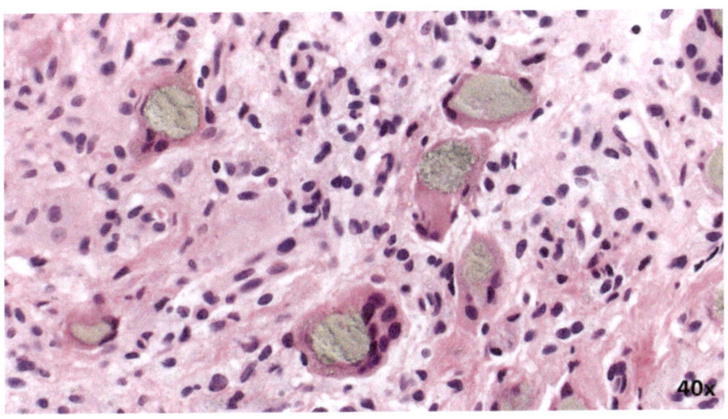

Fig. 34.9 Foreign body granuloma. Dense epithelioid histiocytes with multi-nucleated giant cells associated with varying-sized microspherules of non-birefringent, beige foreign material (cosmetic material: calcium hydroxyapatite (Radiesse)) (magnification 400×)

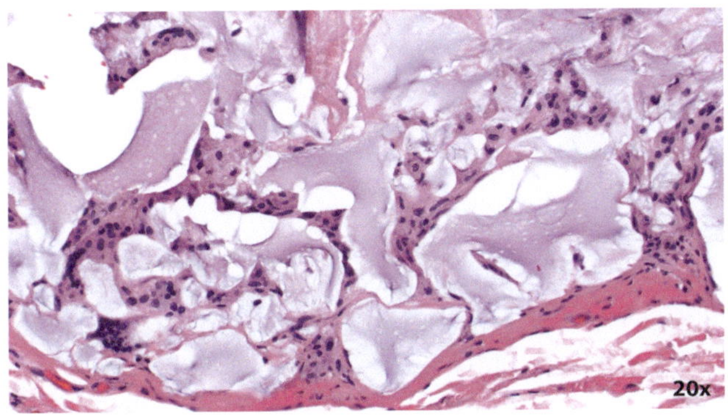

Fig. 34.11 Foreign body granuloma. Pools of non-birefringent, amorphous amphophilic material (cosmetic material: polyacrylamide (Aquamid)) surrounded by epithelioid histiocytes and associated with some multi-nucleated giant cells (magnification 200×)

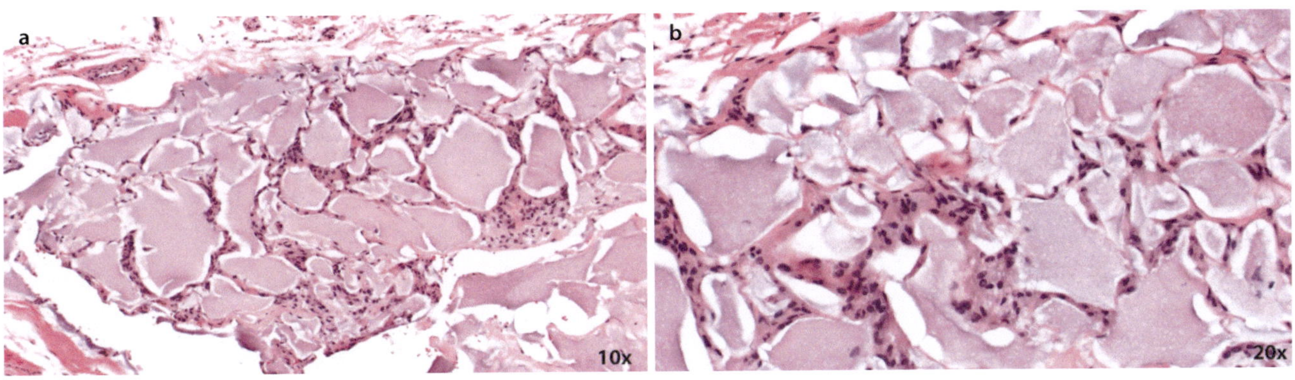

Fig. 34.10 **a** and **b** Foreign body granuloma. **a** Pools of non-birefringent, amorphous amphophilic material (cosmetic material: polyacrylamide (Aquamid)) surrounded by epithelioid histiocytes with chronic inflammatory cells (magnification 100×). **b** Higher magnification showing the foreign material surrounded by epithelioid histiocytes (magnification 200×)

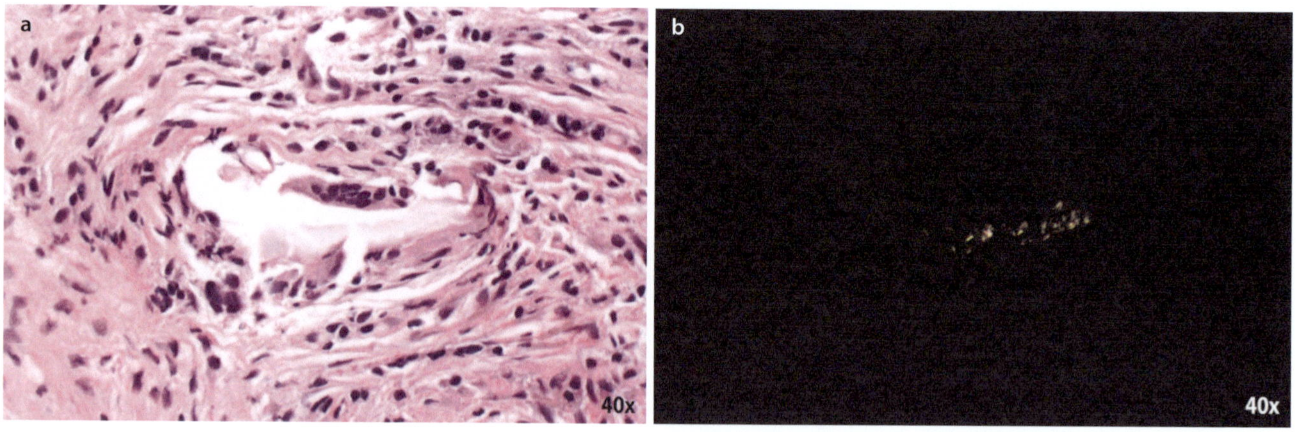

Fig. 34.12 a and b Foreign material. a Multi-nucleated giant cells surrounding bi-refringent, pale basophilic foreign material (suture) (magnification 400×). b The foreign material showing birefringence under polarised microscope (magnification 400×)

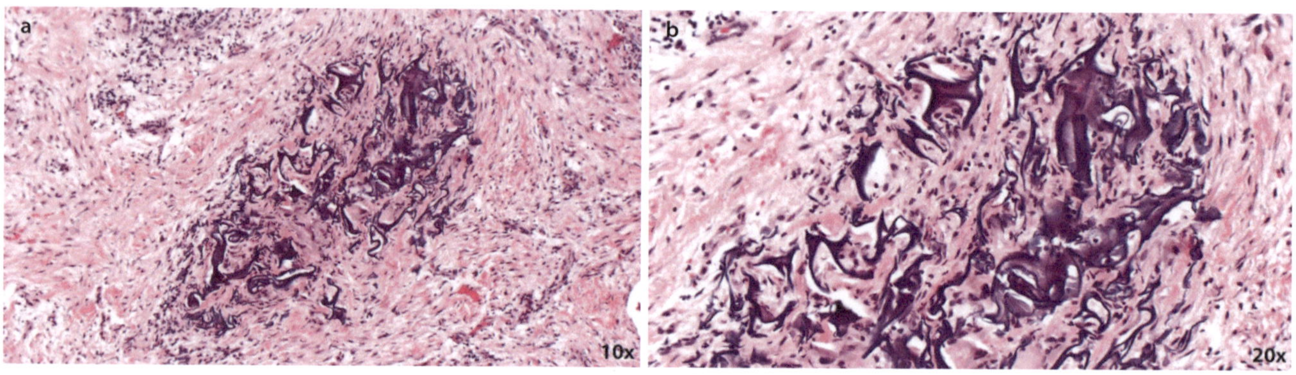

Fig. 34.13 a and b Foreign material. Multiple non-birefringent, irregularly shaped, dark basophilic foreign material (polyvinyl alcohol (PVA) sponge). a magnification 100× and b magnification 200×

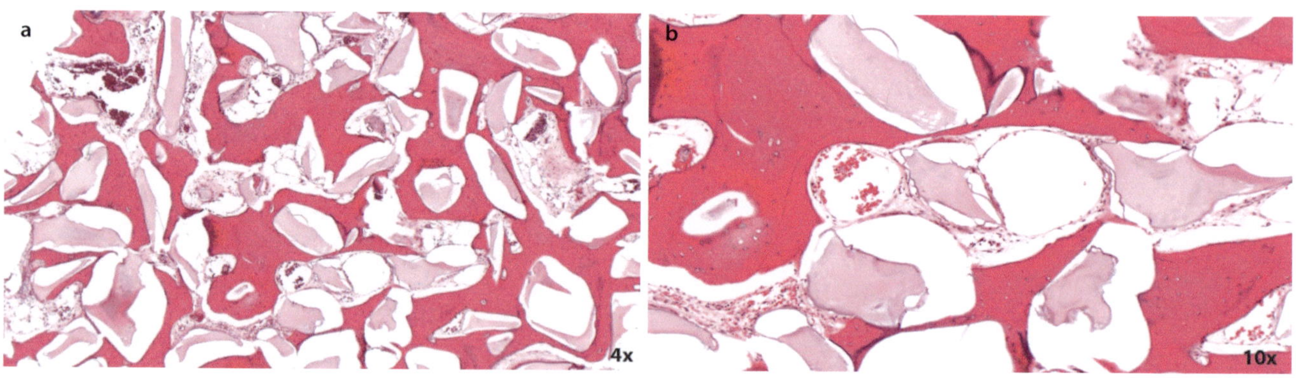

Fig. 34.14 a and b Foreign material. Multiple areas of non-birefringent, amorphous eosinophilic foreign material (bone graft material: deproteinised sterilised bovine bone (Bio-Oss)) associated with vital bone trabeculae. a magnification 40× and b magnification 100×

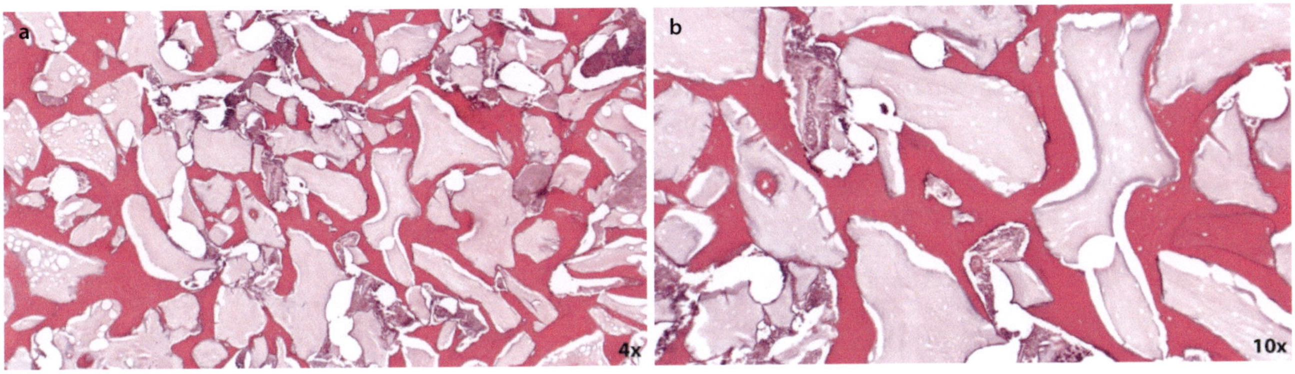

Fig. 34.15 **a** and **b** Foreign material. Multiple areas of non-birefringent, amorphous eosinophilic foreign material (bone graft material: deproteinised sterilised bovine bone (Bio-Oss)) associated with vital bone trabeculae. **a** magnification 40× and **b** magnification 100×

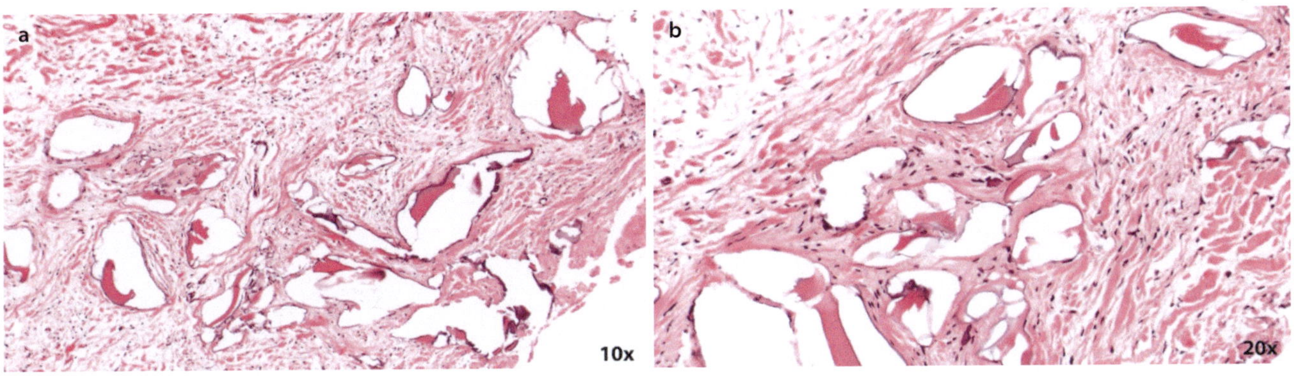

Fig. 34.16 **a** and **b** Foreign material. Multiple non-birefringent, irregularly shaped cavities with eosinophilic to amphophilic foreign material (bone graft material: bioactive glass particles (BioGran)). **a** magnification 100× and **b** magnification 200×

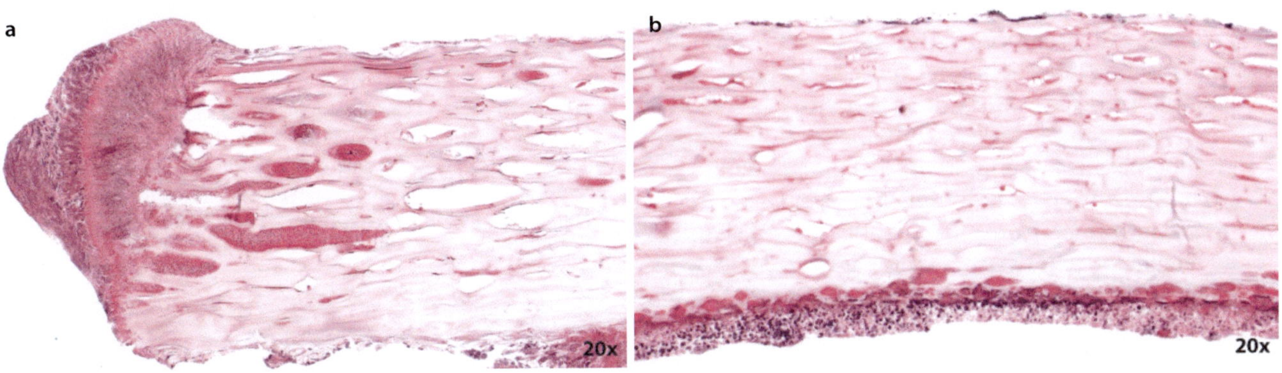

Fig. 34.17 Foreign material. **a** and **b** Non-birefringent food material (popcorn hull) (magnification 200×)

34.3 Orofacial Granulomatosis

Non-specific granulomatous inflammation with varied clinical presentations appears to represent an abnormal immune reaction to several possible triggers. Exact etiologic is not well understood, but allergies to dental materials, toothpaste, food additives, dairy products, cinnamic aldehyde, eggs, wheat, chocolate, etc., have been reported as possible local inciting agents. Some systemic conditions like Crohn's disease, sarcoidosis, tuberculosis, chronic granulomatous disease, and therapeutic medications (e.g., interferons, checkpoint inhibitors, antiretrovirals, etc.) could trigger a granulomatous reaction. The younger the patient who presents with granulomatous inflammation, the more likely to develop Crohn's disease. A diagnosis of idiopathic orofacial granulomatosis is rendered when other known local and systemic causes of orofacial granulomas are ruled out.

34

Key Features

- Highly variable, but the most common site is lips (>90%).
- Non-tender, soft tissue swelling of days/weeks duration, involving partial/complete lip or both lips.
- Long-standing labial swelling may be rubbery, firm, and indurated on palpation.
- Involvement of lips only—cheilitis granulomatosa of Miescher.
- Involvement of lips, facial paralysis and fissured tongue—Melkersson-Rosenthal syndrome.
- Intraoral—hyperplastic folds, ulcerations, fissures, cobblestone appearance, and oedematous mucosa.
- Diagnosis of exclusion—after appropriate stains to rule out infectious aetiology and no allergen/foreign material identified. Medical work-up to rule out sarcoidosis, Crohn's disease, and medication-induced granulomatous inflammation is recommended.
- Management is based on triggering agent—intervention can range from therapeutic pharmaceutical management (e.g., steroids, biologics, etc.) to local surgical intervention.

Histopathology

Microscopic features do not typically show involvement of surface epithelium. However, acanthosis may be noted. The presence of oedema in the superficial lamina propria, along with dilation of vascular channels and lymphatic vessels, may be present (Fig. 34.18a–c). Chronic inflammatory infiltrate, mainly lymphocytes, may be seen as part of interface mucositis or in clusters in deeper connective tissue.

Non-necrotising granulomas composed of epithelioid histiocytes and lymphocytes, with or without multinucleated giant cells, are observed (Fig. 34.18, 34.19, 34.20, 34.21, and 34.22). The inflammatory infiltrate

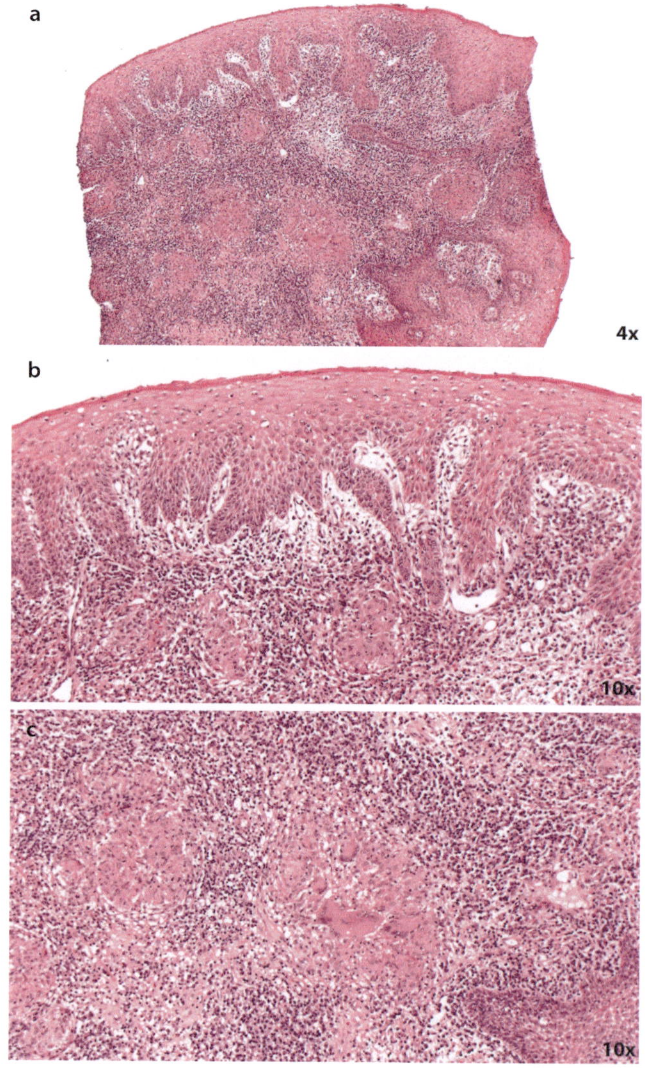

Fig. 34.18 a–c Orofacial granulomatosis. **a** Oral mucosa with underlying granulomas associated with chronic inflammatory cell infiltrates (magnification 40×). **b** Higher magnification showing oedema in the superficial lamina propria (magnification 100×). **c** Granulomas consisting of epithelioid histiocytes and some multinucleated giant cells (magnification 100×

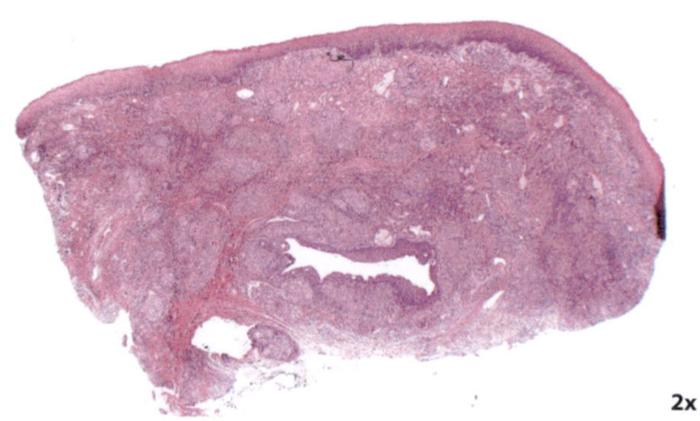

Fig. 34.19 Orofacial granulomatosis. Oral mucosa with multiple granulomas associated with inflammatory cell infiltrates and residual salivary glands and ducts (magnification 20×)

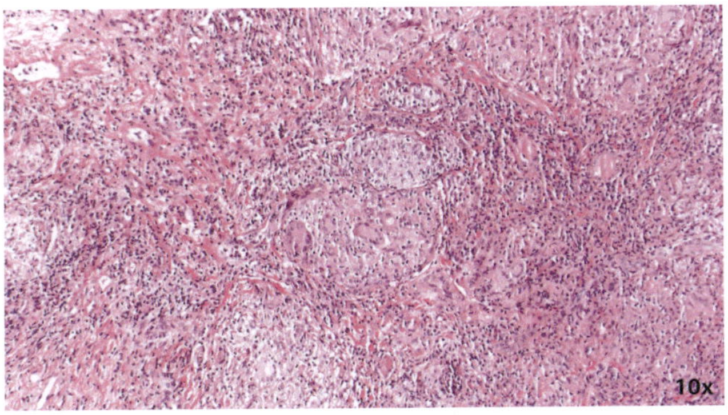

◘ **Fig. 34.20** Orofacial granulomatosis. Granulomas consisting of epithelioid histiocytes admixed with some multi-nucleated giant cells and surrounded by chronic inflammatory cell infiltrates (magnification 100×)

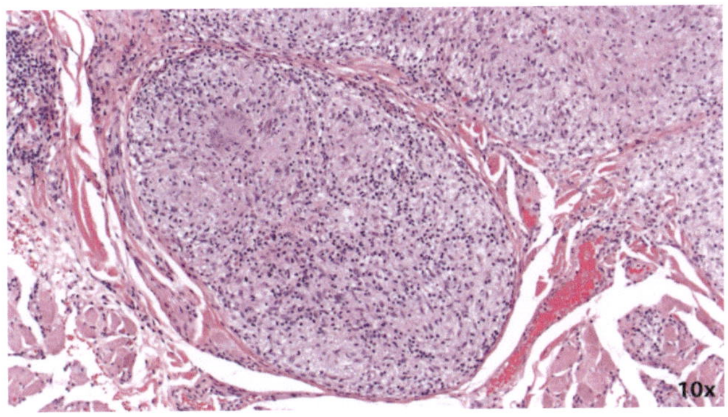

◘ **Fig. 34.22** Orofacial granulomatosis. Granulomas consisting of dense epithelioid histiocytes with some multi-nucleated giant cells (magnification 100×)

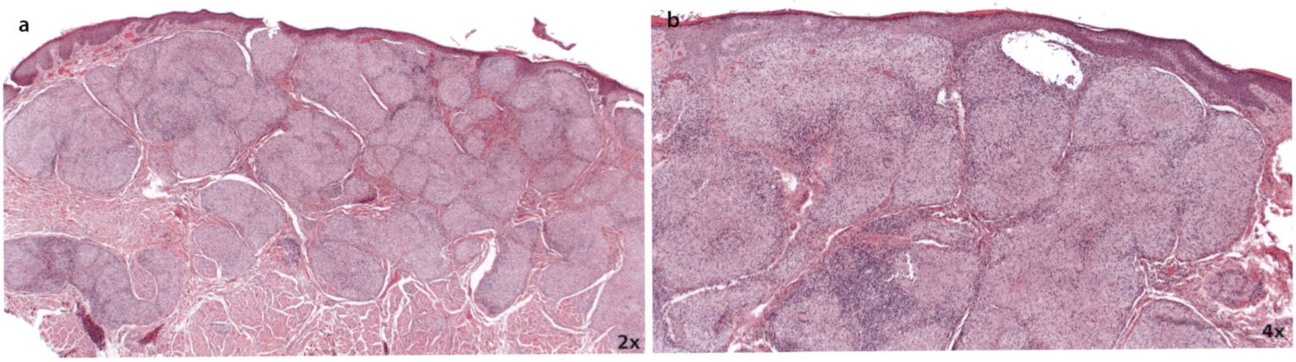

◘ **Fig. 34.21** (**a** and **b**) Orofacial granulomatosis. **a** Oral mucosal mass with underlying numerous granulomas (magnification 20×). **b** High magnification showing well-formed granulomas associated with some lymphocytic infiltrates (magnification 40×)

associated with the granulomas may show plasma cells, lymphocytes, and occasional eosinophils. These granulomas are typically present near vascular channels and can extend into the deeper muscle and salivary glands. In some instances, the granulomas are seen only in the deeper connective tissue, so a superficial biopsy may not show evidence of granulomatous inflammation. It must be emphasised that granulomas associated with orofacial granulomatosis, sarcoidosis, and Crohn's disease have multiple overlapping histologic features. Thus, a definitive diagnosis without clinicopathologic correlation may be challenging. Clinical and imaging studies for systemic disease confirmation are recommended.

34.4 Tuberculous Granuloma

Orofacial tuberculosis is a rare form of extrapulmonary tuberculosis caused primarily by Mycobacterium tuberculosis and can present as a granulomatous disease.

Key Features

- Most common extrapulmonary, head and neck sites are cervical lymph nodes (calcifications).
- Primary orofacial tuberculosis is rare and often seen in children.
- Most oral lesions represent secondary infection with internal organ tuberculosis and subsequent autoinoculation orally.
- Oral cavity involvement is rare, with the most common location being the tongue. However, any part of the oral cavity, including lips and bones, may be involved.
- Clinical presentation is variable—persistent, painful, chronic ulcerations, swellings, gingivitis, sialadenitis, lymphadenitis (scrofula), osteomyelitis, and periapical pathosis.
- Often, oral ulcerative lesions are seen in conjunction with palpable lymph nodes and can mimic malignancy.
- Positive tuberculin (purified protein derivative) skin test does not distinguish active disease from infec-

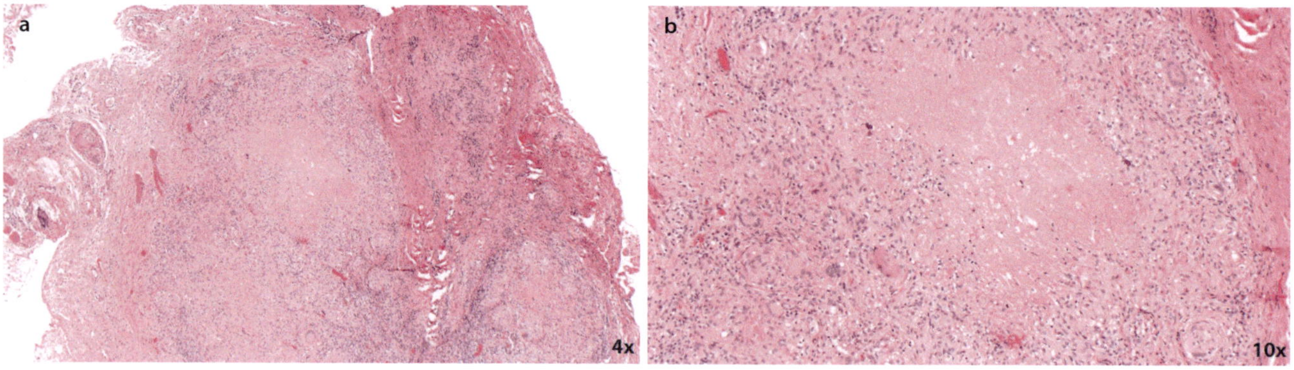

Fig. 34.23 **a** and **b** Tuberculosis. **a** Granulomas with central necrosis (magnification 40×). **b** Higher magnification showing the necrotising granuloma consisting of epithelioid histiocytes admixed with some multi-nucleated giant cells, as well as central necrosis (magnification 100×)

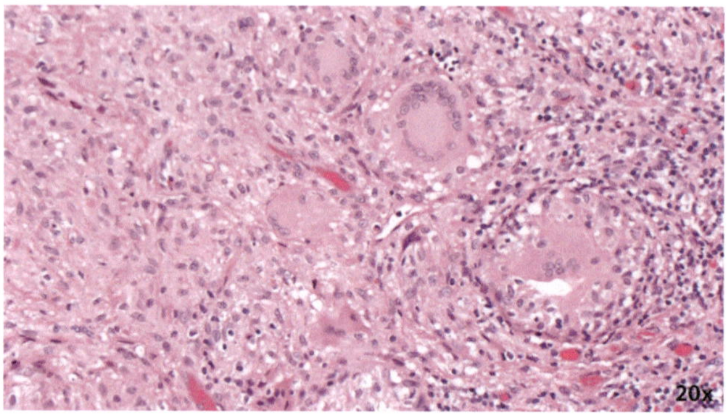

Fig. 34.24 Tuberculosis. Epithelioid histocytes admixed with multi-nucleated giant cells, some of which are Langhans type (magnification 200×)

tion. This is being replaced by interferon-gamma release assay (IGRA). With the assay, the bacillus Calmette-Guerin (BCG) vaccination does not cause a false-positive as seen with the skin test.
- Management is typically under the care of infectious disease physicians, which involves multi-agent therapy for active disease for several months to years.

Histopathology

Granulomatous inflammation associated with tuberculosis shows well-formed, deep granulomas composed of epithelioid histiocytes, lymphocytes and multi-nucleated giant cells. The granulomatous inflammation is often necrotising (grossly caseous necrosis) in nature (Fig. 34.23). Sheets of histiocytes with multinucleated giant cells and areas of necrosis are typically seen. Langhans-type multi-nucleated giant cells with nuclei aligned in a horseshoe pattern are often noted (Fig. 34.24). The term tubercle represents one of these granulomas in a patient with tuberculosis. Special stains, such as Ziehl–Neelsen or other acid-fast stains, may highlight rod-shaped bacilli and mycobacteria. However, due to the scarcity of organisms within the tissue, they may not always be evident. Thus, the lack of acid-fast bacilli does not completely rule out the possibility of this disease.

34.5 Sarcoidosis

Sarcoidosis is a chronic granulomatous inflammatory disorder involving multiple systems and of unknown aetiology.

Key Features

- Multi-organ involvement, mainly lungs (90%), followed by skin, lymph nodes, eyes, liver, etc.
- Bilateral hilar lymphadenopathy, lupus pernio, and uveitis.
- Oral involvement rare—mainly buccal mucosa and gingiva.
- Clinically—papule, granular, ulcerated, violaceous, or hyperkeratotic areas.
- Affects salivary glands in 1 of 20 cases—bilateral, painless enlargement.
- Elevated angiotensin-converting enzyme (ACE) levels (~60% of patients).
- Diagnosis of exclusion—based on a combination of clinical, radiographic, and histopathologic findings.
- Management—spontaneous resolution in approximately 60% of patients within 2 years without treatment. Oral lesions may not require treatment. In disseminated, progressive disease and medical management (systemic corticosteroids, TNF inhibitors, etc.) are recommended.

Histopathology

Granulomatous inflammation shows the presence of aggregates of epithelioid histiocytes intermixed with foreign body-type or Langhans-type multi-nucleated giant cells. These non-necrotising granulomas have been termed "naked" granulomas due to the lack of associated lymphocytic infiltrates (◘ Fig. 34.25 and 34.26). This, however, may not always be the case, and lymphocytic infiltrate within the granuloma and along the periphery ("collarette") may be present (◘ Fig. 34.27).

Even though non-specific concentric calcifications (Schaumann bodies) and stellate inclusions (asteroid bodies) may be seen within the multi-nucleated giant cells, they are not considered diagnostic. Schaumann (conchoidal) bodies are lysosome-derived, large, concentric, calcified, basophilic, and laminated bodies made up of calcium oxalate crystals. The stellate or asteroid bodies are spicule-shaped and represent entrapped collagen (◘ Figs. 34.28 and 34.29). These structures may be seen in other granulomatous conditions.

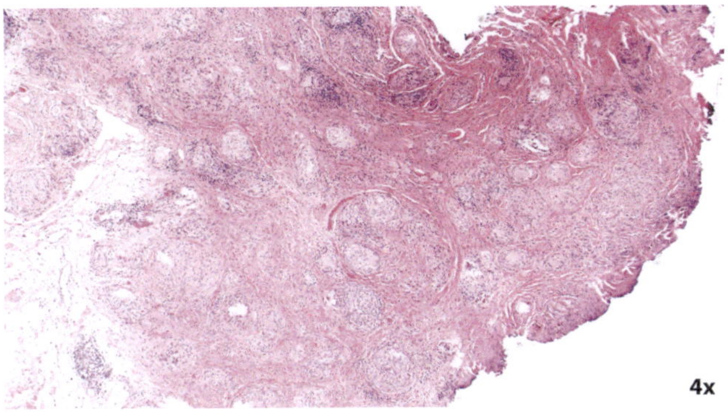

◘ **Fig. 34.25** Sarcoidosis. Multiple granulomas surrounded by a rim of lymphocytes (magnification 40×)

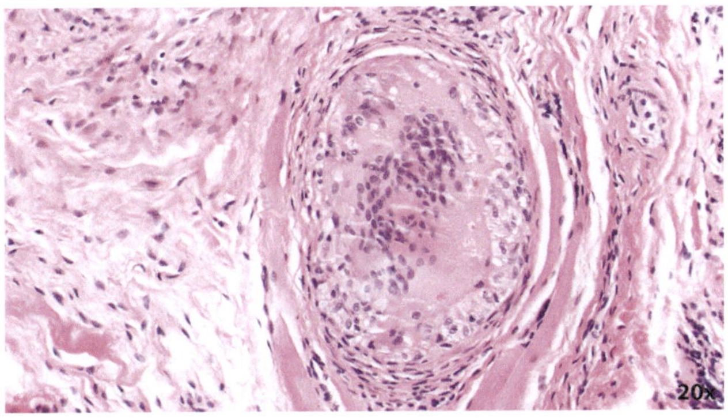

◘ **Fig. 34.27** Sarcoidosis. A granuloma consisting of epithelioid histiocytes with a multi-nucleated giant cell (magnification 200×)

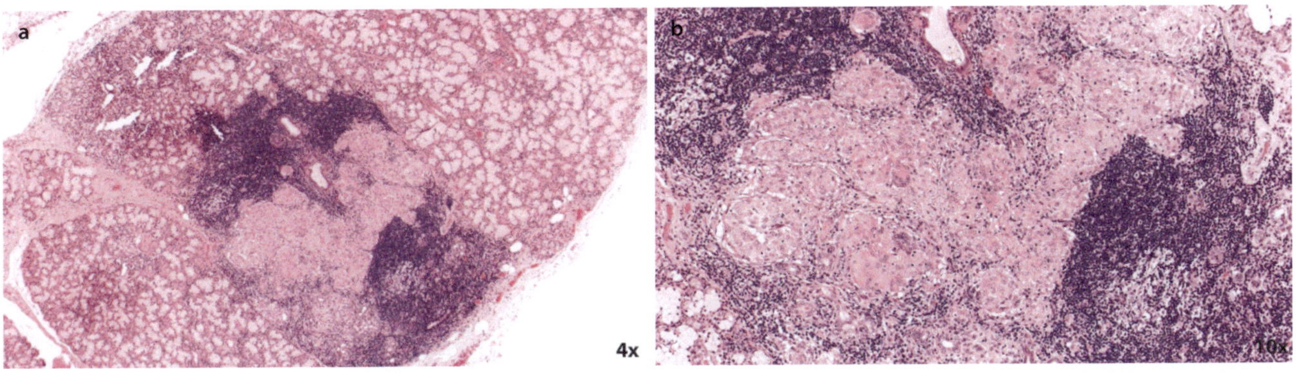

◘ **Fig. 34.26** **a** and **b** Sarcoidosis. **a** Lobules of mucous salivary glands associated with granulomas surrounded by dense lymphocytes (magnification 40×). **b** Higher magnification showing the granulomas consisting of dense epithelioid histiocytes admixed with some multi-nucleated giant cells and surrounded by dense lymphocytes (magnification 100×)

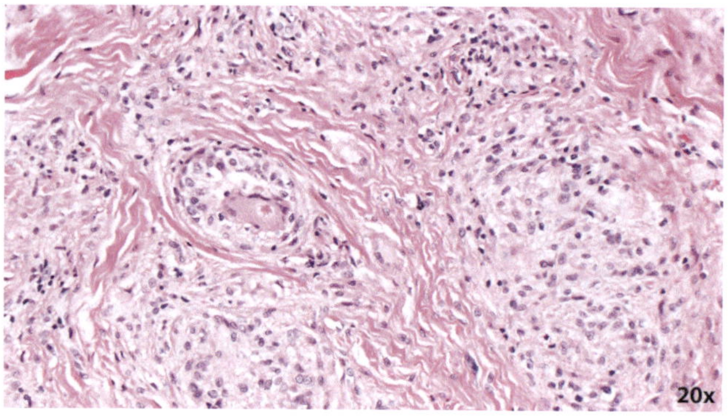

Fig. 34.28 Sarcoidosis. Granulomas consisting of epithelioid histiocytes with a multi-nucleated giant cell containing asteroid body (magnification 200×)

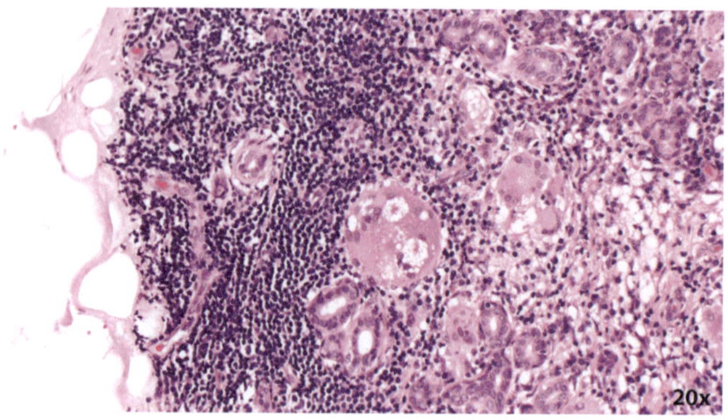

Fig. 34.29 Sarcoidosis. Multi-nucleated giant cells containing asteroid bodies (magnification 200×)

34

34.6 Summary

Oral granulomatous diseases occur due to infectious or non-infectious agents presenting with local or systemic diseases. Histopathological features with special stains and detailed medical work-up are part of the diagnostic process. Sometimes, oral manifestations may be the first sign of the disease. This chapter will discuss the histological features of the granulomatous diseases.

Acknowledgement Dr. Kittiphoj (Sem) Tikkhanarak (University of Iowa) for direct technical help with photomicrographs.

Further Reading

Alawi F, Shields BE, Omolehinwa T, Rosenbach M. Oral granulomatous disease. Dermatol Clin. 2020;38(4):429–39.

Andrade NN, Mhatre TS. Orofacial tuberculosis—a 16-year experience with 46 cases. J Oral Maxillofac Surg. 2012;70(1):e12–22.

Grave B, McCullough M, Wiesenfeld D. Orofacial granulomatosis—a 20-year review. Oral Dis. 2009;15(1):46–51.

Kumar V, Abbas AK, Aster JC, Deyrup AT, editors. Robbins & Kumar basic pathology. 11th ed. Elsevier—Health Sciences Division: Philadelphia, PA; 2022.

Müller S. Non-infectious granulomatous lesions of the orofacial region. Head Neck Pathol. 2019;13(3):449–56.

Neville BW, Damm DD, Allen CM, Chi AC. Oral and maxillofacial pathology. 5th ed. Philadelphia, PA: Elsevier—Health Sciences Division; 2023.

Owosho AA, Bilodeau EA, Vu J, Summersgill KF. Orofacial dermal fillers: foreign body reactions, histopathologic features, and spectrometric studies. Oral Surg Oral Med Oral Pathol Oral Radiol. 2014;117(5):617–25.

Poate TW, Sharma R, Moutasim KA, Escudier MP, Warnakulasuriya S. Orofacial presentations of sarcoidosis—a case series and review of the literature. Br Dent J. 2008;205(8):437–42.

Popescu MR, Pleşea IE, Olaru M, Strâmbu IR, Fronie AI, Petrescu IO, et al. Morphological aspects in tuberculosis of oral cavity—our experience and a review of the literature attempt. Rom J Morphol Embryol. 2015;56(3):967–87.

Santos LG, Jardim LC, Schuch LF, Silveira FM, Wagner VP, Pires FR, et al. Foreign body reactions related to orofacial esthetic fillers: a systematic review. Oral Dis. 2024;30(3):855–64.

Suresh L, Radfar L. Oral sarcoidosis: a review of literature. Oral Dis. 2005;11(3):138–45.

Investigative Oral Pathology

Contents

Oral Soft Tissue Biopsy Techniques: An Overview

Ying Shi Chang

Contents

S R Prabhu et al. (eds.), *Oral Histology and Oral Histopathology*, https://doi.org/10.1007/978-3-031-77481-2_35

35.1 Introduction

An accurate diagnosis is crucial for the effective management of oral mucosal lesions. Tissue biopsy is a common procedure and the gold standard for diagnosing disease, oral or otherwise. It is a surgical procedure in which a tissue sample is removed from a lesion to provide the pathologist with a representative, viable specimen for histopathological interpretation and diagnosis. The word biopsy has its roots in Greek etymology, originating from the words *bio* (life) and *opsin* (to see).

Indications for a biopsy

1. Any lesion with malignant or premalignant features, e.g. rapidly growing, induration on palpation, chronic ulceration, non-homogenous in colour
2. Any unknown lesion in high-risk areas for the development of cancer, e.g. floor of the mouth, ventral surface of the tongue
3. Persistent lesions despite the removal of local irritants
4. Confirmation of clinical diagnostic suspicion
5. Lesion that is causing the patient extreme concern and significant distress (cancerphobia)

There are four main biopsy techniques that can be used for soft tissue lesions.

1. Incisional biopsy
2. Excisional biopsy
3. Punch biopsy
4. Brush biopsy

35.2 Biopsy Fundamentals

35.2.1 History and Examination

A comprehensive history of the lesion and clinical examination are essential initial steps. The history should encompass factors such as duration, preceding events, symptoms, alterations in appearance, as well as any previous diagnostic and therapeutic interventions. Essential components of the clinical examination include assessing the lesion's location, size, colour, and consistency or texture. These should be documented together with good clinical photographs. Assessment of the patient's medical history is important as severe or poorly controlled systemic diseases, inherited coagulopathies, and medications pose an increased surgical risk and may require medical clearance prior to undertaking the procedure.

35.2.2 Consent

Before proceeding with any biopsy, it is essential to obtain both verbal and written informed consent. Patients should be educated thoroughly regarding the surgical procedure, including potential complications such as discomfort, swelling, infection, bleeding, as well as the possibility of temporary or permanent nerve damage if the lesion is in close proximity to nerves. If the lesion is in an area that would affect the appearance of the patient (e.g. vermilion border of the lip) the aesthetic concerns should be addressed.

35.2.3 Armamentarium

The instruments needed for a biopsy procedure are minimal and a well-prepared instrument setup enhances procedural efficiency (Fig. 35.1).

- Syringe and local anaesthetic
- Scalpel handle with #15 blade
- Appropriate tissue retractor
- Fine tissue forceps
- Needle holder
- Small curved haemostat
- Suction tip and hose
- Suture material
- Sterile gauze sponges
- Scissors
- Screw-top, labelled biopsy specimen bottle with transport medium
- Histopathology request form

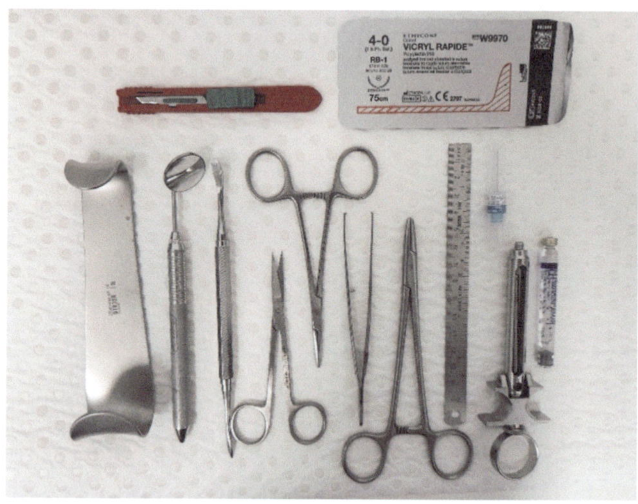

Fig. 35.1 Basic armamentarium for biopsy

35.2.4 Anaesthesia

A local anaesthetic solution containing adrenaline (e.g. 2% Lignocaine with 1:80,000 adrenaline) is preferred as it aids in decreasing surgical bleeding and prolongs the duration of anaesthesia. The area is thoroughly infiltrated with the local anaesthetic, ensuring it reaches deep and surrounds the biopsy site. This will prevent distortion of the cellular architecture of the tissue, which could impede pathological diagnosis.

35.2.5 Tissue Stabilization

The tissue needs to be stabilized as the oral and perioral soft tissue are mobile surfaces. This can be accomplished either by the surgical assistant, chalazion forceps or using retractors. The surgical assistant can stabilize the tissue by grimly grasping the tissue with the thumb and forefinger stretching it into a slightly ovoid appearance. This is the most common technique for stabilizing the tissue. Although Chalazion forceps are especially helpful in the stabilization of the lip and buccal mucosa, it restricts the size and shape of the surgical field due to the size of its aperture.

35.2.6 Incisions

- A biopsy can be performed using either a scalpel or a tissue punch.
- Elliptical incisions, made with a #15 scalpel blade, should have a length-to-width ratio of 3:1 and converge at the ends to facilitate wound closure.
- Care must be taken to avoid iatrogenic injury to the assistant.
- The tissue is excised as a wedge, ensuring an adequate depth to sample tissue from various depths and includes cellular features from the base of the lesion.
- It is important to avoid damaging adjacent significant anatomical structures such as nerves and blood vessels when making the incisions.
- Carefully lift the biopsy specimen with tissue forceps and undermine the ellipse or tissue core (in the case of a punch biopsy) parallel to the mucosal surface using a #15 scalpel blade or curved scissors.
- Ideally, an excisional biopsy should include a 2–3 mm band of peri-lesional tissue. Electrosurgery or laser may cause thermal artefacts that can impede histologic analysis; therefore, these techniques should be used with caution.

35.2.7 Wound Closure

- A tension-free primary closure of the wound is desirable, and the elliptical shape of the wound facilitates this.
- If the wound is very deep, involving multiple tissue layers, each layer should be closed separately.
- Preferred suture materials are 4/0 resorbable, nonreactive, and slowly resorbable (e.g. polyglactin 910 (Vicryl®)).
- Wounds on attached mucosal surfaces (e.g. gingiva) are generally not closed and are allowed to heal by secondary intention.

35.2.8 Biopsy Specimen

- Specimens should always be handled delicately to prevent crush injury, desiccation, thermal damage, or suction-induced harm. Such mishandling can cause tissue artefacts and distortions, compromising pathological diagnosis.
- The specimen should be immediately placed in a screw-capped container with the appropriate transport medium. Typically, this medium is 10% neutral buffered formalin, using at least twenty times the volume of the sample to ensure proper fixation.
- For suspected vesiculobullous lesions, a separate sample should be sent in Mitchel's solution or fresh to the laboratory.
- It is crucial to deliver samples in Mitchel's solution and fresh samples to the laboratory within 24 h, as neither adequately preserves the tissue.
- If multiple biopsy specimens are obtained, each must be sent in separate containers to the laboratory, accompanied by an illustration depicting the location of each specimen.
- If dysplasia or malignancy is suspected, loosely tying a suture at one margin of the specimen to indicate its anatomical orientation relative to the lesion will help the pathologist assess the completeness of the excision.
- The orientation and location of the marker should be illustrated and sent with the specimen to the laboratory.
- Each specimen jar must be labelled with the patient's name, date of birth, the site of specimen collection, the clinician's name, and the date of collection.
- The patient should verify the label to ensure their details are accurate.

- Each pathology laboratory has a unique form that should accompany the specimen container. Relevant clinical details, such as the patient's demographic information, clinical presentation, lesion location, pertinent medical history, and presumptive clinical diagnosis, should be outlined in the form. This information will aid the pathologist in providing an accurate diagnosis. Including a colour photograph of the lesion can be helpful for the pathologist.

35.2.9 Postoperative Considerations and Follow-Up

In general, biopsy procedures usually involve few complications, given thorough assessment and consideration before and during the procedure. Similar to other surgical procedures, swelling and mild postoperative pain are expected. The patient should receive verbal and written standard postoperative instructions covering general guidelines for eating, oral hygiene, pain management, and bleeding control. Providing the patient with emergency contact information is advisable.

A postoperative review should be carried out 1–2 weeks following the procedure to review healing and to discuss the results with the patient, as well as any further management if necessary. If an adverse diagnosis, like cancer, is encountered, patients should receive counselling with sensitivity and the presence of a supportive family member. In such cases it is crucial to emphasize the importance of prompt treatment and diligent follow-up, and a prompt referral to a specialist with the expertise to manage the condition should be arranged.

35.2.10 When to Refer

If the clinician lacks training in biopsy procedures, uncertain of the most appropriate site from which to obtain the biopsy, there is increased surgical difficulty due to the site (e.g. floor of the mouth), complex medical history, or proximity to significant anatomical structures with the potential for significant complications (e.g. bleeding, nerve injury), or is uncomfortable in providing a diagnosis of malignancy referral to a specialist such as an oral surgeon, maxillofacial surgeon, or an oral medicine specialist is advisable.

35.3 Individual Biopsy Techniques

35.3.1 Incisional Biopsy

An incisional biopsy is a biopsy procedure that removes only a small representative portion of the lesion. Thus, the clinician must obtain the sample from the most appropriate site. If the lesion is large or exhibits varying features across different areas, obtaining samples from multiple regions is necessary. It is the biopsy method of choice when a malignancy is suspected or included in the differential diagnosis.

- **Technique**
- Identify the most representative area of the lesion and outline it.
- Stabilize the tissue with fingers or tissue forceps.
- Local anaesthesia.
- Elliptical incisions, with a length-to-width ratio of 3:1, are made with a #15 scalpel blade.
- Carefully lift the biopsy specimen with tissue forceps and undermine the ellipse parallel to the mucosal surface.
- Place the biopsy specimen into a specimen jar with an appropriate transport medium.
- Close the biopsy wound with a few interrupted sutures using resorbable sutures.

35.3.2 Excisional Biopsy

An excisional biopsy is the complete removal of the lesion including a 2–3 mm perimeter of normal tissue surrounding the lesion. This procedure is reserved for small lesions <1 cm in size and often results in definitive treatment of the lesion. An excisional biopsy is not carried out if malignancy is suspected.

- **Technique**
- Stabilize the tissue.
- Local anaesthesia.
- Elliptical incisions, with a length-to-width ratio of 3:1, are made with a #15 scalpel blade.
- Carefully lift the biopsy specimen with tissue forceps and undermine the ellipse parallel to the mucosal surface.

- Place the biopsy specimen into a specimen jar with an appropriate transport medium.
- Close the biopsy wound with a few interrupted sutures using resorbable sutures.

35.3.3 Punch Biopsy

A punch biopsy is a biopsy procedure that utilizes a tissue punch to remove a small lesion in its entirety or to obtain a small representative portion of a larger lesion. It is a quick and easy biopsy technique. Similar to an incisional biopsy if the lesion is large or exhibits varying features across different areas, obtaining samples from multiple regions is necessary. This technique is not suitable for suspected vesiculobullous diseases.

- **Technique**
- Stabilize the tissue.
- Local anaesthesia.
- Place the punch perpendicular to the skin/mucosa.
- Rotate the punch in a twisting motion while applying pressure, until the depth of the punch reaches the connective tissue below the epithelium.
- Gently hold the tissue core with tissue forceps and severe at the base with a #15 blade or curved scissors.
- Place the biopsy specimen into a specimen jar with an appropriate transport medium.
- Close the biopsy wound with one or more interrupted sutures using resorbable sutures.

35.3.4 Brush Biopsy

A brush biopsy is a non-invasive procedure that involves using a stiff wire brush to collect epithelial cells for examination. It does not necessitate any anaesthesia and is quick and straightforward to conduct. This biopsy method might be employed to monitor patients with chronic mucosal changes (e.g. leukoplakia) or as an additional tool in patients with a history of oral cancer to review mucosal alterations. If atypical cells are detected, a conventional biopsy of the lesion is necessary. It is important to note that a brush biopsy serves as an adjunct and does not substitute conventional biopsy techniques.

- **Technique**
- Stabilize the tissue.
- Place the wire brush in contact with the surface of the suspected lesion.
- Rotate with firm pressure 5–10 times.
- Pinpoint bleeding indicated sufficient depth for cell collection.
- Smear the sample onto a glass slide.
- Flood the slide with a fixative solution and send it for analysis.

35.4 Conclusion

Biopsy of tissue plays a vital role in diagnosing soft tissue pathology. Employing the correct technique to obtain a representative tissue sample and ensuring proper handling of the biopsy specimen increases the chances of obtaining an accurate pathological diagnosis. Poor biopsy technique may necessitate further procedures or lead to an incorrect diagnosis. When in doubt, it is recommended to refer the patient to an oral surgeon, maxillofacial surgeon, or oral medicine specialist.

Further Reading

Alsarraf AH, Kujan O, Farah CS. The utility of oral brush cytology in the early detection of oral cancer and oral potentially malignant disorders: a systematic review. J Oral Pathol Med. 2018;47(2):104–16. https://doi.org/10.1111/jop.12660.

Avon S-L, Klieb HBE. Oral soft-tissue biopsy: an overview. J Can Dent Assoc. 2012;78(4):c75.

Babshet M, Nandimath K, Pervatikar S, Naikmasur V. Efficacy of oral brush cytology in the evaluation of the oral premalignant and malignant lesions. J Cytol. 2011;28(4):165–72. https://doi.org/10.4103/0970-9371.86342.

Chen S, Forman M, Sadow PM, August M. The diagnostic accuracy of incisional biopsy in the oral cavity. J Oral Maxillofac Surg. 2016;74(5):959–64. https://doi.org/10.1016/j.joms.2015.11.006.

Jain N. Essentials before sending biopsy specimens: a surgeon's perspective and pathologists concern. J Maxillofac Oral Surg. 2011;10(4):361–4. https://doi.org/10.1007/s12663-011-0234-9.

Jeng P-Y, Chang M-C, Chiang C-P, Lee C-F, Chen C-F, Jeng J-H. Oral soft tissue biopsy surgery: current principles and key tissue stabilization techniques. J Dent Sci. 2024;19(1):11–20. https://doi.org/10.1016/j.jds.2023.09.015.

Logan R, Goss A. Biopsy of the oral mucosa and use of histopathology services. Aust Dent J. 2010;55(s1):9–13. https://doi.org/10.1111/j.1934-7819.2010.01194.

Melrose RJ, et al. The use of biopsy in dental practice. The Position of the American Academy of Oral and Maxillofacial Pathology. Gen Dent. 2007;55(5):457–61; quiz 462–63

Shanti RM, Tanaka T, Stanton DC. Oral biopsy techniques. Dermatol Clin. 2020;38(4):421–7. https://doi.org/10.1016/j.det.2020.05.003.

Diagnostic Methods Employed in Oral and Maxillofacial Pathology

Hannah Walsh

Contents

S R Prabhu et al. (eds.), *Oral Histology and Oral Histopathology*, https://doi.org/10.1007/978-3-031-77481-2_36

36.1 Introduction

A number of diseases and conditions arise in the head and neck and the aetiology of these conditions vary according to the causative agent. Conditions may arise as a result of bacterial, fungal or viral infections (e.g. acute parotitis, primary infection with herpes simplex virus, candidiasis, infection with cytomegalovirus). Other conditions may arise as a result of trauma (e.g. a fibroepithelial polyp, hyperkeratosis of the alveolar ridge), inherited genetics (e.g. white sponge naevus) or as the result of repeated unresolved DNA damage resulting in malignancy (e.g. oral squamous cell carcinoma). With differing causative agents, and a range of diagnostic tests available, the most suitable method must be adopted for clinicians to achieve a diagnosis and formulate appropriate treatment plans for their patients. In this chapter we will take a closer look at the range of diagnostic tests most frequently utilised in oral and maxillofacial pathology, the clinical indications and additional tests that can be used which all combine to give the final report a clinician receives. We will also discuss the importance of histopathological result interpretation and correlation with additional tests in clinicopathological correlation.

36.2 Microbiological Methods of Investigating Disease

A number of infections can arise in the head and neck region. These can be of odontogenic or non-odontogenic origin and can in certain situations result in serious morbidity and the need for patient hospitalisation. Often hospital admission is required for incision and drainage of large facial abscesses and administration of intravenous antibiotics to treat the underlying infective cause. Examination of infections of the head and neck via microbiological methods can be challenging but is paramount to identify the causative microorganism and thus prescribe the correct course of treatment to manage the infection. When undertaking investigative procedures to identify a causative virulent microorganism, one also encounters the rich population of normal flora when trying to obtain a sample. It is therefore paramount that the correct sampling methods are employed and the prescribed procedural steps are followed in order to collect and subsequently analyse the specimen to ensure the clinically relevant information is obtained and the patient can receive the correct course of treatment. There are a variety of methods available for the assessment of microorganisms but is important to consider the differential diagnosis as this will influence the selection of the most appropriate test to collect the sample. Infectious agents in the head and neck can be bacterial, fungal, viral and on rare occasions parasitic in their nature. The various methods of sample collection and assessment methods will be discussed in turn.

Specimen Collection: The collection and transportation of the microbiological sample is a crucial step in the pathway to determine the causative infective agent of the disease process. There are numerous measures that need to be considered when collecting a sample. It is important to consider local anatomy and try as much as possible to avoid contamination with normal commensal organisms. This is a known difficulty within the head and neck environment however clinicians should exercise caution with sample procurement as contamination and overgrowth of the commensal population may obscure examination of the causative infective agent. Once the sample is collected, the specimen must be transported to the laboratory as soon as possible and thus inclusion of the date and time of specimen collection alongside the patient details is important on the request form and specimen receptacle.

Smears: Direct smears using simple stains, such as a Gram stain, are a mainstay of microorganism assessment having been used for over a century. They allow for the rapid assessment of a sample and can give an overview of the number, cellular morphology, arrangement and broad type of microorganisms present. A thin and even spread of the sample is applied onto a glass slide and fixed prior to the application of the stain. The test can give a basic overview as to whether the organisms are commensal or causative and if causative, give a broad overview of the type of microorganism present (e.g. the Gram stain can indicate if the causative agents are Gram-positive or Gram-negative). Although providing a rapid overview of the microbiological landscape and insight into the predominant organisms in the received sample, smears using Gram stain cannot give a definitive diagnosis. It does however guide the most appropriate subsequent tests that should be carried out and allows the laboratory team to continue along the correct line of testing so a definitive diagnosis can be achieved. Additional testing methods are discussed below.

Culture and Antibiotic Sensitivity Tests: Following a smear, a microbiological culture may be employed to identify the type and the abundance of the responsible infectious microorganism. A variety of growth mediums are typically used as all microorganisms cannot grow in one culture medium. Examples include nutrient agar, blood agar, chocolate agar and MacConkey agar to name but a few. For a microorganism to grow and multiply sufficiently to allow for visualisation by eye, the culture medium in which the specimen is placed must provide the required growth environment and nutrition

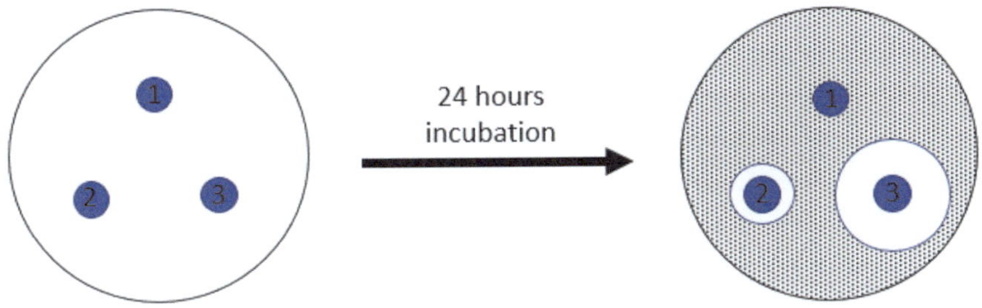

Fig. 36.1 Example of disk diffusion or Kirby–Baur method. Antibiotic disks (i.e. blue circles 1–3) are placed on the culture plate following adequate growth of the bacterial population. The plate is then reviewed after a 24-h incubation period. Disk 1 shows no zone of inhibition and therefore the microorganism is resistant to antibiotic 1. Antibiotic 1 is not an appropriate treatment for the infection. Antibiotic disks 2 and 3 show areas of inhibition of bacterial growth. Disk 3 shows the largest zone of inhibition and has the highest bacterial antibiotic susceptibility, thus is the most appropriate antibiotic therapy to be used for the patient

to support this. Some organisms will not grow in the setting of an artificial culture environment. These organisms are known as obligate organisms. Following adequate growth of the bacteria on the culture plate, a common test known as disk diffusion or the Kirby–Bauer method may be employed to demonstrate the effect of different groups of antibiotic treatments on the cultured microorganisms (Fig. 36.1). Following application of the antibiotic disks, the plate is incubated for up to 24 h. During this time frame, the antibiotic diffuses into the surrounding culture and creates a concentration gradient. The larger the area of no bacterial growth around the disk, the higher the bacterial antibiotic susceptibility. If the bacteria are resistant to a particular antibiotic, no zone of inhibition will be visualised. When discussing antibiotic sensitivity, in broad terms, a microorganism is classified as 'resistant' when they are able to grow in the growth agar and 'sensitive' if they are unable to grow in the growth agar, thus an antibiotic that the microorganism is 'sensitive' to will ensure adequate response to treatment.

Other methods available to assess antibiotic susceptibility include dilution testing and agar dilution. A reliable outcome rests upon the correct handling of the specimen. To ensure a reliable outcome the specimen should be correctly plated in the correct media and the result should be interpreted alongside a Gram stain.

Testing microbiological samples for antibiotic sensitivity is of paramount importance to ensure the patients' infection will be adequately treated with the prescribed antibiotic therapy. Prolonged treatment with inappropriate antibiotic therapy increases the risk of antibiotic resistance, a major issue facing modern medical practice. There are a number of methods in which antibiotic sensitivity can be assessed including; phenotypic methods incorporating manual and automated methods, genetic methods and flight mass spectrometry (matrix-laser desorption ionisation-time of flight mass spectrometry (MALDI-TOF MS)). In-depth discussion of each method is beyond the scope of this book chapter and further reading in the subject area is recommended. Once the antibiotic sensitivity test is completed a final report is issued to the clinician which will document the microorganisms present in the sample and the antibiotics the organisms are sensitive to guiding the appropriate antibiotic therapy for the patient. This chapter gives a brief overview of the challenges of sampling and assessing infections within the head and neck.

36.3 From Patient to Pathologist: The Pathway from Sample to Slide

There are several steps in the pathway to gain a diagnosis from a patient biopsy sample. Within this chapter, an overview of the multiple steps in the process will be discussed. We will look at the different types of biopsy specimens received for histopathological assessment, alternative methods to help with the assessment of the oral mucosa and the laboratory methods used to process the tissue sample effectively for histopathological assessment by a pathologist. A diagrammatic overview of the pathways is seen in Fig. 36.2.

Specimen Types: Several different cellular biopsy sampling options are available and are all suited to specific clinical situations. The most frequently encountered biopsy specimens in oral and maxillofacial pathology are incisional biopsy specimens. This method sees the clinician sample a small amount of lesional tissue and send it for pathological examination in order to obtain a diagnosis and subsequently provide the correct course of treatment. For the most part, a biopsy from the oral mucosa is obtained via the use of a scalpel and forceps. However, in some centres, 'punch' biopsies are also taken. A 'punch' biopsy uses a prefabricated tool with a 5 mm surgical scalpel blade included in the specimen to take the sample.

Although histological examination of conventional biopsy specimens is the gold standard to diagnose diseases of the oral cavity, other less invasive methods of

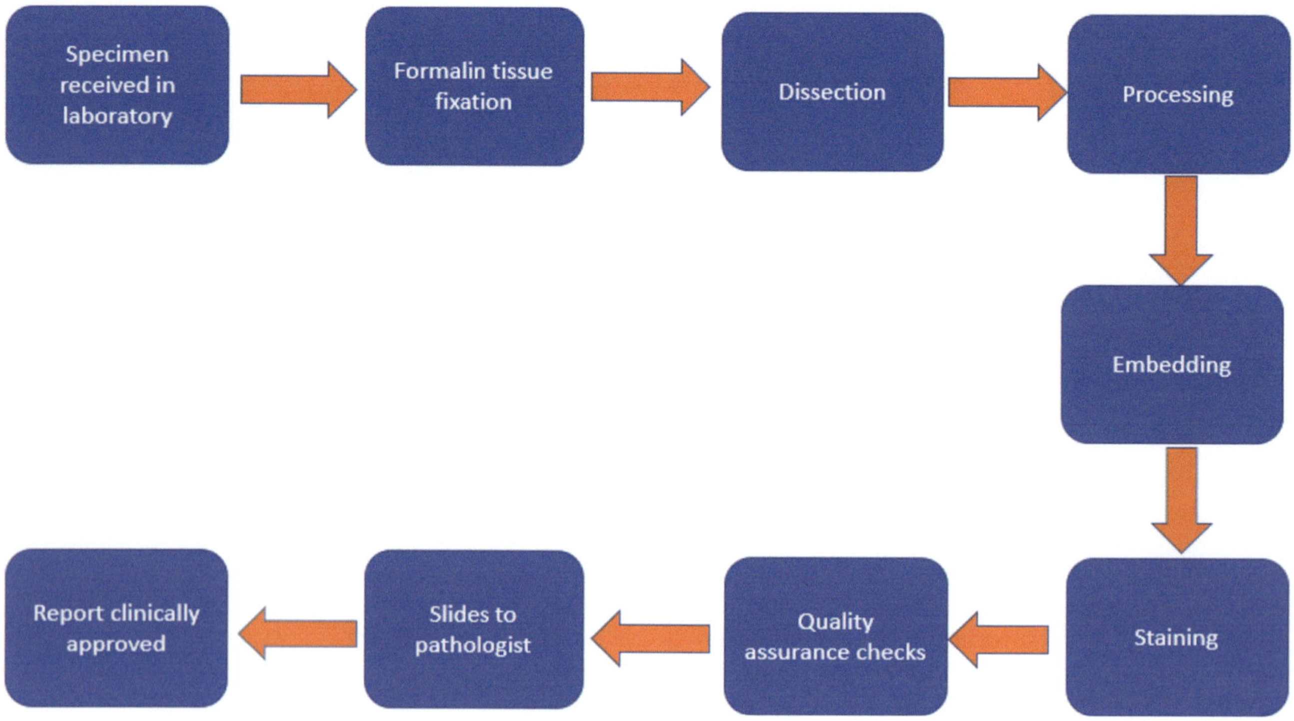

Fig. 36.2 Overview of specimen journey from patient to pathologist

assessing oral premaligant diseases (OPMD) in the oral cavity have been trialled. These techniques include the use of autofluorescence, chemiluminescence and the application of toluidine blue. Autofluorescence is a technique that uses a device which emits blue light of a wavelength between 400–460 nm that causes green autofluorescence of the oral tissues. It is suggested that where there is a loss of autofluorescence in the oral tissues, this may represent an area of non-physiological change. Chemiluminescence involves the patient using a 1% acetic acid oral rinse for 30 s prior to application of the chemilumescent light to aid assessment and identification of altered oral mucosa. Finally, toluidine blue application to the oral tissues can be a helpful adjunct to identify OPMD. The agent is applied to the oral tissues with the excess removed before the oral tissues are reviewed under normal incandescent light. The areas with retained blue staining may be indicative of an area of premalignant change. At present these methods cannot accurately assess and diagnose OPMD, but they may help to provide additional clinical information therefore they should be used in conjunction with the traditional biopsy methods previously discussed.

Another more recently discussed and minimally invasive technique in OMFP is the use of the brush biopsy for OPMD. This method allows for a transepithelial cellular biopsy sample to be obtained without the need for local anaesthetic or sutures. Typically, the result received from this type of sample is either negative or positive. A negative test result indicates that no atypia were identified however a positive result indicates the presence of atypia and warrants further investigations.

Alternative methods are required to sample more deep-seated structures such as suspicious lymph nodes or salivary gland lesions. In these circumstances, a core biopsy is typically carried out under ultrasound guidance. Often the lesions and nodes can only be palpated externally and therefore to ensure the biopsy taken includes representative tissue of the lesion, ultrasound guidance is necessary to ensure the needle core is in the lesion before the sample is taken. A core biopsy is taken with a hollowed needle which is inserted into the mass. When the operator is happy the instrument is in the right location, the instrument is able to cut a sample of the lesional tissue to send for histological examination. Core biopsies can be very useful to a pathologist as they often yield an adequate amount of tissue. The architecture of the lesional tissue is better maintained (vs. a fine needle aspirate (FNA)) and the larger yield of tissue ensures spare tissue for additional tests if required (discussed further in ► Sect. 36.4). An alternative method is an FNA. This method can also be used to sample suspicious lymph nodes or salivary gland masses but this method utilises a finer bore needle than a core biopsy to undertake the sample and thus more limited tissue is retrieved for examination. Often this method retrieves collections of cells only with the architecture disrupted. FNA samples produce a PAP slide and cell block. Although there is theoretically less risk of postoperative complications following an FNA vs. a core biopsy, an FNA yields less tissue for assessment, and therefore less tissue is available if additional tests are required.

Once a diagnosis has been achieved, resection specimens for benign and malignant neoplasms will also be sent for histological examination. The assessment of the specimen margins is very important and often resection specimens will include orientation sutures to assist the pathologist with the anatomical arrangement of the specimen as would be seen in the patient. For example, a parotidectomy for a pleomorphic adenoma may have two orientation sutures, a short suture indicating the anterior aspect of the specimen and a long suture indicating the superior aspect of the specimen. These help the pathologist to accurately report the proximity of the tumour to the surgical margins with meaningful orientation.

Fixation: Typically, all specimens received for histopathological assessment are fixed in a 10% buffered formalin solution. To allow for adequate fixation and to minimise artefactual processing errors as a consequence of insufficient fixation, all tissue should be placed in a volume of buffered formalin solution 10 times its size. For smaller biopsy specimens, 24 h is usually a sufficient amount of time for the specimen to fix in the formalin solution. However, larger specimens (i.e. resection specimens) may take up to 48 h to allow the formalin solution an adequate amount of time to penetrate through the tissue.

Dissection: Once adequately fixed the specimen should be described macroscopically. This description is included in the final report alongside the microscopic report. The specimen should be measured in three dimensions with a description of the mucosal colour, shape, texture and any other relevant features noted. Resection specimens for malignant tumours require additional description and sampling methods to ensure an adequate amount of tissue is examined for the production of the final histopathological report. This ensures the relevant prognostic information is collected and the tumour is staged correctly. This is important as certain histopathological findings (e.g. lymphovascular invasion, tumour size and depth of invasion) can be indicative of an overall poorer prognostic outcome for a patient and may indicate that additional adjunctive treatment such as radiotherapy or chemotherapy are recommended for disease management. An in-depth discussion of each specimen is beyond the scope of this book; however, additional information regarding tissue pathways and datasets can be found from the published guidance from the Royal College of Pathologists and the International Collaboration on Cancer Reporting with sources cited in the recommended reading at the end of the chapter.

Processing: Once specimens have been dissected and macroscopically described, the specimens go through a range of processes including; dehydration, clearing and wax infiltration prior to being embedded. This process sees the fixed tissue embedded in a wax resin within a plastic cassette bearing the unique specimen reference number. Following this, thin ribbons of the tissue embedded in the wax are sectioned on the microtome to be placed on the glass slide ready to be stained with haematoxylin and eosin (H&E). The haematoxylin preferentially stains the nucleus and the eosin in the cytoplasm. Overall, the H&E staining gives a basic overview of the tissue's morphology and is therefore a good starting point for the pathologist to start their initial observations. The slides produced by the laboratory are checked by a member of staff trained in quality assurance to ensure that the material being sent to the laboratory is of a high standard and of use for diagnostic reporting by the pathologist.

H&E slide to pathologist: After the numerous processes are completed in the laboratory, the slide can finally be delivered to the pathologist to be assessed under the microscope. In some cases a single section of the tissue with H&E staining is sufficient for the pathologist to give a diagnosis and a microscopic report with the diagnosis can be issued to the clinical team. In some instances, however, additional tests are required to help the pathologist achieve a final diagnosis and issue a microscopic report. There are a wide range of tests available such as special stains, immunohistochemistry (IHC) and immunofluorescence to name but a few. These additional methods will be discussed in more detail in ▶ Sect. 36.4: *Additional Tests to Aid Histopathological Diagnosis.*

36.4 Additional Aids to Histopathological Diagnosis

As discussed in the previous section, sometimes additional material and tests are required to aid pathologists to achieve a final diagnosis. We will discuss a number of these available methods in this section.

Additional H&E Sections: Sometimes simply additional sections of the current specimen are sufficient for a pathologist to achieve a diagnosis. On occasion, the H&E provided may not have a full intact section of the desired specimen, thus a 'full-face' section can be requested to ensure the specimen is viewed in its entirety. On other occasions, a pathologist may want to see a greater proportion of the tissue of the specimen before reaching a definitive diagnosis, thus 'levels' can be requested. Levels can be requested in multiples with the most common denomination request 3. This is particularly useful when assessing for atypia in OPMD such as dysplasia and when diagnosing malignancy in small biopsy specimens. At specimen dissection, it is possible to request for levels to be cut for the case in the first instance if the clinician is suspicious of an OPMD or malignancy. There may be occasions when a clinician is concerned about malignancy but no evidence of such is visible upon histopathological examination. In these cases, 'levels through the block' can ensure that the tissue from the whole specimen is sampled and thus pathologists can assure the clinician that all available material has been examined.

Special Stains: A wide range of special stains are available for further, more in-depth assessment of histopathological specimens. The mechanism of action for special stains relies on chemical-based reactions as opposed to immunohistochemical tests which rely on antibody-to-antigen binding (see below). Special stains can be used for the detection and identification of numerous structures in specimens. Examples are listed and seen in ◘ Table 36.1 and ◘ Fig. 36.3. As with all additional tests, it is important to view the special test alongside a positive control to ensure that the stain has worked and thus interpretation of the result is correct.

Immunohistochemistry: Alongside additional H&E sections and special stains, sometimes pathologists still require further information to aid arrival at a final diagnosis. Immunohistochemistry (IHC) is a valuable tool in the pathologist's armamentarium. IHC testing relies on antibodies in the test identifying and binding to antigens (i.e. proteins) within the sample tissue. The antigens may have altered expression within the lesional cells of the tumour being investigated and thus are identified following execution of the test. Although some IHCs are specific, a large number of the tests have crossed over

36

◘ **Table 36.1** Examples of common structures that a pathologist may want to try and identify when reporting oral and maxillofacial pathology specimens and appropriate special stains used to do so

Substance	Stain
Fungi	PAS, Grocotts
Bacteria	Gram
Elastic fibres	Elastic Van Gieson (EVG)
Mucins	PAS, alcian blue
Amyloid	Congo red
Mycobacteria	Ziehl–Neelsen (ZN)
Iron	Perls

and are deemed present in several unrelated tumours thus pathologists normally adopt a panel-based approach to the use of IHC to ensure the findings are interpreted correctly and thus the correct diagnosis is achieved. As well as IHC's role in primary diagnostics, IHC can also be used to screen patient's suitability for certain treatments, such as suitability for certain drugs or immunotherapies. In these circumstances, the IHC test can identify if the patients' cells possess the specific target molecules that the drug would target and thus would benefit from the treatment. As with special tests, it is important that a positive control is supplied with the test sample to ensure the test has worked and therefore interpretation of the stained lesional section is correct. Examples of IHC are seen in ◘ Fig. 36.4.

Direct Immunofluorescence: Direct immunofluorescence (DIF) is a less often utilised tool; however, its use is paramount in the assessment of a range of conditions. DIF can be used in histopathology in the assessment of connective tissue diseases, inflammatory skin conditions and, most commonly in oral pathology, the assessment of autoimmune vesiculobullous disorders. The most commonly encountered vesiculobullous disorders identified in the oral cavity include pemphigus vulgaris and mucous membrane pemphigoid. Tissue submitted for assessment via DIF must not be fixed in the conventional buffered formalin solution and instead must be received fresh. The biopsy should be representative of 'normal' appearing mucosa in the oral cavity as successful DIF requires intact epithelium and underling connective tissue to adequately assess the presence and pattern of the autoantibodies expressed. Once received, the tissue is frozen and sectioned prior to the application of the fluorescent autoantibodies. The antibodies bind to abnormally expressed autoantibodies in the patient biopsy specimen and express a fluorescent marker when viewed under a fluorescence microscope. Examples of antibody expression patterns are seen in ◘ Table 36.2.

This subsection gives a basic overview of the utilisation of DIF in diagnostic practice. However, the aetiology and histopathological features of *vesiculobullous disorders are discussed further in Chapter 25.*

Molecular: Whilst IHC allows the pathologist to investigate the types of proteins present within a tumour, advances in molecular medicine and testing methods allow tumours to be examined at the genetic level. A number of techniques are available, but the most commonly encountered tests in histopathology include fluorescent in situ hybridisation (FISH) and sequencing methods such as the use of polymerase chain reaction (PCR) or next-generation sequencing (NGS). Use of such methods in research has helped to identify specific genetic mutations or rearrangements unique to certain tumours and thus aiding diagnosis, (e.g. the presence of

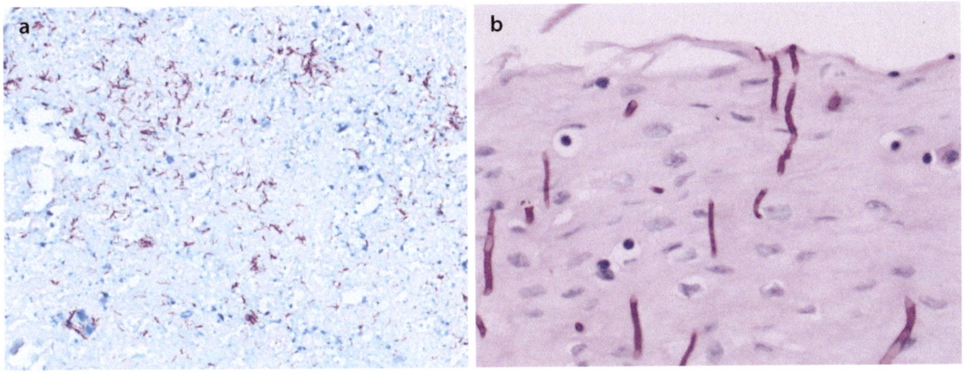

Fig. 36.3 Examples of special stains. **a** A positive control for acid-fast bacilli using Ziehl–Neelsen (ZN) staining. The acid-fast bacilli appear red with the application of this special stain when present. **b** DPAS staining highlights abundant fungal hyphae in the superficial keratin layers of this oral biopsy specimen

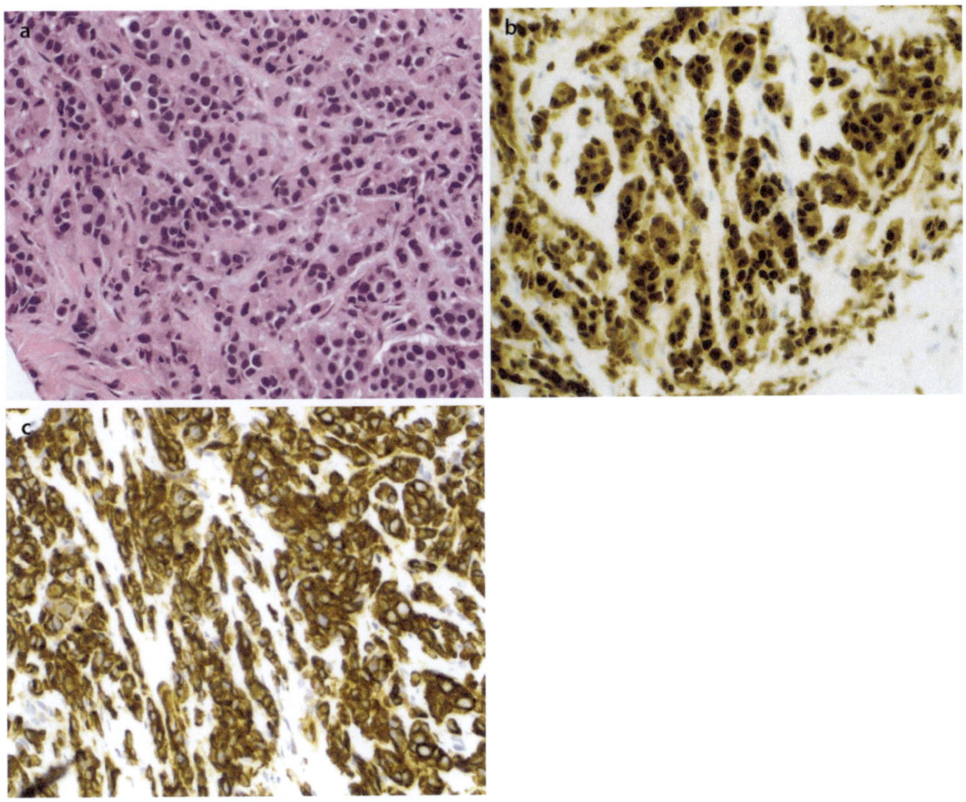

Fig. 36.4 Examples of how IHC is used in diagnostic practice. **a** An H&E stain shows a core biopsy containing metastatic adenocarcinoma. **b** Androgen Receptor (AR) IHC shows diffuse nuclear expression in the tumour, whereas **c**. AE1/AE3 (a pan-cytokeratin stain) shows diffuse cytoplasmic expression

Table 36.2 Patterns of DIF antibody expression in a number of vesiculobullous disorders

Condition	Antibody	Pattern of expression
Pemphigus vulgaris	IgG	Intercellular 'fishnet' pattern
Mucous membrane pemphigoid	IgG, C3	Linear pattern at basement membrane zone
Paraneoplastic pemphigus	IgG, C3	Granular linear pattern at basement membrane zone
Linear IgA disease	IgA	Linear pattern at basement membrane zone
Dermatitis Herpetiformis	IgA	Granular linear pattern at basement membrane zone

MAML2 rearrangements in mucoepidermoid carcinoma). Of course, some genetic alterations are not specific to one disease process therefore identification of the alteration on its own is not sufficient to make a diagnosis. The genetic alteration must be considered alongside the morphological and immunohistochemical profile of the lesion for a definitive diagnosis to be achieved.

36.5 Clinicopathological Correlation

As discussed throughout this chapter, several investigative tests are utilised when trying to achieve a diagnosis for a patient. Histopathology is just part of the 'investigative jigsaw' and is often used in conjunction with clinical information, clinical photography, radiology and when appropriate, multi-disciplinary team meeting (MDT) discussion. Clinicopathological correlation (CPC) allows for a holistic overview of all of a patient's relevant investigations to be considered to achieve the final diagnosis and allow for the formulation of the most appropriate treatment plan. The contributory elements of CPC are discussed in the following paragraphs.

Clinical Information: It is useful to remember that the request form completed by the clinician may contain vital information which may aid arrival at the diagnosis. Relevant clinical medical history including family history, genetic inherited conditions as well as a history of current or previous diseases can be extremely helpful, especially in the setting of metastatic malignancies. A history of the presenting complaint can also be extremely helpful. Factors such as the time frame and clinical course of the presenting complaint as well pattern of distribution can also allude to certain diagnoses. It is also prudent to note that if salient information has been missed from a request form, a simple call or email to the relevant clinician may allow for the acquisition of additional information that may aid the histopathological interpretation of the case and allow for a diagnosis to be achieved. ◘ Figure 36.5 shows an example of a specimen request form.

Clinical Photography: The importance of clinical photographs as an adjunct to diagnosis should not be overlooked. Clinical photography is often utilised as part of patient clinical records to document the presentation of lesions and can be used for comparison to monitor lesions over a period of time and assess response to treatment. This may be of greatest benefit for patients with OPMD such as dysplasia, especially proliferative verrucous leukoplakia (PVL), and other conditions such as lichen planus, recurrent aphthous stomatitis or vesiculobullous disorders. Comparison of photographic records allows clinicians to assess if lesions have progressed or changed in their clinical appearance over time and can help to guide clinical management strategies

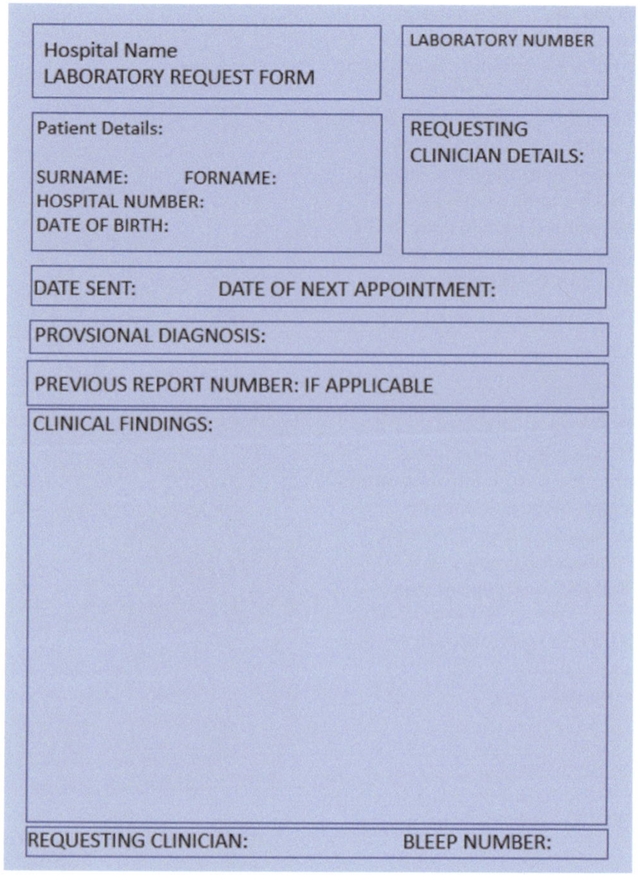
Hospital Name
LABORATORY REQUEST FORM
LABORATORY NUMBER
Patient Details:
SURNAME: FORNAME:
HOSPITAL NUMBER:
DATE OF BIRTH:
REQUESTING CLINICIAN DETAILS:
DATE SENT: DATE OF NEXT APPOINTMENT:
PROVSIONAL DIAGNOSIS:
PREVIOUS REPORT NUMBER: IF APPLICABLE
CLINICAL FINDINGS:
REQUESTING CLINICIAN: BLEEP NUMBER:

◘ **Fig. 36.5** An example of a clinical biopsy request form. The form allows for the acquisition of the correct patient data for submission of the specimen. It also gives the clinician performing the biopsy the opportunity to give additional details regarding the patient's medical history and the presentation of the lesion being sampled

such as considering a new representative biopsy of a lesion if it has changed over time. They may also be of use within the patient's clinical notes to indicate the site of sampling for biopsy specimens.

Radiology: Radiological examination is a core investigative measure when considering lesions of head and neck, in particular those arising in the craniofacial bones and those of odontogenic origin. A number of odontogenic lesions arise in the craniofacial bones, namely cysts and tumours. Often radiographic imaging is one of the first investigative measures used in the preliminary diagnosis of odontogenic lesions. Radiology can help locate the cyst or tumour and its relation to local anatomy (i.e. cyst located at the apex of an extensively carious tooth, multi-locular lesion extending from the body of the mandible to the ramus of the mandible). Radiological assessment is also fundamental in the diagnosis of certain entities such as fibro-osseous lesions. The histological findings of fibro-osseous lesions of the craniofacial bones are very similar and often cannot be differentiated upon histology alone,

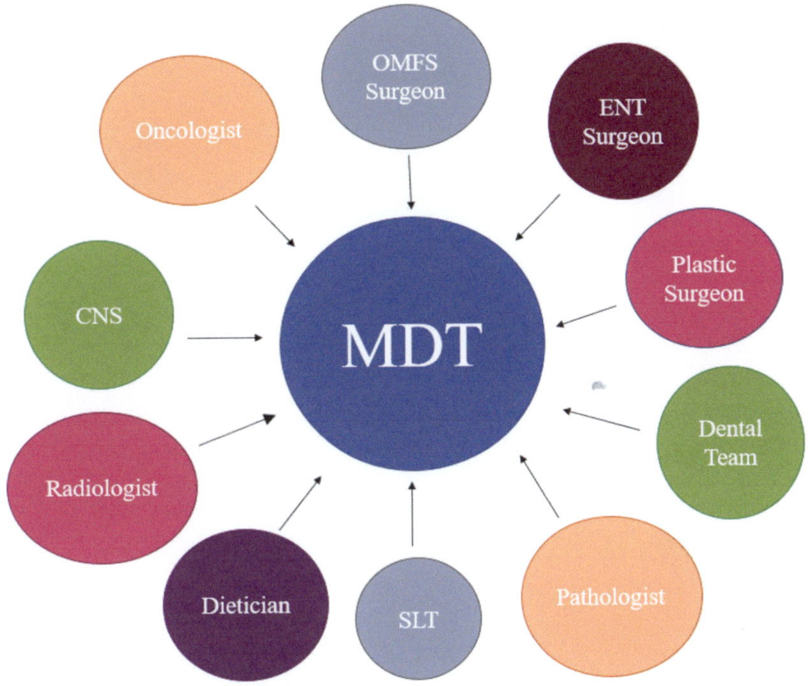

Fig. 36.6 Diagram showing the many members from multi-disciplinary teams present at head and neck MDT oncology meetings/tumour boards. *OMFS* oral and maxillofacial surgery, *ENT* ear, nose and throat, *SLT* speech and language therapist, *CNS* clinical nurse specialist

thus correlation with radiographical findings is paramount in achieving a diagnosis. ***This is discussed more in part 2,*** ► ***Chap.*** 23. Radiology, magnetic resonance imaging (MRI) and positron emission tomography (PET) images are also utilised when patients are diagnosed with malignant disease within the head and neck. These images alongside other investigative tests are discussed at oncology MDT meetings (see below). The results of these images provide the clinical team with important information such as the extent of the tumour (maximum diameter and depth of invasion), invasion into local structures (i.e. bones, adjacent organs) and the presence of locoregional or distant metastases. PET images can also be extremely useful in the setting of patients presenting with metastatic disease to a lymph node from an unknown primary source.

MDT: The MDT (or tumour board) meeting is a key stage in the discussion of patients with malignancies of the head and neck. An MDT meeting brings together the core members involved in the investigation, treatment and management of oncology patients. Core members of the team include surgeons, radiologists, pathologists, oncologists, dieticians, speech and language therapists, restorative dentists and specialist cancer care nurses (Fig. 36.6). The meeting allows patients to be presented in an open forum with all relevant investigations available and discussed by specialists in each respective field with a custom treatment plan compiled for each patient taking their medical history and extent of disease into account. Patients are rediscussed at the MDT following their definitive treatment. The pathologist can then inform the clinical team of the histopathological findings of the tumour and if any poor prognostic findings are identified (e.g. close surgical margins to the tumour, lymphovascular invasion, extranodal extension of metastatic disease) as these findings may mean that the patient requires adjuvant treatment (e.g. chemotherapy, radiotherapy, targeted drug therapies etc.) for appropriate management of the disease process.

Further Reading

Awan KH, Morgan PR, Warnakulasuriya S. Assessing the accuracy of autofluorescence, chemiluminescence and toluidine blue as diagnostic tools for oral potentially malignant disorders—a clinicopathological evaluation. Clin Oral Investig. 2015;19(9):2267–72.

Elvers D, Braunschweig T, Hilgers RD, Ghassemi A, Möhlhenrich SC, Hölzle F, Gerressen M, Modabber A. Margins of oral leukoplakia: autofluorescence and histopathology. Br J Oral Maxillofac Surg. 2015;53(2):164–9.

International Collaboration on Cancer Reporting Datasets. https://www.iccr-cancer.org/datasets/published-datasets/.

Roscoe DL, Hoang L. Microbiologic investigations for head and neck infections. Infect Dis Clin North Am. 2007;21(2):283–304.

Royal College of Pathologists: Cancer Data Sets and Tissue Pathways. https://www.rcpath.org/profession/guidelines/cancer-datasets-and-tissue-pathways.html.

Rekhtman N, Baine MK, Bishop JA. Quick reference handbook for surgical pathologists. Cham: Springer; 2019.

Robson A, et al. Pre-treatment clinical assessment in head and neck cancer: United Kingdom National Multidisciplinary Guidelines. J laryngol Otol. 2016;130(S2):S13–22.

MIX
Papier aus verantwortungsvollen Quellen
Paper from responsible sources
FSC® C105338

If you have any concerns about our products,
you can contact us on
ProductSafety@springernature.com

In case Publisher is established outside the EU,
the EU authorized representative is:
Springer Nature Customer Service Center GmbH
Europaplatz 3, 69115 Heidelberg, Germany

Printed by Libri Plureos GmbH
in Hamburg, Germany